APPLIED
Pharmacology

For Mosby:

Commissioning Editor: Jill Northcott
Head of Project Management: Ewan Halley

APPLIED
Pharmacology

**An Introduction to Pathophysiology
and Drug Management for Nurses
and Healthcare Professionals**

Sylvia Prosser

Barbara Worster

Janet MacGregor

Kate Dewar

Pauline Runyard

Julie Fegan

All at Faculty of Nursing, Midwifery and Social Work,
Canterbury Christ Church College, Canterbury, Kent, UK

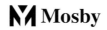 Mosby

EDINBURGH   LONDON   NEW YORK   PHILADELPHIA
ST LOUIS   SYDNEY   TORONTO 2000

MOSBY
An imprint of Harcourt Publishers Limited

© Harcourt Publishers Limited 2000

M is a registered trademark of Harcourt Publishers Limited

The right of Sylvia Prosser, Barbara Worster, Janet MacGregor, Kate Dewar, Pauline Runyard and Julie Fegan to be identified as authors of this work has been asserted by them in accordance with the Copyright, Designs and Patents Act 1988

First published 2000

ISBN 0 7234 2588 4

British Library Cataloguing in Publication Data
A catalogue record for this book is available from the British Library

Library of Congress Cataloging in Publication Data
A catalog record for this book is available from the Library of Congress

Note
Medical knowledge is constantly changing. As new information becomes available, changes in treatment, procedures, equipment and the use of drugs become necessary. The authors and the publishers have, as far as it is possible, taken care to ensure that the information given in this text is accurate and up-to-date. However, readers are strongly advised to confirm that the information, especially with regard to drug usage, complies with the latest legislation and standards of practice.

The
publisher's
policy is to use
**paper manufactured
from sustainable forests**

Printed in Italy

Contents

Authors

Kate Dewar RN RM RNT MSc
Senior Lecturer, Faculty of Nursing, Midwifery and Social Work,
Canterbury Christ Church University College, Canterbury, Kent, UK
2   *Introduction to pharmacology*
6   *Drugs and neoplastic disorders*
18   *Pharmacological management of pain*

Julie Fegan RGN NDN PWT DNEd MA
Senior Lecturer, Faculty of Nursing, Midwifery and Social Work,
Canterbury Christ Church University College, Canterbury, Kent, UK
1   *Introduction to the nature and causation of disease*
4   *Legal aspects of drug administration*
5   *Drugs and immunological disorders*
9   *Drugs and head and neck disorders*

Janet MacGregor RGN OND(Ophth) RSCN BEd MSc
Principal Lecturer, Faculty of Nursing, Midwifery and Social Work,
Canterbury Christ Church University College, Canterbury, Kent, UK
11   *Drugs and respiratory disorders*
14   *Drugs and gastrointestinal disorders*
16   *Drugs and reproductive disorders*

Sylvia Prosser RGN RNT BEd(Hons) MSc PhD
Principal Lecturer, Faculty of Nursing, Midwifery and Social Work,
Canterbury Christ Church University College, Canterbury, Kent, UK
3   *Classes of drugs*
7   *Drugs and psychological disorders*
15   *Drugs and urological disorders*
17   *Drugs and dermatological disorders*
19   *Pharmacological management of medical emergencies*

Pauline Runyard RGN BEd(Hons) ENB 928
Senior Lecturer, Faculty of Nursing, Midwifery and Social Work,
Canterbury Christ Church University College, Canterbury, Kent, UK
8   *Drugs and neurological disorders*
10   *Drugs and endocrine disorders*
17   *Drugs and dermatological disorders*

Barbara Worster RGN BSc(Hons) RCNT PGCE
Senior Lecturer, Faculty of Nursing, Midwifery and Social Work,
Canterbury Christ Church University College, Canterbury, Kent, UK
12   *Drugs and cardiovascular disorders*
13   *Drugs and musculoskeletal disorders*

Preface

This book has been written with the aim of helping students of nursing to link theory with practice. In the context of this book, the 'theory' consists of concepts of disease states and principles of pharmacology and therapeutics. The 'practice' is the work that nurses undertake observing, caring for and informing their patients. During the course of our work helping students to learn, the need for this book became clear to us. Without our students, this book would not have been written, so we acknowledge here their contribution to this text.

Sylvia Prosser
Barbara Worster
Janet MacGregor
Kate Dewar
Pauline Runyard
Julie Fegan

Canterbury 1999

Acknowledgements

The authors would also like to acknowledge the following people:

Ms Maggie Banning, Lecturer in Life Sciences, Royal College of Nursing, for technical help and advice

Ms Julie Johnstone, Nurse Fellow and Mr Roger Goldsmith, Senior Lecturer, both at Canterbury Christ Church University College, for material related to cardiac and trauma care, respectively.

1

Julie Fegan

INTRODUCTION TO THE NATURE AND CAUSATION OF DISEASE

THE PLACE OF THE BIOMEDICAL SCIENCES IN NURSING PRACTICE

A strength of nursing, and sometimes its weakness, is the breadth of the knowledge base upon which practice draws. The breadth of the knowledge base could be viewed as a weakness because breadth may preclude depth, and this is sometimes difficult for 'specialist' professionals to appreciate. In order to be a good nurse, it is important to have empathy and psychomotor skills. However, these are attributes that may also be possessed by lay carers. Possession of these characteristics alone will not ensure that the patient or client receives the help and support that may be expected from a health professional. The scope encompassed by nursing practice seems capable of infinite expansion as professional roles become blurred. Activities that were previously considered the prerogative of medical practitioners may in some circumstances be delegated to nurses. With the inception of the restriction of the junior doctors' hours (NHS Management Executive, 1991), nurses, who have historically been more consistently 'with' the patient, now have greater demands upon their expertise than ever before. The odds are that, if a patient's condition changes, either as a result of a developing illness or because of the intentional or unintentional effects of pharmacological treatment, it will be the nurse who is in a prime position to detect this, and influence the subsequent clinical management.

The authors of this book accept absolutely that nursing knowledge draws from a range of knowledge disciplines; that an understanding of sociology, psychology, ethics and health promotion, for example, is necessary to help ensure that the patient or client receives appropriate care informed by current thinking. Nurses have to span the 'whole', but in order to do this, they need the relevant information, which has to be learned in 'parts'. One challenge is that, unlike some of their more 'scientifically' based colleagues, a student nurse may commence his or her course with a minimal background in the sciences. In turn, this poses

a challenge for those who, like the authors of this book, teach biomedical subjects to these students. In order to be an effective nurse in today's healthcare context, the nurse needs to have a working understanding of some highly complex information, which has been generated and traditionally is taught by people who are well established in the professional and academic traditions of their disciplines. Such teachers may be unable to remember a time when they did not use biochemical terminology or understand the basic principles of chemistry. The students are left with a sense that they are lacking; they are being asked to 'read the book' when they have not had the opportunity first to learn to 'speak the language'.

BIONURSING

A useful framework for examining the dilemma of these nurses in the making, and also of some of those who are already qualified, was devised by Akinsanya and Hayward (1980). These researchers identified a series of levels at which nurses might use biomedical knowledge as they cared for their patients. The levels they identified were task operational, task specific, task contextual and personal and professional development.

Task operational

At the task operational level, a nurse could undertake an activity for a patient correctly, but have no idea of any of the scientific principles for so doing. An illustrative example here could be giving a patient medication: the nurse might know the name of the drug and the recipient, how to store the drug and how many tablets were needed to administer the correct dose, but be totally unable to explain to the patient what the preparation was for or what common adverse effects might be encountered.

Task specific

At this level the nurse might have a small level of knowledge about the agent in question, for example, an understanding that the tablets being given were diuretics. She might explain this to the patient, and not be surprised that the patient subsequently needed to visit the toilet.

Task contextual

The nurse with task contextual knowledge would have sufficient information about the patient and his diuretic therapy to know that he needed to maintain an adequate fluid intake to prevent dehydration. She would also know why the diuretic agent in question carried a risk of potassium depletion, what potential problems that posed and how other treatment the patient was receiving contributed to the prevention of such risks.

Personal and professional development

This level indicates that the nurse has sufficient knowledge to act as a professional resource on a wide scale. A nurse with such knowledge might be working as a cardiac nurse practitioner, advising patients with a specific range of problems, acting as a resource for colleagues from other health disciplines or researching new problems and communicating findings to others through writing papers and conference presentations.

For the aspiring 'bionurse', there is an array of challenges. A huge amount of knowledge must be learned. Not only must the knowledge be acquired in the first place, it must then be transformed into useful knowledge, which can be added to her armoury of expertise to help the patient. Rote learning is of no help here. She needs to be able to sift through her knowledge to be able to answer the patient's questions in a manner appropriate for that patient's own knowledge and experience. In order to do that, she needs to be able to weigh up information and select what is useful. The knowledge must become part of her, rather than part of the content of a lecture or textbook that is inaccessible.

In this book, the authors are concerned to promote 'useful knowledge'. In real life, a nurse does not spend her time doing 'pharmacology' or 'pathophysiology' to a patient. The nurse cares for patients as part of a multiprofessional team and needs to play her part as an interpreter of what she sees before her, and of what the patient experiences. For these reasons, we have put together information from pharmacological and biomedical science in a way that might be unfamiliar to those who view these topics as separate entities which require the student to have a 'starter collection' of what they term elementary knowledge in order to 'pass go'. Our aim has been to provide an explanation of what has 'gone wrong' in commonly encountered conditions, and to discuss how medication prescribed works on the disordered function in order to correct or contain the disorder. Our reason for selecting the pathophysiological content of this book is that the conditions discussed are treated – or the symptoms are controlled – by pharmacological products, and the nurse is likely to encounter patients with these biomedical problems in the course of her clinical practice.

The book is divided into two main subsections: the first four chapters consider general principles; the remaining chapters discuss what it is hoped will be useful knowledge in specific contexts. The book is not meant to supplant other more conventional texts of pharmacology or pathophysiology, but to provide the initial 'useful knowledge' that can then be augmented as appropriate by reference to other more specialised texts.

THE NOTIONS OF ILLNESS AND DISEASE

Disease cuts off the young life with promise and ends the long life, because everyone must die of something. Humankind refers to disease, the scientist to pathophysiology: the scientific study of disease. The word comes from two Greek words: $\pi\alpha\theta o\xi$ (pathos) 'suffering or distress' and $\lambda o\gamma o\xi$ (logos) 'a treatise or study'. Vardaxis (1995) says that disease is an abnormal variation in the structure or function of any part of the body – a 'departure from ease' – adding that conditions that the lay person may not consider to be 'disease' may be disease to a pathologist.

DIFFERING CONCEPTS OF ILL HEALTH: AN OVERVIEW

In order to understand disease, much time has been devoted to the study of human anatomy and physiology. The interdependence of structure and function became apparent early on and the dissecting room was a learning laboratory for medical students and pathologists. There is a range of ways of viewing disease. These are introduced here to provide a context within which the biomedical approach that we use can be seen as a part of a whole. Seedhouse (1986) says that disease is a deviation from a species norm causing a biological disadvantage or is a medical disorder associated with disability, distress or other types of disadvantage. Seedhouse summarises theories of health and recognises three approaches designed to increase health: sociological, medical science and humanist. The common factor in all three approaches is provision of conditions necessary for achievement of potentials or removal of obstacles to achieving chosen goals.

The sociological approach

This is concerned with unequal distribution of disease and illness and unequal use of health services by different sections of the community, and it explains causes of inequality in terms of socioeconomic, political, personal, environmental, biological and chance factors. It tries to provoke changes in society.

The medical science approach

This approach has its emphasis on clinics, hospitals, biology, statistics and measurement of conditions against 'normal' standards. It does research into causes of disease, effects of drugs and surgical techniques to increase understanding and allow preventive, curative and educational measures.

The humanist approach

Here, health is regarded as a positive goal to be achieved personally. Disease, illness and other problems can coexist with health. It recognises that people are complex wholes, living within and permanently influenced by a constantly changing world. It sees interconnections between physical, spiritual and intellectual factors and recognises a latent ability for self-development in all human beings who have the ability to understand the implications of their actions (the ability may be actual or potential).

Those who seek the roots of health problems often find them in social, economic and political factors. MacKinlay underscored the dangers of reacting to outward manifestations of illness when he described the continuous and frustrating process of dragging a succession of drowning victims from a fast-flowing river and hastily applying artificial respiration (Tones, 1981, p. 3).

Again and again, without end, goes the sequence. I am so busy jumping in and pulling them to shore, applying artificial respiration, that I have no time to see who the hell is pushing them all in.

Health scientists are advised to follow MacKinlay's advice and 'refocus upstream'. Most will then find that at source major social problems such as poverty and disadvantage cause disease and ill health. There is as big a gap between the health of social classes I and V today as there was 30 years ago and this applies to all diseases. However, there is not a lot health personnel can do about these huge social problems that large charitable organisations and governments struggle to overcome. The individual health practitioner can only help the individual patient to focus on the aetiology of their own particular disease process and see the individual causes in their own illness. Doing this is not 'victim-blaming' but can help that person next time the same circumstances occur perhaps to 'do things differently' and to understand and avoid or take different actions sooner to avert or overcome illness. This is called education for health and is part of the role of every nurse, health visitor and midwife.

The language of pathology legitimately belongs to the pathologist who tends to use four terms to describe disease: morphology, topography, aetiology and function. **Morphology** is the appearance of the disease or injured tissue to the naked eye and under the microscope. **Topography** is the site of the body in which the disease appears, for example, cirrhosis typically occurs only in the liver, fractures only in bone. **Aetiology** means the cause of the disease and **idiopathic** is used when the cause is unknown. **Function** is used to describe how the individual is affected. Other terms related to disease are listed in **Box 1.1**.

1.1 DESCRIPTIVE TERMS RELATED TO DISEASE

- Aetiology: the study of disease causation
- Epidemiology: the study of patterns of disease in a population
- Prevalence: the numbers of established cases of a given disorder in a population
- Incidence: the numbers of new cases of a given disease process in a population
- Morbidity: the amount of illness caused in the population by the condition
- Mortality: the amount of death caused in the population by the condition
- Pathology: the study of a disease process
- Pathogenesis: description of the manner in which a disease develops
- Pathophysiology: the description of disordered physiological processes
- Sign: what the observer sees in a patient
- Symptom: change in the bodily function perceived by the patient
- Acute: a condition which is of rapid onset
- Chronic: a condition which is of slow onset. The effects are usually permanent
- Diagnosis: identification of the patient's disease by means of formal assessment
- Exacerbation: acceleration of the disease process
- Remission: a reversal or improvement of the disease process, which may or may not be temporary
- Prognosis: the outlook

NATURE AND CAUSATION OF DISEASE

Many have tried to define the nature and causation of disease. It has been described as an inadequate adaptation to alterations in the external and internal environment, as an interruption or disorder of function, or as homeostasis gone wrong. Atheroma, cancer and thrombosis are examples:

- **Atheroma** – the inner walls of arteries receive nourishment by diffusion of nutrients from the blood flowing through these arteries. In some cases the inner wall becomes infiltrated by fat to form atheroma, the major killing disease of Western nations.
- **Cancer** – if organs contained no stem cells capable of mitosis, cancer would be rare; but, if there were no stem cells, cell renewal would be impossible and our life span would be enormously shortened.
- **Thrombosis** – platelet clumping arrests bleeding. Thrombosis along with atheroma is a major cause of death that results from platelet clumping. Again, fatal pathology is an inevitable consequence of a process essential for life (Spector, 1989).

The conceptual problem is to reconcile two opposites such as antibodies defending and attacking the body. The double-edged nature of many survival mechanisms happens because natural selection can act only on individuals young enough to reproduce. What happens to individuals in later life cannot be influenced by natural selection; for example, sickle cell disease helped many African and West Indian children to survive malaria until they could reproduce and pass on the gene. Now from childhood sickle cell disease causes much morbidity and mortality. In middle age most disease consists of the unwanted side effects of homeostatic mechanisms, but what ill effects nature fails to achieve, humans introduce by way of environmental hazards such as cigarettes, industrial pollutants and medicines (Spector, 1989).

Throughout human memory people have been born, lived and died – of something. Human beings have often tried to account for why people have died. Sometimes the cause was obvious and weapons became ever more effective because they 'stilled' forever an opponent. Some traumatic injuries are now treated with drugs to reduce the resulting inflammation and infection, such as infected wounds or rising intracranial pressure in head injuries. Other causes were less obvious. People blamed weather conditions and no doubt today cold and fog seem to go together with colds and flu. The notions of miasmas and mists that seemed to contain contagion were no less logical than today's air pollution or viruses from comets. The idea that spirits possessed individuals and were exorcised is not too different from today's stress-caused emotional or physical illnesses.

Once lay people realised that diseases could be 'caught', the idea of infection spread to other diseases such as neoplasm, causing a great deal of ostracism and fear. Pathophysiology could be regarded as the opposite of health but many people live quite fulfilling lives within or in spite of the confines of a disease. It is of help to both the lay person and the scientist to be able to classify a disease: 'What do I have, Doctor? Why?' It also helps to organise scientific material around a classification into which manageable chunks can be arranged to help understanding.

In this book, we have organised our material mainly into chapters that consider the bodily systems. A patient may initially present complaining of a problem of breathing, sleeping or some other activity of daily living, but after consultation with a medical practitioner and having received the initial diagnosis, may well confide in the nurse, 'I have trouble with my heart…' or 'I have ovarian cancer, why are they giving me these tablets?'. The nurse needs to consult her store of knowledge about the heart or ovarian cancer and the treatments offered in order to be able to share useful knowledge with the patient.

PROBLEMS OF 'PIGEONHOLING' ILLNESS

Many diseases are caused by the 'one thing after another' syndrome, when many different factors combine to cause

illness. Radiation, for example, can cause trauma in the form of burns or may cause cells to mutate and thus cause neoplasm. Some neoplasms may be a result of ageing or degeneration, which may be a natural progression in life or be caused by a specific agent. Ageing impairs the body's ability to deal with healing, repair and replacement of damaged or faulty cells, but is usually not thought of as a disease, however much people try to avoid it. However, ageing combined with another cause may speed up the disease process. Oddly, many malignant neoplasms may be kinder to the ageing body than the young one; the latter may deteriorate more rapidly than the older body that cannot cooperate and allow the neoplasm to spread wildly. Some forms of ill health are caused by medication itself. This is called iatrogenic illness, such as when, through overuse of nasal decongestant drops, the patient's nasal passages suffer a reactive overdilatation of the blood vessels. The result is nasal congestion, which the patient was trying to relieve in the first place.

HISTORICAL VIEWS

Currer and Stacy (1986) say that anthropologists have traced the origins of theories of causes of disease. Medical and lay explanations have long attributed importance to air, climate and seasons. Hippocrates did not see disease as only divinely caused but integrated into the natural order of things. Today, environmental and occupational causes of disease are better understood.

As early as the mid sixteenth century a theory of contagion had developed and three kinds were recognised: person to person, indirect by means of objects, and at a distance without human contact or exchange of objects. Doctors at that time did not support the idea of contagion although it was widespread among people, giving rise to various hygiene and isolation practices not unlike cross-infection prevention measures taken today.

Doctors did recognise the links between plagues and famine. The debate lasted until Pasteur discovered the microbe and demonstrated the model of specific aetiology. Since that time the popular concept of the specific cause of disease being a germ has gone unchallenged and has been accepted as the major cause of biological illness – so much so that people with cancer have had to cope with mistaken notions of contagion.

Diet has long been viewed as a cause of disease, for example, food famine and scarcity; today overeating is considered by many to be responsible for many ills. Modern life has transformed food production so that now chemical fertilisers and pesticide sprays worry people who would like to return to a natural or 'organic cycle' of producing food.

The perception of the link between illness and work has developed differently. Today work, like diet, constitutes an essential element of our way of life as a cause of illness. The physical effects of work were known from the Middle Ages onwards. Much of industrial and trade union legislation and the Health and Safety at Work Act (1974) look at the effects of work on health.

Holistic health care is not new, as Hippocrates advanced this idea over 2000 years ago: 'It is more important to know what sort of person has a disease than to know what sort of disease a person has.' There is a famous medical slogan striven for by all good doctors: 'First do the patient no harm.' Iatrogenesis is derived from *iatro* meaning doctor and *genesis* meaning cause. Many modern drugs, although they save pain and lives, can damage all parts of the body. Part of the nurse's role is to recognise those signs and symptoms caused by treatment.

KEY POINTS

- Biomedical knowledge assists the nurse to address patients' problems.
- Health depends upon normal adaptive physiology and interactions with others in society.

- Holistic understanding is necessary to understand the complex interactions of health and disease.
- The notion of disease has developed concomittantly with advancing psycho-socio-physiological knowledge.

REFERENCES

Akinsanya J, Hayward J. The biological sciences in nursng education: the contribution of bionursing. *Nurs Times* 1980; 76(10) 6.3.80, 427–432.

Currer C, Stacey M. *Concepts of health, illness and disease: a comparative perspective*. Leamington Spa: Berg, 1986.

NHS Management Executive. *The New Deal*. London: NHSME, 1991.

Seedhouse D. *Health: the foundations for achievement*. Chichester: John Wiley and Sons, 1986.

Spector WG. *An introduction to general pathology, 3rd ed*. Edinburgh: Churchill Livingstone, 1989.

Tones K. Health education: prevention or subversion? *R Soc Health J* 1981; 3:1–4.

Vardaxis NJ. *Pathology for the health sciences*. Edinburgh: Churchill Livingstone, 1995.

2 Kate Dewar
INTRODUCTION TO PHARMACOLOGY

MEANING OF 'DRUG' AND 'MEDICINE'

Inbis the healthcare professions, the word 'drug' is often used in place of 'medicine'. In this context, both refer to any substance used in the prevention, diagnosis and treatment of disease; or in the alleviation of disease-derived symptoms or problems. Any substance administered to replace a deficit is also encompassed within this therapeutic term 'drug'. For example, if a vitamin or hormone is taken to overcome a deficiency of the specific item, then it is being used in a therapeutic way, as a drug (Grahame-Smith and Aronson, 1992).

A separate definition of 'drug' involves any substance taken to produce a specific feeling. This may be euphoria or an extra alertness (a 'high'), or alternatively a calm state, depending upon the category of drug involved. In this case continued use of the drug is not directed at influencing the disease or health of the individual, but at continuation of the 'feel-good' and prevention of the 'feel-bad' symptoms. An adverse and particularly damaging effect of this type of chronic usage is dependence, and these important issues are discussed further in Chapter 7 *Drugs and psychological disorders*.

CATEGORIES OF DRUGS DEFINED BY VARIOUS SOURCES

Patients, doctors, nurses, pharmacists, pharmacologists, government bodies and international regulatory agencies all view drugs from slightly different perspectives, on the basis of their distinct relationship with, or responsibility for, pharmacological agents. Drugs can be classified in many ways, depending upon the specific audience for which the naming of drugs is aimed. However, it is worthwhile to identify the variety of drug categories so that nurses can use the system that best fits in with the needs of a specific situation (**Table 2.1**). For further detail on legal aspects of drug categorisation, see Chapter 4 *Legal aspects of drug administration*.

CATEGORIES CHOSEN FOR THIS TEXT

The aim of this book is to help nurses make reasoned connections between drug usage and specific pathophysiological changes and disease outcomes. A mixed generic effect- and use-related approach seems appropriate. This allows nurses to identify the links between the therapeutic effects and side effects of each drug and the body system(s) influenced by drugs and disease processes. Further discussion of these issues can be found in Chapter 1 *Introduction to the nature and causation of disease*.

FORMULATION OF DRUGS FOR ADMINISTRATION

Manufacturers prepare drugs in a variety of formulations that contain a reliably consistent dosage and are easy to use. In the manufacturing process, ingredients are added to improve taste, to give a distinctive colour to the product or to alter the rate of drug absorption. The common preparations are included in **Tables 2.2–2.5** with a brief description of each and a rationale for choosing each route of administration. For further information on the nurse's legal accountability related to drug prescription, administration and storage responsibilities, see Chapter 4 *Legal aspects of drug administration*.

There are special considerations affecting the safety and comfort of patients that must be taken into account when giving drugs via each route and when using complex drug infusion delivery systems (Giuliano *et al.*, 1993; Wood and Gullo, 1993). For further information consult a textbook of nursing practice.

NEW FORMULATION

A recently developed vehicle for transdermal absorption of a drug involves a gas-drug formulation. This has many potential advantages over injection or other transdermal methods and is in trial at present. This new format is as follows: a powdered drug is delivered in a compressed helium 'gun'. When the 'gun' is fired, under high velocity

Categories of Drug Names	
Generic name	The 'approved' or official name. This is often one that has been sanctioned by the World Health Organization or some other, usually nationally recognised, body e.g. the British Pharmacopoeia Commission.
Trade or brand name	This 'proprietary' name is given to a drug by its pharmaceutical producer. It is the name by which it is marketed by the company, therefore it is, generally, short and 'snappy' and easy to remember for potential prescribers. As a consequence a drug marketed by several manufacturers will have several 'trade' names. A brand name refers to a particular preparation manufactured by a particular company. In this book, preparations will be identified by their generic names only.
Chemical name	Each drug has been identified according to its chemical structure and given an appropriate chemical name. These are often long and complex, and of primary interest to chemists, particularly those working in pharmaceutical companies or in toxicology units.
Use name	Commonly drugs are categorised according to the use for which they are prescribed e.g. antihypertensives, contraceptives, anti-inflammatory agents.
Effect name	For some drugs, the categorisation relates to the physiological or biological response in the body e.g. diuretic, cytotoxic agent, beta-blocker.
Legal name	National, legal restrictions are imposed on the sale and use of various categories of drugs, based on judgements about their relative safety and potential for misuse. There are 'over the counter' drugs and those that can only be (legally) obtained via prescription. Prescribers have various controls that determine their prescribing activities; in the United Kingdom, the Misuse of Drugs Regulations leglislation imposes restrictions on drugs according to the class or schedule in which they are placed e.g. Class A, B or C drugs, or Schedule 1–5 (see Chapter 4 *Legal aspects of drug administration* for more detail).

Table 2.1 Categories of drug names

the helium molecules bounce off the skin surface and the drug is delivered at high speed through the skin. It is painless and leaves no puncture site. Injection phobia and infection risk are not a problem

PLACEBO

The word 'placebo' denotes 'an inactive substance administered to a patient ... sometimes for the psychological benefit to the patient through his believing he is receiving treatment' (Knight, 1997, p. 868). It is, therefore, any drug given knowingly that will not have a direct pharmacological benefit to the recipient. That there is a potential for misuse of placebo is without doubt. In the type of health professional–patient relationship implied in the above definition, the power and decision-making are in the hands of the health professional. It is not shared and there can be scant openness or trust in the relationship. The judgement about a potential therapeutic benefit from deception rests entirely with the health professionals (Grahame-Smith and Aronson, 1992). However, it is extremely difficult for anyone to understand the world from another person's perspective. A health professional would have to be extraordinarily sure

of the patient's thoughts and feelings in order to be able to justify the administration of placebo.

Many years ago, placebos were administered far more commonly than today, particularly to patients with 'inappropriately high' levels of pain. However, the judgements may well have been based on faulty and incomplete knowledge about the patient, their disease process and pain physiology. As a result, placebo administration was often inappropriate and probably caused unnecessary suffering to many patients.

The notion that a patient who demands drug therapy, despite doctor or nurse insistence that no medication is required, should be given a placebo is difficult to support. This suggests that placebo administration will placate the patient and save carers' time, and therefore it is justified. Any 'feel better' outcome of placebo action may be temporary and could be far outweighed by the 'feel worse' outcome that would result from a patient suspecting that they had been given inactive medication. It seems best to conclude that the administration of a placebo is morally suspect and should always be questioned, except when it is given as part of a properly organised clinical trial. If health professionals adopt this type of response the occurrence of placebo misuse will be minimised.

Oral preparations	
Tablet	• A pressed powder form. • Manufacturers often 'personalise' the shape of the tablet of a particular drug. • Sometimes mixed with colorant. • When formula tastes bitter, the powder can be covered in sugared coating. • A few drugs can be absorbed from the sublingual and buccal areas of the mouth.
Capsule	• A gelatine covered form. • After ingestion, the gelatine slowly dissolves releasing the active drug. • Cylindrical or oblong in shape. • Slow-release formulations are available, in which small capsules within the main capsule contain the drug and release it slowly.
Liquid	• Drugs that can be manufactured in this form are mixed with a fluid component, which allows the drug to be taken orally in one of the following ways: solution, mixture, syrup or elixir.
Solution	• The active constituent(s) (solute) is dissolved in a solvent, often water. • Additives to alter the colour and/or flavour may be present.
Mixture	• This is generally used when drugs do not dissolve in solution, but remain as particulate matter in suspension. • In order to disperse the drug evenly through the liquid, and ensure accurate dose delivery, the liquid must be shaken before use.
Syrup	• The drug is delivered in a strong sugar solution.
Elixir	• The drug is contained in a flavoured and mixed solvent, usually water and alcohol.

Table 2.2 Oral preparations

Injectable preparations
Some drugs can be stabilised in one or more of the following injectable forms: Intra- or subcutaneous • Solutions that are absorbed slowly from within or under the skin. Intramuscular • Drugs which are absorbed most evenly from a site in skeletal muscle Intravenous/intra-arterial • Administration directly into the circulation allows for quick delivery to sites of drug action

Table 2.3 Injectable preparations

HOW THE BODY DEALS WITH DRUGS AND HOW DRUGS AFFECT THE BODY

Drug action depends upon complex interactive processes involving the drug and the body. It is therefore important to understand the mechanisms by which the body interacts with the drug and vice versa. Pharmacologist researchers working for drug manufacturers undertake exhaustive experiments in the laboratory and in field trials. They identify the normal variability of these interactive processes applied to each drug in various experimental situations and at each stage of the life cycle (Rang *et al.*, 1995). See Chapter 4 *Legal aspects of drug administration* for further details of drug trials.

As a consequence, appropriate drug information can be supplied to healthcare professionals. The range of information made available in this way is identified in **Table 2.6**. Armed with this information, healthcare professionals can prescribe, administer and evaluate the response to drug therapy. They can also give accurate drug-related health education information and advice to patients.

HOW THE BODY DEALS WITH DRUGS

The effects that the body has on drugs depend on the processes of absorption, drug distribution, metabolism and elimination. Study of these biological mechanisms is called pharmacokinetics. A diagrammatic outline of pharmacokinetic processes and the ways in which they inter-relate is presented in **Figure 2.1**. Various factors influence how the body can use drugs, and of these one important consideration is the age of a patient (Parker *et al.*, 1995). The main effects on pharmacokinetics that are related to life span are outlined in **Table 2.7**. An equally important factor is the interaction of one drug with another when a patient is taking two or more drugs. The potential for drugs to interfere with each other is widespread, and occurs in all drug categories. Various mechanisms may be involved, affecting any of the pharmacokinetic processes (Laurence and Bennett, 1992). Before administering patient medication, it is important for the nurse to check that factors influencing pharmacokinetics have been taken into account appropriately, including the potential for drug interactions.

HOW DRUGS ARE TAKEN INTO THE BODY

As discussed previously, drugs can be taken in through different routes. Each of these has certain advantages and disadvantages as far as administration is concerned, and there are pharmacokinetic implications associated with each route (Whitman, 1995; Professional Development Unit, 1994a). Some of a drug, whether taken orally, transdermally or by subcutaneous or intramuscular injection, may

Table 2.4 Topical preparations

Topical preparations	
These preparations can be used alone to cool, soothe or moisten an area of skin. They can also be used as vehicles to deliver a drug to the skin.	
Lotion	• A fluid that may be a solution or a mixture. • Water or alcohol based. • Applied to the skin for quick but brief local effect.
Cream	• A composite of water with grease and an emulsifier. • It soothes and prevents drying of the area. • Some cooling is brought about by evaporation of the water component.
Ointment	• Grease based, and thicker and stickier than a cream. • Prevents drying of the treated skin surface.
Paste	• Grease and powder formulation. • The thickest vehicle of all, so has a protective function. • Moisturises by preventing surface evaporation.

Table 2.5 Special local preparations

Special local preparations	
Transdermal	• An adhesive 'patch' is loaded with the drug and positioned on the skin. • The drug is slowly absorbed through the skin.
'Drops'	• A sterile solution. • Introduced locally by a pipette or 'dropper'. • Common sites for this type of application: ear, eye and nose.
Inhalations	• Various devices can be used to deliver a drug to the airways; these are generally nebulisers or pressurised aerosols. • Drugs selectively have a local effect on the airways or are absorbed for a more generalised effect.
Pessaries	• Relatively large, elongated smooth-surfaced, solid formulations. • For insertion into vagina using fingers or special device. • The active drug is usually mixed with a fatty compound. • As the body heat melts the fat, the drug is slowly liberated.
Suppositories	• Cone or bullet-shaped and smooth-surfaced solid formulations. • For insertion through the anus, into the rectum. • The active drug is usually mixed with a fatty compound. • As body heat melts the fat, the drug is slowly liberated.

be changed or metabolised before it reaches the systemic circulation; therefore the amount available for distribution to the tissues – the bioavailability of the drug – is less than 100%. When a drug is given intravenously or intra-arterially, it all enters the circulation and therefore has a 100% availability. This may influence the calculation of the amount and timings of dosage (Schwertz, 1991).

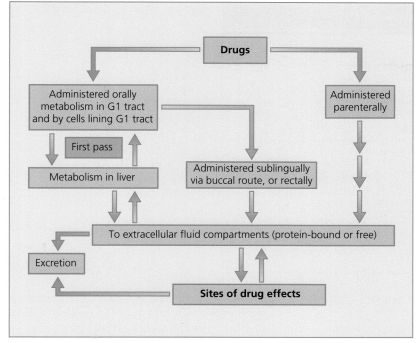

Fig 2.1 A diagrammatic outline of the pharmacokinetic process.

Drug information for health professionals
Formulations of the drug
The expected drug effects
Acceptable routes and rate of administration
Frequency of administration
Dosages
Special precautions
Contra-indications
Drug interactions and incompatibilities
Side-effects

Table 2.6 Drug information for health professionals

Age implications of drug formulations and administration

Ageing and its implications for drug formulations and administration should be taken into account when deciding what is appropriate for an individual patient, and the main considerations are identified in **Child Box 1** and **Elderly Box 1** below.

DRUG ABSORPTION

Drugs are most commonly given orally, so must first be absorbed through the gastrointestinal tract wall to get into the blood and be carried to their site of action (Rang *et al.*,

1995). Drugs are transported through the wall in one of three main ways: passive diffusion, active transport and filtration (**Fig. 2.2**).

Passive diffusion

The drug molecules are dissolved in gastrointestinal tract fluid and pass across the lining cell membranes and into the bloodstream, down a drug concentration gradient. The efficiency of this process depends not only on the degree of drug concentration (the concentration gradient) but also on the lipid solubility of the drug. As cell membranes have many lipoprotein elements, drugs that are relatively soluble in lipids can use these lipoprotein elements to quicken their progress across membranes. This characteristic influences not only absorption in the gastrointestinal tract but also distribution of the drug throughout the body.

Active transport

A few drugs can make use of physiological mechanisms already in existence for the transport of selected substances across membranes, for example levodopa (L-dopa) is actively transported via a mechanism usually used to transport amino acids.

Filtration

A small number of drugs can be absorbed though a pressure gradient via 'pores' between cells. This capacity is restricted to only the smallest of drug molecules, as most drugs are too large to pass through the pore.

Table 2.7 Age and pharmacokinetics

Age and pharmacokinetics		
	Children	Elderly
Absorption	Unreliable in neonates	In general unchanged
Distribution	Fat component of body mass tends to be proportionately greater, acting as drug reservoir so relatively large drug dose required	
Metabolism	Reduced capacity due to immature liver in infants, so drug effects prolonged/excessive	Slight reduction due to impaired liver function, so drug effects more pronounced and longer lasting
Excretion	Reduced capacity due to immature kidneys in infants	Reduction due to impaired glomerular filtration rate

Factors influencing absorption through oral route

The absorption of drugs can be influenced by many mechanisms. These include the nature of the drug formulation, natural interactions within the alimentary tract, disease states and altered gut motility.

2.1 DRUG ADMINISTRATION AND THE YOUNG

Children do not like to take bitter-tasting medicine and their normal response is to spit it out. So, if possible, sweet-tasting medicine should be used, while trying to avoid the risk of dental caries. Otherwise, perhaps the bitter taste can be disguised in sweet-tasting food, if the presence of food does not adversely affect absorption. A problem of providing medicines in a sweet-tasting formulation is that the child may mistake the medicine for sweets, therefore safe storage is particularly important.

Some children also find it difficult to swallow tablets, and may need to have powdered tablets crushed.

Children often have a fear of injection and this fear can persist into adulthood. When giving intermittent injections is unavoidable, 'magic patches' can be used to anaesthetise the site before each injection.

It is important to attend to psychological aspects of injection in order to prevent or minimise distress to children, particularly to those who may require injections daily all their life.

Transcutaneous absorption is greater in children than in adults, resulting in higher levels of drug in the blood than with a similar drug dose given to an adult; therefore application of drugs to the skin should be used in a reduced dose.

Some drugs are broken down by enzymes or are inactivated by the pH environment in the gastrointestinal tract, for example insulin, and therefore cannot be given orally. Special chemical packaging of drugs can affect their absorption rate such as slow-release potassium (slow K). The presence of food may reduce, quicken or slow absorption, for example milk impairs absorption of tetracycline, and food of any sort limits absorption of rifampicin, whereas propranolol is absorbed more quickly

2.1 DRUG ADMINISTRATION AND THE OLDER PERSON

Part of the ageing process includes the production of less saliva, which may result in a dry mouth. This may make the swallowing of tablets difficult. It is important, therefore, to moisten the mouth before introducing a tablet, and provide a large volume of fluid (at least 100 ml or a half-full tumbler) to help swallow the tablet and prevent it sticking to the wall of the oesophagus.

Compliance in the elderly is a potential problem for several reasons. For example, some elderly people are taking several drugs and find it difficult to remember the correct therapy schedule.

Older people have increasing difficulty sorting out in their memory whether they actually took their drug or just thought about taking the drug. As a result, they may mistakenly believe they took it – so missing a dose – or mistakenly believe they did not take it – so taking double the prescribed dose.

Safety caps on bottles are, by their nature, difficult to open, and this may present a particular problem for weakened, possibly arthritic, elderly hands and wrists. On request, pharmacists will supply non-safety caps.

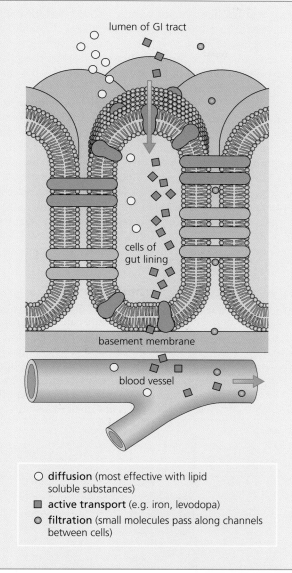

diagram labels:
lumen of GI tract

cells of
gut lining

basement membrane

blood vessel

○ **diffusion** (most effective with lipid
  soluble substances)
■ **active transport** (e.g. iron, levodopa)
◉ **filtration** (small molecules pass along channels
  between cells)

Fig 2.2 Absorption of drugs from the alimentary tract.
GI, gastrointestinal.

in the presence of food. As most drug absorption happens in the first part of the small intestine, any change in gastrointestinal motility will influence it. If gastric emptying is delayed, as happens for example in migraine, then absorption of analgesic agents, for instance, may consequently be delayed. Also, the gastric emptying rate in young babies is unreliable, and as a result absorption is likely to be uneven and unpredictable. Disease that affects the gastrointestinal tract wall may cause malabsorptive problems. Logically it might be expected to be associated with impaired drug absorption, but, rarely, it can cause an increase. For example, infective diarrhoea results in reduced absorption,

whereas, in coeliac disease, some drugs (such as cephalexin) are absorbed more efficiently.

Factors affecting absorption through injection (subcutaneous, intramuscular, intravenous)

The blood supply to muscle is greater than that to subcutaneous tissue, so it is generally the case that absorption is quicker from intramuscular sites. However, sometimes drugs are incompletely and unpredictably absorbed through both these routes (John and Stevenson, 1995). Similarly, intramuscular absorption should be quicker than through the oral route, but this is not the case for a few drugs, phenytoin for instance. Absorptive rates can be modified deliberately, by changes to the nature of the drug and/or its solvent. For example, insulin can be injected in soluble form, which is quickly distributed throughout the body, or attached to protein, which delays its uptake and availability to the tissues. Intravenous drugs are introduced into the circulation directly and are therefore available for quick and efficient distribution to target tissues.

DRUG DISTRIBUTION

Once into the bloodstream, a drug must be distributed to body tissues in order to have an effect. Drugs travel bound to plasma protein, mostly an alpha glycoprotein. It is the drug not bound to the protein or other carrier molecules that is available for binding to cell membrane receptors and therefore responsible for activating cellular responses. Factors modifying protein-binding may affect the proportion of unbound drug. Examples include renal disease, hypoalbuminaemia (e.g. in liver failure), displacement by other drugs and saturation of binding sites. In such cases dosage may need to be correspondingly adjusted (Grahame-Smith and Aronson, 1992).

Distribution throughout the fluid compartments of the body depends on the lipid solubility of the drug, as mentioned previously. Drugs that are highly lipid soluble are distributed freely in all fluid compartments because they pass easily through cell membranes. Those with limited lipid solubility are able to pass into interstitial tissue spaces or are retained in the plasma, but only pass in a minor way into intracellular compartments. Obesity affects distribution of drugs, particularly very lipid soluble ones such as the anaesthetic agent thiopentone, by acting as a drug trap or reservoir.

Variability in blood circulation to parts of the body influences the ability of the drug to get to target tissues. Tissues with a good blood supply, for example kidneys and liver, tend to receive more of the drug than those with a poorer blood supply. In shock, when perfusion is reduced, there can be a major effect on the efficiency of drug delivery to even the 'vital' organs. In pregnancy, many drugs are effectively distributed, through increased blood flow in the uterine wall, to the placental and fetal circulation.

The availability of cell membrane receptors is a factor that must also be taken into account when considering drug distribution. They may already be saturated with the drug or the medication may have to compete with another drug for the receptor binding site. Finally, in some cases, the presence of active transport mechanisms that drugs can utilise to get into cells may be important (Rang *et al.*, 1995).

Metabolism

Drugs are mostly metabolised in the liver, although the gastrointestinal tract, lungs and kidneys may also be involved. Cytotoxic drugs, however, are designed to be metabolised in many different body cells, whereas neurotransmitters undergo their chemical changes at nerve endings only. Metabolic reactions consist of two types: phase 1 and phase 2.

Phase 1 involves various chemical reactions (hydrolysis, oxidation, reduction) that change the chemical structure of a drug to produce, generally, equally active, or more active, metabolites. The group of enzymes facilitating phase 1 reactions commonly are called cytochrome P450 and are situated in the smooth endoplasmic reticulum of liver cells.

Phase 2 involves various conjugation reactions, in which a drug is chemically combined with a more water-soluble substance (e.g. sulphate, glucuronide, acetyl CoA). As a result, the more water-soluble product is generally an inactive compound and it is in a form that can be easily excreted.

Drugs that are absorbed through the gastrointestinal tract pass via the hepatic portal circulation to the liver where many are metabolised before reaching the general, systemic circulation.

This 'first pass' metabolism may result in a more active drug metabolite product, or more commonly a relatively inactive one (John and Stevenson, 1995). In either case, first pass metabolic effects must be known when working out the dosage of oral drugs, since a larger or smaller dosage may be needed compared with, for example, intravenous dosage requirements. Without metabolic reactions, drugs would persist in the body possibly for months or years.

Half-life

This is a measure of the rate at which the active drug is removed from the body. It is a variable and depends upon the particular mix of pharmacokinetic properties characteristic of each drug. For example, if the peak plasma level of a drug is 10 mg/l and this is reduced to 5 mg/l after 3 hours, then the half-life of that drug is 3 hours. This is an important consideration in determining dosage and dose intervals necessary to maintain therapeutic plasma levels of the drug.

Excretion

Most drugs must be metabolised to more water-soluble metabolites before they can be excreted. All body fluids, including breast milk, saliva and sweat can be used to excrete drugs; however, the urinary system offers the main drug excretion route (**Fig. 2.3**). In the kidney, those drugs that are active in relatively water-soluble form can be excreted unchanged through filtration. Drugs can also be passively reabsorbed in the proximal tubule down a concentration gradient. The third process important to drug clearance is secretion, carried out by cells lining the proximal tubules. Any variability in the effectiveness of these processes influences the rate of excretion (Laurence and Bennett, 1992). For example, in the first 6 months of life, the immature kidneys have a reduced drug clearance ability. After the age of 40 years, kidney function deteriorates so drug excretion becomes less efficient. Various disease processes also affect excretion, such as renal failure caused by glomerular or tubular pathology. If drugs are excreted in a metabolically active form, then these factors will necessarily have an influence on dosage considerations (White, 1994).

HOW DRUGS AFFECT THE BODY

Study of the ways in which drugs can affect body tissues is termed pharmacodynamics. As the purpose of drug administration is to achieve a certain, predicted effect within the body, it is essential for nurses to have a level of knowledge about drug actions sufficient to support safe

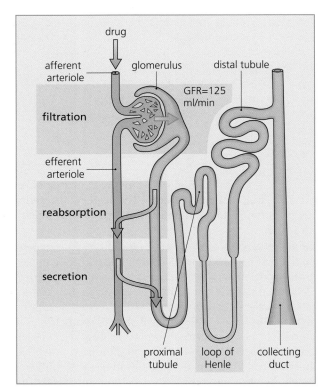

Fig 2.3 Route of drug excretion. GFR: glomerular filtration rate.

practice. This is particularly relevant as experienced nurses are, increasingly, expanding their practice into new areas of prescribing, administration and evaluation of drug therapy (Kelly, 1995).

It is perhaps not surprising that many factors can influence the ability of drugs to have their therapeutic effect at target tissues, given the precision of targeting required. As well as unpredictable idiosyncratic responses in individuals, various diseases may have pharmacodynamic effects; for example, in nephrotic syndrome there is a reduced sensitivity to frusemide because of abnormal influences of albumin in the kidney tubule lumen. Drug interactions can also have various pharmacodynamic effects in target tissues. In patients taking digoxin and diuretics, hypokalaemia brought about by diuretic action in the kidney may increase the effect of digoxin on the heart. Age also offers potential for variation in the effects of drugs on tissues because ageing tissues have a changed sensitivity to some drugs. Before administration of drugs it is important, therefore, to check that pharmacodynamic considerations have been taken into account (Professional Development Unit, 1994a and 1994b).

Drugs exert their effects by binding to molecules in body cells. Through this chemical reaction they bring about some modification of the cell physiology because the 'new' bound elements function differently to the original unbound cell molecules. This 'difference' amounts to the drug effect. Generally, drugs are formulated to have a targeted effect on specific cells rather than to have their therapeutic effect operate equally on all body cells. As a consequence, therefore, a drug must have an unequal uptake in the body, being bound only to targeted molecules in specific tissues (Rang *et al.*, 1995). An outline of the main target mechanisms for drugs is presented in **Figure 2.4**.

Receptor-targeted mechanisms

Although much about pharmacodynamic processes cannot be explained as yet, it is clear that many drugs produce therapeutic effects at the cell by binding with a receptor either on the cell surface or in the cell cytoplasm. The drug–receptor interaction then produces the drug effect, and the drug is called an agonist. The degree of drug effect is proportional to the number of receptors with which it interacts.

Alternatively, when some drugs bind to their receptor molecules they block the receptors so that these receptors cannot be occupied by any other chemical. The result in this case is a negative one because a biological response is prevented by the presence of the drugs. In this type of interaction, the drug is termed an antagonist. If the antagonist does not completely block the receptors, it is termed a partial agonist, so the relationship between agonist and antagonist is a competitive one. (For examples see Chapter 8 *Drugs and neurological disorders*.) Four categories of receptors have been identified (**Fig. 2.5**). To bring about their actions, these receptors may be linked with other

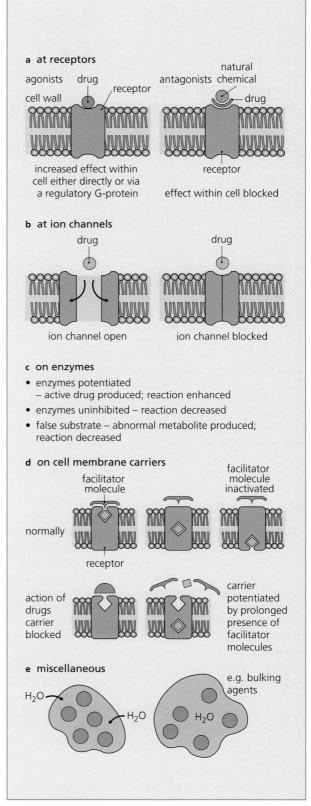

Fig 2.4 Mechanisms of drug action.

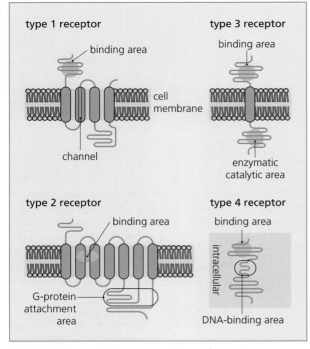

type 1 receptor

binding area

cell membrane

channel

type 2 receptor

binding area

G-protein attachment area

type 3 receptor

binding area

enzymatic catalytic area

type 4 receptor

binding area

intracellular

DNA-binding area

Fig 2.5 Diagrammatic representation of receptor structure. (From Rang et al 1995, with permission.)

molecules in the cell in an organised way to cause a series or cascade of processes (receptor–effector links) that eventually lead to the desired effect.

Type 1 receptors are situated in cell membranes, with the binding site positioned on the outside, and are linked directly with an ion channel through which the receptor-specific drug can pass into the cell extremely quickly (Lombard, 1992). For example, many excitatory neurotransmitters such as acetylcholine use this mechanism and as a result may provoke the influx of 10^7 ions per second through just one ionic gate into the cell.

Type 2 receptors are also situated in cell membranes but their binding site is within the cell membrane layers. Many hormones and some slow neurotransmitters use this type, which exerts its effects more slowly than the type 1 receptors. The type 2 activated receptor becomes receptive to a group of proteins labelled G-proteins inside the cell. As a result the G-protein locks into the receptor molecule. This in turn causes an enzymatic change to part of the G-protein complex, which then breaks off from the receptor and travels to another part of the cell membrane; here it exerts its effect by bringing about activation or inhibition of an ionic channel or a membrane enzyme. The complex nature of this series of activities understandably produces a time delay between receptor activation and effect.

Type 3 receptors are used by several hormones, including insulin and cell growth factors. The receptor site on the outside of the cell membrane is connected to a tyrosine

enzyme component lying inside the cell membrane. When a receptor binding site is occupied, the tyrosine itself is then converted into a binding site for compatible intracellular proteins. Proteins that are compatible have a great variety of effects; some, for example, in turn trigger proteins influencing cell division and differentiation. It is known that many growth factors can activate oncogenes to bring about persistent, repetitive cell division cycles. In other words, the cell growth factors each trigger transcription of targeted strips of chromosomes and in this way control growth and replication of the cell.

Type 4 receptors are part of a pathway by which DNA transcription is regulated through the stimulus of, for example, thyroid and steroid hormones. Although these hormones all have very dissimilar effects in different tissues, it has recently been discovered that they operate through the same cellular mechanism. Each triggers transcription of particular genes, which in turn provokes production of specific proteins which in their turn have specific functions within the cell.

Iodine-containing thyroid hormones and many steroid hormones are very lipid-soluble, so pass across cell membranes readily. Once inside the cell, they bind to the receptor, which in this case is situated within the nucleus. Binding stimulates the receptor molecule to change shape so exposing the previously hidden DNA-specific component. This area of the receptor then binds to its targeted area of DNA. The outcome is the transcription of selected mRNA, which is then translated by the cell ribosomes to produce specific proteins.

Although the mechanism is the same for all hormones that bind type 4 receptors, each hormone affects different genes, so different proteins are produced, and this explains the diversity of hormonal action. The effects of type 4 reactions are very slow to appear compared with the results of types 1–3. The explanation rests in the protein synthesis part of the mechanism, as achieving an increase in protein production is a relatively slow and laborious process.

Any of these receptor-mediated processes can be used by drugs operating as either agonists or antagonists. However, the specific receptor mechanisms utilised by drugs are incompletely identified or understood, and much research is currently going on in this area. As well as these important receptor-linked pathways, there are other mechanisms that drugs can use.

Ion channel targets

Some drugs can operate directly on ion channels, without the process being regulated via receptors. For example, amiloride blocks kidney tubule sodium channels, preventing the influx of these ions (see Chapter 15 *Drugs and urological disorders*); vasodilator drugs such as nifedipine influence calcium channels directly by binding to protein in the channel wall (see Chapter 12 *Drugs and cardiovascular disorders*); sulphonylureas moderate the activity of potassium channels in the pancreatic β cells, causing electrical change across the cell membrane, which consequently stimulates insulin production (see Chapter 10 *Drugs and endocrine disorders*). Drugs acting to stop the action of ion channels are termed 'blockers' and those that change the channel operation in some way are termed 'modulators' (Rang *et al.*, 1995). Of all the possible drug activation mechanisms in body tissues, it is the processes involving ion channels, both the receptor-mediated and the direct action ones, that are the most common and important processes.

Enzyme-targeted mechanisms

Several drugs have their effect by acting directly on enzymes to enhance or, more commonly, to inhibit their actions (Kelly, 1995). These drugs may act as competitors (or 'inhibitors') to the enzyme, for example neostigmine competes with cholinesterase and thus reduces its effective action (see Chapter 8 *Drugs and neurological disorders* for further details). Because heparin interferes with enzymes in the blood coagulation cascade, it reduces the efficiency of the clotting mechanism (see Chapter 12 *Drugs and cardiovascular disorders*). The actions of monoamine oxidase enzymes are inhibited by the antagonistic effects of selegiline (see Chapter 7 *Drugs and psychological disorders*). In this case, the blocking action is irreversible, and the drug effects only diminish when more enzyme is synthesised. This inhibition causes an increase in the availability of noradrenaline and serotonin in central nervous system neurons, which then (in some way not yet well understood) have an antidepressant effect (see Chapter 7 *Drugs and psychological disorders*). Azathioprine acts as a cytotoxic agent through its ability to inhibit enzymes involved in DNA synthesis.

Alternatively, drugs may mimic an enzyme's own target molecules (acting as 'false substrate'), preventing the normal metabolic pathways from operating. For example methyldopa inserts itself into noradrenaline production processes, so reducing the effectiveness of sympathetic nervous system action, and as a consequence causes reduction in arterial blood pressure (see Chapter 12 *Drugs and cardiovascular disorders*).

Carrier molecule targets

Many molecules require some assistance to cross through a cell membrane. This help can be provided by carrier molecules of (generally) protein. Each type of carrier seems to be specific to a particular type of molecule requiring assistance. The specificity of carrier systems operates through recognition sites on the carrier molecule. Some drugs can target these sites, so inhibiting the influx or outflow of specific molecules (Rang *et al.*, 1995). For example, tricyclic antidepressants such as imipramine inhibit uptake of nor-adrenaline at nerve endings by targeting and blocking the carrier for noradrenaline.

Miscellaneous targets

Some drugs have idiosyncratic actions not easily categorised because they depend on the site of administration of the drug and/or its particular physical and chemical properties. For example, bulk aperients act by retaining a larger volume of water within the lumen of the gastrointestinal tract than normal, adding 'bulk' to the contents; this stimulates peristalsis.

UNWANTED DRUG EFFECTS

Although extensive pre-marketing trials of drugs aim to establish the range of dosage within which it is safe to prescribe, and the potential for unwanted effects in a variety of experimental situations and in different age groups, it is impossible to be 100% sure that every possible ill effect is identified before the drug appears on the market. Thalidomide is an excellent example of a drug with many advantages over the drugs it was planned to supersede, but with devastating teratogenic properties that had not been recognised.

All drugs are capable of bringing about harmful effects. These may relate to the main therapeutic function of the drug and therefore be, to some extent, predictable. Rarely, drugs can cause harm through overdosage, or because of some action that is not related to their main therapeutic function. Thus damage can occur as a result of pharmacokinetic or pharmacodynamic reactions. One drug can bring about an alteration in the effects of another drug, and sometimes the outcome is beneficial to the patient. Occasionally, however, drug combinations can have a detrimental effect.

Adverse effects related to pharmacological function

This is the commonest category of adverse reactions, and may result in severe symptoms. Clinically important ones often result from a narrow 'therapeutic margin'. This relates to the difference between the therapeutic dose range of a drug and the toxic level. When there is little leeway between the two, adverse effects are more likely (John and Stevenson, 1995).

Tolerance, or a decrease in the body's response to a drug, eventually leading to ineffectual treatment, is a potential problem in various drug–body interactions. For example, long-term pain management using opiates produces less and less pain relief though the drug dose is unchanged. As a result, to maintain a consistent level of pain control, increasing dosages are required (Grahame-Smith and Aronson, 1992).

Occasionally, tolerance may not be identified until the drug is stopped, the dose reduced, or an antagonist drug prescribed. At this point, symptoms of 'withdrawal' may become obvious. Several categories of drug may provoke this type of adverse effect, not only opiates; these are discussed in the appropriate system chapters. However, the ability of the body to make 'tolerance' adjustments is not, in all cases, a maladaptive response, but can be used therapeutically. For instance, vaccination relies on such an outcome and is explained in more detail in Chapter 5 *Drugs and immunological disorders.*

Other examples of drugs that have unwanted effects linked to the pharmacological action of the drug include anticoagulants, aspirin and cytotoxic agents.

Anticoagulants

Anticoagulants such as heparin and warfarin can cause excessive bleeding, therefore careful observation of patients for evidence of subcutaneous blood loss (abnormal bruising), and/or occult or frank blood in excreta is an important aspect of nursing care.

Aspirin

Aspirin is an anti-prostaglandin agent and it is through this counteraction of the prostaglandins that it exerts an anti-inflammatory effect. However, this mechanism can be harmful when it involves the gastrointestinal tract. In the stomach, prostaglandin synthesis brings about inhibition of gastric acid secretion. Aspirin inhibits the action of an enzyme necessary for prostaglandin production. Excess acid secretion results, and gastritis, stomach wall erosion and bleeding are the unwanted outcomes. Although these effects are usually minor, occasionally bleeding may be torrential and life threatening.

Cytotoxic agents

These operate by interfering in various ways with the synthesis of DNA and RNA, so that malignant neoplastic cells can be killed. It is not surprising that normal cells may be affected in a similar way, particularly cells with short cell cycles such as stem cells in the bone marrow and epithelial tissues.

Adverse effects unrelated to pharmacological function

These unwanted drug effects are not dose dependent, and are unpredictable. They are associated with a higher mortality than the adverse reactions related to pharmacological action (McPherson, 1993). The commoner responses are often the result of some type of allergic reaction to the drug. Examples of drugs that might provoke an idiosyncratic effect include glucocorticoids, allopurinol and penicillins.

Glucocorticoids

The therapeutic properties of this class of drugs are attributable to their anti-inflammatory effects; these are achieved through interaction with inflammatory cells, mediators and blood vessels. Unwanted effects are interference with collagen synthesis and inhibition of osteoblast activity, which may cause osteoporosis.

Allopurinol

Pharmacological effects of allopurinol involve a reduction in the amount of insoluble urates produced, by inhibition of an enzyme in the pathway of synthesis, so that insoluble crystals of urate are not deposited in the kidneys and other tissues. It is therefore used as a gout preventative agent. However, toxic effects include a generalised 'rash', erythema multiforme, which may prove fatal.

Penicillins

Therapeutically, penicillins are used to interfere with the enzyme systems of a microorganism, eventually leading to its death. Rarely, penicillin metabolites may react abnormally with body cells and provoke some type of hypersensitivity reaction. Such reactions are generally minor, but an uncommon, potentially fatal, response is anaphylactic shock.

Drug interactions

These may account for up to 20% of all unwanted drug reactions. The greater the number of drugs taken by a patient the more likely is a risk of interaction (Hussar, 1993). As the elderly tend to suffer more disease than younger age groups, polypharmacy (multiple drug therapy), and the potential for adverse drug interactions is more common in these patients (Drake and Romano, 1995). As with other drug effects, unwanted effects from interaction between drugs can involve pharmacokinetic or pharmacodynamic processes. To avoid, as far as possible, the potential for initiating this type of response, it is important for the nurse to check the drug literature supplied by the manufacturer and/or source texts containing the relevant information before administering combined drug schedules (Nicholson, 1993).

As well as toxic interactions in the body, when drugs are mixed together in a solution to prepare them for administration, there is the potential for the drugs to change chemically, and so alter their efficacy. To minimise this risk, nurses should follow a few safety principles as a guide to administering intravenous therapy and these are listed in **Warning Box 1**. Discussion on the legal aspects of adverse reactions and monitoring requirements is taken further in Chapter 4 *Legal aspects of drug administration.*

DOSAGE CONSIDERATIONS

The main practical nursing consideration when seeking to identify appropriate dosage for an individual patient is that the drug information leaflet or other relevant pharmacological text is checked and the recommended dose applied. The therapeutic range and margin of each drug and its dosage schedule is meticulously identified through research by pharmaceutical companies as the drug is being developed. As a result, overall dose recommendations are produced that are based on data about a variety of component elements.

2.1 GUIDELINES ON AVOIDANCE OF INTRAVENOUS DRUG INTERACTIONS

Read the drug manufacturer's leaflet.

Do not add drugs to intravenous solutions if possible.

Administer drugs in bolus intravenous injection as an alternative if possible.

Avoid adding more than one drug to a solution.

Check the drug is compatible with the intravenous fluid you wish to mix with it.

Use only dextrose or saline solutions as diluents, depending on compatibility with drug.

Mix the drug thoroughly with the intravenous fluid before attaching the giving set.

Secure a label to the infusion bag detailing the drug, dose and infusion times.

Protect infusion solutions from the light if appropriate.

If you have remaining, unanswered doubts, contact a pharmacist for advice.

Calculation of drug dosages is often by estimating the body surface area, particularly in children. Except for single-dose preparations given for a specific short-term effect, for example a premedication, consideration of the appropriateness of dosage is linked with the frequency of administration. Drugs have different rates of absorption, metabolic pathways, distribution patterns and excretion profiles. As a consequence, different dose–frequency schedules are required to maintain the required therapeutic levels in the plasma.

The nurses' accountability for safe practice requires them to assess the relevance of potential influences on the dosage of a drug, relating each of these to the individual patient's particular situation. The main issues to consider are listed in **Table 2.8**. Once she has identified the influences operating on a patient, the nurse can then judge the dose appropriate in that specific circumstance. In the United Kingdom, only selected groups of nurses who have undergone a specialist preparation programme can prescribe drug therapy. Nevertheless, all nurses are accountable for assessing the appropriateness of each aspect of a drug regime (Giuliano *et al.*, 1993; UKCC, 1992; Parker, 1993). Discussion of these important nursing care issues as they relate to legal accountability is to be found in Chapter 4 *Legal aspects of drug administration*.

A recent addition to knowledge about drug–body interactions stems from the increasing understanding of the relationships between the biorhythms of the body and the environment. It is now recognised that both pharmacokinetic and pharmacodynamic processes are influenced by normal daily physiological variations in body systems. These variations are controlled through pulsed melatonin production by the pineal gland. Melatonin secretion, in turn, is moderated by external light cues from the environment. By delivering drugs to fit in with the natural biorhythms, the effectiveness of drugs may be improved and the onset and severity of side effects can be limited (TPS Drug Information Centre, 1992). Numerous current research projects are focused in this area and evidence to support the relevance of chronopharmacology is being identified. For example, some biorhythm scheduling of anti-cancer therapy has been shown to produce beneficial

Table 2.8 Factors influencing dosage

Factors influencing dosage	
• Patient's condition	Physical/cognitive/emotional/social problems, e.g. patient's ability to understand and comply
• The drug	Category of drug Specific pharmaco-kinetic and -dynamic consideration of the drug
• Route of adminstration	Formulation of drug Consideration of patient's preference
• Age of patient	Young and old may require modified dosage Drug may have particular unwanted effects in young/old
• Nature of patient's disease	Severity Tissues/systems involved in pathophysiological changes Other, concomitant disease state affecting drug absorption Metabolism/distribution/excretion/potential beneficial effects
• Financial	The smallest dose/shortest course therapy likely to result in therapeutic effects. The cheapest drug available

outcomes (Kmietowicz, 1997). As the body of evidence about a greater variety of drugs increases, it is likely that chronopharmacological considerations will become an important element in planning many drug regimes.

DRUG MONITORING

It is part of the nurse's role to monitor the effects of therapy, make judgements about its effectiveness and identify possible reasons for a lack of, or unexpected, results (Kelly, 1995). A useful approach to evaluation is to have a series of questions in mind, each of which addresses an aspect of the 'drug choice to drug effect' pathway. This helps to cover all the potential areas of variability.

Prescribing drugs for children

There are differences in the absorption, distribution and elimination of drugs between adults and children. Major implications for monitoring are outlined below:

- Absorption of drugs given orally to the neonate and infant is unpredictable because of variable gastric emptying times, gastric acidity, gut motility and the effect of milk in the stomach.
- The rectal route is more reliable than the oral route.
- The intravenous route is the best option to ensure adequate blood and tissue concentrations.
- In the first few months of life the plasma protein is low so more of the drug may be unbound and pharmacologically active.
- The intramuscular route should be avoided as there is small muscle bulk, absorption is variable and this route is painful.
- There is significant systemic absorption across the skin surface. This can sometimes be used therapeutically but it is a potential cause of toxicity, for example alcohol and iodine from skin cleansing preparations.
- The older child may need liquid rather than tablet preparations; these are sugar free but the child has to be persuaded to swallow them.
- Because water constitutes a larger percentage of the body in the neonate (80%) than the older child (55%), drugs that distribute within the extracellular fluid require a larger dose relative to body weight.
- As extracellular fluid correlates with body surface area, this measurement is used when accurate drug dosage is needed; however, body weight is useful for drugs with high therapeutic indices as it is easier to manage.
- Drugs may also be prescribed on the basis of the average age and weight of children. In children over 12 years of age this weight-related dose should not be extrapolated as the dose will be toxic.
- Elimination in the neonate is slower than in older children and adults; the drug biotransformation is reduced as the microsomal enzymes in the liver are immature. This results in the prolonged half-life of drugs metabolised in the liver.

2.1 A FRAMEWORK OF QUESTIONS FOR EVALUATING DRUG THERAPY

Does the patient's condition warrant continued therapy?
Is this the right drug?
Is the route of administration appropriate?
What does the patient and/or carer say?
Is the drug being taken; is compliance a possible problem?
Are any patient symptoms likely to be linked to the drug's beneficial or adverse actions?
Should dosage be modified because of some change in patient or disease?
Are frequency or timings of administration appropriate?
Have relevant monitoring tests been carried out and results used appropriately?

- Renal excretion in the young is reduced by a low glomerular filtration rate, which increases the half-life of some drugs.
- Thus plasma concentrations particularly in neonates must be regularly checked (Campbell and Glasper, 1995).

MONITORING THERAPEUTIC AND TOXIC DOSAGE

Some drugs have a narrow therapeutic range and it may be vital to ensure the range is maintained, particularly in acute, severe illness when pharmacokinetic and/or pharmacodynamic problems may be suspected. Below the therapeutic dose, the drug is ineffective and the patient's condition remains unchanged; if the therapeutic range is exceeded, the drug may have toxic effects (Grahame-Smith and Aronson, 1992). It is therefore an important part of drug regimens that the serum level of the drug is intermittently estimated as accurately as possible during a course of therapy. For example, gentamicin has severe dose-related toxic effects; it is particularly damaging to inner ear sensory cells and kidney tubule cells. Tissue levels of the drug rise throughout the course of therapy and, as the drug is excreted in a relatively active state via the kidneys, it is important to check that kidney damage is not inhibiting excretion; were this to be so, blood tissue levels would quickly rise, causing further damage in an upwardly spiralling way. As part of the monitoring programme plasma and urine samples should be tested for evidence of abnormal levels, and the urine should be further tested for signs of kidney damage.

In order to achieve a therapeutic level of drug distribution, some drugs must first be given in an extra large, bolus dose called the loading dose. Plasma samples are tested before, during and after the loading phase in order to check that a therapeutic effect has been reached (and not exceeded). The anticoagulant warfarin is monitored in this way. Unfortunately, with warfarin the results are difficult to interpret because the fibrin effects take a few days to develop. The picture is further complicated by, usually, prior administration of heparin therapy. However, a standardised international time test is used to measure the action of warfarin on plasma prothrombin. In this way, its effectiveness can be maximised while the risk of potential bleeding resulting from overdose is restricted.

For patients with insulin-dependent diabetes mellitus, it is important to test how their insulin therapy is affecting the β pancreatic cells. An outcome of the activity of insulin, that is, blood glucose levels are therefore assessed. By intermittent monitoring, the insulin dose can be titrated against blood glucose level and modified appropriately. In this way, an approximation to the normal homeostatic regulation of blood glucose can be attempted. If this is carried out, not only will it prevent the major acute metabolic disturbance of hypoglycaemia, but it will lessen the occurrence of chronic, disabling complications.

Knowledge of the basic pharmacological and therapeutic issues discussed in this introductory chapter is essential to help the nurse make appropriate judgements about patients' drug requirements.

 KEY POINTS

- The formulation of a drug is specific to its method and route of administration.
- Pharmacokinetics involves drug absorption, distribution, metabolism and elimination.
- Drug absorption, distribution and metabolism are influenced by age, the nature of the drug and disease.
- The relationship between drug absorption, distribution and metabolism determines the blood levels of drug available to body tissues.
- Pharmacodynamics is the study of effects of drugs on the body.

- Targets for drugs vary; receptor molecules and cell enzymes are two examples.
- Side effects of drug therapy can involve either pharmacokinetic or pharmacodynamic processes.
- Drug characteristics and their interaction with the patient's condition determine dosage and frequency of administration.
- The nurse must evaluate the effectiveness of drug therapy.

REFERENCES

Campbell S, Glasper EA. *Whaley and Wong's children's nursing.* London: Mosby, 1995.

Drake AC, Romano E. How to protect your older patient from the hazards of polypharmacy. *Nursing* 1995; **25**:34-39.

Giuliano KK, Richards N, Kaye W. A new strategy for calculating medication infusion rates. *Crit Care Nurse* 1993; **13**:77-81.

Grahame-Smith DG, Aronson JK. *Oxford textbook of clinical pharmacology, 2nd ed.* Oxford: Oxford University Press, 1992.

Hussar DA. Reviewing drug interactions. *Nursing,* 1993, 23(9):50-57.

John A, Stevenson T. A basic guide to the principles of drug therapy. *Br J Nurs* 1995; **4**:1194-1198.

Kelly J. Pharmacodynamics and drug therapy. *Professional Nurse* 1995; **10**:792-796.

Kmietowicz Z. Chemotherapy better tolerated when matched to body's rhythm. *BMJ* 1997; **315**:627.

Knight L. *Collins English dictionary and thesaurus.* Glasgow: Harper Collins, 1997.

Laurence DR, Bennett PN. *Clinical pharmacology, 7th ed.* Edinburgh: Churchill Livingstone, 1992.

Lombard JC. Update on pharmacology. *Nursing RSA Verpleging* 1992; **7**:43-44.

McPherson G. Absorbing effects. *Nurs Times* 1993; **89**:30-32.

Nicholson SH. Infusion therapy programme requires nursing skill and knowledge. *Provider* 1993; **April**:38-40.

Parker BM, Cusack BJ, Vestal RE. Pharmacokinetic optimisation of drug therapy in elderly patients. *Drugs Ageing* 1995; **7**:10-18.

Parker S. Trading places. *Nurs Times* 1993; **10**:42-43.

Professional Development Unit. 8 Part 1, Medication – knowledge for practice. *Nurs Times* 1994a; **90**:1-4.

Professional Development Unit. 8 Part 3, Medication – revision notes. *Nurs Times* 1994b; **90**:9-14.

Rang HP, Dale MM, Ritter JM. *Pharmacology, 3rd ed.* Edinburgh: Churchill Livingstone, 1995.

Schwertz DW. Basic principles of pharmacological action. *Nurs Clin N Am* 1991; **26**:245-263.

TPS Drug Information Centre. The right time? Chronopharmacology – a new science. *Nursing RSA Verpleging* 1992; **7**:23-27.

UKCC. *Standards for the administration of medicines.* London: UKCC, 1992.

White A. Pharmacology for nursing practice. *Br J Nurs* 1994 **3**:506-509.

Whitman M. The push is on – delivering medications safely by IV bolus. *Nursing* 1995, **25**:52-54.

Wood LS, Gullo SM IV. Vesicants: how to avoid extravasation. *Am J Nursing* 1993; **93**:42-50.

Sylvia Prosser

CLASSES OF DRUGS

INTRODUCTION

Drugs can be classified according to the effects they have or to the physiological mechanisms they enhance or inhibit. The main groups presented here are discussed later in the specific chapters; to avoid duplication, only the major modes of action are outlined below. The information that follows here should therefore be read in conjunction with the specific system chapters.

Some pharmacological agents have a range of functions, although they are primarily described as being within a specific class. For instance, beta adrenergic blockers, henceforth referred to as beta-blockers, work by inhibiting the uptake of nerve impulses from the β receptors of the sympathetic nervous system. These agents can be used to reduce blood pressure by decreasing the cardiac output and peripheral resistance; in addition, they reduce subjective anxiety and relieve palpitations and migraine. Aspirin may be taken to relieve pain and is most popularly known as an analgesic; but, in low doses, it also has the effect of relieving platelet stickiness by its action upon prostaglandins and is therefore used as prophylaxis against thrombotic episodes.

ADRENOCORTICOSTEROIDS

These are the hormones that are secreted by the adrenal cortex: hydrocortisone (cortisol); aldosterone; some of the androgens and oestrogens, and corticosterone. The corticosteroids are mainly subdivided into glucocorticoids and mineralocorticoids. Glucocorticoids, as the name implies, have influence upon glucose handling within the body, and mineralocorticoids, in the form of aldosterone, are largely responsible for sodium homeostasis by influencing renal sodium reabsorption in the distal tubule of the nephrons. Because the distal tubule excretes potassium in exchange for the conserved sodium, aldosterone also reduces serum potassium levels.

The term adrenocorticosteroid is most frequently used to describe hydrocortisone. This hormone mediates the long-term stress response by mobilising glucose for muscle fuel and allowing the effects of sympathetic nervous system stimulation to be sustained. The result is that the initially increased cardiac drive is maintained, and a vasopressor effect elevates the arterial blood pressure. This is augmented by the sodium-retaining properties of aldosterone, which is also secreted as part of the natural long-term stress response. Adrenocorticosteroids may be given as replacement therapy in cases of adrenal failure, as in Addison's disease or adrenal failure caused by septic shock, or may be prescribed to inhibit cellular activity, as in the treatment of leukaemia, or to suppress the immune system, as in anti-rejection treatment after organ transplantation. The cells of the body have steroid receptors in their cytoplasm. Steroids combine with these receptors and the resulting compound passes into the cell nucleus, where protein replication is subsequently inhibited. For this reason, patients receiving corticosteroids have impaired wound healing and tissue regeneration.

THE EFFECTS OF PROLONGED CORTICOSTEROID THERAPY

There is a balance to be maintained between the benefits of steroid therapy and the adverse effects. Benefits include an enhanced sense of wellbeing; increased appetite; the reduction of symptoms of inflammatory disorders, such as pain, joint dysfunction and swelling in severe arthritic disease; reduction of bronchospasm in chronic obstructive airways disease and reduction of symptoms associated with steroid-sensitive tumours. Although the administration of corticosteroids may produce what can seem a miraculous improvement for the patient, there are, however, costs of long-term steroid therapy (see **Table 3.1**). Patients receiving sustained corticosteroid therapy should be observed and taught to recognise signs of the adverse effects.

Problems which may be encountered when nursing patients taking high dose corticosteroids for prolonged periods of time	
Problem	**Need**
Risk of suppression of the hypothalamus, pituitary or adrenal glands due to loss of normal homeostatic feedback systems	Monitoring of blood pressure for hypotension; increase steroid therapy to cover physiological stresses such as surgery or infection. Patients carry steroid cards for this reason
Risk of Cushing's syndrome	Observe for fat accumulation on face ('moon face') and trunk; hypertension; hirsutism of face; abdominal striae; bruising; acne; muscle wasting; oedema; pathological fractures due to osteoporosis
Steroid-induced diabetes	Observe for glycosuria; blood sugar monitoring
Immunosuppression	Observe for signs of infection
Risk of peptic ulceration	Enteric coated corticosteroids to protect gastric mucosa; antacid therapy; observe for signs of gastro-intestinal bleeding
Impaired wound healing	Particular care of pressure areas and incisions and skin trauma
Mental instability	Heed relatives' and friends' reports of altered mood states such as depression, changes in thinking patterns or insomnia
Cataracts	Report complaints of altered vision

Table 3.1 Problems which may be encountered when nursing patients taking high dose corticosteroids for prolonged periods of time

Steroid preparations

These include:

- **Hydrocortisone** is given orally, intramuscularly or intravenously for replacement therapy, allergic or hypersensitivity disorders.
- **Prednisolone** and its precursor drug, prednisone, are given to reduce inflammation.
- **Methylprednisolone** is given as an anti-inflammatory and for anti-rejection transplant therapy.
- **Triamcinolone** is given as an anti-inflammatory; it has no sodium-retaining effect.
- **Dexamethasone** is given as an anti-inflammatory.

Corticosteroids suppress the natural homeostatic stress response when taken over a prolonged period. For this reason, patients receiving long-term treatment carry warning cards to inform personnel of this in a medical emergency. Sudden withdrawal of the corticosteroid would put the patient at risk of developing adrenal failure and hypotension. For this reason, treatment is never curtailed dramatically, rather it is reduced gradually.

ANAESTHETICS

This group of chemicals is given, as the name implies, to diminish sensation. The desired effect may be loss of sensation within a discrete area of the body, for which a local anaesthetic is used, or complete loss of consciousness, in which case a general anaesthetic is required. Anaesthetics are given to enable toleration of an invasive procedure, and therefore anaesthetic agents may be administered in combination with additional preparations to obtain specific effects. For example, in order to suture a bleeding wound on the head, a vasoconstrictor such as adrenaline may be added to the local anaesthetic. Vasoconstrictors must not be used as part of local anaesthesia for extremities such as fingers and toes, as the encircling ring of local anaesthetic and vasoconstrictor may interrupt the arteriolar circulation, causing localised ischaemia and a risk of necrosis. In the case of surgery to the internal viscera, in addition to the lack of pain and sensation, muscle relaxation is required to enable surgical access to deep structures that would otherwise be made inaccessible by muscle spasm.

Anaesthetics work by interrupting the generation of action potentials along the nerve tracts conveying pain information to the cerebral cortex. Local anaesthetics impede transmission within the nociceptor fibres in the peripheral tissues or the ascending tracts of the spinal cord. General anaesthetics impede transmission within the central nervous system, thus producing a loss of consciousness. In these circumstances, the patient loses not only consciousness, but also the protective cough and swallow airway reflex, so a general principle of care for an anaesthetised patient is to preserve the airway until such time as recovery enables the patient once more to resume this function. Muscle relaxation and the loss of the protective proprioceptor input require that staff caring for an unconscious anaesthetised patient assume responsibility for that patient to ensure that damage does not occur as a result of unsuitable positioning during the operative procedure. The removal of pain perception will form part of a strategy for anaesthesia as, clearly, in addition to being unaware of events, the patient would wish to feel no pain. Medication for anaesthesia will incorporate, therefore, substances that remove the perception of pain.

ANALGESICS

Algesia means 'pain', so analgesics are substances that remove the perception of pain. Because they are not general anaesthetics, the perception of pain is removed without causing the patient to lose consciousness. In a manner similar to local anaesthetics, analgesics work by interrupting the transmission between the peripheral nociceptor fibres and the sensory cortex of the brain. Depending upon the cause of the pain, reduction of overall awareness may be desirable. Some strong analgesics also produce sedation, which is helpful when treating patients with traumatic injuries in whom fear would otherwise amplify pain perception.

Pain may be of a chronic nature and in such cases analgesia that causes drowsiness would produce an undesirable disruption to everyday living, possibly provoking accidents because of reduction in vigilance and reaction times. It would be inconvenient to be precluded from driving a car because one had taken analgesia for a headache or dysmenorrhoea! For these reasons, there are a range of pharmacological agents used in the treatment of pain; some are relatively mild in their overall effects and these can be bought without prescription. Others are potent analgesics causing sedation and, in susceptible subjects or in large sustained doses, chemical dependency. In the case of these latter preparations, distribution is subject to legal restrictions (see Chapter 4 *Legal aspects of drug administration*).

ANTI-INFLAMMATORY DRUGS

In addition to the adrenocorticosteroids discussed above, the unwanted effects of inflammation such as pain and dysfunction may be treated with non-steroidal anti-inflammatory drugs (NSAIDs). These drugs exert their effect by inhibiting the chemical chain reaction that takes place in response to tissue damage caused by toxins, infection or mechanical trauma.

Non-steroidal anti-inflammatory drugs inhibit the production of prostaglandins. This group of chemical mediators is produced as a result of interaction between arachidonic acid and the enzyme cyclo-oxygenase. The arachidonic acid molecule is converted to a prostaglandin by cyclo-oxygenase. Prostaglandins enhance the inflammatory reaction and are also algesic (pain-producing) substances in their own right. By blocking prostaglandin synthesis, therefore, the inflammatory process is suppressed and the transmission of nociceptor (pain) nerve impulses is diminished. Pain is thus reduced by both means. Non-steroidal anti-inflammatory drugs are classed according to the strength of their action. Paracetamol is an example of a weak NSAID; ibuprofen is a moderate NSAID and salicylic acid (aspirin) is a potent agent. All of these agents have the advantage of reducing pain without causing undue sedation or producing the adverse effects associated with adrenocorticosteroid therapy for painful inflammatory conditions. The weaker preparations are most commonly used for simple pain relief, but aspirin has more widely ranging effects and is therefore used as treatment for a variety of conditions.

ACTIONS OF ASPIRIN
- Mild analgesic (blocks prostaglandin synthesis).
- Antipyretic: the temperature-regulating centre in the hypothalamus is controlled by prostaglandins. By blocking the action of these, raised temperature caused by inflammatory processes is controlled by re-instituting the normal heat loss mechanisms that were temporarily suspended as a result of the pathological process. Aspirin only influences thermoregulation in infective states and has no other effect upon temperature control (Laurence and Bennett, 1992).
- Effects upon blood coagulation: aspirin affects the process of haemostasis in two ways. The main effect is by blocking platelet cyclo-oxygenase. Aspirin forms an irreversible bond with cyclo-oxygenase and prevents thromboxane A_2 production for the duration of the life of the platelets. This prolongs the bleeding time. Large doses of aspirin compete chemically with vitamin K within the clotting cascade, and thus inhibit clot formation.
- Moderate doses of aspirin increase the excretion of urates from the kidney. Low-dose aspirin therapy causes the kidney to retain urates.

In excessive doses, such as in aspirin overdose, aspirin causes an increase in the metabolic rate, with increased cellular oxygen consumption and carbon dioxide secretion. The increased acidic load of carbon dioxide and salicylic acid produces a stimulant effect upon the chemoreceptor system and the respiratory centre, so hyperventilation is notable in aspirin poisoning.

ANTIARRHYTHMIC DRUGS

Cardiac arrhythmias may result from altered impulse formation or conduction. Action potentials within nerves or muscle fibres are produced as a result of shifts in positively charged ions in and out of the nerve or muscle cells. As the positively charged particles enter the cell via ion pumps in the muscle cell membrane, the interior of the cell becomes positively charged. The action potential thus created causes an increase in the affinity of actin and myosin for each other in the muscle fibres. Calcium is released from store; this release makes the binding sites available between the two molecules, and they combine transiently and repeatedly, thus moving over each other. During this process, the muscle fibre shortens. Drugs given to reduce cardiac arrhythmias usually act by blocking the movement of sodium, potassium or calcium across the muscle cell membrane (**Fig. 3.1**); fewer action potentials are generated and thus the muscle cells do not respond and fibre length remains unchanged. A detailed discussion of this class of drugs is to be found in Chapter 12 *Drugs and cardiovascular disorders*.

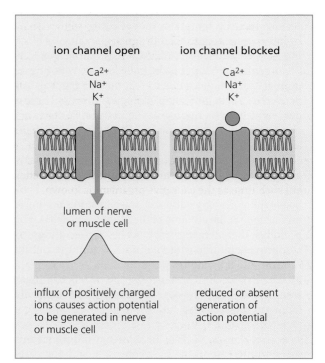

Fig 3.1 Action of ion channel blockers on nerve and muscle fibre.

ANTIBIOTICS

As their name implies, this class of drugs acts against life – the life in this context being that of microorganisms. For this reason, these drugs are also known as antimicrobials. Antimicrobial drugs may be antibacterial (acting upon bacteria); antiviral (acting upon viruses); antifungal (acting upon fungi); antiprotozoal (acting upon protozoal infections) or anthelmintics (acting upon parasitic worms). Antibiotics may act primarily by stopping cell division (bacteriostats) or by killing the microorganisms directly (bactericides). The cells most susceptible to the effects of bacteriostats and bactericides are those that divide rapidly (**Fig. 3.2**).

For the antimicrobial drug to be effective, it must be present in sufficient concentration within the patient's bloodstream, and therefore the interstitial fluid.

BACTERICIDAL PREPARATIONS

Penicillin is an example of an antibiotic that kills bacteria by damaging the structure of the bacterial wall. In this way, the bacteria lose the ability to maintain their normal internal environment: water enters the structure as a result of uncontrolled osmosis and the bacterium swells and finally bursts. Penicillin-based antibiotics need to be in the presence of dividing bacterial cells to be effective as they disrupt the newly formed cell walls. Another group of antibiotics that work in a similar manner are the cephalosporins. Some bacteria are penicillin-resistant, in that they have synthesised an enzyme that breaks the structure of the antibiotic, thus preventing interference with the structure of the bacterial wall.

Aminoglycosides produce a bactericidal effect within the cell by binding onto the bacterial ribosomes and causing the formation of incorrect amino acid sequences that are lethal to the bacterium. This class of antibiotics tends to cause toxic effects that may involve the auditory and vestibular branches of the eighth cranial nerve, or which may cause damage to the kidneys or nerves. Examples of aminoglycosides include gentamycin, neomycin and streptomycin. Nalidixic acid causes its bactericidal effect by inhibiting an enzyme that maintains the twisted shape of the bacterial DNA molecule.

BACTERIOSTAT PREPARATIONS

These preparations prevent bacterial cell division. Sulphonamides work by interfering with the steps by which DNA and RNA are formed. The tetracycline group bind onto bacterial ribosomes, thus impeding normal protein synthesis. Tetracyclines must not be given to pregnant women, because permanent damage to the teeth of the fetus may occur because of removal of calcium phosphate. Photosensitivity and rashes may also occur. Metronidazole acts to prevent the replication of anaerobic microorganisms by binding to the bacterial DNA to inhibit the synthesis of nucleic acids.

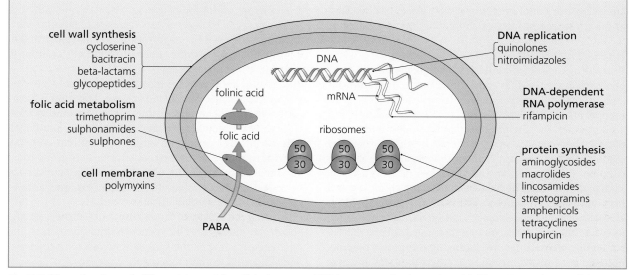

Fig 3.2 Sites of action of different types of antibiotic agent. PABA, para-aminobenzoic acid. (From Page 1997, with permission.)

THE RANGE OF ACTIVITY

Antibiotics are classed as **broad spectrum** or **narrow spectrum**. Broad-spectrum antibiotics are effective against a range of different microorganisms such as cocci and bacilli. The manner in which different bacteria take the staining substances used by microbiologists to identify them causes them to be subdivided into Gram-positive and Gram-negative groups. A broad-spectrum antibiotic may be effective against Gram-positive and Gram-negative groups. Narrow-spectrum antibiotics are highly effective against a specific microorganism.

Antibiotic resistance

Over time, antibiotics may become ineffective against a specific microorganism. This is brought about by a protective change occurring within the microorganism. One such change could be the microorganism becoming able to synthesise an enzyme that inactivates the antibiotic. The change in susceptibility to an antibiotic occurs in one of two ways: natural selection or spontaneous mutation.

- **Natural selection**: an antibiotic may eradicate all but a small number of the infecting organisms within that species, in which case the survivors replicate and develop natural resistance.
- **Spontaneous mutation**: a resistant strain may emerge as a result of a mutation, and this strain may then become dominant over more vulnerable strains.

Resistant strains of microorganisms may develop as a result of feeding livestock with fodder that routinely contains antibiotics.

Prevention of antibiotic resistance is achieved by avoiding the overexposure of microorganisms to a given antibiotic through unnecessary prescribing; by encouraging patients to continue with a complete course of antibiotics even though the symptoms of the infection have disappeared and, lastly, by avoiding the use of antibiotics 'just in case' an infection develops. An example of antibiotic resistance is the appearance of methicillin-resistant *Staphylococcus aureus* within hospitals.

Unless it is likely that an infection is caused by a common organism that is known to be sensitive to a given antibiotic, a specimen is cultured in the microbiology laboratory to establish the identity of the organism and its sensitivity to antibiotics. With potentially lethal infections such as bacterial meningitis, a combination of broad-spectrum antibiotics that are effective against a substantial range of microorganisms is prescribed. This avoids the risks of leaving the patient with a dangerous unchecked infection until such time as the causative organism is known.

OPPORTUNISTIC INFECTION

The body has its own natural defences against infection. These are usually sufficient to control the number and site of commensals – microorganisms such as Döderlein's bacilli, which maintain the normal pH in the vagina, or *Escherichia coli*, which synthesises vitamin K in the bowel. Commensals may become uncontrolled and colonise areas of the body inappropriately in cases in which the natural defences become weakened; this occurs in immunosuppressed states such as AIDS, and may result in disease. The commensals normally protect the body against other microorganisms. However, when the commensal colonies are lost as a result of medication their place may be taken by other pathogenic (disease-producing) microorganisms.

HYPERSENSITIVITY

When drug molecules combine with body proteins or complex carbohydrates, they may stimulate the immune system to mount a hypersensitivity reaction. This is an inappropriate form of the normal inflammation that accompanies the formation of antigen–antibody complexes. Hypersensitivity may accompany many types of medication, but because of the frequency of their administration, it is a particular concern when patients are prescribed antibiotics. The hypersensitivity may manifest as a rash with urticaria (itchy swellings of the skin). More severe hypersensitivities may cause angioneurotic oedema, in which the periorbital tissues become swollen; the tissues of the pharynx may swell causing respiratory obstruction and generalised increased capillary permeability may cause anaphylactic shock. The potentially fatal effects of anaphylaxis may require adrenaline to support the cardiovascular system, antihistamines to block the inflammatory process and an emergency trachaeostomy to prevent asphyxia. For these reasons, patients who have once had a reaction to a given agent should be advised to avoid the substance in future, and may wear a warning bracelet or medallion. Nurses giving antibiotics should take care to check with the patient that, to their knowledge, they have not before experienced an adverse reaction to that substance.

ANTICONVULSANTS

These preparations are also described as anti-epileptic drugs and work by a variety of means to reduce the excitability of nerve cells. Epileptiform attacks occur as a result of an overall overexcitability in the central nervous system that causes the neurons to depolarise inappropriately, producing focal (localised) or generalised seizures. Anticonvulsants interfere with the generation or spread of action potentials within the neurons. Not all convulsive seizures are indicative of epilepsy: small children with infection may suffer febrile convulsions for which anticonvulsants may be given, and convulsions in the older person may occur as a result of biochemical abnormalities such as hypoglycaemia, hypoxia or hepatic or renal failure, or space-occupying lesions in the brain. Most anticonvulsants exert some level of sedative effect, so advice must be given that vigilance is likely to be impaired and activities requiring fine control, such as driving or operating machinery, should be avoided.

ANTIHYPERTENSIVES

In health, systemic blood pressure is held within normal boundaries by the interaction of an array of homeostatic mechanisms, and stability is maintained despite variables such as postural changes or varying levels of physical activity. Antihypertensive agents work by antagonising one or more of the homeostatic mechanisms that combine to maintain blood pressure, by:

- **Increasing the size of the blood vessel circuit** by altering the muscle tone of the blood vessels. The lumen of the arterioles may be increased, thus reducing arteriolar resistance. The venous capacitance vessels may be dilated, thus reducing the venous return and consequently the cardiac output. The vasopressor effect of converting renin to angiotensin II via the use of angiotensin-converting enzyme inhibitors also reduces vasomotor tone, as does blockade of the sympathetic nerve ganglia.
- **Reducing the activity of the cardiac muscle** by decreasing heart rate and force. This reduces the cardiac output and particularly reduces the sympathetic response to stress. Beta-blockers work in this manner.
- **Reducing the fluid volume within the vascular compartment**. Diuretics achieve this by causing the kidney to excrete more water from the body. Reduction of serum sodium levels, through the use of angiotensin-converting enzyme inhibitors to block aldosterone production, will also reduce the water load in the body.

Because of their modes of action, antihypertensive agents tend to reduce exercise tolerance and diminish the homeostatic adaptation to changes in body posture; the preparations that reduce blood pressure by increasing water excretion produce a risk of dehydration and renal impairment, particularly in those concurrently taking NSAIDs.

ANXIOLYTICS

The normal arousal response can in some people produce dysfunctional anxiety that requires pharmacological control. Anxiety may cause some sufferers to complain of altered bodily sensation or functioning, such as gastro-intestinal symptoms or palpitations; these may need specific symptomatic control in addition to counselling, psychotherapy and drugs that act upon the central nervous system to reduce the reactivity of the neurons. Inhibition of the sympathetic nervous system by the use of β-adrenergic blockers produces a reduction in subjective anxiety, particularly when there are other symptoms associated with the anxiety. Benzodiazepines work by potentiating the inhibitory central nervous system neurotransmitters, thus diminishing neuronal responsiveness. Anxiolytic agents may also act as sedatives, producing a mood of tranquillity, and when anxiety is associated with sleep interruption hypnotic agents may be needed to produce drowsiness. People taking anxiolytics therefore need advice related to the overall effects of their medication, and when significant alteration of the arousal state and therefore the reaction times makes activities such as driving unsafe, this should be clearly understood. In general, alcohol and anxiolytics are not compatible because of the enhanced sedative effect that is produced.

BRONCHODILATORS

Bronchodilators are prescribed for conditions in which the calibre of the respiratory airways is reduced, such as bronchial asthma and chronic obstructive airways disease. In health, the bronchioles are expanded during inspiration, and constrict slightly during expiration. Any decrease in the lumen of the respiratory passages is therefore likely to cause an outflow obstruction, which inhibits exhalation. Bronchodilators work by correcting the outflow obstruction, either by relaxing the smooth muscle of the bronchiolar walls by altering the actions of receptors that constrict the bronchiolar muscles or by reducing inflammatory swelling in the respiratory mucosa.

RELAXATION OF BRONCHIOLAR MUSCLE

In health, when the sympathetic nervous system is activated as part of the 'fright, fight, flight' mechanism, the airways dilate to enable maximum ventilation and therefore oxygen uptake and carbon dioxide excretion. This enables the body to respond to the increased metabolic needs associated with physical exercise. The airways are activated by β-adrenergic receptors and, if these are stimulated by giving a β agonist, there will be a corresponding increase in the bronchiolar diameter. Because β agonists stimulate activation of the sympathetic nervous system, these preparations tend to produce other effects consistent with sympathetic stimulation such as mental arousal and increased cardiac drive. The muscular walls of the airways can be relaxed by the use of xanthines such as theophylline. Theophylline appears to act as a bronchodilator in two ways: it counteracts the potent bronchoconstrictor effect of adenosine, and it may inhibit prostaglandin synthesis, therefore exerting an anti-inflammatory effect (Herfindal and Gourlay, 1996).

REDUCTION OF INFLAMMATION

The action of bronchodilators is enhanced by further increasing the bronchiolar lumen by reducing the swelling of the mucosa that results from inflammation. For this reason, treatment with bronchodilators may be augmented by the use of anti-inflammatory drugs such as corticosteroids or sodium chromoglycate.

DIURETICS

The diuretics increase the removal of water, sodium and other solutes from the body. Diuretics may work by increasing the filtration pressure within the glomeruli; by increasing the osmotic pressure of filtrate within the Bowman's capsule; by altering the concentration mechanism of the loop of Henle; by altering the sodium load within the distal and collecting tubule filtrate; by opposing the sodium-sparing effect of aldosterone or by opposing the action of antidiuretic hormone. The normal renal excretion may be influenced by increasing water loss as a result of glomerular filtration, as in the administration of osmotic diuretics; by impeding the mechanism of the loop of Henle (the loop diuretics antagonise the concentration of urine); or by antagonising aldosterone and thus increasing the loss of sodium and therefore water within the urine. As increased sodium excretion from the distal tubule takes place at the expense of potassium, hyperkalaemia is a hazard in such therapy.

Loop diuretics such as frusemide have additional vasodilator action, which makes these preparations useful in reducing the circulatory load in cardiac failure. By increasing the efficiency of cardiac function, renal perfusion is accelerated. In a similar manner, inotropic drugs given as cardiac support will produce a diuresis by increasing the blood supply to the kidneys. Diuretics that operate by altering the sodium load at the distal tubule may reduce the sodium available for excretion, causing excessive potassium loss in consequence. In such cases, patients require monitoring for hypokalaemia and may need to take potassium supplements. Alcohol acts as a diuretic by opposing the effect of antidiuretic hormone.

Water and electrolyte control in health is a finely balanced series of operations, which diuretic therapy will only be able to mimic in a crude way. Those prescribed diuretic therapy need, therefore, to be monitored for the adverse effects of diuretic drugs, particularly dehydration and possible renal dysfunction and electrolyte imbalance.

ENZYME BLOCKERS AND AGONISTS

Many of the body's functions take place because they are facilitated by enzymes. Communication between neurons (thinking); detoxifying metabolites; transport of carbon dioxide in the blood and the breaking down of fatty acids for use as long-term muscle fuels all rely on the capacity of the body to function as a chemical 'factory'. Pharmaceutical chemicals may influence biochemical reactions, thus enhancing or inhibiting enzyme cascades. In some cases, these interactions are used for their therapeutic effect, as when anticholinesterases are given to combat the rapid muscle fatigue of myasthenia gravis. In this case, diagnosis is made when the characteristic muscular weakness is abolished when a test dose of edrophonium is given. Edrophonium is an antagonist of cholinesterase, the enzyme that removes the transmitter acetylcholine from neuromuscular junctions. Administration of edrophonium enables communication between the motor nerve and the muscle to be sustained for sufficient length of time for the drug to be established as the cause of the transient improvement, thus allowing subsequent prescription of a longer lasting anticholinesterase as treatment. Another example of an enzyme inhibitor is acetazolamide, which inhibits carbonic anhydrase and is used to treat glaucoma (**Fig. 3.3**).

A less useful example of enzyme blocking occurs in paracetamol overdose. The liver inactivates paracetamol by adding part of its limited store of glutathione to it. If there is so much paracetamol to metabolise that the store of glutathione is exhausted, the paracetamol is oxidised instead into a metabolite that is a lethal cellular poison. The poison n-acetyl-p-benzoquinone-amine inactivates the thiol groups of hepatic cellular enzymes by oxidation. Death occurs as a result of liver failure a few weeks after the overdose was taken.

Some preparations enhance enzyme actions and this is an important cause of drug interactions. For example, anticonvulsants inhibit the formation of active vitamin D by breaking it down prematurely, causing dietary calcium to be insufficiently absorbed, and this has subsequent ill effects upon the formation of bone (Laurence and Bennett, 1992). Medication may be metabolised prematurely, making it therapeutically ineffective, erratic or toxic. Chronic alcohol abuse causes enzyme induction, thereby predisposing to decreased tolerance of certain drugs as a result of the production of toxic metabolites.

HISTAMINE AND ANTIHISTAMINES

The inflammatory response is in part mediated by histamine, which is stored in inactive form in the body tissues and the mast cells (basophils). Histamine contributes to the body defences; it has a role as a local tissue hormone, communicating between cells, as in the gastric mucosa

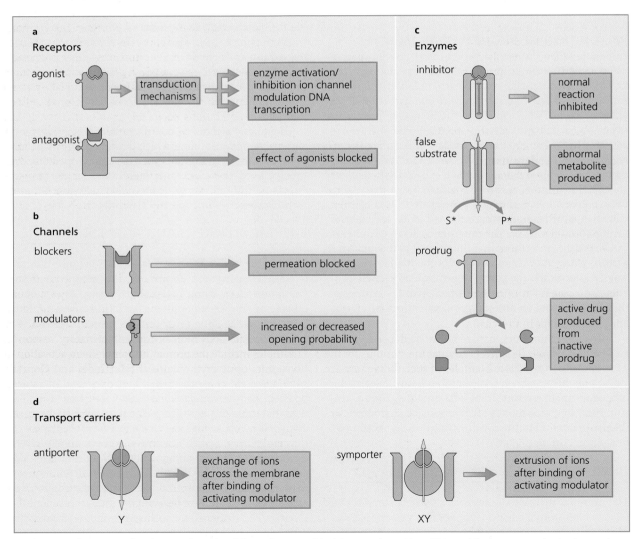

Fig 3.3 Protein targets for drug action. S*: false substrate; P*: false product; X and Y: positively or negatively charged ions. (From Page 1997, with permission.)

where histamine release and binding to H_2 receptors causes the secretion of hydrogen ions which combine with chlorides to produce hydrochloric acid. Histamine binds to H_1 receptors to cause the smooth muscle fibres of the bronchioles to constrict producing bronchospasm. Arterioles dilate, increasing the blood flow through tissues, and capillaries become more permeable, enabling movement of water into the tissues to dilute toxins and migration of phagocytic white cells to combat bacterial infection. The binding of histamine to H_1 receptors is responsible for anaphylactic shock.

Histamine is generally produced in adequate amounts to mobilise the body's defences and therefore is not administered therapeutically. Pharmacological treatment is more commonly needed to antagonise the effects of histamine. Histamine antagonists are classed according to the receptor (H_1 or H_2) that is blocked. H_1 receptor antagonists are used in hypersensitivity states and compete with histamine for the receptor sites. If the H_1 receptor antagonist crosses the blood–brain barrier, drowsiness is a hazard of treatment. H_2 receptor blockers, generally used to correct gastric hyperacidity states, do not tend to produce drowsiness as a side effect.

HORMONES

Hormones may be used therapeutically as replacement therapy in deficiency states or to alter the functioning of a hormone-dependent tissue. For example, (female) hormone replacement therapy is given to combat the sequelae of ovarian failure in post-menopausal women, and thyroxine is given for hypothyroidism. Less ethically, androgens may be administered to produce increased muscle bulk and improved physical performance in athletes. In the latter cases, because there was no original deficiency state, those taking anabolic steroids will gradually exhibit the signs of hormone excess, the most obvious being virilisation in women. An important example of hormone therapy is the administration of adrenocorticosteroids, which is discussed earlier in this chapter.

To control tumours that are hormone dependent, hormone therapy may be given to counter the stimulus for the tumour cells to replicate. Examples of such therapy are the use of female hormone stilboestrol to inhibit the development of tumours derived from the prostate gland.

People who undergo gender reassignment will require the appropriate male or female sex hormone to complete the secondary sexual characteristics appropriate to their new persona. This constitutes a form of replacement therapy to augment the adrenal sex hormones as the original gonads will have been removed surgically.

HYPNOTICS

Hypnotics are preparations that produce sleep. Normal sleep has a cyclical pattern characterised by the different wave forms seen on the electroencephalogram during a typical period of sleep. Levels of sleep can also be assessed by the appearance of the sleeper; in the early stages of sleep (stages 1 and 2), drowsiness and the occasional myoclonal (muscular) jerks occur and the person may be easily aroused to full consciousness. As the sleep cycle continues, progressive relaxation occurs and the sleeper passes into non-rapid eye movement (NREM) sleep. As the sleep period proceeds, NREM sleep is interspersed by increasing periods of rapid eye movement (REM) sleep. The scientific evidence for the physiological need for sleep is scanty, but sleep disruptions are perceived by sufferers as a source of a diminished sense of wellbeing. Sleep disruptions may accompany a range of conditions, particularly those associated with pain or altered mental health.

A range of medications such as narcotics and monoamine oxidase inhibitors may impair sleep. In general, it is better for patients to try simple remedies to promote their normal sleep patterns before seeking hypnotic medication from their family doctor. This is because hypnotics generally produce a diminishing effect (tolerance) and dependence. Cessation of long-term hypnotic therapy needs to be gradual and is itself characterised by sleep disturbances such as nightmares. In order to take effect, hypnotic preparations must be capable of crossing the blood–brain barrier. Hypnotics tend to produce a hangover effect the following day and are potentiated by alcohol. Care should be taken, therefore, when driving or operating dangerous machinery. The sustained use of some hypnotics can suppress REM sleep, and rebound insomnia is a problem for people withdrawing from the use of hypnotics (Herfindal and Gourlay, 1996).

IMMUNOSUPPRESSIVES

The use of drugs to diminish the immune response has increased as the immunological basis of a range of conditions has become better understood. Immunosuppressant therapy may be given for conditions caused by excessive or inappropriate activation of the inflammatory response. Examples include the premature complement activation in systemic lupus erythematosus (Herfindal and Gourlay, 1996) and the presence of antigen–antibody complexes, particularly in small blood vessel systems, found in some forms of vasculitis, Wegener's granulomatosis, Goodpasture's syndrome, acute glomerulonephritis and systemic lupus erythematosus (Wilson et al.,1991). The tissue damage caused by macrophage activity in infective conditions may cause pathological changes that complicate the original disorder. An example is the apparently paradoxical administration of immunosuppressives in serious infections such as meningitis. This is done to minimise the additional cerebral damage that may result from the activation of immune defences in response to the original infection.

The immune system has a role in the detection of abnormal body cells. Healthy lymphocytes 'scan' tissue cells and activate cytotoxic killer cells if mutations or abnormal cell contents are present. Immunosuppressive therapy is necessary for recipients of allograft organ transplant to prevent tissue rejection of 'non-self' cells. Adrenocorticosteroids such as hydrocortisone or prednisone (see above) may be used for their immunosuppressant properties, and specific immunosuppressives such as azathioprene or cyclosporin (originally developed as an antibiotic) may be prescribed.

COMPLICATIONS OF PROLONGED IMMUNOSUPPRESSANT THERAPY

Suppression of the immune reaction, by its nature, decreases the individual's resistance and this makes them susceptible to opportunistic infection. Bone marrow depression and infertility may occur. Care must be taken with immunising immunosuppressed patients; the use of live vaccines brings a risk of overwhelming infection by the organism, so vaccination is avoided in immunosuppressed patients. Additionally, patients on long-term immunosuppressant therapy tend to have an increased risk of malignant disease because of the inhibition of lymphocyte vigilance.

MUSCLE RELAXANTS

Breathing, movement and posture is dependent upon the presence of muscle tone and the ability to institute muscle contraction at will. Muscle relaxation is achieved by interrupting the communication between the motor cortex and nerve and skeletal muscle. It is needed during endotracheal intubation for the induction of general anaesthesia, and in abdominal surgery to enable access to deeply sited structures that would otherwise be protected by the 'guarding' action of the musculature. Muscle relaxants may also be used in disorders such as tetanus, in which muscle contraction is unwanted because it increases the metabolic work of the body and causes skeletomuscular damage; respiratory obstruction and malignant hyperthermia, in which muscle relaxation is sought to exclude thermogenesis by shivering during artificial cooling.

Muscle relaxation can be achieved by two major means: by the blocking of acetylcholine or by its potentiation. In either case, the normal flux of positively charged ions into the muscle fibre is interrupted and so depolarisation is either prevented or prolonged. The end result is the same: muscle fibres are unable to shorten rhythmically and so lose the ability to initiate movement. Such action may be short or long acting. It is important to remember that muscle relaxants effectively produce paralysis, therefore asphyxia will occur unless respiratory effort is compensated by artificial ventilation. In addition, although muscle relaxants prevent movement and therefore stop the patient from being able to express himself by speech, movement or facial expression, they do not alter consciousness so, unless potent sedation is administered, for the duration of the muscle relaxation the individual is left with a 'locked brain': consciousness but no means of expressing it.

PSYCHOTROPIC AND PSYCHOACTIVE DRUGS

Disorders of thinking and mood present a range of disabling conditions for the sufferer. Thinking and mood generation occur in a similar way to neuromuscular communication: the action potentials from one neuron arrive at synapses and cause release of various groups of neurotransmitters in discrete locations in the central nervous system, thus activating other neural structures. Thought, perception and emotion can be altered by influencing the biochemical balance in the brain. Although the natural central nervous system transmitters exert specific effects within the relevant structures, pharmaceutical preparations tend to be less discriminating in their effects, and side effects and chemical interactions, some of them potentially dangerous, occur. This makes psychotropic therapy hazardous, particularly when potentially lethal preparations are used in patients who are at risk of taking an overdose. Interest in altered states of perception has caused some people to take psychoactive substances in the absence of medical need, sometimes with tragic outcomes.

DRUGS THAT INFLUENCE THE AUTONOMIC NERVOUS SYSTEM

DRUGS AFFECTING THE SYMPATHETIC NERVOUS SYSTEM

These groups of drugs have a spectrum of functions that depend upon whether they stimulate the sympathetic nervous system (sympathomimetics or sympathetic agonists) or compete with natural sympathetic neurotransmitters for attachment to receptors (sympathetic blockers).

The sympathetic transmitters are adrenaline and noradrenaline. Their chemical precursor is dopamine, and these three transmitters are collectively termed catecholamines. All three neurotransmitters are also found in the central nervous system, where they sustain mood and arousal. In the autonomic nervous system, they mediate arousal by producing the physiological changes consistent with activating the 'fright, fight, flight' response to perceived threat, a role shared with the adrenal medulla, which also secretes adrenaline and noradrenaline. A sympathomimetic such as salbutamol may be described as a bronchodilator because of the effect upon the calibre of the bronchi, although to a lesser degree, it also increases the cardiac rate and force, so could be used as a cardiac stimulant. A sympathetic nervous system agonist such as dopamine may be classed as an inotropic cardiac drug because of its effect in increasing the rate and force of the heart beat. Although it exerts a sympathomimetic effect in the autonomic nervous system, dopamine is also a central nervous system transmitter; in the central nervous system it produces a totally different series of effects, depending upon the location of the synapse in the brain. Propanolol, a beta-blocker, may be described as an antiarrhythmic, an antihypertensive and an anxiolytic substance or a migraine-relieving agent, because it exerts effects in all these areas.

The sympathetic adrenoceptors are classed as α or β receptors. Examples of activation and blockade of the sympathetic receptors are described below.

Alpha$_1$ receptors are present in the iris of the eye. When these receptors are **activated**, the pupil dilates, allowing more light into the eye. When these receptors are **blocked**, the pupil constricts (miosis).

Alpha$_1$ receptors are present on arteriolar smooth muscle. When **activated**, vasoconstriction occurs and the venous return is increased and blood pressure rises. When **blocked**, smooth muscle relaxes, the lumen of the arterioles increases and peripheral resistance and arterial blood pressure falls. The coronary and cerebral circulations are largely spared from these effects. Alpha$_1$ blockers are therefore used to control hypertension, although they tend to produce postural hypotension as a result of the loss of the homeostatic response to alterations in body position.

Alpha$_1$ receptors are present in uterine muscle fibres, where they produce contraction in pregnancy; they are also found in sweat glands, bladder sphincters and the male ejaculatory system.

Alpha^2 receptors are present on the presynaptic nerve endings, where they are involved with the feedback mechanism for controlling the release of noradrenaline (Laurence and Bennett, 1992).

β_1 and β_2 receptors are present in the heart in the sino-atrial node, where **activation** of the receptors increases cardiac rate. **Blockade** reduces heart rate.

In the atrioventricular node β_1 and β_2 receptors increase the responsivity of the cardiac muscle to action potentials. **Blockade** therefore renders the cardiac muscle less reactive to stimuli.

Stimulation of cardiac β_1 and β_2 receptors increases the contractility of the myocardium, the speed of impulse transmission and the myocardial metabolic rate and decreases the duration of the diastolic phase. **Blockade** of these receptors results in reduction of cardiac rate force and myocardial oxygen demand. Beta-blockers are consequently useful as a treatment for hypertension and some forms of tachycardia.

In the arterioles, stimulation of β_2 receptors causes vasodilatation. In the bronchi, relaxation and therefore bronchodilatation occurs. **Blockade** consequently produces a risk of bronchospasm, which is a sign of excessive treatment with beta-blockers. For this reason, beta-blockers should not be given to asthmatic patients.

Beta$_2$ receptors are also present in the uterus, where they produce relaxation of the pregnant uterus, in skeletal muscle, in which their activation increases skeletal tone, and in the detrusor muscle of the bladder, which they cause to relax.

Depending upon the receptor affected, sympathetic blockers produce a range of effects that diminish the normal sympathetic response to stress. Sympathomimetics enhance the natural physiological response to stress and are therefore useful when support of the cardiovascular system is needed.

DRUGS THAT ACT UPON THE PARASYMPATHETIC NERVOUS SYSTEM

The nerve endings of the parasympathetic system contain cholinergic receptors for which acetylcholine is the neurotransmitter. Parasympathetic drugs that oppose acetylcholine are termed antimuscarinic substances because they block receptors that also combine with the poison muscarine. Most antimuscarinic drugs work by competing with acetylcholine at the parasympathetic nerve endings and within blood vessels. Atropine is an example of a substance that blocks the parasympathetic nervous system, causing quickening of the heart rate in bradycardic states; reduction of gastric, respiratory and glandular secretions; relaxation of gastrointestinal and bronchial smooth muscle and dilatation and paralysis of the iris.

VITAMINS AND MINERALS

Vitamins are substances that generally cannot be synthesised by the body. An exception to this is vitamin D, which is activated from its inert form in the skin by the effect of sunlight. Vitamins are needed for metabolic processes. They are usually taken to remedy deficiency states, often as a result of dietary inadequacies, and are divided into two subgroups: the water-soluble vitamins C and the B group, which need regular replacement because the body is unable to store them, and fat-soluble vitamins A, D, E and K, which can be stored by body tissues. A misconception has arisen that, because they are necessary for health, vitamins taken in increased doses must produce enhanced effects; this is largely without foundation, and some vitamins such as vitamins A and D are toxic when taken in excess.

Minerals are necessary for the formation of healthy tissues and to maintain a correct biochemical balance. In normal health, and with an adequate balanced diet, sufficient vitamins and minerals are taken to enable normal homeostasis. Some substances interact with the absorption of vitamins and minerals, for example, excessive dietary fibre inhibits the absorption of calcium, iron, magnesium and zinc (Herfindal and Gourlay, 1996).

KEY POINTS

- Some pharmacological agents such as aspirin produce a range of diverse effects.
- Long-term corticosteroid treatment has deleterious side effects.
- When muscle relaxants are used in general anaesthetic, the patient must receive adequate sedation and analgesia.
- The inappropriate use of antibiotics may result in the development of antibiotic-resistant strains of microorganism.
- Beta-blockers may cause bronchospasm in patients predisposed to bronchial asthma.
- Diuretic therapy provides at best a crude substitute for natural mechanisms of water homeostasis.
- Antihistamines may cause drowsiness.
- Patients prescribed hypnotics may develop tolerance and dependence.
- Vaccination may not be safe for patients who are receiving immunosuppressant therapy.
- Some vitamins are toxic in excess; 'more' does not therefore necessarily mean 'better'.

REFERENCES

Herfindal ET, Gourlay DR, eds. *Textbook of therapeutics*. Baltimore: Williams & Wilkins, 1996.

Laurence DR, Bennett PN. *Clinical pharmacology*. Edinburgh: Churchill Livingstone, 1992.

Page C. *Integrated Pharmacology*. London: Mosby, 1997

Wilson JD, Braunwald E, Isselbacher KJ, Petersdorf RG, Martin JB, Fauci AS, Root RK, eds. *Harrison's principles of internal medicine*. New York: McGraw-Hill, 1991.

4 Julie Fegan
LEGAL ASPECTS OF DRUG ADMINISTRATION

INTRODUCTION

When a person becomes a health professional rather than a lay carer a whole new set of expectations over and above those of civil law as applied to any citizen arise. Nurses are bound by the **Code of Professional Conduct** (UKCC, 1992a) as a profession. This is administered by the **United Kingdom Central Council for Nursing, Midwifery and Health Visiting** (UKCC). The UKCC is responsible for guaranteeing to the public that those registered as nurses, midwives and health visitors are safe to practice. As such the council sets standards for the profession that must be met in order to practise, and every nurse, midwife and health visitor is **accountable** to the UKCC, the profession and the public to maintain his or her professional knowledge and practice. In the context of this book, the nurse needs to be aware that she will be judged according to what is considered reasonable performance for the grade of practitioner who usually performs a given activity for the patient. It is reasonable to expect a nurse to be able to interpret changes in a patient's condition and implement action or alert the appropriate colleague to do so. An important point is that the nurse needs a clear understanding of the limits and the potential of her knowledge.

The document Standards for the Administration of Medicines (see Appendix 1) sets out the responsibilities of nurses, midwives and health visitors for their knowledge and practice. It states that administration of medicines
is not solely a mechanistic task to be performed in strict compliance with the written prescription of a medical practitioner. It requires thought and the exercise of professional judgement…
(UKCC, 1992a, p. 2)

Thus this textbook intends to increase every nurse, midwife and health visitor's knowledge of the pathophysiology and pharmacology related to conditions commonly seen in practice and the drugs that are given for those conditions. The nurse, midwife and health visitor should therefore be able to exercise intelligent professional judgement.

DIFFERENCES BETWEEN LAW, ETHICS AND MORALS

Defining these guiding principles of nursing and midwifery practice is important for understanding accountability. The law sets out what a nurse, midwife and health visitor can do in relation to the administration of medicines. The UKCC then explains and defines what those responsibilities mean in law. The nurse, midwife and health visitor are accountable in law for understanding the legal responsibilities of administering medicines. As an important legal principle, **ignorance of the law is no excuse**. Professional accountability means that every practitioner is responsible and accountable for knowing how far his or her responsibilities extend.

Morality may or may not be part of the nurse's thoughts as she assists in administering abortion drugs. Ethics plays an important role when administering strong pain relief in terminal illness to alleviate suffering. However, **morality** and **ethics** aside, the **law** about giving prescribed drugs is clear that the nurse is **wrong** in the following instances:
- If she gives an inappropriate dosage of drug in relation to a particular patient's age and size, for example to a child or an elderly patient.
- If she gives prescribed drugs to a patient when she knows or should know that the patient has experienced side effects in the past (such as allergy).
- In giving a prescribed drug to a patient who is now having side effects that have hitherto gone unnoticed (for example if she omits to take the pulse before giving a patient digoxin).

The exercise of professional judgement includes:
- Confirming the correctness of the prescription.
- Judging the suitability of administration at the scheduled time of administration.
- Reinforcing the positive effect of the treatment.
- Enhancing a patient's understanding of their prescribed medication.

- The avoidance of misuse of these and other medicines.
- Assisting in assessing the efficacy of medicines and the identification of side effects and interactions.

In assessing a patient's physical condition and being involved with their medication, a nurse must adhere to the requirements of the UKCC *Code of Conduct* (1992a) that

> *As a registered nurse, midwife or health visitor you are personally accountable for your practice and, in the exercise of your professional accountability, must:*
>
> *1. act always in such a manner as to promote and safeguard the interests and well-being of patients and clients;*
>
> *2. ensure that no action or omission on your part, or within your sphere of responsibility, is detrimental to the interests, condition or safety of patients and clients;*
>
> *3. maintain and improve your professional knowledge and competence;*
>
> *4. acknowledge any limitations in your knowledge and competence and decline any duties or responsibilities unless able to perform them in a safe and skilled manner* (UKCC, 1992a, p. 1).

These requirements extend to the activities of storing, calculating and giving drugs.

It is important for the nurse to be conversant with certain key pieces of legislation. The main legislation governing the supply, storage and administration of medicines is in The Medicines Act 1968 and 1971; The Misuse of Drugs Act 1971 and The Misuse of Drugs Regulations 1985.

The Medicines Act 1968 and 1971 controls the licensing, packaging and labelling of medicines and the conditions for the sale and supply of 'pharmacy only' and 'prescription only' medicines. The Misuse of Drugs Act 1971 lists and classifies controlled drugs, makes it a criminal offence to manufacture, supply or possess controlled drugs unless authorised and empowers the Secretary of State to make regulations relating to drug misuse. In addition, the Act created an Advisory Council on Misuse of Drugs and gives the power of search, arrest and forfeiture under criminal law.

The Misuse of Drugs Regulations 1985 divides drugs into five schedules. The level of control relates to the potential for abuse of the substance:

- Schedule 1: High potential for misuse e.g. cannabis.
- Schedule 2: High potential for dependency; prescriptions cannot be renewed, includes stimulants, narcotics and depressants e.g. opiates and amphetamines. These are listed as Controlled Drugs.
- Schedule 3: Subject to special prescription requirements, but are not recorded in Controlled Drug registers e.g. barbiturates.
- Schedule 4: Limited potential to abuse e.g. benzodiazepines (temazepam).

- Schedule 5: Low potential to abuse, that is, they contain only small amounts of narcotics e.g. codeine linctus, DF118 tablets and kaolin and morphine which makes it difficult to extract the narcotic present (Jason-Lloyd, 1998).

The purpose of legislation is to prevent misuse of drugs by making professionals responsible for safe control and administration. All medicines must undergo rigorous testing – usually 6–10 years – before they can be prescribed. Medicines must be stored appropriately (this may refer to temperature or access). The drugs must reach the patient in a stable condition. They must be labelled according to law and be given out under properly written instructions, a medical prescription or in the case of nurse prescribing, a properly qualified nurse (UKCC, 1991).

Controlled Drugs are very closely monitored. Waste must be accounted for in a strict manner. They must be ordered in the Controlled Drug book. They must be delivered to the ward in a locked box and stored in a locked cupboard inside another locked cupboard. The keys to the drug cupboard must be held by the nurse in charge. There is a clearly defined role of the nurse in relation to giving drugs: prescribing, knowledge of appropriate administration, side effects and special precautions.

For safe administration of drugs the nurse must:

- Be aware of the patient's allergies.
- Ensure that the drug is correctly prescribed.
- Understand the action of the drug, any interactions or side effects.
- Be aware of the appropriate range of dose for the specific drugs. If there is any doubt in the nurse's mind she should check, for example, with the British National Formulary.

The **Five Rights** provide a useful aide memoire for nurses administering drugs:

- The right drug.
- The right dose.
- The right time.
- The right route.
- The right patient.

Nurses are human and capable of making mistakes. However, a drug error is a potentially serious matter that may be detrimental to the patient's wellbeing and must be reported immediately to the nurse in charge, the doctor and the nurse manager. Although in the past drug errors were a cause for disciplinary action, nowadays it is acknowledged that in the event of a drug error occurring, the most important thing is that the error is made known so that the patient's condition can be observed and corrective steps taken if appropriate. To this end, a record must be made in the patient's notes and an incident form must be completed, according to local protocol. Ideally, errors with medication would never happen, but should they occur, the patient's wellbeing must be paramount. Then and only then, a debrief should occur so that potential errors and mishaps are avoided for the future. Although the severity of an error should not be trivialised, it is more serious to conceal or collude with suppression of the incident as there would then be insufficient factual knowledge available upon which to base future decisions about the patient's management.

PATIENT SELF-MEDICATION

Self-medication is in use in some clinical areas. It encourages patient independence, empowers the patient and increases drug compliance. Some parents are encouraged to give their children their medications in hospital and in patients approaching discharge self-medication is similarly encouraged. The nurse is still responsible for ensuring the necessary security and storage arrangements for the patient's drugs (Dimond, 1995).

EXTENDED ROLE
(ROUTES OF ADMINISTRATION)

Administering medication via the intravenous route has classically been the preserve of physicians, but has now become an all but essential skill among nurses. Certificates in extended roles such as administering intravenous drugs and intravenous cannulation are often stated as required or at least 'desirable' in job advertisements. To be a safe practitioner in this respect the nurse must possess recent relevant knowledge of the agents being administered

5.1 GOOD PRACTICE POINTS

Check all calculations.
Whenever possible the patient should understand what their medication is for.
Do not leave the drug trolley unlocked and unattended.
Always take the prescription sheet to the patient.
Always positively identify the patient.
Do not leave medicines at the bedside – stay with the patient until medicine is taken.
Do not handle tablets and capsules.
Do not give drugs unless taken directly from pharmacy-labelled container.
Do not give any drug that you have not checked.
If the patient refuses a drug, this must be recorded.
Do not return unused drugs to stock.
When given, all drugs must be recorded on the prescription sheet.
Always observe the patient for effect.
Be aware of local drug policy.
If in doubt ALWAYS ASK.

intravenously. The whole issue of professional accountability becomes increasingly important when professional boundaries become indistinct (Nursing Standard, 1996).

EXTENDED ROLE (NURSE PRESCRIBING)

The legislative process that culminated with the passage of the Medicinal Products Act 1992, passed in 1994, empowered suitably qualified nurses, midwives and health visitors to undertake the independent activity of prescribing from the Nurses' Formulary. Together with named specialist nurses they are also to be able to alter the timing and dosage of medications prescribed by medical practitioners within clearly defined protocols.

In 1993 limited nurse prescribing was introduced in the community under the Medicinal Products: Prescription by Nurses etc. Act 1992 (Commencement No. 1) Order 1994. As a result for certain nurses practising in the community there is a Nurses' Formulary, which is listed in the British National Formulary (George, 1999). Nurses who assume this responsibility must develop and maintain their knowledge of pharmacology, physiology, disease and illness processes, therapeutics and practical prescribing. It is clear that such nurses empowered to prescribe must have undergone the necessary education and training and have a record to that effect on the UKCC Register (Hunt and Wainwright, 1994).

Factors that the prescribing nurse must consider include the patient's past health history, current and anticipated health problems and knowledge of the underlying illness. Thorough knowledge of the item to be prescribed, its actions, side effects, dosage and frequency of use in a variety of circumstances is essential. Then the nurse must take account of the socioeconomic and psychological needs of the patient as well as her legal and administrative responsibilities as a prescriber (Hunt and Wainwright, 1994).

Under this Act the nurse must ensure that the prescription is **legible** and states the correct dose, frequency of administration and route of administration and is signed by the prescriber.

Permitted abbreviations in prescriptions are g for gram; mg for milligram and l for litre; **microgram must not be abbreviated**. When decimals have to be used they must always be preceded by a zero, for example 0.5 ml. In some circumstances prescribing over the telephone is allowed, but local policy should be checked. Usually there must be two nurses who hear and repeat the message back to the doctor to check.

EXTENDED ROLE (VACCINATION)

Health visitors are often involved in giving advice to mothers about the immunisation of children as part of their role in promoting health and preventing illness. The UKCC sets out guidelines for nurses, midwives and health visitors involved in vaccination programmes, including advance 'direction' for the administration of vaccines for people who meet certain criteria. In the case of particular community nurses, practice nurses or health visitors giving advice to patients going abroad, a single telephone conversation with a medical practitioner is sufficient authorisation for a one-off vaccination (Dimond, 1995).

The Royal College of Nursing produces a 'green book' that includes the following information:
- Details of drugs that can be given by nurses.
- Circumstances in which vaccines can be given.
- Procedure for checking that a patient is suitable for vaccination.
- Procedure for action in anaphylactic shock.
- Necessary equipment for vaccination.

The importance of ascertaining the suitability of the patient for vaccination cannot be overemphasised. If a nurse, midwife or health visitor, knowing there is a history of convulsions, fails to take this into account in advising a mother to have a child vaccinated, and also fails to advise the doctor of this, then the nurse, midwife or health visitor may well share some liability for any harm that befalls a child as a result of undergoing vaccination.

DRUGS AND THE MIDWIFE

Rule 41 of the Midwives Rules details legally binding regulations in relation to the administration of medicines by midwives and Rule 42 requires the midwife to keep records in relation to medicines. Paragraphs 24–27 of the Midwife's Code of Practice expands upon the midwife's duty in relation to medicines and analgesics (see Appendix 2).

Midwives are recognised as an exception for the supply and administration of specific drugs. They had special dispensation for prescribing and giving drugs even before nurse prescribing, in a limited sense, was started in 1993. It rests with the individual midwife to become familiar with and have a working knowledge of the preparations she works with in order to exercise her extended role of limited prescribing. This may be via **Standing Orders**, a list of drugs that are approved by local obstetric consultants and that the midwife can administer without prescription by a doctor, including opioid analgesics for use in labour. There are also approved drugs that can be administered by community midwives such as antiseptics, laxatives, oxytocics and opioid antagonists (Dimond, 1994a).

The Midwives Rules 1993, the Midwives Code of Practice 1994 and the UKCC guidelines for the administration of medicines (1992b) – see Appendix 1 – should be adhered to when any drug is administered, as should local policy and protocols agreed between obstetric consultants and pharmacists, such as the administration of magnesium sulphate or ritodrine hydrochloride (Banister, 1997). Paragraph 33 of the *Standards for the administration of medicines* (1992b)

sets out the UKCC guidelines for midwifery practice (see Appendix 1). Controlled drugs such as pethidine and pentazocine may be obtained and used by midwives in their practice. The controlled drug legislation requires that strict control over supply, storage, use and destruction of these drugs must be maintained (Jenkins, 1995).

The midwife's job description may be defined by the employer so that she may administer antibiotics and other medications not presently covered by the midwives' powers of prescribing and medication under Rule 41. The employed midwife has an implied duty to obey the reasonable orders of the employer (Dimond, 1994b). When the midwife becomes aware that an order may conflict with her first duty to the patient's or mother's rights, she should bring this to the attention of the supervisor of midwives and senior managers so that it can be resolved before it gives rise to problems in practice.

DRUG TRIALS

Clinical trials are an essential part of the development of new and better drug therapies. For trials involving human patients, respect for individual patient autonomy requires that research participants give informed consent. The European Good Clinical Practice guidelines (Molin, 1996) insist that:
- Information should be given in oral and written form wherever possible.
- Individuals must be allowed sufficient time to decide whether they wish to participate.
- If the individual consents to participate after a full and comprehensive explanation of the study, this consent should be appropriately recorded.
- Consent must be documented either by the individual who should sign and date the document, or by the signature of an independent witness who records the individual's assent. In either case the signature confirms that the consent is based on information that has been understood and that the individual has freely chosen to participate.

Nurses assume a shared responsibility in the management of research protocols and are often integral members of the research study. Although it may not be the nurse's responsibility to obtain consent, clarifying the information given certainly falls within the nursing role (Molin, 1996). The scientific concepts of clinical trials are difficult and time consuming to explain to research participants. For this reason, increased reliance may be placed on written informed consent, which should be designed according to the reading level of the participants, with the backup of the nurse to supplement written materials with verbal explanations.

KEY POINTS

- The nurse must act within the limits of reasonable knowledge and action.
- Protocols and procedures do not replace the need for professional judgement.
- Ignorance of the law is no excuse.
- When working in an 'extended role', the nurse will be judged according to reasonable practice for a member of the professional group whose role she is assuming.

- If an error with medication occurs, it is important to inform the appropriate people.
- The responsibilities of the nurse in relation to the patient's medication are based upon legal principles.
- Midwives have additional roles and responsibilities for drug administration during labour and childbirth.

REFERENCES

Banister C. *The midwife's pharmacopoeia.* Hale: Books for Midwives Press, 1997.

Dimond B. Medication and the modern midwife: statutory control. part 1 *Modern Midwife* 1994a; **4**:34-35.

Dimond B. *The legal aspects of midwifery.* Hale: Books for Midwives Press, 1994b.

Dimond B. *Legal aspects of nursing.* London: Prentice Hall, 1995.

George C. *British National Formulary,* No 37. London: British Medical Association and the Royal Pharmaceutical Society of Great Britain, 1999.

Hunt G, Wainwright P. *Expanding the role of the nurse: the scope of professional practice.* Oxford: Blackwell Scientific, 1994.

Jason-Lloyd L. Controlled drugs: the legal framework. *New Law Journal* 1998; **148**: 1387-8, 6857

Jenkins R. *The law and the midwife.* Oxford: Blackwell Scientific, 1995.

Molin C. The special case of clinical trials. *Eur J Cancer Care* 1996; **5 (suppl 1)**:5-6.

Nursing Standard Editorial Taking on Junior doctors' roles: who is accountable? *Nurs Standard* 1996; 10/39 **19.6.96**:32.

UKCC. *Report on the proposals for the future of community education.* London: UKCC, 1991.

UKCC. *Code of professional conduct for the nurse, midwife and health visitor.* London: UKCC, 1992a.

UKCC. *Standards for the administration of medicines.* London: UKCC, 1992b.

5 Julie Fegan
DRUGS AND IMMUNOLOGICAL DISORDERS

INTRODUCTION

The immune system is both primitive and quite sophisticated in its endeavours to protect the human body from infection. **Infection**, once considered to be conquered by antibiotics and vaccines, is now on the rise again worldwide. Infection is an important stimulus to the immune system and so the process is discussed in this chapter. Individual infections are discussed in the systems chapters as they affect each system differently and are part of the disorders of each system of the body. **Inflammation** was originally the first line of defence against assault from the outside world but now appears to cause more problems than it solves. Acute inflammation affects each system and its function differently and is therefore discussed in each systems chapter. Chronic inflammation seems to become a different disorder, affecting the whole body and is therefore discussed in this chapter. **Hypersensitivities**, which arise from the immune response, result in allergy and autoimmunity. **Allergy** and **autoimmunity** tend to affect the whole body and are discussed in this chapter, although individual disorders such as diabetes may have autoimmune causes and these are discussed in the systems chapters. **Immunodeficiency** has many causes. These are all

discussed in relation to the drugs used to treat or prevent immunopathology. The disorders that are given as examples are those that are found throughout the body and will not be found in the individual systems chapters. Specific disorders of the immune system are to be found at the end of this chapter with the pathophysiology and the pharmacological treatment of each.

INFECTION

Infection implies that microorganisms capable of causing disease have gained access into body tissues; subsequent establishment and multiplication produces clinical signs of infection. **Endogenous** infection is literally 'from within', that is, the causative organism comes from another part of the victim's own body. For example, *Escherichia coli*, normally a harmless resident of the gut, causes infection in a wound or the urinary tract. **Exogenous** infection is infection originating outside the body, that is, it is acquired from another person or object. Many infections are considered to be **opportunistic** infections and are most prevalent in people who are immunodepressed. Many factors are needed to cause an infection (see Table 5.1). Any organism can cause severe disease if the conditions are right and almost any

Genesis of infection as related to host and microbial determinants		
Genesis of infection	Host determinants	Microbial determinants
Specificity	Susceptibility	Commensalism, mutualism
Epithelial attachment	Immunodeficiency	Toxins
Multiplication	Undernutrition	Adherence factors
Colonisation	Predisposing factors	Evasive factors
Invasion	Precipitating factors	Invasive factors
Initiation of immune response		Opportunism

Table 5.1 Genesis of infection as related to host and microbial determinants

pathogen can live in peaceful symbiosis in a disease-free host (Spector 1989). Today many infectious diseases are under control because of improvements in sanitation and housing, improvements in nutrition and extensive immunisation programmes.

THE CAUSATIVE ORGANISMS
Viruses
Viruses are very small and simple organisms. They range in size from 28 nm up to 450 nm [a nanometre (nm) is one-millionth of a millimetre]. They are composed of either RNA or DNA, but never both, and with a protein coat called a capsid. They can only multiply within the cells of a host but can survive outside cells in a resting form for long periods and even under very unfavourable conditions. They are the cause of many diseases, from the common cold to smallpox, and are now believed to cause some cancers.

Rickettsiae
Rickettsiae are larger than viruses and contain both RNA and DNA plus proteins. Like viruses they can only multiply within the cells of a host. They can survive for months outside the body and can cause many severe diseases, notably typhus.

Prions
Prions are proteinaceous infectious particles or 'slow viruses' that cause nervous system diseases in livestock and humans, such as scrapie in sheep and goats, bovine spongiform encephalitis (BSE) in cattle and kuru and Creutzfeldt–Jakob disease (CJD) in humans.

Bacteria
Bacteria are larger and more highly organised, containing DNA, RNA and a cell wall. With their complex chemical structure, they have the capacity to proliferate outside cells by binary fission (dividing into two) and are not obliged to multiply within the host cell. Many bacteria survive in a resting form in unfavourable conditions as spores with a waxy coat, for example in dust. It is traditional to divide bacteria into the two broad categories of Gram positive and Gram negative on the arbitrary basis of whether they retain a Gram stain. They are also subdivided by virtue of shape, for example the round cocci or the rod-shaped bacilli. They can also be aerobes (requiring oxygen) or anaerobes (damaged by oxygen).

Mycoplasma
Mycoplasma are similar to, but less organised than, bacteria. An example is *Mycoplasma pneumoniae*, which causes atypical pneumonia.

Protozoa
Protozoa are unicellular organisms that cause many tropical diseases, including malaria, amoebic dysentery and sleeping sickness.

Fungi
Fungi are plants devoid of roots, stems or leaves. They reproduce by spores. Fungi rarely produce more than superficial disease except in the immunodeficient.

Helminths
Helminths are worms. They may cause disease at a variety of stages of their life cycle. Examples are tapeworm, roundworm and threadworm. Helminths may remain in the circulation or lymphatic system for many years.

THE RESERVOIR OF INFECTION
The continuance of infectious diseases in the human population requires reservoirs of infection. They may come from sources external to the human body (exogenous) or may be normal inhabitants of the body (endogenous). Reservoirs are shown in **Table 5.2**.

PORTALS OF ENTRY
The route by which an organism enters its host is called the portal of entry. To be an effective pathogenic agent an organism must be able to invade a susceptible host (**Box 5.1**). It can do no harm if it cannot get into the tissues no matter how potentially lethal it may be. The main portals of entry are:
- The respiratory tract, through **inhalation** of organisms (e.g. tuberculosis, diphtheria and mumps).
- The alimentary tract, through **ingestion** of contaminated food or water (e.g. dysentery, hepatitis A and salmonellosis).
- The skin and mucous membranes, either by the passage of organisms through damaged skin as with infected wounds (**penetration**), or the **inoculation** of organisms (e.g. hepatitis B transferred from contaminated needles).
- The **placenta**, via the transfer of organisms from the maternal to the fetal circulation (e.g. rubella, cytomegalovirus and syphilis).

Endogenous and exogenous reservoirs of infection		
Human	skin nasopharynx intestinal tract	staphylococcus meningococcus *Giardia* *Escherichia coli* *Entamoeba histolytica*
Animals	Chicken Cattle	salmonella tuberculosis and brucellosis

Table 5.2 Endogenous and exogenous reservoirs of infection

5.1 FACTORS ESSENTIAL TO THE PROCESS OF INFECTION

- A reservoir for the infective agent.
- An entry route into the host.
- Establishment of multiplication within the host, i.e. a way for the organism to spread within the body; the type of tissue and conditions in which it can grow and multiply; and the susceptibility of the host to infection.
- An exit route and means of transmission from the host to a new victim.

5.2 MODES OF TRANSMISSION FOR INFECTIOUS AGENTS

Direct personal contact with contaminated body secretions or excretions (e.g. skin diseases, sexually transmitted diseases) particularly via the hands – handwashing is the most important way of preventing cross infection.

Endogenous spread from one part of a person's body to another e.g. faecal–oral route in hepatitis A.

Insect vectors such as cockroaches, fleas, flies, mosquitoes (malaria) and other insects that harbour infectious agents.

Airborne spread (e.g. of contaminated skin scales of organisms and spores) directly by the wind or through an aerosol of contaminated droplets from patients sneezing and coughing.

Spread by food and water.

Spread by fomites i.e. transmission of infection via an inanimate object such as a book or bed linen.

SUSCEPTIBILITY TO INFECTION

Many factors may influence the susceptibility to infection. The very **young** and **old** are less able to resist infection because of immaturity and ageing of the immune system, respectively. Diabetics are compromised because phagocytosis, chemotaxis and bactericidal function of neutrophils is diminished by **hyperglycaemia**. People who are **immunodeficient** or **immunocompromised** have increased susceptibility. Those with sickle cell trait (an example of a **genetic trait**) are actually more resistant to malaria.

Undernutrition impairs host defences through alterations in the epithelial integrity and ability to repair these tissues. It also leads to a decrease in gastric secretion and abnormalities of immunological proteins, and the ability to form antibodies is reduced.

Exposure to **radiation** in large doses reduces the patient's defence mechanisms because leucocyte and antibody production are suppressed. **Exposure to cold** causes the body temperature to drop below normal, which is thought to decrease ciliary movement in the respiratory tract, reduce blood supply to superficial tissues and suppress antibody formation – all natural defence mechanisms.

ESTABLISHMENT OF INFECTION

An organism that has passed a portal of entry stimulates the immune response and may be destroyed or may produce an infectious lesion by further progressive invasion of tissues or by the production of toxins, that is, chemical poisons. Tissue invasion may lead to destruction of tissue cells or mechanically important structures; in some cases infection spreads through the lymphatic channels to the bloodstream and once there it may be carried to other organs such as the kidneys or central nervous system to cause further foci of infection. The presence of bacteria in the bloodstream is called bacteraemia; the presence of virus in the bloodstream is viraemia; and multiplication of bacteria in the bloodstream is septicaemia. Many microorganisms produce certain virulence factors that enhance their ability to establish themselves in the host and cause disease. These are toxins, adherence factors, evasive factors and invasive factors and can be found in the section on characteristics of bacteria. When an infection is established it will follow a fairly predictable course.

Course of infectious disease

- The **incubation period** is the phase when the pathogen begins active replications without producing recognisable symptoms in the host.
- The **prodromal phase** describes the initial appearance of symptoms; these may only be a vague malaise. Disease is called insidious if it has a protracted prodromal phase; a **fulminant** illness is characterised by abrupt onset of symptoms with little or no prodrome.
- During the **acute stage** the host experiences the maximum impact of the infection; subclinical or subacute illness progresses from infection to resolution without clinically apparent symptoms.
- The **convalescent stage** describes the containment of infection, the progressive elimination of the pathogen, repair of damaged tissues and the resolution of associated symptoms. It depends on the efficiency of the immune system.
- **Chronic disease** has a protracted and irregular course; patients may experience continuous or sporadic symptoms for months or years.
- **Fatal infections** are variants of the typical disease course.

Infection does not always occur once an organism has entered its host; conditions may not be favourable. Some examples are listed below:
- Microbe in **wrong place** and unable to multiply, e.g. respiratory pathogen landing on skin.

- Microorganisms must attach to **specific host receptor sites** before they can multiply.
- **Antibacterial factors** that destroy or inhibit growth of microbes may be present in tears, saliva and perspiration (IgA and lysozyme).
- **Normal flora** in areas such as the mouth, vagina and intestine occupy the space and use the available nutrients.
- **Microbes** already growing in a region produce antibacterial factors (bacteriocidins) that have a local antibiotic effect, e.g. streptococci inhibit diphtheria pathogen.
- **Antibodies** may be present to attack and destroy specific pathogens, i.e. active and passive immunity (IgG).
- **Phagocytes** present in mucous membranes may engulf and destroy the invader.

VACCINES, SERUMS AND OTHER IMMUNISING AGENTS

ACQUIRED IMMUNITY
Acquired immunity is gained after birth through the immune response. It is distinct from innate or nonspecific immune mechanisms such as lysozyme in tears and saliva, or competition from the normal gut flora, which act in a nondiscriminating way. It can be active or passive.

Active acquired immunity
This is also called adaptive or specific immunity, and is produced by the host after natural exposure to an antigen or from immunisation. The individual produces antibodies to **specific** bacterial or viral infections, which then destroy this specific agent when recognising it on future exposures without damaging the host cells. The common cold unfortunately is caused by a number of viruses so the individual may be re-infected many times throughout their life. In the primary response IgM antibody is evident in the blood with lesser amounts of IgG, which indicate that the immune system has now been primed. On a second challenge by the same antigen a secondary immune response produces many IgG antibodies very rapidly, so the individual suffers no illness (McCance and Huether, 1998).

There are different types of antigen used in immunisation programmes but all aim to stimulate an immune response in the host. Toxoids are preparations of a bacterial exotoxin that causes no disease state; they have been killed with formalin. Killed vaccine is a dead organism such as pertussis, typhoid, paratyphoid and influenza. Both these preparations are given in three doses, with the number of organisms contained therein decreasing each time.

Attenuated vaccine is a weak strain of the organism that is not pathogenic but mimics a natural infection response, for example smallpox, polio, measles, rubella and tuberculosis. The polio vaccine contains three strains of virus; three doses are given to ensure that all three 'take'. Measles has to be given after 1 year of age as the maternal

IgG destroys the vaccine organisms before they are able to elicit an immune response. Rubella is given at 18 months or 2 years for the same reason. Pregnant women must take care to be protected 4 months before conception as rubella will damage the growing fetus in its early stages of development. There are protocols to advise on the giving of vaccines (see Chapter 4 *Legal aspects of drug administration*). The Royal College of Nursing have produced a 'green book' that provides the following information:

- Details of drugs that can be given by nurses.
- Circumstances in which vaccines can be given.
- Procedure for checking that a patient is suitable for vaccination.
- Procedure for action in anaphylactic shock.
- Necessary equipment for vaccination.

The immunisation schedule for most children is outlined in **Table 5.3**.

IMMUNISATION
The immunisation of children and adults aims to increase the 'herd' protection against transferable infections that cause morbidity and suffering within a population. Most parts of the world have similar schedules; differences are usually a response to local need. For example, some boroughs in London routinely offer vaccination against tuberculosis for all newborn babies. Vaccines are available for hepatitis A and B, rubella, anthrax, yellow fever, rabies, influenza, meningococcal and pneumococcal infection, typhoid, smallpox and varicella. Immunoglobulins can be given for rabies, hepatitis B, varicella zoster, cytomegalovirus, tetanus and Anti-D (Rh_o) The debate continues concerning the extent of programmes required for childhood safety and for international travel, for example cholera vaccine is now considered to be ineffective.

Some common contraindications for vaccination
A viral vaccine is not effective if interferon is present, for example if the individual has a cold or other acute illness. If oral polio vaccine is given to an individual with diarrhoea, it will not be absorbed. In these cases vaccination should be postponed. If chemotherapy treatment is being given or the patient is immunosuppressed for other reasons, the immune response will be suppressed and the patient may suffer the illness. This is especially dangerous with chickenpox and measles vaccines. It is therefore recommended that children are vaccinated in the 'well' phase of their disease. Measles, mumps and rubella vaccine may be given 6 months after chemotherapy and 3 months after steroids are completed, otherwise contacts may be given passive immunity with specific immunoglobulins. Those who have a history of severe reaction to previous vaccines, those who have severe allergy to eggs and those who have an evolving neurological condition will not usually be vaccinated.

Vaccination schedule	
1 week (if vulnerable to exposure)	**BCG (bacillus Calmette–Guérin) vaccine:** infants aged under 3 months, 0.05 ml; older children, 0.1 ml; intradermal. Serious reactions with BCG are uncommon but prolonged ulceration or subcutaneous abscess formation may occur as a result of faulty injection technique.
During first year of life	**Adsorbed diphtheria, tetanus, pertussis toxin (DTP),** which must be stored at 2–8°C. The dose is 0.5 ml intramuscular or deep subcutaneous injection at 2 months of age followed by two or more doses at 4-week intervals.
	Polio: oral 0.35 ml (3 drops) live attenuated strain vaccine contains three strains of polio virus. This vaccine is grown in the kidney cells of monkeys, so patients may develop allergies. The vaccine is supplied in a 10-dose multidose vial. For those for whom live vaccine is inadvisable, 0.5 ml subcutaneous inactivated vaccine is available. First dose at 2 months with two more doses at 4-week intervals. **Haemophilus influenza type B (HiB):** three doses at 4-week intervals with first dose at 2 months of age: 10–25 µg, depending on the combination of DTP it is administered with. This vaccine is produced in a double vial, the fluid DTP element(s) is used to dissolve the HiB 'powder'. Thus the child receives only one injection of 0.5 ml fluid deep subcutaneous or intramuscular.
During second year of life	**Measles, mumps, rubella (MMR):** single dose (0.5 ml) at 12–15 months of age. **Haemophilus influenza type B:** single dose at age 13 months to 4 years if not previously immunised.
On entry into school or nursery school	**Adsorbed diphtheria, tetanus (DT):** single booster dose, given after MMR in separate limb. **Polio:** single booster dose. **Measles, mumps, rubella:** single booster dose. It is given at same session as DT but using a separate syringe and needle; MMR should be given first as it is less painful, in separate limb, or a second appointment should be made.
Between 10–14 years	**BCG:** if tuberculin negative to Heaf test and if not given in first week of life – record keeping is therefore very important. May be given simultaneously with another live vaccine or 3 weeks apart.
On leaving school, before employment or further education	**Adsorbed diphtheria and tetanus** vaccine for adults and adolescents – single booster dose. **Polio:** single booster dose.
During adult life	**Polio:** 3 doses at intervals of 4 weeks if not previously immunised and single booster dose if not immunised within last 10 years **Rubella:** susceptible women of childbearing age should be tested for rubella antibodies and offered rubella immunisation if seronegative; pregnancy must be excluded before immunisation. All those who might put pregnant women at risk, e.g. nurses and doctors in obstetric units, should also be seropositive to antibodies or be vaccinated if seronegative **Adsorbed tetanus:** if not previously immunised, 3 doses at 4-week intervals. Booster dose 10 years after primary course and 10 years later maintains satisfactory level. If diphtheria cover also needed use Adsorbed Diphtheria and Tetanus for adults and adolescents. **Adsorbed diphtheria** for adults and adolescents: if not previously immunised, 3 doses at 4 week intervals. Booster dose 10 years after primary course. If tetanus needed, give Adsorbed Diphtheria and Tetanus for adults and adolescents.

Table 5.3 Vaccination schedule

Do we need to 'jab'?

Few developments in public health create more debate than child mass vaccination programmes. The effectiveness was graphically demonstrated in the United Kingdom when the uptake of whooping cough vaccine fell to 30% in the 1970s. One result was two large outbreaks of the disease during 1977–1978 and 1981–1982 when notifications reached 100 000 in each period and 51 children died. Since uptake has resumed, deaths and morbidity have declined. In 1988 MMR (measles, mumps and rubella) was introduced. In 1992 no deaths from measles virus was reported and the lowest recorded numbers, 10 264, were seen. Also only 2–4% of fetuses were affected by rubella, compared with the years before 1970 when approximately 15% were severely damaged (Parker, 1996). *Haemophilus influenzae* type B (HiB) produces meningitis (70%), epiglottitis (15%), cellulitis, septic arthritis and pneumonia. Mortality from this virus was seen in 5% of children; 65 died each year and 150 were left with neurological sequelae such as sensorineural deafness, hemiparesis and mental retardation. In 1995, after the introduction of HiB vaccine in combination with diphtheria, pertussis and tetanus (DPT) and polio, no deaths were recorded.

A 95% uptake of vaccine is required to provide 'herd immunity' so that very young babies and those immunosuppressed are protected within a society. It has been found recently that earlier vaccination with DPT with polio is effective in 90% of children at 2, 3 or 4 months after birth and that preterm infants born at 28 weeks' gestation also produce an immune response.

Influenza is a potentially lethal condition, especially in 'at risk' patients, that is, those with diabetes, chronic bronchitis, renal impairment or heart disease and those who are elderly. The composition of vaccine for this disease is changed almost every year so that it contains protection against the strains most likely to be prevalent in a society. The vaccine can now be formulated as a 'surface antigen' that contains the haemagglutinin and neuraminidase antigens but not the extraneous protein particles that produce adverse effects (Henderson, 1991). Use of this vaccine has cut death rates by 75% in those routinely vaccinated (Ahmed *et al.*, 1995).

The success of the vaccination programme appears to have sown the seeds of its own downfall as public perception has changed in the United Kingdom; the risk associated with the vaccine is now considered to be higher than the rarely seen disease. But, perhaps the success *is* wildly exaggerated and inaccurately reported. It may be that the seriousness of the side effects is played down and the long-term health damage never properly investigated. Death rates from diphtheria, for example, had dropped from 900/million to 300/million by the 1940s, before the introduction of vaccination programmes.

It has been noted that infections are generally less severe among those with a high standard of living. The factors that contribute to this are good nutrition, housing, hygiene in food and waste handling and professional care in periods of vulnerability e.g. childbirth (Meers *et al.*, 1995).

Live measles vaccination has been linked to the development in later life of Crohn's disease, an inflammatory condition of the bowel (Thompson *et al.*, 1995). The mass MMR vaccination programme of 7 million UK school-age children in November 1994 was criticised as being an experiment (Day, 1995a). As all children since 1988 had been offered MMR, it was believed that all primary school children should be immunised to increase the levels of immunity as the mean age of infection had increased. Many infected children were now over ten years of age and in this age group measles was often more severe (Lissauer & Clayden, 1997). Many parents refused to cooperate as they felt their older children could safely experience rubella and that they needed more information to comply and give informed consent. It is felt that insufficient information was given to the parents by the general practitioners, who appeared to be rushing to achieve their quotas to gain their cash incentives (Day, 1995b) and delight the drug industry. There are many stories of vaccine-induced damage; some children suffer brain damage, paralysis and seizures from the single and combination immunisations. We do not know the extent of the morbidity in the long term of present programmes; the debate over the 'Gulf War Syndrome' reported by UK and US military personnel continues. As hepatitis B vaccine is being piloted with a view to it being added to the expanding 'menu', the public is challenging the need for mass protection from diseases restricted to small isolated groups (Day, 1995c). The question exists as to whether the United Kingdom will follow the USA and use vaccination certificates as social 'passes' without which children are barred from schooling and adults are barred from insurance and work. This in turn raises issues related to the feasibility of exercising free choice as human numbers increase in our overcrowded world.

Passive acquired immunity

This is a protection that is imported in the form of ready-made antibodies from outside the system. This type of immunity only lasts a few weeks or months. The fetus receives maternal antibodies across the placenta and the neonate from breast milk. Passive acquired immunity can also be conferred by transfer from a previously sensitised host. Today many of these antibodies are manufactured artificially; in the past they may have been drawn from horses, for example antibodies to tetanus. The 'foreign' protein, in this case from horses, may have caused some anaphylactic reactions. Today's artificial antisera are also used in other circumstances. They can neutralise rabies infections before the virus enters the tissues, neutralise blood-borne antigens before they have a devastating effect, for example bacterial toxins of *Clostridium botulinum* found in improperly preserved food, and prevent the immune response of a rhesus-negative woman to her rhesus-positive fetus (Nowak and Handford, 1994).

PERSON CENTRED STUDY 1

Mrs Bailey has come to see the health visitor about having her new baby daughter immunised. She has recently read that vaccination may cause many future problems and is probably not necessary anyway as she is breastfeeding and they live in a bright, clean new house in a rural village. Her mother has told Mrs Bailey that she survived without any vaccination. Mr and Mrs Bailey also like to travel and have thus far avoided catching 'anything nasty' without injections as Mr Bailey hates needles.

1. Does she really need to put her baby through all the pain of injections?
2. How can you put her mind at rest about the dangers of vaccination?
3. What could you tell Mr and Mrs Bailey about preventing the pain of injections?

INFECTIOUS DISORDERS

The disorders that follow are examples of infections attributable to each type of causative organism. The most common and important may be covered within the systems chapters; those that affect the entire body of the individual, such as influenza and malaria, are discussed in this chapter.

CREUTZFELDT–JAKOB DISEASE

Creutzfeldt–Jakob disease is a slowly progressive dementia characterised pathologically by spongiform encephalopathy caused by a prion. Kuru is a similar dementia, characterised by cerebellar ataxia and it is believed to be caused by ritual cannibalism of victims of kuru. Prions are even smaller than viruses and are resistant to sterilisation processes. Infection has been transmitted from post mortem, surgical specimens, corneal grafts and human growth hormone (obtained from human pituitary glands at autopsy).

Pathophysiology

The mechanism of action is under intense study after recent apparent transmission from cattle to humans in beef nervous tissue and possibly bones. Cattle, who have the special capacity and digestive systems to transform cellulose into protein without ingesting meat, developed BSE after being given cattle feed containing sheep carcasses (including brains and nervous tissue) in order to speed up meat production (Prusiner, 1997). Most ingested microorganisms are dealt with by the resident macrophages in the gastrointestinal tract or liver (or they cause gastrointestinal tract symptoms of food poisoning or, in the liver, of hepatitis). Immunity should result, but in the case of a prion, long-term damage is caused and no immunity can develop.

Pharmacological Management

There is as yet no treatment for CJD.

VIRAL INFECTIONS

Mature virus particles, virions, are so small and simple in structure that they do not fit the living cell classification of most microorganisms. However, there are viruses, called bacteriophages or simply phages, that infect bacteria, that are living cells. These phages may be able to be exploited for new treatments for bacterial infections that no longer respond to antibiotics. Viruses also seem able to cause genetic changes, acting as carcinogens, in addition to causing infection. Viruses, excluding bacteriophages, have five specific properties that distinguish them from living cells and are classified according to the characteristics listed in **Table 5.4**.

Some important human viral diseases include the common cold, influenza, mumps, measles, chickenpox, smallpox, rabies, cold sores, venereal herpes, warts, poliomyelitis, encephalitis and HIV. Smallpox is now considered to be eliminated worldwide by universal vaccination. Others of these viral diseases are controlled by immunisation.

Antiviral drugs

Viruses are only susceptible to antiviral drugs when they multiply. They use the metabolic systems of the cells they invade to achieve this so they are difficult to attack without damage to the host (**Fig. 5.1**). To succeed, antiviral drugs need to be backed up by effective host defence mechanisms. Today's antiviral drugs attack virus multiplication at one of three points. The first is as the virus enters the cell and is uncoated to release its nucleic acid; the second is when new viral nucleic acid is manufactured and the third is the production of the protein units used to form viral capsids (the protective layer of protein molecules).

Amantadine stops **viral entry** into cells and uncoating. Aciclovir, foscarnet sodium, ganciclovir, idoxuridine, ribavirin and zidovudine stop **synthesis of viral nucleic acid** and interferon and protease inhibitors prevent **synthesis of viral protein**.

Zidovudine, a nucleoside reverse transcriptase inhibitor, was the first of the anti-HIV drugs; it penetrates the blood–brain barrier and may be useful in preventing AIDS dementia. Other nucleoside reverse transcriptase inhibitors include **didanosine**, **lamivudine**, **stavudine** and **zalcitabine**. Side effects include blood disorders, gastrointestinal disturbances, headache, rash, fever, myalgia, neuropathy, insomnia, malaise and asthenia with pancreatitis,

Table 5.4 Characteristics of viruses

Characteristics of viruses	
Properties of viruses	**Classification by**
1. They possess either DNA or RNA, never both.	a) The type of genetic material.
2. Their replication is directed by viral nucleic acid within a host cell.	b) Shape of the capsid and number of capsomeres.
3. They do not divide by binary fission or mitosis.	c) Presence or absence of an envelope.
4. They lack the genes and enzymes necessary for energy production.	d) The host that it infects and the kind of disease produced.
	e) The target cell.
5. They depend on the ribosomes, enzymes and nutrients of infected cells for protein production.	f) Immunological properties.

peripheral neuropathy, eye changes and diarrhoea. Protease inhibitors are specific to particular viruses. As they have been produced for HIV, hepatitis C protease inhibitors are now being developed. Protease inhibitors inhibit the cytochrome P450 enzyme system and therefore have a potential for significant drug interactions. At present, protease inhibitors are used in combination with nucleoside reverse transcriptase inhibitors, but combination trials based purely on different types of protease inhibitors are underway. Protease inhibitors include **indinavir**, **ritonavir** and **saquinavir**. The side effects are similar to those experienced with the reverse transcriptase inhibitors but may include hepatic disorders as well. Nausea is very severe and can last for up to 3 months. Indinavir may possibly affect the clotting cascade, which would limit its usage in haemophilia.

Specific therapy of virus infections is usually unsatisfactory and is therefore mainly symptomatic. As each virus infection differs slightly, drugs are changed until a tolerable combination is found for the individual. In the immunocompetent patient, the majority of infections resolve spontaneously. The development of chemotherapy for viral diseases has been difficult because by the time signs and symptoms appear viral multiplication is usually ended. To be clinically effective antiviral drugs must be administered prophylactically (McKenry and Salerno, 1995) before the disease appears. The limiting factor in antiviral drugs is that the virus is a true parasite and replicates within the human cell using the cell's own enzyme system. Because it has no enzyme system of its own for internal metabolism, antibiotics are ineffective. Therefore drugs strong enough to stop replication would damage the host cell.

For eye infections please see Chapter 9 *Drugs and head and neck disorders*. Antiviral therapy for skin infections is discussed in Chapter 17 *Drugs and dermatological disorders*. Major systemic viral infections such as hepatitis B or the 'childhood' illnesses (measles, mumps, whooping cough, and polio) are best prevented with vaccines or treated with immune sera.

Aciclovir is active against herpes viruses but does not eradicate them. It is selectively taken up by the herpes simplex virus and is then converted to an active triphosphate form that is incorporated into growing viral DNA chains, thus ending chain development (McKenry and Salerno, 1995). It has been used systemically for varicella zoster (chicken pox/shingles) and topically and systemically for herpes zoster. Oral aciclovir is used to treat and manage genital herpes, and to treat chickenpox in children if it is used within 24 hours of the rash appearing. It is given by injection to patients with severe herpes zoster and genital herpes and to those unable to absorb the oral form. Otherwise, the oral form is poorly absorbed (15–30%) but therapeutic serum levels are achieved in relevant bodily fluids, including cerebrospinal fluid, vaginal mucosa and herpetic vesicular fluid. The half-life is about 2.5 hours and the peak serum level at steady state is about 0.6 µg/ml after an oral dose of 200 mg every 4 hours, or 9.8 µg/ml after a parenteral dose of 5 mg/kg. Aciclovir is metabolised by the liver and excreted in the urine. The most frequent side effects with chronic usage of the oral form are diarrhoea, dizziness, headache, pain in joints, nausea and vomiting; less frequent side effects are acne, anorexia and insomnia. In the injectable form dizziness is the most common and headache and sweating are less frequent side effects. **Famciclovir** and **valaciclovir** are similar to aciclovir and are used for varicella zoster and genital herpes. **Idoxuridine** is only effective at the start of an infection and is too toxic for systemic use. Although used orally for

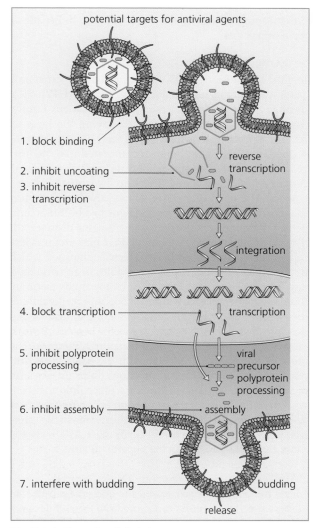

potential targets for antiviral agents

1. block binding

2. inhibit uncoating

3. inhibit reverse transcription

reverse transcription

integration

4. block transcription

transcription

5. inhibit polyprotein processing

viral precursor polyprotein processing

6. inhibit assembly

assembly

7. interfere with budding

budding

release

Fig 5.1 Action of antiviral drugs

antiviral is 100 mg twice daily (McKenry and Salerno, 1995). Dosage is not established for neonates or infants up to 1 year of age. For children aged 1–9 years the dosage is 1.5–3 mg/kg orally every 8 hours with a maximum dose of 150 mg daily; for children aged 9–12 years, it is 100 mg orally every 12 hours and for children aged 12 years and older the adult dosage is used. Most frequent side effects are anorexia, nausea, anxiety, red-purple skin spots, increased irritability, dizziness, insomnia, difficulty concentrating and nightmares. The most frequent adverse reactions are mood changes, hallucinations and confusion in the elderly.

Interferons, α, β and γ, are produced by leucocytes, fibroblasts and T lymphocytes when the cells are infected by certain viruses, chlamydias, rickettsias or other protozoa; they are also produced in response to certain tumours and cancers. The interferons are secreted into the surrounding cells where they inhibit the synthesis of proteins essential for the production of viruses and other pathogens within those cells, inhibiting the spread of infection. Thus many viral diseases are self-limiting. Similarly, the acute phase of the herpes simplex cold sore is of limited duration but the virus can hide in the nerve ganglion where it is protected until the individual's defences are down and the cold sore cycle can begin again. The chicken pox virus, herpes zoster, can also hide in the nerve ganglion and reappear in the form of shingles when the individual's defences are down.

Interferons are not pathogen specific but they are species specific, which means that human interferon is only effective in humans. Human interferons are produced artificially by bacteria in which interferon genes have been inserted using recombinant DNA techniques. These interferons are used for some viral infections, cancers, tumours and immunodeficiency diseases.

Interferon α preparations are used for Kaposi's sarcoma, various leukaemias, lymph or liver metastases, chronic active hepatitis B and chronic active hepatitis C, and as an adjunct in malignant melanoma and for the maintenance of remission in multiple myeloma (see Chapter 6 *Drugs and neoplastic disorders*). Side effects are dose related and include nausea, flu-like symptoms, hypotension or hypertension and arrhythmias, lethargy, ocular side effects and depression (suicidal behaviour reported). Myelosuppression may affect granulocyte counts, and hepatotoxicity has been reported. Other side effects include hypersensitivity reactions, thyroid abnormalities, rash, coma and seizures (mainly in the elderly).

INFLUENZA

The influenza virus belongs to the orthomyxovirus group and exists in two forms – A and B. Influenza B is associated with localised outbreaks of a milder nature whereas influenza A is responsible for worldwide pandemics. Influenza A has the additional ability to develop new

herpes simplex, the effectiveness of **inosine pranobex** has not been established.

Amantadine has been used orally for herpes zoster and is used prophylactically during outbreaks of influenza A only in those who are at risk and have not been immunised, in those who are at risk and cannot be immunised and in healthcare workers and other key personnel during an epidemic. Amantadine should not be used for both prophylaxis and treatment in the same household because of the risk of resistance to the drug. Amantadine is believed to prevent influenza A by penetrating respiratory epithelial cells to block the encoding of the virus and the release of viral nucleic acid into host cells. It is rapidly absorbed orally and distributed to saliva and nasal secretions. It has a half-life of 11–15 hours and reaches peak serum levels within 2–4 hours of administration. Amantadine is excreted mostly unchanged by the kidneys. The adult dose as an

antigenic variants at regular intervals. Human immunity develops against the H and N antigens on the viral surface. In 1957 a major shift in the antigenic make-up of the virus led to a pandemic of influenza A2 type H2N2. A further pandemic occurred in 1968 owing to the emergence of Hong Kong influenza type H3N2. Secondary bacterial infections particularly with *Streptococcus pneumoniae* and *H. influenzae* commonly follow influenza virus infection. Rarer but more serious is pneumonia caused by *Staphylococcus aureus*, with a mortality up to 20%.

Pathophysiology

The main route of infection is by inhalation of the influenza virus. Infection begins when the virion, the viral material, attaches itself to the receptor site on a vulnerable cell (one which cannot resist viral invasion and replication). Once bound the virus penetrates the plasma membrane by receptor-mediated endocytosis: the cell 'eats' the virus. The viral DNA or RNA is released into the cytoplasm and takes over the cell's protein synthesis to replicate more viruses, which spill out of the cell into the surrounding extracellular fluid by budding. The progression from infection to disease follows predictable stages but the symptoms mainly result from the host's immune and inflammatory response. The fever, headache, muscle and joint pain, fatigue and malaise and loss of appetite are typical. Unfortunately, the infection does not produce immunity except to that very specific virus type and the influenza virus is noted for its ability to mutate, called antigenic shift, to a new form against which the host will not be immune the following year.

Pharmacological management

Protection by influenza vaccines is only effective in up to 70% of people and only lasts for about 1 year. It should not be given to people who are allergic to egg proteins, as some vaccines are manufactured in chick embryos. As new vaccines have to be prepared to cover each change in viral antigenicity, vaccine is in short supply at the beginning of an epidemic. Therefore, routine vaccination is reserved for susceptible people with chronic heart, lung or kidney disease, and the elderly. In pandemics key hospital and health service personnel are also vaccinated (George, 1999).

Amantadine hydrochloride 100 mg daily for 4–5 days may attenuate influenza A and should be reserved for individuals with chronic respiratory or cardiovascular disease who have not been previously immunised. Treatment is bed rest and aspirin, with antibiotics for individuals with chronic bronchitis, heart or renal disease. Amantidine hydrochloride is given for prophylaxis, 100 mg daily for 6 weeks; in those aged over 65 years the dosage is less than 100 mg daily or 100 mg at intervals of more than 1 day. It should not be used for prophylaxis and treatment of influenza in the same household because of the risk of resistance. It should not be given in epilepsy, when there is a history of gastric ulceration or during pregnancy and breastfeeding, and should be used with care in hepatic or renal impairment.

HUMAN IMMUNODEFICIENCY VIRUS

In 1983 the cause of **AIDS** was identified as a virus, now called the **human immunodeficiency virus** (**HIV**). HIV belongs to the lentivirus group of the retrovirus family; these viruses are characterised by having the enzyme reverse transcriptase, which allows viral RNA to be transcribed into DNA and thence incorporated into the host cell genome. Other human pathogens in this group cause certain kinds of leukaemia. There are two, possibly three, types of HIV – HIV-1 and HIV-2 – and another rarer form found in Cameroon. They are distinguished by minor antigenic differences, but they produce the same disease with the same epidemiology, although HIV-2 may progress less rapidly. Each variant may have different genotypes, which may produce different resistance profiles in antiviral therapy. The AIDS virus is carried in bodily fluids (seminal fluid, vaginal secretions, lymph, blood, cerebrospinal fluid, breast milk), although this can vary among individuals, so it is spread in exactly the same way as the hepatitis B virus. However, in comparison with a hepatitis B infection, the blood of an individual infected with the AIDS virus contains perhaps 100 000 fewer infectious doses in each unit of volume. The amount of blood (or other fluid that contains the virus) that must pass from an HIV-positive person to infect someone else is significantly greater so the infection is transmitted much less easily. The AIDS virus is more easily destroyed than the hepatitis B virus.

PATHOPHYSIOLOGY

Inside the body the virus attaches to and enters cells that possess specific receptors called the CD4 (cluster designation 4) antigens, which are found primarily on T-helper cells (otherwise known as T4 cells because of the presence of CD4), monocytes, macrophages and other antigen-presenting cells, including dendritic cells in the cerebrospinal fluid, Langerhans' cells in the skin and follicular dendritic cells in the brain and lymph nodes where much of the early infection and replication of HIV takes place (Meers *et al.*, 1995; Kumar and Clark, 1994). The disorganisation or destruction of these cells prevents the development of an effective immune response. The virus thus persists and infected individuals are considered to be infectious for the rest of their lives. However, one of the goals of antiviral therapy is to lower the viral count so that it is negligible and individuals may be regarded as noninfectious.

As HIV infection progresses, the number of CD4 lymphocytes in the circulation falls. Counts of these cells made at intervals allows the condition of patients to be monitored. A normal count of CD4 lymphocytes is $800–1300/10^{-6}$/l. At some point in the progress of the disease the immune competence is reduced to the point that microbes, usually of little importance, begin to cause infections. This is thought to happen when the CD4 count is below $200/10^{-6}/l$. In the USA two consecutive CD4 counts below $200/10^{-6}/l$ classifies the patient as having AIDS. As a marker, however, it is not necessarily that accurate and many people are asymptomatic with extremely low, or uncountable, CD4 counts.

A new laboratory test for viral counting, the polymerase chain reaction, is able to attract or exclude genetic material and then multiply the material so that it can be examined. This enables only the virus material to be counted. It is probably more important than the CD4 count alone as the viral load used in combination with the CD4 count gives a more accurate picture. The polymerase chain reaction is now used for all the viruses that can be tested for and is a most important new test for measuring viruses quantitatively. Treatment can therefore be evaluated immediately.

Opportunistic infections occur because the CD4 counts are so low. Microbes may already exist within the body, for example the herpes viruses, *Toxoplasma gondii* and sometimes the tuberculosis bacillus, or they may be a part of the normal flora such as *Candida albicans*. When these opportunistic infections are treated, the immune systems of HIV-positive individuals fail to provide the assistance antimicrobial drugs need to be effective. By the same token, a variety of malignancies that are normally kept at bay by the immune system take hold. These opportunistic infections and malignancies usually mean the transition from HIV infection to the clinical illness of AIDS. Immunodeficiency and the opportunistic infections of AIDS are discussed in the section on immune suppression below.

Pharmacological management

Treatment for HIV is aimed at boosting the immune system or reducing the plasma viral load as much as possible and for as long as possible.

5.3 TREATMENT STRATEGIES FOR HIV

Direct therapy for the opportunistic infection or malignancy.
Secondary prophylaxis for the opportunistic infection or malignancy.
Primary prophylaxis.
Antiviral treatment.
Vaccine (as a stimulus for immune function).
Dietetics (elemental diet encourages regrowth of villi in intestine).
Psychoneuroimmunology; the aim is to create a protective coping mechanism which helps the immune system's function, i.e. CD4 counts are directly affected by stress; reducing stress boosts the immune system.

Most of the advances in chemotherapy have been based on attacking the virus. Treatment should be started before the immune system is irreversibly damaged, but this needs to be balanced against concerns about resistance developing.

PERSON CENTRED STUDY 2

George is 45 years old and a haemophiliac; he was diagnosed HIV positive in 1984 after being a recipient of contaminated blood, possibly as early as 1978. When he was first told about his antibody status, he was misinformed and told that although he was antibody positive he had developed antibodies against a dead virus. When he was subsequently informed about the true picture, he had by that point developed a degree of denial as a coping mechanism. HIV was a non-issue for him as far as prognosis was concerned. He did, however, maintain safe practices for other people around him and did accept medical advice related to treatment, but very passively.

He was enrolled on the MRC Concorde Trial and had been on the AZT treatment wing, rather than placebo (see Figure 5.1 for the HIV replication and potential site of action of antiviral drugs). Therefore when his CD4 count began a further decline in 1995, he was placed on dual therapy of zidovudine with didanosine (King, 1996). George did not tolerate the treatment very well and there was a query of pancreatitis developing with didanosine, which was therefore stopped. He then started on lamivudine, which was effective at reducing his viral load with no side effects.

In early 1997 George's CD4 count started to dip again. Use of the new polymerase chain reaction technology indicated an increase in viral load. George is, however, asymptomatic but his disease progress suggests that he may need a protease inhibitor. Although George has been compliant with therapy, he has not always taken his medication as scrupulously as he should have done.

1. What do you need to tell George about protease inhibitors?
2. How will you explain to George that his nausea can be controlled?
3. Could you give an explanation of the new treatments and how they work to help boost his morale and ensure his compliance with treatment?

The need for early drug treatment is balanced against possible toxicity. The development of drug resistance is prevented by using a combination of drugs that should have a synergistic or additive activity but their toxicity must not be additive.

The optimum time for initiation of treatment will depend on the CD4 cell count, the plasma viral load and clinical symptoms. Initiation treatment is with zidovudine, with either didanosine or zalcitabine or lamivudine. Combinations of three drugs (including a protease inhibitor or a non-nucleoside reverse transcriptase inhibitor) have been recommended and may be appropriate in high plasma viral load. Deterioration of the condition may mean switching treatment or adding another antiviral drug. The choice of alternative regimens depends on factors such as the response to previous treatment, tolerance and the possibility of cross-resistance.

Zidovudine, a nucleoside reverse transcriptase inhibitor (or nucleoside analogue) was the first of the anti-HIV drugs. It penetrates the blood–brain barrier and may prevent AIDS dementia. Other nucleoside reverse transcriptase inhibitors are didanosine, lamivudine, stavudine and zalcitabine. The protease inhibitors (indinavir, ritonavir and saquinavir) have been introduced recently to inhibit the cytochrome P450 enzyme system, and therefore they have a potential for significant drug interactions. Non-nucleoside reverse transcriptase inhibitors are not on the UK market but may be available on a named-patient basis (George, 1999).

In the event of a healthcare worker requiring prophylactic treatment for an injury involving HIV-infected blood a 'triple therapy' regime is recommended. For further information, please see the section on anti-viral drugs.

Occupational prophylactic treatment for HIV infection

Zidovudine 200 mg three times a day or 250 mg twice daily is given with **lamivudine** 150 mg twice daily, preferably without food, and **indinavir** 800 mg three times a day.

Once it is established that the individual has been substantially exposed to HIV-infected bodily fluids, such as by needlestick injury, these three drugs are given for 4 weeks to prevent HIV infection. Zidovudine and lamivudine are nucleoside reverse transcriptase inhibitors and indinavir is a protease inhibitor. These drugs have a potential for severe drug reactions, and side effects include blood disorders, gastrointestinal disturbances, headache, rash, fever, myalgia, neuropathy, insomnia, malaise and asthenia. Indinavir also has skin and renal side effects, with possible liver disorder. There is only a fairly short time to institute treatment to prevent HIV infection and advice should be sought at once in the event of a needlestick injury (Easterbrook and Ippolito, 1997). There is a growing debate about the effect of this prophylaxis on the development of HIV-specific antibodies, which actually do protect against the disease.

BACTERIAL INFECTIONS

Bacteria range in size from 0.5 to 10 µm in their greatest dimension, so are small even by microscope standards. They are grouped by shape into spheres (cocci) and rods, which can be curved like a comma (vibrio) or form tightly or loosely coiled spirals. Bacteria reproduce by binary fission and in cocci the daughter cells may remain together to form pairs called diplococci or chains. A few, usually soil bacteria, are able to form spores when there is a need to survive drought.

The differences between prokaryotic bacterial cells and human eukaryotic cells (**Fig. 5.2**) are exploited in order to destroy bacteria that cause infections without damaging host cells.

Prokaryotic cells do not have their nuclear DNA enclosed within a special membrane as human eukaryotic cells do. Instead it floats free in the cytoplasm. All bacteria are prokaryotes and are tiny cells bound by a rigid cell wall with an inner cell membrane. Bacterial cell walls contain a polymer called peptidoglycan, which gives strength and rigidity. There is so much pressure within the bacterium that with sufficient damage to the cell wall, it will split open and the bacterium will die. Because peptidoglycan is unique to bacteria it provides a target for substances that in theory are poisonous to bacteria and nothing else.

Bacterial metabolism

Bacteria differ in their metabolism. A byproduct of metabolism is hydrogen and most living organisms get rid of it by combining it with oxygen to make water. These forms of life will therefore die without oxygen and are called **obligate aerobes**. Other organisms are more flexible and use a variety of chemicals in addition to oxygen as hydrogen acceptors. A few have developed these alternatives to the point that oxygen is a poison; such organisms are called **obligate anaerobes**. Between the two extremes lie the great mass of bacteria, which are **facultative anaerobes**. Most of these prefer to grow in oxygen but can manage without, usually with reduced efficiency.

Staining methods

In 1884, a Danish scientist called Christian Gram discovered that bacteria could be distinguished by staining with dyes to make them easy to see under a microscope. Bacteria pick up these dyes differently so they can be more easily identified. The method has been called Gram stain ever since. Although much more is now known about bacterial cell walls it is still not known why they stain as they do. Mycobacteria, the mycoplasmas, the rickettsias and some of the spiral bacteria do not stain by the Gram method and another staining method called Ziehl–Neelson (ZN) or acid-fast is used.

Bacterial genetics

Bacteria have made a fundamental contribution to the study of heredity and the science of genetics, mainly because they are small, breed rapidly and are easy to handle in large numbers. The time for a newly formed bacterial cell to grow and divide is called generation time. This varies between bacteria and also depends on the temperature and appropriate available nourishment. For rapidly growing *E. coli* it may only be 20 minutes; for slower growing *Mycobacterium tuberculosis* it is as long as 24 hours.

The DNA that makes up the genetic blueprint may be altered in two ways: by mutation and by recombination. A mutation changes the structure of DNA and the offspring may not be viable. Recombination is the transfer of preformed functional DNA, thus it is more likely to be inherited. It is supposed that by recombination or mutation some bacteria pick up a fragment of DNA that gives acquired resistance to some antibacterial drugs. The mechanism of resistance may be, for example, an alteration of cell wall permeability so that the antimicrobial is excluded from the cell. Two or more fragments of DNA may be acquired so that the microbe becomes resistant to several drugs at the same time. Any large population of microbes

is likely to include a few that by chance have acquired one or more of these resistance mechanisms. If the population is then exposed to an appropriate drug the sensitive majority are wiped out and the resistant minority multiply to fill the gap. In this way an apparently 'sensitive' population of bacteria become resistant.

The organism must be able to find a suitable place to multiply before it is killed by the defence mechanisms of the body. For example, *Clostridium perfringens* is a normal inhabitant of the faeces and soil and frequently gets into wounds. It causes disease comparatively rarely because it can multiply only under anaerobic conditions. In penetrating injuries, such as in farming or road traffic accidents, with dirt and dead muscle involved, the conditions become anaerobic and the disease gas gangrene is produced. Some organisms, like the haemolytic *Streptococcus*, can grow and multiply using any tissue in the body as a source of food. Others are more selective and can find the materials for growth only in a particular type of tissue, such as brain tissue in encephalitis.

Table 5.5 Differences between prokaryotic cells and eukaryotic cells

Differences between prokaryotic and eukaryotic cells		
SITE	EXPLOITABLE DIFFERENCES	ANTIBACTERIAL DRUGS
Peptidoglycan cell wall	Peptidoglycan cell walls are a uniquely prokaryotic feature not shared by eukaryotic (mammalian) cells. Drugs that act here are therefore very selective.	penicillins cephalosporins glycopeptides
Cytoplasmic membrane	Bacteria possess a plasma membrane within the cell wall, which is a phospholipid bilayer, as in eukaryotes. However, in bacteria the plasma membrane does not contain any sterols and this results in differential chemical behaviour that can be exploited.	polymyxins
Protein synthesis	The bacterial ribosome (505+30S subunits) is sufficiently different from the mammalian ribosome (60S+40S subunits) that sites on the bacterial ribosome are good targets for drug action.	aminoglycosides tetracyclines chloramphenicol macrolides fusidic acid
Nucleic acids	The bacterial genome is in the form of a single circular strand of DNA plus ancillary plasmids unenclosed by a nuclear envelope, in contrast to the eukaryotic chromosomal arrangement within the nucleus. Drugs may interfere directly or indirectly with microbial DNA and RNA metabolism, replication and transcription.	antifolates quinolones rifampicin

In order to continue its life cycle the microorganism must have an exit route, called the portal of exit. The exit route may be the same as that of entry, such as the respiratory tract in tuberculosis, or a different route, as in salmonella infections for which the route of entry is via the mouth and the exit route is in the faeces. Once it has produced the disease in one host, a pathogen, if it is to continue, it must be transmitted to another host or the race will die out. Transmission (or communicability) depends on:
- Site of lesion in the infected host.
- Place of maximum concentration of the organism; for example a haemolytic *Streptococcus* infection can cause tonsillitis in which case the bacterium can be coughed or breathed into the surrounding air and transmitted to another host. The same organism can cause a mastoid infection in which case it is much less likely to be transmitted because it is confined in the bone of the mastoid process.
- The length of time an organism capable of causing disease can live outside the human body.

Bacteria vary enormously in the length of time they can spend in unfavourable conditions and their communicability is profoundly affected by this. The organism of tuberculosis can live for many months protected by mucus in sputum even after it has dried, such as in dust away from sunlight, therefore tuberculosis can be caught by inhalation of dust from a room that has previously housed a tuberculosis patient. The gonococcus bacterium is killed in minutes in dry atmospheric air. Gonorrhoea can therefore be transmitted only by direct person-to-person contact.

Characteristics of bacteria associated with infection

Slime **capsules** of polysaccharides (some have a protein layer) enable bacteria to attach to tissues and resist phagocytosis. The cell envelope of group A *Streptococcus pyogenes* has an antiphagocytic 'protein M'. **Flagella** make bacteria motile thus they may invade aqueous areas. **Pili** and **fimbriae** adhere to cells in mucous membranes where others cannot, for example *Neisseria gonnorrhoeae* with pili attach to urethral cells and multiply.

Specific bacteria produce toxins and enzymes. For example:
- **Haemolysin**, which damages host red blood cells, e.g. β-haemolytic streptococci.
- **Leucocidin,** an enzyme-like exotoxin secreted by some staphylococci and streptococci, which destroys white blood cells.
- **Lecithinase**, the α-toxin of *Clostridium perfringens*, destroys cell membranes of red blood cells and other tissues.
- **Exotoxins**, described by the target organ affected, are proteins secreted by living pathogens.
- **Neurotoxins** cause nerve destruction e.g. in botulism, diphtheria and tetanus.

- **Enterotoxins** secreted by *S. aureus*, *Vibrio cholerae* and *Shigella dysenteriae* affect the vomiting centre.
- **Endotoxins** are contained in the cell walls of some Gram-negative bacteria and cause disease when the bacteria are present in large numbers. Destruction of bacteria in the gut releases endotoxins, e.g. in dysentery, typhoid, meningitis, gonorrhoea and cholera.

Enzymes associated with invasiveness
- Pathogenic staphylococci can clot plasma using **coagulase** to form their own fibrin 'coat' for protection; it looks like 'self' to the host.
- **Streptokinase** can lyse a fibrin clot covering a wound to invade and spread.
- **Hyaluronidase** enables the spread through connective tissue by breaking down hyaluronic acid in tissues.
- **Collagenase** breaks down collagen in tendons, cartilage and bones, e.g. *C. perfringens* causes gas gangrene and spreads deep within the body by secreting collagenase and hyaluronidase.

Choice of antimicrobial treatment

Antimicrobials can be bactericidal (will kill) or bacteriostatic (stop bacterial multiplication). The clinician first considers the patient and the causative organism. Factors related to the patient may include history of allergy, renal and hepatic function, resistance to infection (i.e. immunocompromised), ability to tolerate drugs by mouth, severity of illness, ethnic origin, age and, if female, whether pregnant, breastfeeding or taking an oral contraceptive. The known or likely organism and its antibiotic sensitivity in association with the above factors will suggest one or more antibiotics. The final choice depends on the microbiological, pharmacological and toxicological properties (George, 1999). An example is the problem of treating a nauseated woman who has a urinary tract infection in early pregnancy. The organism is reported to be resistant to ampicillin but sensitive to nitrofurantoin (can cause nausea), gentamicin (only by injection and best avoided in pregnancy), tetracycline (can cause dental discoloration), cotrimoxazole (folate antagonist therefore theoretically teratogenic) and cephalexin. The safest antibiotics in pregnancy are the penicillins and cephalosporins; therefore it is likely that cephalexin will be chosen for her treatment.

The range of bacteria that are susceptible to a particular drug is spoken of as the spectrum of activity. A **broad-spectrum** drug is effective against a large number of different kinds of bacteria, whereas a narrow-spectrum one acts against only a few. A broad-spectrum drug will do more damage to the host's normal flora than a narrow one. When the bacterial cause is known it is better to use a narrow-spectrum drug to preserve as much as possible of the normal flora. A drug must be available in sufficient concentration and be able to reach the site of infection. Arterial disease or prolonged inflammation may prevent antimicrobials reaching the site. The eye, inside human cells and the brain are sites where microbes are protected from the effects of antibiotics.

Four categories of target are available in bacteria to attack (Meers *et al.*, 1995): cell walls, cell membranes, protein synthesis by ribonucleic acid (RNA) and deoxyribonucleic acid (DNA). The exploitation of these different structures by antibiotics is shown in **Table 5.5**.

Antibacterials against cell walls

The peptidoglycan of bacterial cell walls is not found in human tissues, thus any substance that can interfere with the production of peptidoglycan may have an antibacterial effect without undue toxicity to the host (see **Fig. 5.2**). Formation of peptidoglycan begins inside the bacterial cell with construction of the basic glycan building block; this is then transported through the cell membrane by a carrier molecule, which releases the glycan to form long strands. The carrier molecule is then recycled to repeat the process. **Vancomycin** binds to and inactivates the carrier molecule. Layer upon layer of glycan strands are cemented by their peptide portions, like bricks joined with mortar. The enzymes responsible for cementing the peptides together are situated on the cell membrane. **Penicillin** and the other **beta-lactams** bind to these enzymes so they are no longer effective. There are a number of these so-called penicillin binding proteins, each with a different function. Different bacteria have different permutations of penicillin binding proteins and the various beta-lactams bind preferentially to different combinations of these. Eventually with the cell wall weakened the bacterium ruptures.

Acquired resistance to the beta-lactam antimicrobials may be the result of changes in cell wall permeability, changes in the penicillin binding proteins or may be caused by the development of enzymes that act directly against the beta-lactam antimicrobials, beta-lactamases or penicillinases. **Benzyl penicillin** was the first narrow-spectrum penicillin and is very vulnerable to beta-lactamase. When penicillin is given by injection it is rapidly excreted by the kidneys, therefore it can be given with probenecid to delay excretion and maintain very high tissue levels. **Methicillin** was the first to appear that was resistant to a beta-lactamase and was used to treat penicillinase-producing staphylococci, although it has now been superseded by drugs like **flucloxacillin**, which is used against **MRSA** (methicillin-resistant *S. aureus*). Clavulanic acid is the parent of a group of drugs called clavams, which inhibit the action of many beta-lactamases. They have little or no antimicrobial activity on their own but may be given at the same time as one of the broad-spectrum penicillins to neutralise any beta-lactamase present thus enabling the penicillin to reach its target before being destroyed.

Antibacterials against cell membranes

Cell membranes are basically concerned with what goes in and out of the cell. Agents that act on the cytoplasmic membrane are bactericidal although rather toxic to humans. Colistin is the only antibacterial agent in this category and is usually only used topically in eye drops and the skin. It belongs to the class of polymyxins. It is not absorbed orally and thus needs to be given by injection to obtain a systemic effect. It has been used by mouth for bowel sterilisation, especially in neutropenic patients (usually in conjunction with nystatin) but should not be used for gastrointestinal infections.

Antibacterials against RNA

Bacterial RNA exists in the ribosomes and makes protein for the cell. The information they need is in the bacterial

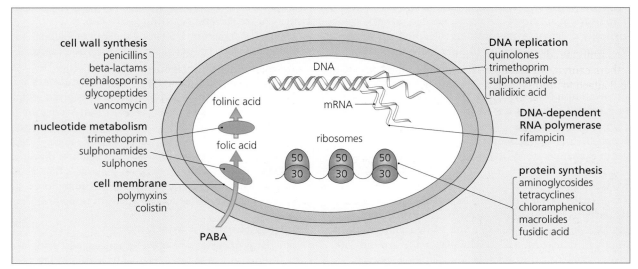

Fig 5.2 Sites of action of antibiotics

DNA and is transmitted to the ribosomes by **messenger RNA (mRNA)**. **Rifampicin** prevents the formation of bacterial mRNA but does not affect human mRNA. The amino acids needed to make the protein are brought to the ribosomes by **transfer RNA (tRNA)**. The **aminoglycosides** (streptomycin, neomycin, gentamicin, tobramycin and amikacin) together with chloramphenicol, tetracyclines, lincomycins (lincomycin, clindamycin) and fusidic acid bind to the ribosome itself. They all act to prevent protein synthesis. Although the ribosomes of most bacteria are sensitive to these antimicrobials, permeability barriers sited at the cell wall exclude the drugs from some bacteria; for example, erythromycin is excluded from Gram-negative bacteria (Meers *et al.*, 1995). The aminoglycosides are bactericidal whereas the others are mainly bacteriostatic.

Antibacterials against DNA

The basic building blocks of DNA are nucleotides; DNA is made up of strings of these molecules formed into long strands. Without these individual building blocks, no DNA is made and deprived cells cease to multiply and die. The sulphonamides (bacteriostatic) and trimethoprim (bactericidal) interfere with the production of the basic building blocks. They act at different points in the synthesis so they may be more active when taken together. Cotrimoxazole is a mixture of these two drugs.

The quinolones (ciprofloxacin, cinoxacin, nalidixic acid, norfloxacin, ofloxacin) inhibit an enzyme that acts to coil the very long molecules of DNA into neat packages that fit easily inside small microorganisms. Nalidixic acid is taken orally to treat Gram-negative bacteria that cause urinary tract infections. The newer fluorinated quinolone derivatives have enhanced activity and a wide antibacterial spectrum, but bacteria develop resistance to them fairly easily (Meers *et al.*, 1995).

Synergy between antibacterial agents

Two or more antimicrobial drugs are said to work synergistically if, when given together, they produce an effect that is greater than the sum of their individual actions. If the combined action is reduced below that of the more active component they are said to be antagonistic. They may also simply be additive in their joint effect. There are no hard and fast rules but an aminoglycoside with a penicillin, for example, is synergistic. If two bacteriostatic agents that act on the ribosome are used together they may get in each other's way and thus are antagonistic.

MALARIA

Travel in the past few years has increased dramatically, particularly to those regions of the world where control of malaria is poor, for example the Indian subcontinent, South America and Africa. This has led to around 3500 cases of malaria being reported annually and approximately 10 deaths per year have occurred in UK residents returning from abroad. In 1997, malaria risk existed in 100 countries and in 92 of these transmission included the malignant *Plasmodium falciparum*. The incidence of malaria worldwide is 300–500 million clinical cases annually. Some 1.5–2.7 million people die of malaria each year; about one million deaths among children of 5 years of age and under are attributed to malaria alone (WHO, 1998).

Malaria is transmitted by the bite of an infected *Anopheles* mosquito. The pathogenic protozoa of the genus *Plasmodium* are inoculated along with the mosquito's salivary juice and enter the skin's capillary vessels within half an hour. The injected sporozoites are taken up by the parenchymal cells of the liver, where they divide and multiply and are liberated as merozoites into the bloodstream from where they quickly enter the red blood cells. Here they continue to multiply asexually. When the parasites reach maturity the infected red blood cells burst, releasing toxic substances of microbial metabolism. The host's response to this exotoxin is to release chemical mediators such as prostaglandins (McCance and Huether, 1998). The protozoa soon enter fresh red blood cells; after a time these destructive cycles become synchronised (Meers *et al.*,1995) and sharp attacks of fever occur in the host. Each cycle takes 48 or 72 hours to complete. There are four recognised forms of human malaria: *Plasmodium vivax*, *P. falciparum* and *P. ovale* with fever occurring every third day and *P. malariae* with fever occurring every fourth day.

Pathophysiology

The episodes of fever start with a chill and shivering, which are caused by the toxic byproducts of microbial metabolism, cell lysis and the immune response of the host leading to tissue damage and inflammation. The individual becomes hot with headaches, muscle pains and perhaps vomiting ending with a drenching sweat. Long-term signs are progressive anaemia caused by the destruction of the red blood cells, debility and splenomegaly from overactivity of the spleen in clearing up the debris.

With *P. falciparum*, known as 'malignant malaria', the infected red blood cells congregate in the blood capillaries of internal organs, causing their obstruction. When the brain is finally affected, indicated by severe headaches and neck stiffness, unless vigorous treatment is given, coma soon occurs followed by death. *Plasmodium falciparum* is responsible for the majority of malarial deaths and is estimated to affect 1–1.5 million people in Africa alone (Meers *et al.*,1995), the majority of these being children (Payling, 1995). The danger with this form of malaria is that it can manifest in many ways and may be misdiagnosed as influenza because of the nonspecificity of symptoms.

Pharmacological management

Prophylactic measures to prevent malaria occurring are very important; these can be active (covering limbs after dusk, nets and aerosol sprays) or by oral administration, for example proguanil, 200 mg daily, which has few side effects. Orally administered prophylaxis is commenced 1 week before entry into the country and is continued 4 weeks after leaving to ensure full protection. Mefloquine, 250 mg each week, is another prophylactic drug, used for the treatment of chloroquine-resistant *P. falciparum*. This drug is not recommended for people with psychiatric disorders, as it has been found to be associated with post-malaria neurological syndrome, depression and psychoses (Mai *et al.*, 1996). Chloroquine, 300 mg weekly, interacts with the DNA of the parasite and causes its destruction. It was given as a prophylaxis for malaria rather than treatment and this is believed to have caused the resistance now shown by the *P. falciparum*. Chloroquine is effective as treatment for benign malaria, but can cause pigmentary changes, lichenoid lesions of the skin and diplopia, and in 10% of black men who have a genetic decrease of glucose-6-phosphate dehydrogenase, severe haemolytic anaemia occurs (Matthewson-Kuhn, 1994). Both mefloquine and chloroquine are contraindicated during pregnancy and lactation. Other treatments for *P. falciparum* are quinine and halofantrine.

Quinine, 600 mg every 8 hours for 7 days, can be given intravenously if the patient is very ill. Side effects are tinnitus, headache, visual disturbances, blood disorders, nausea, abdominal pain and rashes.

Halofantrine is given for chloroquine-resistant falciparum malaria: three doses of 500 mg 6 hours apart on an empty stomach repeated 1 week later. It is contraindicated in pregnancy, cardiac disorders and electrolyte imbalance, or with other drugs that may cause arrhythmias. Side effects are diarrhoea, nausea, vomiting and gastrointestinal pain (George, 1999). Qinghaosu (or artemisinin), an extract from *Artemesia annua* or wormwood plant, has been shown to have potential as a powerful antimalarial agent but needs further development (Hein and White, 1993). As yet there is no vaccination for malaria, as unfortunately trials of SPf66 malaria vaccine in Gambia and Thailand in 1995 and 1996 failed to show any preventive effect against the protozoan, although the subjects had seroconverted (Child Health Dialogue, 1998).

FUNGAL INFECTIONS

It has been difficult to produce drugs that are active against fungi and not toxic to humans at an unacceptable level (Meers *et al.*, 1995). Most of the drugs being used act against fungal **cell membranes**. The azole group (**miconazole, ketoconazole, fluconazole, itraconazole**) interfere with the manufacture of the cell membrane, whereas amphotericin B and nystatin cause the cell membrane to leak. Amphotericin B is fairly toxic. Griseofulvin, taken by mouth for severe skin infections, and flucytosine, used in serious generalised fungal infections, act on fungal DNA. Thus far, no drugs have been produced that act against fungal RNA.

The azole group, flucytosine and griseofulvin, tend to cause gastrointestinal disturbance, with occasionally some abnormalities of liver enzymes, headache, dizziness, rashes and possibly blood disorders. Amphotericin, the only anti-fungal that can be given parenterally, can cause gastro-intestinal disturbance, febrile reactions, headache and muscle and joint pain.

CANDIDIASIS

Candida albicans infection is a common opportunist in transplant centres, oncology units and in immunocompromised HIV-positive patients. *Candida albicans* is a yeast-like fungus that normally lives harmlessly on the skin or mucous membranes of the mouth, intestine and reproductive tract. When the chemical balance is upset and the number of normal bacteria are reduced, this yeast flourishes to cause infections. It becomes an AIDS-related opportunistic infection when it is suspected of involving the oesophagus or in recurrent episodes in the vagina. This usually occurs when CD4 counts fall below 250/μl, which may occur at seroconversion.

Pathophysiology

Candidiasis typically involves the mucous membranes and produces white adherent patches commonly seen in infants with 'thrush'. They cause soreness, inflammation and discharge. Severely immunodeficient patients can suffer from serious generalised infections involving lungs, kidneys or the heart as a part of *Candida* septicaemia. The diagnosis is made when the yeasts are seen by microscopy.

Pharmacological management

As yeasts and fungi are considered to be weakly infective except as opportunists, the immunodeficiency needs to be addressed or the drug therapy may fail (George, 1999). Several agents are well established for the treatment of candidiasis, and show high success rates and a low incidence of adverse events. **Ketoconazole**, one of the first imidazole antifungal agents, has been shown to be effective when administered twice daily for 10–14 days. Studies with daily dosage regimes are in progress; they appear to be less successful, with cure rates of only 50–75% after 28 days. Ketoconazole induces hepatic enzymes so there are several important drug interactions. It has anti-androgenic effects and prolonged use may be associated with gynaecomastia and testicular atrophy. The most serious potential adverse reaction is hepatotoxicity, which occurs most commonly in middle-aged women. Amphotericin is not absorbed from the gut and is given parenterally. It is active against most fungi and yeasts, but toxicity (renal, neurological and cardiac) and side effects are common.

INFLAMMATION

Inflammation is a local reaction to injury or irritation. It is a biochemical and cellular process that occurs in vascularised tissues. Most of the essential components of the inflammatory process are found in the circulation, and most of the early mediators of inflammation act on the vascular bed to increase the movement of plasma and blood cells from the circulation into the tissue surrounding the injury. These substances, known collectively as exudate, defend the host against infection or injury and facilitate tissue repair and healing.

The inflammatory response is nonspecific in that it occurs the same way no matter what the stimulus and occurs in the same manner on subsequent exposure to the same stimulus. Inflammation comes from the Latin *inflammare*, meaning to burn. The cardinal signs of inflammation, as described by Celsius in AD 35, are CALOR (heat), RUBOR (redness), TUMOR (swelling) and DOLOR (pain). There is also a fifth sign – loss of function and movement.

Inflammation and repair can be divided into several phases. Cellular injury leads to acute inflammation, which may result in resolution and healing of the injured site or progress into chronic inflammation. In turn, chronic inflammation may result in healing or progress into the development of a granuloma. The final step of the process is usually healing and reconstruction of the damaged tissue.

Acute inflammation begins after lethal or nonlethal cellular injury. It is self-limiting and will only continue until the threat to the host is eliminated (approximately 8–10 days). Cellular injury may be caused by trauma (mechanical forces), oxygen or nutrient deprivation, chemical agents, microorganisms (infection), temperature extremes, ionising radiation, the presence of dead cells that may be host cells to microorganisms or cells of dead parasites.

There are three major responses that characterise the inflammatory process: the **vascular response**, the **cellular response** and the **chemical response.**

The vascular response

The vascular response occurs in seconds. The arterioles near to the site of injury constrict briefly (vasoconstriction). Then the arterioles dilate (vasodilatation), which increases the blood flow to the area and results in redness and heat. This leads to the flushing of the capillary network with blood and the opening up of dormant capillary channels. Arteriolar dilatation increases pressure in the microcirculation and venules. There is also dilatation of venules and lymphatics. The capillaries and venules, which are normally only permeable to water and small solutes, become more permeable. This is because biochemical mediators stimulate the endothelial cells that line the capillaries and venules to retract, creating spaces at junctions between the cells. Large molecules such as plasma proteins and blood cells can now move into the tissues. This leads to swelling of the tissues, known as oedema, and the fluid itself is the fluid exudate (**Fig. 5.3**). The pressure of this fluid on nerve endings can cause pain. The blood remaining in the microcirculation flows more slowly and becomes more viscous (thick and sticky).

In mild injuries the inflammatory exudate resembles serum, in more acute inflammation the exudate contains fibrin and red blood cells. It causes great discomfort to the invading organisms and to the host. It may last for less than 1 hour or for several days. The inflammatory exudate is caused by three factors: hyperaemia occurring after injury, increased capillary permeability and increased filtration pressure. The inflammatory exudate has three functions: to dilute the toxins released by bacteria; to bring to the site certain nutrients necessary for tissue repair and to carry the protective cells that will phagocytose and destroy bacteria. Although very useful it causes problems as the increased fluid causes pressure, pain and immobility. It is especially dangerous for people with head injuries or infective conditions of the central nervous system.

The cause of these events is believed to be chemical mediators that are manufactured and discharged when cells are damaged; these include histamine, serotonin, bradykinin, prostaglandins and the complement system which, in this instance, acts as a chemical mediator (see *The chemical response* below).

The cellular response

While vascular permeability is occurring the leucocytes leave the centre of the bloodstream and move to the edge, forming a layer against the inner surface of the cells lining the blood vessel walls. This is known as pavementing or margination and occurs in readiness for migration through the vessel wall into the adjacent tissues. As a result of the increased vascular permeability the white blood cells are able to squeeze out through the spaces created by endothelial retraction into the tissues. This is known as emigration or diapedesis. Chemotaxis is a directional orientation that occurs because white blood cells appear to be called to the injury site by chemical signals produced by infectious agents, damaged tissue and even protein changes in the blood. Neutrophils are the first phagocytic leucocytes to arrive at the inflamed site. They phagocytose bacteria, dead cells and cellular debris, then die and are removed as pus through the epithelium or lymphatic system.

The next phagocytes on the scene are monocytes and macrophages, which perform many of the same functions as neutrophils but for a longer time and later in the inflammatory response. Other cells found in inflamed tissues are eosinophils, which help to control the inflammatory response and act directly against parasites; basophils, which have a function similar to that of mast cells, and platelets, which are cytoplasmic fragments that stop bleeding if vascular injury has occurred.

The chemical response

The biochemical mediators and cellular components of the acute inflammatory response form a complex system of interactions that frequently begins with degranulation of mast cells and ends with healing. The mast cells are

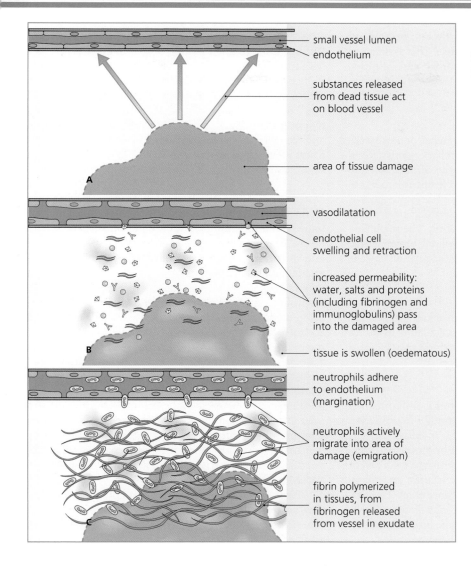

— small vessel lumen
— endothelium

substances released from dead tissue act on blood vessel

— area of tissue damage

A

— vasodilatation

endothelial cell swelling and retraction

increased permeability: water, salts and proteins (including fibrinogen and immunoglobulins) pass into the damaged area

— tissue is swollen (oedematous)

B

neutrophils adhere to endothelium (margination)

neutrophils actively migrate into area of damage (emigration)

fibrin polymerized in tissues, from fibrinogen released from vessel in exudate

C

Fig 5.3 Formation of inflammatory exudate (From Stevens & Lowe 1995, with permission.)

probably the most important initiators of the inflammatory response. They activate the response in two ways: by degranulation and by the synthesis of leucotrienes and prostaglandins.

Degranulation is the release of granular contents into the extracellular matrix. These granules contain histamine, neutrophil chemotactic factor and eosinophil chemotactic factor. A chemotactic factor is a biochemical substance that attracts a specific leucocyte to the site of inflammation. These mediators are released in seconds and exert their effects immediately. Serotonin is another potent mediator released by platelets. Histamine and serotonin appear to act in the same way and initiate the vascular response. As with most defence systems of the body, the acute inflammatory response is only required in a specific area for a limited time. Therefore control mechanisms are required to prevent the biochemical mediators from evoking more inflammation than is needed. Eosinophils contain several enzymes

that destroy serotonin and histamine, hence the importance of attracting these cells to the site of inflammation.

Leucotrienes produce similar effects to that of histamine but appear to be important in the later stages of the inflammatory response as they stimulate a slower and more prolonged response. **Prostaglandins** cause increased vascular permeability and neutrophil chemotaxis, but they also induce pain. They can inhibit some aspects of inflammation by suppressing the release of histamine from mast cells and release of lysosomal enzymes from neutrophils. Enhancement or suppression of the inflammatory response may be related to the concentration of prostaglandins. Prostaglandin inhibitors used to treat inflammation are aspirin, indomethacin, ibuprofen and other non-steroidal anti-inflammatory drugs (NSAIDs).

Inflammation is also mediated by three key plasma protein systems: the complement system, the clotting system and the kinin system. The complement system is a nonspecific mechanism that, once activated, participates in virtually every inflammatory response. This system not only activates and assists inflammatory and immune processes but also plays a major role in the direct destruction of cells (especially bacteria).

The clotting system

The clotting system forms a fibrinous exudate or mesh work at the inflamed site to trap exudates, microorganisms and foreign bodies. This prevents the spread of infection and inflammation to adjacent tissues and keeps microorganisms and foreign bodies at the site of greatest phagocytic activity. It also forms a clot that stops bleeding and provides a framework for future repair and healing. The main substance in this fibrinous mesh is an insoluble protein called fibrin, which is the end product of the coagulation cascade (see **Figure 5.3**).

The kinin system

The primary kinin is bradykinin, which at low doses causes dilatation of vessels and acts with prostaglandins to induce pain; it increases vascular permeability and may increase leucocyte chemotaxis.

CHRONIC INFLAMMATION

The difference between acute and chronic inflammation is purely one of duration, in that chronic inflammation lasts for 2 weeks or longer, regardless of cause. Chronic inflammation is sometimes preceded by an unsuccessful acute inflammatory response. For example, if infection or foreign objects persist in a traumatic wound, an inflammatory response will continue for more than 2 weeks. Suppuration, pus formation and incomplete wound healing may characterise this type of chronic inflammation.

Pathophysiology

Chronic inflammation is characterised by a dense infiltration of lymphocytes and macrophages. If tissue damage is inevitable, the body attempts to wall off and isolate the infected site by forming a granuloma. The latter are formed if neutrophils and macrophages are unable to destroy microorganisms during the acute inflammatory response. Granuloma formation begins when some of the macrophages differentiate into large epithelioid cells that are incapable of phagocytosis but are capable of taking up debris and other small particles. Other macrophages fuse into multinucleated giant cells, which are active phagocytes and can engulf particles too large to be engulfed by single macrophages. The decay of cells within the granuloma results in the release of acids and the lysosomes of dead phagocytes. In this inhospitable environment the cellular debris is broken down into its basic constituents and a clear fluid remains in the granuloma. Eventually this fluid diffuses out and leaves a hollow, thick-walled structure in the tissue that may remain for the life of the individual.

Pharmacological management

Chronic inflammation is often treated in the first instance with anti-prostaglandins such as aspirin and paracetamol to reduce pain and fever. A variety of NSAIDs are used on a wide range of disorders that cause pain and loss of function (see Chapter 3 *Classes of drugs*). Treatment for acute and chronic inflammation involves the use of NSAIDs, aspirin and the salicylates, corticosteroids and some miscellaneous drugs that suppress the rheumatic disease process in rheumatoid arthritis and psoriatic arthritis.

Non-steroidal anit-inflammatory drugs

Non-steroidal anti-inflammatory drugs counteract or reduce inflammation by inhibition of prostaglandin synthesis. They are not glucocorticoid in nature. Non-steroidal anti-inflammatory drugs are divided by chemical group into fenamates, indoles, oxicams and derivatives of propionic acid, pyroleacetic acid and salicylic acid. They include ibuprofen, naproxen, fenbufen, fenoprofen, flurbiprofen, ketoprofen, tiaprofenic acid, azapropazone, diclofenac and aceclofenac, diflunisal, etodolac, indomethacin, ketorolac, mefenamic acid, meloxicam, nabumetone, phenylbutazone, piroxicam, sulindac, tenoxicam, tolfenamic acid and tolmetin. Their analgesic and anti-inflammatory activity is mainly attributable to the inhibition of arachidonic acid metabolism. In response to the stimuli that cause inflammation, arachidonic acid is released from the cell membrane phospholipids. This is then metabolised by two major pathways: the leucotriene pathway and the prostaglandin pathway. Both routes result in inflammation and both may be blocked by NSAIDs.

Absorption of NSAIDs is very good orally, although it may be delayed by food. To decrease the gastrointestinal side effects, certain NSAIDs should be administered with antacids or food. In some cases of long-term therapy, drugs such as a prostaglandin analogue (misoprostol), H_2 receptor antagonists (cimetidine, famotidine, nizatidine, ranitidine) or proton pump inhibitors (omeprazole, lansoprazole, pantoprazole) can prevent NSAID-induced gastric and duodenal ulceration. Protein binding is very high and most of the agents are metabolised by the liver and excreted by the kidneys.

Side effects may include gastrointestinal discomfort, nausea, diarrhoea, possible dizziness, headache, vertigo or hearing disturbances. Blood disorders have also occurred. Non-steroidal anti-inflammatory drugs should be used **with caution in the elderly** and are **contraindicated** in patients with a history of hypersensitivity to aspirin or any other NSAID, particularly individuals in whom attacks of asthma, angioedema, urticaria or rhinitis have been precipitated by aspirin or any NSAID, or in those with renal impairment.

Aspirin and the salicylates

Aspirin was the traditional first choice anti-inflammatory analgesic. Now other NSAIDs are used as there is little anti-inflammatory effect with doses of less than 3 g daily. Larger doses, that is anti-inflammatory doses, are associated with a high incidence of gastrointestinal bleeding and may also cause mild chronic salicylate intoxication characterised by dizziness, tinnitus and deafness. Benorylate is an aspirin–paracetamol ester that has similar side effects to aspirin and paracetamol.

Corticosteroids

Glucocorticoid activity is of no advantage in anti-inflammatory treatment unless the effects of fluid and electrolyte retention can be avoided. Dexamethasone has insignificant mineralocorticoid activity and thus is suitable when water retention would be a disadvantage (cerebral oedema). Beclomethasone has low mineralocorticoid activity and a marked topical effect, therefore it is used for skin applications and asthma and nasal inhalations.

Systemic corticosteroids

Systemic corticosteroids should be reserved for specific indications when other anti-inflammatory drugs are unsuccessful. In severe and possibly life-threatening situations, a high initial dose is given to induce remission; this is then gradually reduced to the lowest dose possible for maintenance. Patients can become physiologically dependent on corticosteroids. For this reason pulsed doses of corticosteroids (e.g. methylprednisolone), up to 1 g intravenously on 3 consecutive days, are used to suppress highly active inflammatory disease while longer-term and slower-acting medication is being commenced.

Prednisolone is used for most purposes because it has the advantage, as do the more potent corticosteroids, of permitting finer dose adjustments. To minimise side effects the maintenance dose is kept as low as possible, usually 7.5 mg daily. Diseases usually treated with prednisolone include **polymyalgia rheumatica** (10–15 mg daily); giant cell (temporal) arteritis (40–60 mg daily); and **polyarteritis nodosa** and **polymyositis** (initial dose of 60 mg with a maintenance dose of 10–15 mg daily). **Systemic lupus erythematosus** is treated with corticosteroids when necessary. Acute severe asthma may be treated with oral prednisolone 30–60 mg or intravenous hydrocortisone 200 mg.

Recent evidence has suggested that prednisolone, 7.5 mg daily, may substantially reduce the rate of joint destruction in moderate to severe rheumatoid arthritis. Ankylosing spondylitis should not be treated with long-term corticosteroids; rarely, pulse doses may be needed when the disease is very active and not responding to conventional treatment.

Overdosage or prolonged use of systemic corticosteroids may exaggerate some of the normal physiological effects of glucocorticoid and mineralocorticoid activity:

- Glucocorticoid side effects include diabetes and osteoporosis, avascular necrosis, mental disturbances, muscle wasting and peptic ulceration. High doses may lead to Cushing's syndrome. In children high doses may result in suppression of growth and in pregnancy they may suppress fetal adrenal development. Infection may spread rapidly through suppression of symptoms, allowing tuberculosis or septicaemia to reach an advanced stage.
- Mineralocorticoid side effects include hypertension, sodium and water retention and potassium loss.
- Adrenal atrophy can persist for years after stopping prolonged corticosteroid therapy. Therefore in any illness or surgical emergency temporary re-introduction of corticosteroid therapy may be needed to compensate for lack of sufficient adrenocortical response. Patients should carry cards giving details of their dosage and possible complications.

The suppressive action of a corticosteroid on cortisol secretion is least when it is given in the morning. Thus a single dose in the morning should reduce pituitary–adrenal suppression. Alternate day administration has not been very successful but pituitary–adrenal suppression can be reduced by intermittent therapy with short courses.

Local corticosteroid injections

In inflammatory conditions of the joints corticosteroids may be given by intra-articular injection to relieve pain, increase mobility and reduce deformity in rheumatoid arthritis. They can also be given for 'tennis' or 'golfer's' elbow or compression neuropathies. In tendinitis, injections are given into the tendon sheath and not directly into the tendon. These drugs may also be injected into soft tissues for treatment of skin lesions such as keloid scars or hypertrophic lichen planus. Injections used include dexamethasone, hydrocortisone, methylprednisolone acetate and triamcinolone. Flushing has been reported with intra-articular corticosteroid injections and Charcot-like arthropathies have been reported after repeated intra-articular injections. The risk of necrosis and muscle wasting may be slightly greater with triamcinolone.

Immunosuppressants

Immunosuppressants are used in severe rheumatoid arthritis, systemic lupus erythematosus and polymyositis. **Cyclosporin** may retard the erosive damage seen on X-ray in rheumatoid arthritis, but it can be nephrotoxic. **Azathioprine** (can cause bone marrow suppression and hepatic and renal impairment) and **methotrexate** (severe haematological, pulmonary, gastrointestinal and other toxicity) are used in the treatment of psoriatic arthropathy. They are often given in conjunction with corticosteroids for patients with severe or progressive renal disease, although their benefit has not been proved. Cyclophosphamide may be used for severe systemic rheumatoid arthritis manifestations (unlicensed indication) and other connective tissue disease, especially with vasculitis. It is toxic and regular blood counts (including platelet count) should be carried out.

Miscellaneous

Drugs such as gold, penicillamine, hydroxychloroquine, chloroquine, immunosuppressants and sulphasalazine may suppress the disease process in rheumatoid arthritis as may gold and immunosuppressants in psoriatic arthritis. Unlike NSAIDs, they may take 4–6 months to achieve a full response. They improve not only the inflammatory joint disease but also the extra-articular manifestations such as vasculitis. They reduce the erythrocyte sedimentation rate and sometime the titre of rheumatoid factor. Chloroquine, an antimalarial drug, is sometimes used to treat discoid and systemic lupus erythematosus.

IMMUNODEFICIENCY

Immunodeficiency exists when there is a lack of normal immune functioning, primary or secondary. Primary immunodeficiency is generally seen congenitally and manifests in the newborn or the infant with deficiencies in T cell, B cell, or both T and B cell, function. Secondary immunodeficiency exists in conjunction with and often as a consequence of other disease states, generally appearing later in adult life.

Primary immunodeficiency

This includes agammaglobulinaemia, congenital thymic aplasia and combined immunodeficiency – a rare congenital lack of lymphocyte stem cell precursors in the bone marrow.

Agammaglobulinaemia

This is an X-linked genetic disorder know as Bruton's disease; B cells and functioning plasma cells are lacking but there are adequate and functioning T cells. The infant is most at risk of bacterial infections, which are treated with antibiotics and gamma globulin from pooled, donated human blood. The life expectancy of patients with agammaglobulinaemia is much reduced.

Congenital thymic aplasia

Also known as Di-George syndrome, this congenital thymic aplasia is a very rare congenital anomaly characterised by the absence of the parathyroid and thymus glands. Neonates who survive the hypocalcaemia exhibit a total lack of cell-mediated immunity; in these individuals viral, fungal and protozoal infections are likely to become systemic. Without helper T cell function, which is important in antibody synthesis, the susceptibility to bacterial infections is slightly increased. Treatment of these children is very difficult; administration of interferon injections with antimicrobial drugs orally or by injection and the prevention of infection are the only means available.

Combined immunodeficiency

This consists of a congenital lack of lymphocyte stem cell precursors in the bone marrow. In order for these children to survive they must be placed in sterile rooms. The only treatment is a bone marrow transplant, which is limited by the difficulty of matching donor and recipient marrow tissue type and by the graft versus host response (the functioning immune cells mount an attack on the recipient's tissues). For this reason, marrow banks are now in existence; normal healthy donors have a minor operation by which a small amount of bone marrow is removed and frozen, the tissue type having been recorded. When needed it is thawed and transplanted into the recipient (Vardaxis, 1995).

Secondary immunodeficiency

Many disease states are associated with secondary immunodeficiency, which is generally not as severe as seen in primary immunodeficiency. **Ageing** causes the thymus gland to involute (it becomes a tiny remnant in old age) and many elderly people suffer from recurrent infections, having had a previously normal immune response. This decreased efficiency may have a more complex aetiology and be linked with decreased cellular mitosis, cumulative environmental toxins, and increasing susceptibility caused by the breakdown of nonspecific defences to infection.

Aplastic anaemia

Aplastic anaemia is a rare condition in which there is a reduction or absence of haemopoietic elements in all the cell lines in the bone marrow, leading to peripheral blood pancytopenia. Fanconi anaemia which appears in children between the age of 5 and 10 years, is the most common inherited cause; this is an autosomal recessive condition that is accompanied by other constitutional malformations. It is a DNA repair disorder and is associated with an increased risk of developing acute leukaemia and other malignancies. Acquired aplastic anaemia is similar to primary aplastic anaemia and is often caused by drugs such as chloramphenicol or chemicals such as benzene. The condition is progressive and children are usually treated with allograph or antihuman thymic globulin from horses or rabbits together with cyclosporin and cytokines (see Chapter 6 *Drugs and neoplastic disorders*) (Lissauer and Clayden, 1997). Adults may be given androgens or corticosteroids which can stimulate mitotic activity of the bone marrow.

Infections

Infections with some microorganisms can lower the immune response and allow secondary infections to occur. An example is the influenza virus. Early researchers looking for the cause of influenza isolated a bacterium from nearly every case of 'flu and named it *H. influenzae*. The bacterium was of course only the secondary bacterial infection in the disease caused by the influenza virus. The mechanisms by which this secondary immunodeficiency is produced are not clear (Vardaxis, 1995).

Malignant tumours

These are associated with secondary immunodeficiency, especially tumours affecting the bone marrow, thymus or lymph nodes. Thymomata are thymus tumours that cause a decrease in T cells. Hodgkin's disease is another malignancy associated with T-cell deficiency. In multiple myeloma, a tumour of plasma cells, decreased humoral immunity is observed. Leukaemia generally leads to secondary immunodeficiency, as do secondary (metastatic) tumours in bone.

Immunosuppressive drugs

These drugs are meant to suppress the immune reaction; they include corticosteroids and azathioprine, which generally suppress the cell-mediated response and therefore patients are likely to get viral and fungal infections. In certain cases drugs lead to a secondary immunodeficiency by causing an allergic reaction – a hypersensitivity to the drug – and this immunodeficiency is reversible on cessation of the drug.

Radiation

Radiation for malignant tumours or exposure to radioactivity in the wake of bomb blasts or nuclear accidents may produce a secondary immunodeficiency caused by destruction of the stem cells in the bone marrow. In general, the doses of radiation required to cause such serious effects on the bone marrow will kill the individual before they develop extensive life-threatening infections (Vardaxis, 1995).

AIDS

AIDS was first described in groups of homosexual men in 1981. The cause of this new disease was found by French and US researchers to be the human immunodeficiency virus (HIV, see section *Viral infections* earlier in this chapter). Between 2 and 10 years after becoming infected the person goes into the **persistent generalised lymphadenopathy** phase in which lymph nodes around the body swell and become prominent. This indicates the second phase of virus replication and release. The persistent generalised lymphadenopathy phase is associated with the **AIDS-related complex** phase. In the AIDS-related complex phase the first indications of immunodeficiency begin to occur. Weight loss, fatigue, weakness, headache, night sweats, diarrhoea, anaemia and decreased T-cell counts in the blood with more suppressor T cells than helper T cells.

The last phase is full-blown AIDS, which is associated with multiple infections and cancers, with debility, emaciation, enlarged lymph nodes, severe continual dry cough, severe diarrhoea, purplish skin lesions, sore throat and fever. AIDS-associated dementia may occur with replication of the virus in the brain. Treatment continues with antiviral drugs (see immunodeficiency virus section above) and symptomatic treatment of opportunistic infections (see *Choice of antimicrobial treatment and fungal infections* above). Opportunistic infections and their incidence are seen in **Tables 5.6** and **5.7**.

Spectrum of opportunistic conditions at different levels of immunodeficiency	
CD4 + counts/mm^3	Opportunistic conditions
>250	Tuberculosis
250–100	Pneumocystosis Oesophageal candidiasis Toxoplasmosis Cryptococcosis Other fungal infections
100–50	Cryptosporidiosis Microsporidiosis
50–0	Cytomegalovirus infection Disseminated non-tuberculous mycobacteriosis
Table adapted from Youle, 1993, p 4	

Table 5.6 Spectrum of opportunistic conditions at different levels of immunodeficiency

Pyrexia in immunosuppressed children

Pyrexia is defined as a temperature above 38°C on two occasions and 38.5°C on one occasion, with a neutrophil count lower than 10 million/ml. At this stage an attempt is made to identify the foci of infection. These children will usually then be considered septic and samples of line bloods, urine, stool, sputum, throat and cerebrospinal fluid are taken as appropriate for analysis in the laboratory. Children are usually assessed and treated as three distinct groups; those immunosuppressed and taking prophylactic medication, those being treated by a course of chemotherapy and those of the preceding two groups who have had recent contact with chickenpox or measles.

For those children receiving prophylactic medication such as septrin, this is stopped and **first-line** treatment is initiated with a broad-spectrum antibiotic, such as piperacillin, in combination with gentamicin, which widens the antibacterial cover of this anti-pseudomonal penicillin. If, after 48 hours, the temperature is not subsiding, a **second-line** antibiotic is added such as teicoplanin, which is bactericidal against most Gram-positive organisms. If symptoms continue, a **third-line** addition is an antifungal agent, as candidiasis may be indicated, and/or aciclovir if herpes lesions are evident.

Children on chemotherapy will have the infection, for example a urinary tract infection or, commonly, *Pneumocystis* respiratory infection, treated with appropriate

Opportunistic infections and their incidence in different populations

Opportunistic infection	Incidence	
	High	Low
Tuberculosis	Intravenous drug users	Gay men
	Developing world	BCG vaccinated
	Poor social conditions	
	Prisons	
Pneumocystosis	Developed world	Prophylaxis
	No prophylaxis	Developing world
Toxoplasmosis	Countries where raw meat is frequently consumed	
Cryptococcosis	Developing world	Europe
Other fungal infections	Endemic areas (USA, South America	
Cryptosporidiosis	Endemic areas (UK)	
Microsporidiosis		
Cytomegalovirus infection	Gay men	Developing world
Non-tuberculous mycobacteriosis		Developing world

Table adapted from Youle, 1993, p 5

Table 5.7 Opportunistic infections and their incidence in different populations

antibiotic therapy and continue their chemotherapy if their neutrophil count is satisfactory.

Passive immunisation with human immunoglobulins is given to children who have been in contact with measles and chickenpox. These are produced from pooled plasma of a large group of donors, which contains antibodies currently prevalent in the population. Specific immunoglobulin such as varicella zoster immunoglobulin is produced from pooled blood of convalescent patients, recently immunised donors or donors who have a sufficient antibody titre.

HYPERSENSITIVITY: ALLERGY, AUTOIMMUNITY AND ISOIMMUNITY

Hypersensitivity is an altered immunological reaction to an antigen that results in an abnormal immune response after re-exposure. Allergy, autoimmunity and isoimmunity differ in the source of the antigen. Allergy is hypersensitivity to environmental (exogenous) antigens and auto-immunity is the disturbance of immunological tolerance to self-antigens, which results in the destruction of host tissues. Isoimmune diseases occur when the immune system produces an immunological reaction to tissue from another individual such as with transfusions, grafted tissue or the fetus during pregnancy. Some infertility is believed to be caused by an immunity of the woman to the man's sperm.

It is generally believed that genetic, infectious and possibly environmental factors contribute to hypersensitivity and include at least three variables: an original insult, which alters immunological homeostasis, the genetic make-up, which alters susceptibility to the insult, and an immunological process, which amplifies the insult. Hypersensitivity reactions are immediate or delayed, depending on the time required for the reaction to appear after re-exposure. The most rapid reaction is anaphylaxis, which can be local or systemic and may result in death.

Although difficult to define taxonomically, hypersensitivities such as allergies, hay fever, asthma and eczema appear to be familial traits and fall into the category of congenital. No specific gene has been found to distinguish hypersensitivity but these diseases tend to 'run in families', although they are also modulated by environmental factors. Hypersensitivity responses can also be divided into two groups: group 1 hypersensitivities (type I, anaphylactic; type II, cytotoxic; type III, immune complex mediated and type V, receptor mediated), which are antibody mediated; and group 2 hypersensitivities, that is type IV, which are cell mediated.

Immunoglobulins

Antibodies are very large proteins made up of polypeptide chains and are produced and secreted in response to the presence of antigens. As they are a part of the immune response they are referred to as immunoglobulins. They are found in all bodily tissues, but in greatest concentration in the blood. **Immunoglobulin G (IgG)** protects the extravascular compartments (outside the blood and lymph vessels) from microorganisms and their toxins. **Immunoglobulin M (IgM)** is the first line of defence against microorganisms in the bloodstream. **Immunoglobulin A (IgA)** protects mucosal surfaces and is found, for example in saliva and tears. **Immunoglobulin D (IgD)** is believed to influence lymphocyte functions and **immunoglobulin E (IgE)** protects against intestinal parasites and is responsible for many of the symptoms of allergy.

Group 1 hypersensitivities

Type I (anaphylactic) hypersensitivity is **IgE** or **mast cell-mediated**, produces histamine and involves various disorders such as urticaria, atopy (allergic rhinitis e.g. hay fever), food allergies, bronchial asthma and systemic anaphylaxis (**Fig. 5.4**). In 1902 Richet coined the term anaphylaxis for the severe and sometimes fatal reaction of animals to a second injection of a foreign protein. The original contact with the foreign protein stimulates the formation of IgE antibodies instead of IgG or IgA, which is what occurs when immunity develops (Kumar and Clark, 1994). The treatment for type I hypersensitivity involves antigen avoidance, antihistamines, corticosteroids (usually topical) and sodium cromoglycate (see Chapter 9 *Drugs and head and neck disorders*). For anaphylaxis, systemic antihistamines and corticosteroids are necessary (see Chapter 19 *Pharmacological management of medical emergencies*).

Type II (cytotoxic) hypersensitivity is tissue specific and is limited to those cells with tissue-specific antigens such as erythrocytes and platelets. Type II reactions are therefore commonly the cause of anaemias and thrombocytopenias (**Fig. 5.5**). The first mechanism is the binding of antibody to the cell surface, which activates complement. Cell lysis occurs and neutrophils and macrophages then ingest the opsonised, antibody-coated cells. Many important diseases are caused by such hypersensitivity reactions: isoimmune reactions such as **erythroblastosis fetalis** (haemolytic disease of the newborn) and incompatible **transfusion reactions**. Close control of transfusion procedures means that transfusion reactions are now rare. In the course of

pregnancy some fetal blood cells get into the maternal circulation but these will be destroyed by maternal killer cells and phagocytosis. Erythroblastosis fetalis occurs when considerable numbers of fetal erythrocytes from a rhesus-positive baby enter the mother's rhesus-negative circulation during labour and delivery. Therefore at the end of the first pregnancy the mother has been sensitised and has rhesus antibodies and anti-rhesus lymphocytes in her bloodstream. In subsequent pregnancies the maternal IgG antibodies cross the placenta into the fetal circulation where they begin to react with the rhesus-positive fetal erythrocytes.

Type III (immune complex mediated) hypersensitivity results when there are large amounts of soluble antigen in the body. The antigens combine with large numbers of antibodies to form large numbers of immune complexes. These form microthrombi, which circulate and lodge in small vessels, causing vasculitis (**Fig. 5.6**). Farmer's lung is an example of a type III reaction to sensitising allergens contained in dust from mouldy hay. Post-streptococcal glomerulonephritis, systemic lupus erythmatosus, rheumatoid arthritis, rheumatic fever, various drug reactions and some manifestations of leprosy, syphilis, malaria, hepatitis B and measles are other examples of type III reactions. Treatment is for the inflammatory and allergic effects.

In **type V cellular receptor hypersensitivity** antibodies are formed to receptor proteins on cell surfaces. Instead of destroying the cell these antibodies stimulate the cell into activity as if they were the signal molecules that normally attach to the receptor. An example is thyroid-stimulating hormone, which attaches to receptors on the thyroid cell. In a type V hypersensitivity reaction antibodies attach to the thyroid cells and stimulate them to overproduce thyroxin, resulting in thyrotoxicosis. In many of these patients the antibodies, which are called LATS (long-acting thyroid-stimulating), can be demonstrated in their blood. Another manifestation of type V hypersensitivity is when the antibody attaches to the receptor site but instead of stimulating the cell it destroys the receptor site, reducing the number of functioning receptor sites on the cell and thus making the cell less responsive to stimulation. An example of this is myasthenia gravis in which antibodies form against the

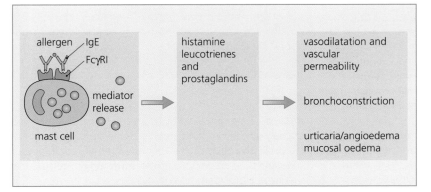

Fig 5.4 Mechanism of type I anaphylactic hypersensitivity reaction. (From Page, 1997, with permission.)

acetylcholine receptors on the skeletal muscle end plates. This makes the muscle cell less responsive when acetylcholine reaches the motor end plate and the result is muscle weakness and fatigue.

Group 2 hypersensitivities

Type IV cell-mediated delayed hypersensitivity includes transfusion and graft rejection. The prototype is the tuberculin reaction in the Mantoux test. Tissue damage in type IV reactions occurs because the antigens that cause them persist in the tissues for long periods, leading to large numbers of inflammatory cells in the area. Mosquito and flea bites induce a type IV reaction, whereas bee stings induce anaphylactic type I reactions. Allergic treatments such as antihistamines with anti-inflammatory drugs are used. In graft rejection immunosuppressive drugs are used. Examples of hypersensitivity reactions are given in **Table 5.8**.

Antihistamines

Antihistamines are frequently used for hypersensitivity reactions; they compete with histamine for its receptor sites. With the discovery of two histamine receptors, H_1 and H_2, antihistamines should be divided into H_1 receptor

antagonists and the H_2 receptor antagonists. The H_2 receptor blocking agents include cimetidine and ranitidine, which are used in the treatment or prevention of peptic ulceration. H_1 receptor antagonists have the greatest therapeutic effect on nasal allergies, particularly on hay fever. These are palliative and do not immunise the individual, so their benefits are short-lived. In asthma antihistamines act only as supplements to other more specific remedies.

Antihistamines compete with histamine for H_1 receptor sites on smooth muscle of the vascular system, bronchioles, and lacrimal, salivary and respiratory mucosal glands. They do not inhibit the histamine already attached so they are better given before histamine is released. Antihistamines are indicated for the treatment of allergies, vertigo, motion sickness, cough (diphenhydramine), and sedative and local anaesthetic effects in dentistry. Their oral absorption pattern is good and onset of action is 15–60 minutes. The antihistamine dosage varies with each drug's chemical classification and pharmacokinetic profile. The newer agents that have been released are generally longer-acting drugs with fewer sedative side effects. Older agents that exhibit sedation are usually labelled with

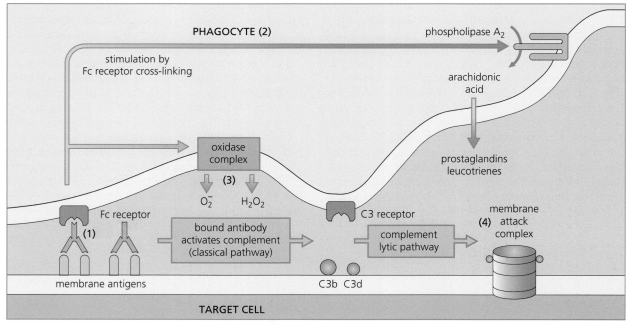

Fig. 5.5 Mechanism of type II hypersensitivity reaction. (From Page 1997, with permission.)
Antibodies become attached to cell surface antigens (1). The linkage of the antibodies to the cell surface antigens attracts phagocytic white cells (2). Within the phagocyte, arachidonic acid is produced which is made into prostaglandins and leucotrienes. The phagocytic cell also produces oxygen free radicals and hydrogen peroxide (3). The presence of antigen/antibody complexes also causes complement to be activated (4). The end result is the formation of membrane attack complex which perforates the target cell membrane and, because it is not possible to repair the lesion, cell death ultimately occurs. The damaged or dead cell is ingested by the phagocytes (not shown in this figure).

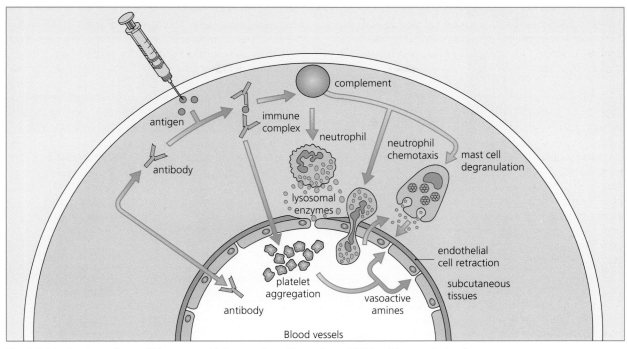

Fig 5.6 Mechanism of type III hypersensitivity reaction. (From Page 1997, with permission.)
Antigens injected into the skin combine with a specific antibody to form immune complexes. These activate complement and cause platelets to release vasoactive amines. The immune complexes also cause macrophages to release tumour necrosis factor and interleukin 1 (not shown in this figure). Complement 3a and 5a cause mast cells to degranulate and to attract neutrophils into the tissues. The substances released by the mast cells (which include histamine and leucotrienes) increase blood flow and capillary permeability. The polymorphs release lysosomal enzymes which augment the inflammatory reaction. The immune complexes become coated with complement 3b, which encourages their ingestion by phagocytic white cells.

warnings about drug use in the elderly, who may be more sensitive.

Antihistamines should be used with caution in those with asthma, as the drying effect may thicken secretions and diminish expectoration, in those with prostatic hypertrophy or a predisposition to urinary retention, and in those with a predisposition to narrow-angle glaucoma, as the drug may precipitate an acute episode. Concurrent use of alcohol, monoamine oxidase inhibitors or central nervous system depressants may enhance central nervous system depression. Increased cardiotoxic effects have been noted when terfenadine is administered with erythromycin. Ketoconazole administered with terfenadine, astemizole or loratidine may lead to increased levels of antihistamines and so concurrent administration should be avoided. With the administration of antihistamines, the patient should be assessed for drowsiness, dry mouth and throat, rash, tinnitus, blurred vision, hypotension, urinary retention, unusual bleeding and restlessness. The patient should have a reduction in symptoms of allergy or motion sickness.

AUTOIMMUNE DISEASE
The function of the immune system is to distinguish between self and non-self. Once this distinction has been made, what is recognised as belonging to the body is tolerated. However, it is apparent in some diseases that this system has broken down and the immune system is mounting an immune response against components of the body. In these diseases the body's normal proteins, complex carbohydrates and other macromolecules function as antigens and are called **autoantigens**, thus giving rise to **autoantibodies**. They may also stimulate a cell-mediated immune response with sensitised T cells reacting with and destroying tissues. Many diseases for which the cause was previously unknown are now seen to be essentially attributable to an autoimmune response. Therefore, human autoimmune diseases have various features in common, as outlined below.

Aetiology of autoimmune disease
It appears that a multifactorial aetiology exists.

Relative incidence and examples of hypersensitivity reactions				
	Mechanism			
Target antigen	Type I (Immunoglobulin E mediated)	Type II (Tissue specific)	Type III (Immune complex)	Type IV (Cell mediated)
Allergy	++++	+	+	++
Environmental antigens	Hay fever	Haemolysis in drug allergies	Gluten (wheat) allergy	Poison ivy allergy
Autoimmunity	±	++	+++	+
Self-antigens	May contribute to some type III reactions	Autoimmune thrombocytopenia	Systemic lupus erythematosus	Hashimoto's thyroiditis
Isoimmunity	±	++	+	++
Other person's antigens	May contribute to some type III reactions	Haemolytic disease of the newborn	Anaphylaxis to IgA in intravenous γ-globulin	Graft rejection
* The frequency of each reaction is indicated in a range from rare (±) to very common (++++). An example of each is shown.				

Table 5.8 Relative incidence and examples of hypersensitivity reactions

12.4 COMMON FEATURES OF HUMAN AUTOIMMUNE DISEASES

Most common in women.
A positive family history (relatives may show similar genetic trends e.g. HLA genotype).
Autoantibodies in blood (some without clinical effect) e.g. thyroid antibodies without thyroid disease.
Circulating harmless autoantibodies in healthy relatives.
Lymphocytes and macrophages abundant in target tissues, especially around blood vessels.
Vasculitis and arthritis are especially common in autoimmune complex disease.
Immunoglobulin and complement are detectable in sites of tissue damage.
Disease responds to immunosuppressive treatment.

Cross-reaction of self tissues with foreign antigens
This occurs when a microorganism that enters the body possesses some of the body's own proteins. The immune system reacts with the microbe and produces antibodies that, after the infection is overcome, react with those body proteins that share some of the antigenic properties. Rheumatic fever is one example in which some strains of *Streptococcus* species give rise to an autoimmune reaction against the connective tissues and heart valves.

Failure of 'self tolerance' mechanisms
The immune system's recognition of 'self' is poorly understood. It is believed that this may be connected with the suppressor T group of lymphocytes, which normally suppress immune responses when there is no need of them. They appear to interact with the virgin T cells specific to the body proteins that are present in the body from birth (Vardaxis, 1995). A reduction in suppressor T-cell levels in animals is associated with an increase in autoimmunity.

Emergence of normally 'hidden' antigens
Occasionally tissue damage or death can release small fragments of cell proteins that have remained sequestered inside the cell and therefore 'out of sight' of the immune system. Once released into the tissue fluid they may stimulate an immune response. Such a response results in immunity directed against all proteins that bear the same antigenic determinants.

Modification of self antigens
This may be an important factor, as the incidence of autoimmunity increases with age and the cumulative tissue

damage and alteration of body proteins. If body tissues become sufficiently different from what the immune system recognises as 'normal', there may be an autoimmune state. Another similar mechanism operates when one becomes hypersensitive after drug administration.

Polyclonal activation

Some specific types of microbes such as *Mycobacterium leprae* (leprosy) and Epstein–Barr virus infection (glandular fever) can induce a nonspecific activation of humoral and cell-mediated immunity, with many different clones of antigen-reactive cells in the immune system leading to autoimmunity.

Genetic factors

Genetic factors are believed to exist because many autoimmune diseases are seen as running in families or are more commonly encountered in some races. Also, as women are more affected by autoimmunity than men, there may be effects of the double X genotype.

Formation of autoantibodies

An autoimmune disease may have a hypersensitivity component. Autoantibodies are found after infectious diseases such as syphilis and other granulomatous diseases (tuberculosis and leprosy). The frequency with which they are found increases with age. Autoantibodies are found against several antigens. Examples are rheumatoid factor (anti-IgG) seen in rheumatoid arthritis; antinuclear factors seen in systemic lupus erythematosus (anti-DNA); and antibodies against thyroid, adrenal, gastric cells or intracellular organelles (Vardaxis, 1995).

Autoimmune disease can be divided into the organ-specific, confined to one tissue type or one specific organ, and the systemic, in which autoimmunity is seen in many tissues and organs, sometimes with quite severe effects. Organ-specific autoimmune disease is usually found in glandular tissues of the thyroid and pancreas and stomach mucosa. The systemic diseases commonly affect the connective tissues, mainly the muscles, joints and loose connective tissues. Most of these autoimmune states are associated with the presence of sensitised T cells or autoantibodies. In apparently healthy blood relatives of people with autoimmune disease, autoantibodies will be found, thus indicating a genetic cause for this disease.

ORGAN-SPECIFIC AUTOIMMUNE DISEASES

Although most organ-specific autoimmune diseases affect glandular tissues, some may affect other epithelia such as the skin or blood cells. Specific autoantibodies are formed against the specialised parenchymal (functioning) cells of the affected tissue. The antibodies react with these parenchymal cells and, through the mediation of cytotoxic T cells and/or complement, the parenchymal cells are destroyed. The tissue appears chronically inflamed, and the organ shrinks as more and more parenchymal cells are replaced by fibrous (scar) tissue (Vardaxis, 1995). Some examples are Hashimoto's disease (chronic autoimmune thyroiditis), which gives rise to hypothyroid symptoms; chronic autoimmune atrophic gastritis, which manifests with dyspepsia and disruption of protein digestion and, occasionally, when there are autoantibodies against intrinsic factor, patients present with atrophic gastritis and severe anaemia. Autoimmune adrenalitis and para-thyroiditis are rarely seen.

SYSTEMIC AUTOIMMUNE DISEASE

SYSTEMIC LUPUS ERYTHEMATOSUS

Systemic lupus erythematosus (SLE) is a chronic, multisystem, inflammatory disease and is one of the most common, complex and serious of the autoimmune disorders. The patient's skin and connective tissues are affected, with characteristic rashes on the face and exposed areas. There is usually serious renal disease and the most common cause of death is renal failure. Most patients have increased infections due to reduced levels of complement. There may also be platelet destruction, with an increased tendency to haemorrhage.

Pathophysiology

Systemic lupus erythematosus is characterised by a large variety of autoantibodies against nucleic acids (found in DNA, RNA and other nuclear materials), erythrocytes, coagulation proteins, phospholipids, lymphocytes, platelets and many other self-components. A genetic predisposition for SLE has been proposed because of the increased incidence in twins and the presence of other autoimmune diseases in families of individuals with SLE. Circulating immune complexes formed by the antibody–antigen complexes are deposited in the tissue and have a high affinity for the basement membrane of the glomerulus, damaging renal function. The deposits of immune complexes cause inflammation wherever they occur, leading to the signs and symptoms used to diagnose this difficult disease (McCance and Huether, 1998).

Pharmacological management

Treatment is with anti-malarials, salicylates, corticosteroids, immunosuppressants in severe cases (azathioprine for psoriatic arthritis and methotrexate for skin manifestations) and possibly renal dialysis. Avoiding the sun and ultraviolet light is essential to prevent photosensitivity. The aim is for control, as SLE is not curable (McCance and Huether, 1998).

RHEUMATOID ARTHRITIS

In this systemic autoimmune disease there is marked damage to bones and joints and other connective tissues. The autoantigen in this case is an abnormal form of IgG to which the immune system forms an antibody, an IgM, called the rheumatoid factor. IgM and IgG react together in atypical antigen–antibody fashion and are deposited in many body sites but mainly around synovial membranes. Destruction of connective tissues in the eyes may lead to impaired vision.

Signs and symptoms are general systemic manifestations of inflammation, including fever, fatigue, weakness, anorexia, weight loss and generalised aching and stiffness. The joints become painful, tender and stiff, with early morning stiffness for about 1 hour after rising. Joint swelling is widespread and symmetric, and initially involves the small joints of the hands and wrists and only later the weight-bearing joints. Joint deformity occurs as the disease progresses.

Pathophysiology

In spite of intensive research the cause of rheumatoid arthritis remains unknown; however, it is thought to be a combination of genetic, environmental, hormonal and reproductive factors. The key genetic element has been localised to the HLA-DR4, HLA-DQ and HLA-DP areas of the major histocompatibility complex. Infectious organisms that may play a role include bacteria (mycoplasmas) and viruses (particularly Epstein–Barr virus). With long-term or intensive exposure to an antigen, the normal IgG become autoantibodies and attack the host's own tissues (self-antigens). The transformed antibodies are called rheumatoid factors. The rheumatoid factors usually consist of two classes of immunoglobulin antibodies (for IgG and IgM) but may involve antibodies for IgA. Their main antigenic targets are part of the immunoglobulin molecules; rheumatoid factors bind with their self-antigens in blood and synovial membrane, forming immune complexes that cause microvascular injury and mild synovial cell proliferation.

Synovitis occurs when the immune complexes trigger the inflammatory response, mainly by activation of complement. Complement causes kinin and prostaglandin release to attract leucocytes and lymphocytes to the synovial membrane to release enzymes which then destroy synovial membrane and articular cartilage. As the newly targeted self-antigens are in relatively plentiful supply, unlike a microorganism, which is killed in the process, the inflammation and formation of immune complexes can continue indefinitely. Inflammation causes haemorrhage, coagulation and fibrin deposition on the synovial membrane, in the intracellular matrix and in the synovial fluid; this forms a granulation tissue called pannus, which appears to extend into adjacent articular cartilage, destroying it. Pannus formation does not lead to healing but to formation of scar tissue that immobilises the joint.

Pharmacological management

Most of the treatment is for inflammation and those drugs are discussed in detail in the section entitled *Inflammation* earlier in the chapter. Drug therapy regimes are complex but analgesics and NSAIDs are the mainstay of treatment. Aspirin and its derivatives remain effective. Gold salts, antimalarials, and penicillamine are used for more recalcitrant cases. Corticosteroids and various immunosuppressive agents are used as a last resort.

SCLERODERMA

Scleroderma causes thickening and damage (sclerosis) to the skin, mainly the dermal collagen and epithelial cells of the epidermis. This rare disease (1 in 400 000) is found in patients with some chromosomal abnormalities. It is caused by an acquired defect that develops because of a damaging plasma factor present in the patient's blood. The patient usually presents with arthritis or Raynaud's phenomenon and this may progress over years to organ damage, namely in the kidneys, gastrointestinal tract and lungs, with systemic scleroderma.

Pathophysiology

Impaired regulation of collagen gene expression probably underlies the persistent fibrosis (McCance and Huether, 1998), but autoimmunity and an immune reaction to a toxic substance are possible initiating mechanisms. Autoantibodies are often found in the skin and serum of those with scleroderma. There are massive deposits of collagen, with fibrosis accompanied by inflammation and vascular changes in the capillary network, namely a reduction in capillary loops and dilatation of the remaining capillaries.

Pharmacological management

Treatment is difficult and patients do not respond well to steroids or immunosuppressive agents. Potassium aminobenzoate has been used to treat the excessive fibrosis but its therapeutic value is doubtful (George, 1999). If malignant hypertension occurs, the prognosis is poor.

KEY POINTS

- Infection is caused by colonisation by microorganisms; the severity depends on the host's susceptibility, the virulence of the microorganism and the concentration of the microorganisms within the host.
- Vaccination programmes raise the immunity of the population against pathogens.
- Antiviral agents inhibit the release of viral nucleic acid from the protective capsid or the synthesis of viral nucleic acid or protein.
- HIV destroys T4 helper lymphocytes, monocytes, macrophages and other antigen-presenting cells. Opportunistic infections develop. Prophylaxis is by immunisation and treatment includes the use of antiviral agents.

- Broad-spectrum antibiotics may damage natural flora.
- Tissue injury leads to inflammation; this causes pain and, when chronic, permanent tissue alteration. NSAIDs used in treatment may alter immunity.
- Immunodeficiency increases susceptibility to infection and, in some cases, to the formation of malignant tumours.
- Overactivity of the immune system may cause hypersensitivity or tissue damage as a result of autoimmunity.

5

MULTIPLE CHOICE QUESTIONS

Choose the correct answers.

1. Antimicrobial treatment is given for infection with which of the following?
   a. prions;
   b. fungi;
   c. viruses;
   d. bacteria spores;
   e. helminths.

2. Susceptibility to infection is increased in which of the following situations?
   a. hyperglycaemia;
   b. gastric hyperacidity;
   c. cold stress;
   d. hypersensitivity;
   e. loss of cellular adherence factors.

3. Which of the following vaccinations are given routinely to school age children?
   a. human immunodeficiency virus;
   b. hepatitis B;
   c. influenza;
   d. tuberculosis;
   e. rubella.

4. In which of the following cases should vaccination NOT be given?
   a. during the administration of cytotoxic chemotherapy;
   b. during growth spurts;
   c. if the individual has an upper respiratory tract infection;
   d. to an atopic individual;
   e. all of the above.

5. For which of the following conditions would passive immunisation be given?
   a. influenza;
   b. hepatitis B;
   c. measles;
   d. tuberculosis;
   e. rubella.

6. Antiviral agents work by
   a. inhibiting reverse transcriptase
   b. inhibiting protease
   c. altering the structure of viral nucleic acid
   d. preventing viral entry into cells
   e. all of the above

7. Patients receiving treatment for human immunodeficiency virus should be observed for which of the following reactions to their medication?
   a. opportunistic infection;
   b. gastrointestinal disturbances;
   c. rash;
   d. insomnia;
   e. all of the above.

8. Non-steroidal antiinflammatory drugs produce their therapeutic effect by
   a. antagonising prostaglandins, thus reducing pain;
   b. stimulating the migration of polymorphonuclear leucocytes into the tissues;
   c. enhancing the action of prostaglandins, therefore increasing capillary permeability;
   d. encouraging complement fixation;
   e. stimulating 'pavementing' within the capillaries.

9. An intra-articular injection of hydrocortisone may cause which of the following adverse effects
   a. localised muscle wasting;
   b. immunosuppression;
   c. hypertension;
   d. hyperglycaemia;
   e. flushing of the skin.

10. The aims of treatment for a patient with auto-immune disease include which of the following?
    a. to increase the activity of helper T-lymphocytes;
    b. to remove marker proteins from cell membranes;
    c. to suppress the activity of cytotoxic T-lymphocytes;
    d. to suppress the fixation of complement;
    e. to suppress the activity of B-lymphocytes.

REFERENCES

Ahmed A, *et al.* Reduction in mortality associated with influenza vaccine during 1989/90 epidemic. *Lancet* 1995; **346:**591-595.

Banister C. *The midwife's pharmacopoeia.* Hale: Books for Midwives Press, 1997.

Child Health Dialogue (1998) *Research Update.* Nairobi, Kenya: Appropriate Resources and Technologies Action Group. Available from: http://www.who.ch/chd/pub/newslet/dialog/6/research.htm [Accessed 21 July 1998]

Day M. Inquiry call over mass measles jabs. *Nurs Times* 1995a; **91/36:**7.

Day M. HVA claims child vaccination rush by GPs jeopardises informed consent *Nurs Times* 1995b; **91/41:**6.

Day M. The needle and the damage done. *Nurs Times* 1995c; **91/39:**14.

Easterbrook P, Ippolito G. Prophylaxis after occupational exposure to HIV. *Br Med J* 1997; **315:**557-558.

George C. *British National Formulary, no. 37.* London: British Medical Association and the Royal Pharmaceutical Society of Great Britain, 1999.

Hein T, White J. Qinghaosu. *Lancet* 1993; **341:**603-608.

Henderson N. Vaccination review. *Practice Nurse* 1991; **Oct:**271-277.

King E. *HIV and AIDS treatments directory.* London: NAM Publications, 1996.

Lissauer T, Claydon G. *Illustrated Textbook of Paediatrics.* London: Mosby, 1997.

Kumar P, Clark M. *Clinical Medicine.* London: Baillière Tindall, 1994.

Mai N, Day N, Chuong L, *et al.* Post-malaria neurological syndrome. *Lancet* 1996; **348:**917-921.

Mathewson-Kuhn M. *Pharmaco-therapeutics.* Philadelphia: FA Davis, 1994.

McCance KL, Huether SE. *Pathophysiology: the biologic basis for disease in adults and children, 3rd ed.* St. Louis: Mosby, 1998.

McKenry L, Salerno E. *Pharmacology in Nursing.* London: Mosby, 1995.

Meers P, Sedgwick J, Worsley M. *The microbiology and epidemiology of infection for health science students.* London: Chapman & Hall, 1995.

Nowak T, Handford A. *Essentials of Pathophysiology.* Dubuque: W.C. Brown, 1994

Page C. *Integrated Pharmacology.* London: Mosby, 1997.

Parker C. Rubella vaccination: why vigilance must continue. *Prof. Care of Mother and Child* 1996; **6/1:**2-3.

Payling K. The prevention and treatment of malaria. *Prof Nurse* 1995; **10/8:**506-507.

Prusiner SB. Prion diseases and the BSE crisis. *Science* 1997; **278:**245-251.

Spector WG. *An Introduction to General Pathology 3rd ed.* Edinburgh: Churchill Livingstone, 1989.

Stevens A, Lowe J. *Pathology.* London: Mosby, 1995.

Thompson NP, *et al.* Is measles vaccination a risk factor for inflammatory bowel disease? *Lancet* 1995; **345:**1071-1074.

Vardaxis NJ. *Pathology for the health sciences.* Edinburgh: Churchill Livingstone, 1995.

World Health Organization (1998) Malaria Prevention and Control: burdens and trends. [on-line] WHO Division of Control of Tropical Diseases. Available from: http://www.who.ch/ctd/cgi-bin/ctd.cgi?f...guest&langue=english&p=&r=malariaburtre [Accessed 21 July 1998].

Youle M. Master Lectures in Opportunistic Infections. Intramed Communications No. 172. 1993; April, Milan

6 Kate Dewar
DRUGS AND NEOPLASTIC DISORDERS

INTRODUCTION

Cancer is a common condition, and is second only to cardiovascular disease as a cause of death in the United Kingdom (Department of Health, 1995). Cancerous conditions are a group of diseases in which the cell growth mechanisms have lost their restraining controls. Our knowledge about cancer is growing quickly and its complexity is being uncovered. It is beyond the scope of this chapter to explore this complexity in detail, but an outline of the relationships between normal cell function (the cell cycle) and cancer are provided so that chemotherapy can be understood in relation to normal cell physiology. Following this, cancers are considered according to the body system from which each arises. There are too many types of cancer to include all in

this text, so those that are common and generally respond well to chemotherapy have been chosen for inclusion. Reference to specific cancers can also be found within the relevant systems chapters.

CELL DIFFERENTIATION

Growth of cells is just one of the cell characteristics controlled and organised by genes. Despite the different characteristics and functions of different cell types (e.g. epithelial and muscle cells), each cell in a single individual has the same genes. Cell differences are produced early on in the life of a cell through differentiation. Differentiation is a process whereby the actions of certain genes are neutralised. The particular mix of genes that are 'switched off' during differentiation gives a cell the limited abilities peculiar to a specific type of cell, for example muscle cells cannot move from their position in the body but they can change their shape in contraction and relaxation, whereas phagocytic leucocytes have retained the ability to move around the body.

The rate of growth and replacement of a cell is another function manipulated during differentiation. As a result, stratified epithelial cells of the skin have a quick growth and replacement cycle (cell cycle) but the ability of muscle cells to reproduce seems to be 'switched off'. Some cells (stem cells) in a particular cell type grow and divide in order to maintain the population of that type of cell at a constant number, whereas other cells are 'resting' rather than actively growing. For example, it is only the cells of the basal levels of skin epithelium that grow and divided to replace the upper layers of skin cells.

CELL CYCLE

The process of cell growth and division involves phases (**Fig. 6.1**). G0 is the resting phase; G1 is a period when protein synthesis occurs, preparing the cell for S phase when DNA is synthesised; then, in G2, there is synthesis of protein components necessary for mitosis; finally, at M, mitosis takes place.

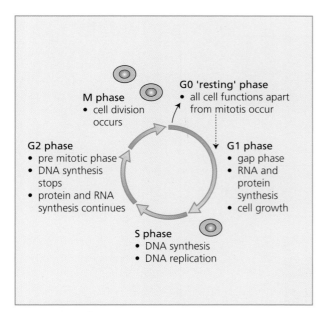

Fig 6.1 The cell cycle. (From Steven & Lowe 1995, with permission.)

Most cells in the G0 phase can be activated to enter G1 when cell damage or death requires the remaining cells of the population to replicate and replace those lost. Some cells in maturity are permanently in G0, such as neurons. Cancer cells go through the same phases of cell cycle as non-cancerous cells.

Each cell contains genes that stimulate growth (proto-oncogenes) as well as those that suppress growth (anti-oncogenes or tumour suppressor genes). The normal rate of growth and replication of a cell is controlled by a dynamic balance of activity in the operation of these genes (Bodmer, 1997). Growth control genes include ones that recognise when mistakes in DNA have occurred and can stop cell growth and division while the DNA is repaired. Similarly when DNA damage is too great for repair, these genes organise the cell to commit suicide (apoptosis).

The functioning of these genes, and therefore the cell cycle, is controlled through interactive processes involving substances such as hormones and growth factors (e.g. platelet-derived growth factor; epidermal growth factor; interleukin-2 and nerve growth factor). As research into growth factors continues, it is expected that more will be discovered and our understanding of their functions will increase.

CARCINOGENESIS

In cancer, some of the functions lost to cells during differentiation are reinstated, and some understanding of these cell features is necessary in order to appreciate the nature of cancer and its treatments.

Neoplasm means new growth, that is, a group of excessive numbers of cells (**Fig. 6.2**). Neoplasms may be benign or malignant. Malignant neoplasms have lost more of their differentiated features than benign neoplasms. So, compared with a 'normal' cell, they have changed their structure and function in many ways, reverting to a more primitive type of cell. In this chapter the emphasis is upon cancerous change and its drug treatment rather than benign change, as the latter is rarely treated with drugs.

Cancer is commonly used as a 'group' name for malignant neoplasms. Cancerous change can happen in any body tissue, and specific cancers are named after the tissue from which each derives. This type of change is the result of alteration in the activity of the growth control genes in a cell. Such changes occur as a result of:
• Naturally occurring 'mistakes' in replication of genes (mutation) when the cell reproduces.

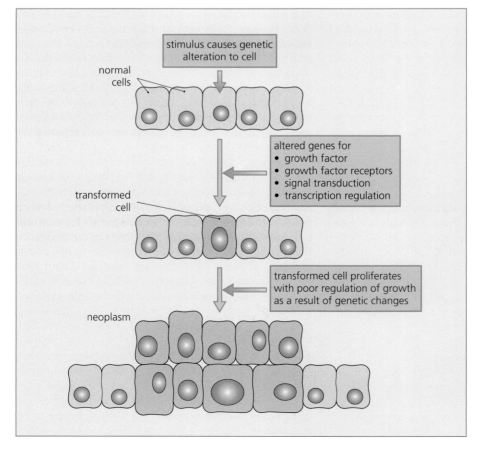

Fig. 6.2 Events in neoplastic transformation

stimulus causes genetic alteration to cell

normal cells

altered genes for
• growth factor
• growth factor receptors
• signal transduction
• transcription regulation

transformed cell

transformed cell proliferates with poor regulation of growth as a result of genetic changes

neoplasm

• External stimuli or trigger factors in the environment, such as tobacco smoke, alcohol, high-fat diet, some viruses, exposure to ultraviolet and other radiation, asbestos and other chemical agents and chronic irritation of an area.

Excessive stimulation of growth genes and reduced stimulation of growth inhibiting genes therefore results in a quicker cell cycle rate. A completed cell cycle involving all the cells in a particular cancer site is called a doubling. Cancers are likely to have undergone around 30 doublings before they are identified clinically (Lind, 1992). Their growth rate is limited in several ways. For example, cells do not all proliferate at the same rate, local blood vessels tend to grow at a slower rate so that food supplies and therefore growth are limited, and continuing mutation in malignant cells can produce some daughter cells that have lost the ability to replicate completely or that develop a slower growth pattern than the parent cell.

MODEL OF CARCINOGENESIS

Various models attempting to explain the complexity of carcinogenesis have been put forward. It seems clear that the process consists of at least two main stages, in each of which successive mutation of genes occurs.

The first stage is initiation, in which cells are subject to one or more attacks by initiating agents, causing them to proliferate. By itself this does not necessarily produce cancerous change, but seems to 'prime' cells to respond to further stimuli. Further, cancerous, change may be prevented at this stage if the cell recognises and repairs its damaged DNA.

The second stage is promotion, in which exposure to promoting agents results eventually in malignant cell changes. Promoters cannot bring about cancerous change alone, they only affect cells that have previously been attacked by initiators. Few agents have so far been identified specifically as initiators or promoters; however, those that have some role in initiating or promoting cancer are commonly called carcinogens (McMillan, 1992).

There are naturally occurring differences in the ability of cells to adapt to carcinogens, so that individuals in a population will have differing abilities to withstand attack by them. This may account for the differences in occurrence of malignancies in a group of individuals who have all been exposed similarly to carcinogenic agents. This model also offers an explanation for the increased incidence of cancer with ageing, as the number of exposures to promoters is likely to build up with increasing age.

SPREAD OF MALIGNANT DISEASE

As cancerous cells grow more quickly than the surrounding non-cancerous ones, tumours will grow locally, so applying increasing pressure to surrounding cells. Eventually the neighbouring cells will die from pressure necrosis, providing space into which cancer cells can grow.

Malignant change is also associated with the ability of cells to move from their site of initial growth (primary site): to travel elsewhere in the body and 'seed' new colonies (metastasis) at one or more secondary sites (**Fig. 6.3**). In order to be able to carry out these activities, genes cause the cancerous cell to produce 'factors' or proteins, including enzymes, which in turn change the cell's behaviour so that the changed cells can invade and metastasise (Bodmer, 1997). Features of invasion, metastasis through blood and lymph channels, and the secondary site are now outlined.

Invasion

The surface of the cancerous cell loses its ability to adhere to neighbouring cells so that it breaks free of them. The cell surface membrane and cytoplasmic structural elements change, enabling the cell actively to move from its position in a particular tissue. The cancer cell develops cell surface receptors that bind with elements in the surrounding intercellular matrix or basement membrane, causing the release of enzymes. These enzymes disrupt the surrounding matrix or basement membrane, easing the passage of the migrating cancer cell. In addition to autocrine motility factors secreted by cancer cells, these enzymes organise the direction in which the cells move, through the process of chemotaxis (see Chapter 5 *Drugs and immunological disorders*). Some tumour cells can populate and block local blood vessels and lymph channels because they produce enzymes that allow invasion through the vessel and channel walls.

Metastasis

As well as growing and spreading through neighbouring tissues, cancer cells from the primary site spread to distant parts of the body via one or more routes. In a body cavity, malignant cells can spread from one organ surface to another. More generally, cancer cells are distributed to other parts of the body in the blood or lymph. Once they have invaded the local vessel wall, the cancerous cells can be swept into the main stream of blood or lymph.

Generally, invasion occurs into capillaries or veins rather than arteries, probably because the thickness of arterial walls acts as a natural barrier. Once in the circulation the embolic cancer cells must withstand being buffeted by the blood cells in the fast-moving swirl of the bloodstream. From here they travel into larger and larger veins, through the right side of the heart, and so into the pulmonary circulation where the blood vessels become smaller and smaller. Tumour cells may become wedged in a capillary there and, using motility factors and enzymes as before, may invade through the thin capillary wall into local lung tissue. As a result, the lung is a common secondary site of tumour growth.

Tumours in the abdominal cavity may spread via the hepatic portal vein to the liver where they may lodge in the small intralobular sinusoids. As a consequence, the liver

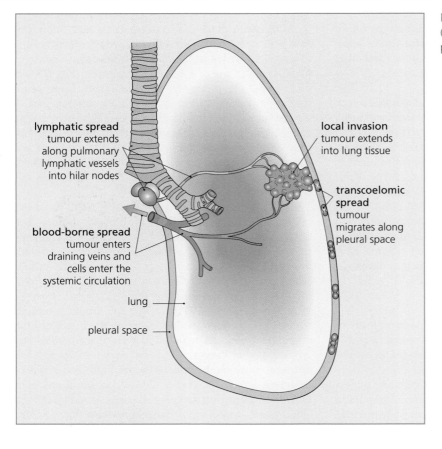

Fig 6.3 Main routes of tumour spread. (From Stevens & Lowe 1995, with permission.)

is a major site of metastasis for primary malignancies within the abdomen.

Cancerous emboli that reach the systemic arterial system, for example from a primary site in the lung, are spread to the whole body and may 'seed' in many different areas.

Cancer cells can also invade local lymph channels, travelling through larger and larger channels with their associated lymph nodes, eventually to join the bloodstream. Those cancer cells that have developed cell surface characteristics that allow them to evade recognition by immune cells can grow successfully in lymph nodes. Here they may block the flow of lymph, which, if it is regional lymph nodes that are blocked, will result in oedema in the area drained by those nodes. From the lymph node, further emboli can break free of the tumour mass, travelling on to join the circulation, with the potential to form metastatic colonies (Darling and Tarin, 1990).

The secondary site

On reaching distant sites, the cells must be able to build a cancer cell colony. This requires production of factors that stimulate local blood vessel growth sufficiently in order to supply its nutrient needs. There is evidence that cancer cells from different primary sites selectively seed at specific secondary sites. A probable explanation is that a particular range of conditions has to be present at the secondary site for seeding to be successful; for example, chemotactic and growth factors that are compatible with the growth requirements peculiar to that type of cancer cell must be present locally.

Given the range of conditions that must be satisfied for a malignant tumour to grow at its primary site and metastasise, it is probably only the very few that succeed, whereas the majority are destroyed through a variety of mechanisms. For example cancer cell membranes may break when the cell is buffeted around the circulation, or the cell may be recognised as abnormal by immune cells and be killed (Holmes, 1997).

INVESTIGATION OF CANCER

The extent of a cancer and its response to treatment can be gauged by staging the tumour, by grading it histologically and by assessing the level of tumour markers in the blood. Clinical classification of tumours by staging or grading them is useful as an extended description of the tumour, and as a basis for assessing prognosis and making decisions about the 'best' treatment option. Staging is applied to solid tumours.

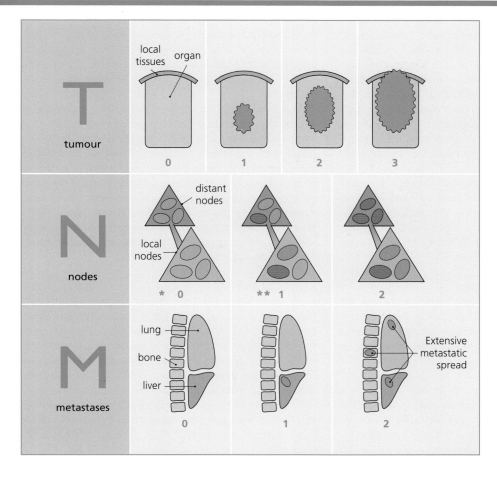

Fig 6.4 Staging of carcinoma by TNM. (From Stevens & Lowe 1995, with permission.)

Legend:

⬭ node infiltration

* No evidence of lymph node metastasis

** n1 & n2: increasing evidence of lymph node metastasis

In the simplest descriptive system, tumour at stage 1 indicates that growth is limited to the primary site; stages 2 and 3 describe progression towards stage 4 in which the tumour has spread to distant sites. Advancing stages are associated with worsening prognosis.

The TNM staging system (see **Figure 6.4**) is recognised and used internationally. In this system the cancer is described in terms of three characteristics: 'T', primary tumour size; 'N', regional lymph node invasion; and 'M', metastases. T, N and M characteristics are further defined by the use of numbers from 0 to 3, where 0 indicates none and 1–3 represent increasing values. For example, T1N1M0 describes a primary tumour of less than 2 cm in diameter with invasion of local lymph nodes but no obvious metastases.

After biopsy of a tumour, it can be graded histologically, classifying it by the degree to which it appears different to the tissue from which it grew. Grade I tumours are very similar to 'normal' cells whereas grade IV tumour cells are very unlike the parent tissue; they are undifferentiated or anaplastic. Grades II and III are in-between categories. Higher grades are generally associated with poorer prognosis (Holmes, 1997).

Malignant tumours produce chemicals that can be used as 'markers' as levels will drop as a measure of the success of treatment (Neal and Hoskin, 1997).

COMMON PATHOPHYSIOLOGY OF MALIGNANT TUMOURS

Some effects may result from the growth of any malignant tumour, whereas others are specific and depend on the site of primary and secondary growths.

Destruction of normal tissue

As the tumour grows, it destroys tissue at primary and secondary sites, through direct invasion or through pressure necrosis of surrounding cells. This reduction in functional tissue mass will eventually result in overt malfunction. Some tumours cause symptom-related problems for the affected individual early in the tumour life cycle, whereas others are asymptomatic until late in their growth and metastatic life, with obvious implications for prognosis.

Obstruction

As it grows, a tumour may block a hollow tube or duct. For example, oesophageal carcinoma may inhibit passage of food and cause difficulty swallowing; a bronchogenic tumour can restrict airflow through the bronchi, making it difficult for the individual to breathe. Obstruction can also arise because the tumour presses on a structure externally. For example, a tumour arising in the rectum can exert pressure on the nearby ureter causing obliteration of its lumen and pressure damage to the kidney. If both ureters are affected then obstruction to urinary outflow results with serious consequences for the excretory capabilities of the body.

Obstruction of lymph nodes by tumour cells can cause slowing of lymph flow from the area drained by those nodes. The slowing may be intensified by surgical removal of the nodes for biopsy purposes. The resulting oedema, termed lymphadenopathy, may be extremely distressing for the patient (Neal and Hoskin, 1997).

Pain

Nerves may be invaded directly by tumour and as a consequence elicit pain sensations. Alternatively, the compression and distortion of tissues neighbouring the tumour may cause stimulation of their sensory nerves which, in turn, will bring about sensations of pain.

Blood and circulatory dysfunction

If a tumour invades a local blood vessel, it may weaken the wall and cause bleeding, which may be minimal or catastrophic. Tumour can also cause bleeding through invasion into the regions of bone marrow involved in platelet production, as platelets are necessary to normal blood coagulation (see Chapter 12 *Drugs and cardiovascular disorders*). The liver produces a range of factors essential to normal blood coagulation. Secondary spread to the liver may reduce production of these factors, increasing the likelihood of bleeding.

Chronic blood loss may also lead to anaemia. In addition, invasion of the bone marrow may affect erythrocyte production, so that less red blood cells than normal are produced and anaemia results. Other causes of anaemia include the excessive uptake by tumour cells of substances vital to bone marrow cells (e.g. folate), so that normal marrow cells are starved of components necessary to their fast-replication function and so cell turnover is slowed. Tumour at sites other than the bone marrow may affect its function by producing marrow suppression factors, which travel to the marrow via the bloodstream. In general, therefore, the cause of anaemia in malignant disease is multifactorial.

Infection

If the bone marrow's white cell production sites or lymphoid tissue is invaded, the body's resistance to infection will be reduced. However, infection may also result from tumour interference with airway function or with urinary drainage, as excessive growth of microorganisms in these areas then becomes possible. Similarly, if normal bowel peristalsis is disrupted, excessive growth of microorganisms will result, which may lead eventually to the spread of infection to the peritoneal cavity and subsequent peritonitis.

Cachexia

This is a syndrome consisting of weakness, anorexia with weight loss, and raised body temperature. It occurs most commonly in advanced malignant disease, probably as a result of all the effects described previously. In addition, the secretion of cachexia-producing cytokines (e.g. tumour necrosis factor-α and interleukin-6) may increase the metabolic rate and therefore the use of nutrients, outstripping supply and leading to weight loss (Espat *et al.*, 1995). However, cachexia remains a somewhat ill understood feature of malignancy, although it may lead to the death of the individual affected.

Miscellaneous

Malignant change can bring about hormonal imbalance. If it occurs in an endocrine gland it can stimulate excessive secretion of that gland's hormones or inhibit their secretion altogether, resulting in endocrine disease. More rarely, when subjected to cancerous change, non-endocrine cells may have genes that cause production of hormones 'switched on'. For example, adrenocorticotrophic hormone (ACTH) may be produced by lung or kidney tumour; and parathyroid hormone may be secreted by tumours of the breast, lung or ovary (see Chapter 10 *Drugs and endocrine disorders*).

There are some little understood sequelae of malignant change, in which an association is evident but the nature of the connection is as yet not well defined. For example, there is a link between deep vein thrombosis of the leg and cancers, particularly those of lung and pancreas.

PHARMACOLOGICAL MANAGEMENT
Use of chemotherapy

Agents used in the treatment of malignant tumours have a variety of group names: 'chemotherapeutic', or 'cytotoxic' or 'anti-neoplastic'. Biological response modifiers are sometimes categorised separately as their action is unlike that of other anti-tumour drugs.

Cytotoxic agents may be used in various ways to support the aim of a particular treatment regime. The latter may aim to:

- Cure the patient, achieving total remission.
- Offer palliative help, reducing the severity of symptoms without necessarily expecting a cure.
- Increase the likelihood of a cure, or prolong remission, as adjuvant with other modes of treatment, i.e. surgery and/or radiotherapy.

Site and action of chemotherapeutic drugs

Chemotherapeutic agents vary in their action and effect. They are classified according to the specificity of their action on the cell cycle. Cell cycle specific agents act during a particular phase of the cell cycle, for example methotrexate works in phase S. These drugs are particularly useful in the treatment of tumours with quickly dividing cells. Drugs that are not cell cycle specific, such as busulphan, can act on resting and replicating cells. Agents are also classified according to their pharmacological effects.

Adverse effects of cytotoxic therapy

Cytotoxic agents kill tumour cells through some disruption to the cell cycle. It is inevitable that they also effect normal non-cancerous cells as their cell cycle consists of the same phased processes. Anti-tumour drugs act most effectively on rapidly dividing cells, denying them, in various ways, the requirements to complete their cell division cycle. These effects are also produced in normal fast-replicating cells. However, side effects can also arise in cells in G0 or in a cycle of slow growth as these drugs, by their nature, are toxic to all cells (Holmes, 1997).

Because of the risk of bone marrow suppression with any cytotoxic regime, bone marrow function is assessed before therapy begins. If the white cell count is below $4 \times 10^9/L$ or the platelet count below $100 \times 10^9/L$ the therapy will be deferred. Less common side effects include confusion, memory loss, hallucination, fluid and electrolyte imbalances, hypersensitivity reactions and damage to kidneys, bladder, lung, heart, sight and hearing.

Some adverse effects are associated with most cytotoxic agents, such as those of bone marrow suppression, whereas others are known to occur more commonly or more severely with specific chemotherapeutic agents. Identification of those agents most likely to cause specific side effects is important in the prevention or early recognition of the occurrence of these side effects, so that the premature termination of therapy is avoided and prompt, appropriate nursing interventions are made. Unwanted effects of chemotherapy may be temporary or permanent, mild or disabling, and there is considerable variation in individual response. However, in general, the occurrence of side effects depends on the route and duration of therapy as well as the total dose of cytotoxic agent (Hollinger, 1997).

The frequency of occurrence of cytotoxic therapy side effects and their unpleasantness sometimes cause patients to refuse potentially life-saving therapy (Klopvitch and Clancy, 1985; Bleiberg, 1996). As a result, chemotherapeutic regimes are constructed to minimise the occurrence of side effects, as illustrated in the following examples.

Emesis

Antiemetic therapy is given as part of a regime containing emetic chemotherapeutic agents. When the patient is at moderate risk of vomiting, oral dexamethasone 8 mg and domperidone 20 mg may be given 2 hours before treatment. For those with high-risk emetic regimes, dexamethasone 24 mg and ondansetron are given intravenously 30 minutes before treatment. Dexamethasone can be topped up during treatment, 2–4 mg orally or intravenously 3 times daily, and ondansetron likewise, 8 mg intravenously 2–4 hourly for two further doses then 8 mg orally twice daily for a maximum of 5 days. If emesis is not controlled, in place of ondansetron, granistron 3 mg may be prescribed, given by intravenous infusion over 5 minutes followed by two further doses each separated by at least 10 minutes. It can also be given orally 1 mg taken 1 hour before treatment and twice daily thereafter for a total maximum dose of 9 mg (see Chapter 14 *Drugs and gastrointestinal disorders* and Chapter 10 *Drugs and endocrine disorders*).

Bone marrow suppression

Severe bone marrow suppression can be a cause of premature termination of chemotherapy, so evaluation of bone marrow function is an important part of the nurse's role. Methotrexate in high doses acts in S phase by interfering with an enzyme involved in DNA synthesis. In methotrexate therapy, partial protection or 'rescue' of normal bone marrow cells can be achieved by administering folinic acid. This allows the cell to circumvent the drug-induced enzyme inhibition. It is given intramuscularly or intravenously to a maximum dose of 120 mg in divided doses over 12–24 hours. Then an intramuscular dose of 12–15 mg or orally 15 mg is given 4 times daily for up to 3 days.

Increasingly colony-stimulating factors (a type of biological response modulator) are given in an attempt to prevent dose-limiting bone marrow suppression. These include granulocyte-, macrophage- and erythrocyte-stimulating factors.

Drug interactions

During a course of chemotherapy, other drugs should be given concurrently only with caution as cytotoxic agents interact adversely with many drugs. Consequently, nurses should check for interaction risks before administering other drugs.

Extravasation

Extravasation is a particular risk associated with intravenous administration. Nurses need to be aware of these risks so that they can be prevented or recognised early and appropriate care can then be given to minimise the worst effects. Some agents can cause a severe local reaction, which, if unrecognised, may lead to amputation of the affected limb or skin grafting. The reaction produced may be one of pain and inflammation (irritant drug) or of tissue death associated with blistering (vesicant drug).

Tumour lysis syndrome

When a large tumour mass is broken down by radiotherapy or more commonly chemotherapy, the cells release minerals and proteins that provoke the metabolic imbalance associated with hypocalcaemia, hyperkalaemia, hypophosphataemia and hyperuricaemia. Nursing implications include encouraging the patient to maintain a reasonable fluid intake and keeping a record of intake and output. Oral allopurinol should be given, starting before commencement of anti-cancer therapy, to counteract hyperuricaemia.

Resistance

Some tumours do not respond to a chemotherapeutic treatment, whereas others, after an initial good response, have a progressively poorer response. Initial **unresponsiveness** may be caused by several factors. For example, large solid tumours tend to have a relatively poor blood supply, which limits the distribution of the drug to the tumour. Also tumours that have a slow mitotic rate have few cells at any one time undergoing replication, which is the time in the cell cycle at which cancer cells are most vulnerable to chemotherapy. As a result few cells will be damaged or killed following the first or subsequent exposure to chemotherapy.

Resistance that increases with sequential doses of chemotherapy seems to be the result of successive mutations in the DNA of cancerous cells. As a consequence these cells adapt to levels of chemotherapeutic agents that would normally be cytotoxic (Skeel and Lachant, 1995). This type of resistance probably causes most failures in chemotherapeutic response. Drugs are given in combination in most first-line therapeutic regimes to minimise the capacity of malignant cells to adapt in this way.

Drug regimes designed for second-line therapy, that is treatment that follows failure of first-line drugs or recurrence of the tumour, are usually modified to take into account the risk of resistance.

Administration of cytotoxic therapy

Some drugs can be administered orally, and some may be given directly into a body cavity, but chemotherapeutic agents given subcutaneously or intramuscularly may provoke an intense local inflammatory response. Research continues into intra-arterial perfusion of cytotoxic agents as therapy for advanced localised primary tumour or for localised treatment of metastasis, and several studies have demonstrated a higher tumour response than that achieved with intravenous therapy (Chang *et al.*, 1997). However, most cytotoxic drugs are generally given intravenously.

Dosage

Cytotoxic dosage can be calculated in relation to kilograms of body weight. A more accurate formula is based on height and weight figures, producing a measure of body surface area in metres squared. Calculation of dosage in children is based on the same principles. Dosage for premature and newborn babies should be based on weight. In this chapter adult doses are given except where specified.

Combined cytotoxic therapy

Cytotoxic drugs are usually delivered in combination with others. These combined schedules are designed to include agents from different classes with differing actions and side effects. The aim is to minimise the risk of resistance and improve tumour cytotoxicity without increasing the incidence of dose-limiting side effects. Work continues to understand the complex ways in which these combinations have their positive effects on treatment outcome. Efforts to discover further synergistic combinations that are not associated with increased incidence of side effects also continue (Hollinger, 1997).

Timing of chemotherapy

Recent work indicates the importance of timing in administration of chemotherapy in line with the body's biorhythms. It is likely that immune system activities and hormone release in the body vary according to the pattern of the daily rhythms. These varying levels may well influence the effectiveness of concomitant chemotherapy. For example, in one trial, tumour shrinkage rates were increased by up to 50% when chemotherapy was given according to the patients' biorhythms, whereas only a 30% shrinkage rate was achieved with constant rate chemotherapy (Van de Velde, 1993).

Future developments

Efforts persist to improve drug delivery because, if methods could be found that allowed drugs to be targeted more specifically at cancer cells while sparing normal cells, side effects could be minimised and therapeutic outcomes would be improved.

CYTOTOXIC REGIMES IN SELECTED CANCERS

The examples of cytotoxic therapy included in this section are mainly ones aimed at cure, usually through adjuvant use. A few examples are also given of cancers in which palliative cytotoxic therapy may be useful. Cancers that are relatively unresponsive to chemotherapy, such as those of head and neck, pancreas, bladder and bone, are not included. There is little national standardisation of chemotherapeutic regimes and they therefore tend to vary between different cancer regional treatment centres. Consequently, the cytotoxic agents presented in this chapter are offered only as examples of those which might be used as treatment for each type of cancer.

CANCERS OF THE REPRODUCTIVE SYSTEM

BREAST CANCER

Breast cancer is defined as a malignant neoplastic disease of breast tissue and is the most common malignancy in women in the United Kingdom.

Pathophysiology

Benign tumours of the female breast are much more common than malignant ones, nevertheless breast cancer is very common, affecting 1 in 12 women in the United Kingdom at some time in their life. Worldwide, the incidence has been increasing since the 1930s, and it is the commonest cancer in women, accounting for 31% of all malignancies in women (Hortobagyi, 1997). Although it is rare in those under 25 years old, the incidence rises after that age to peak in menopausal and postmenopausal women. It is associated with early menarche, nulliparity or having a first child late (after the age of 30 years) and late menopause, indicating a link between carcinogenesis and oestrogens. It is also linked with socioeconomic category one, obesity and a high saturated fat intake. Although the causative explanation is unclear, it may also relate to oestrogen produced by fat cells (Risch *et al.*, 1994).

Most breast cancers are adenocarcinomas as they arise from glandular tissue, that is the breast lobules along with their terminal ducts. There are two main categories of malignant breast tumour: invasive and noninvasive. Noninvasive tumour may be termed carcinoma *in situ* and is confined to the layer of cells first affected. It is likely that approximately one-third of these will progress to become invasive. Invasive tumours eventually produce distortion in the structure of the breast such as a localised swelling, and dimpling and reddening of the skin, termed peau d'orange. When the tumour is near to the nipple, distortion may invert the nipple and invasion into ducts, local lymphatic channels and capillaries may cause a usually watery, and sometimes blood-stained, discharge from the nipple. Spread into the nipple and areola (Paget's disease of the nipple) is accompanied by erythema and ulceration of the area (Stevens and Lowe, 1995).

Response to treatment varies partly because of the different types of breast malignancy: prognosis is worst for women with fast-growing tumours. Tumours that produce cell surface receptors for oestrogens and progesterones are associated with a better prognosis than those that do not. When tumour spread is localised and does not involve lymph nodes the prognosis is good, with 85% of patients surviving for 10 years after initial diagnosis (Stevens and Lowe, 1995). It is expected that by the time of diagnosis, at least 50% of primary breast tumours will have metastasised; because of this, one model of breast cancer identifies it as a systemic disease with local (breast tumour) manifestations (Jatoi, 1997).

Pharmacological management

Removal of the primary growth is generally accompanied by treatment aimed at eliminating secondary sites of tumour growth. Treatment, therefore, generally involves surgical removal of the tumour along with adjuvant radiotherapy and/or chemotherapy.

There are several chemotherapeutic regimes in use. **Cyclophosphamide** is an alkylating agent useful in treatment of some lymph and solid tumours. It is not a cell cycle specific agent so has its effect throughout the growth cycle of the cell. By the destruction of cells in various stages of the growth cycle, cells in G0 may be stimulated into G1 and active growth to replace cell losses. Once in active growth they become more vulnerable to attack by chemotherapeutic agents.

In order for the double helix strands of DNA to link together normally and to part when required to code for cell proteins and to replicate, the strands are joined by special hydrogen bonds. Cyclophosphamide and other alkylating agents replace hydrogen with 'alkyl' groups, causing the DNA, and therefore the cell, to malfunction and die. Cyclophosphamide can be given orally or parenterally 100 mg–600 mg/m^2 administered within a 28-day cycle of cytotoxic therapy.

Side effects include risk of vomiting and moderate risk of bone marrow suppression. The patient should be advised that alopecia is likely, usually commencing after 2 weeks of cyclophosphamide therapy. In some individuals hair loss is total whereas in others it is minimal and patchy. Several treatments to limit hair loss are available, such as scalp tourniquet and cooling the scalp. These rely on reducing blood supply to the scalp and therefore limiting the drug dose to the basal cells in the hair follicle. Their efficacy remains controversial and they are uncomfortable for the patient; therefore, having informed the patient about these treatments, the nurse should support the patient's decision on whether to try out one of these options (Holmes, 1997).

There is also high risk of teratogenic change, and part of the nurse's role is to discuss with the patient the importance of avoiding pregnancy during treatment. Similarly, infertility is a likely outcome and it is important to identify those patients who might wish to have children. The possibility of undertaking oocyte harvesting before chemotherapy, followed by in-vitro fertilisation measures after the treatment cycles are complete, might be discussed in addition to other options.

A specific and severe side effect associated with cyclophosphamide is haemorrhagic cystitis. Fluid intake should therefore be encouraged and the patient advised to report suprapubic discomfort and any evidence of blood in her urine. There is also risk of pulmonary toxicity, therefore the patient should be assessed for dyspnoea and cough. Because another dose-limiting side effect involves myocardial toxicity, assessment of cardiac function before and during treatment should be carried out.

5-Fluorouracil is a cell cycle specific (S stage) anti-metabolite that acts as a pyrimidine antagonist.

Pyrimidine compounds are one of the two types of building blocks of DNA and RNA. Specifically, these molecules are cytosine (DNA and RNA), thymine (DNA) and uracil (RNA). 5-Fluorouracil mimics uracil but is inactive, so that when the cell uses it in place of uracil, RNA cannot be synthesised and the cell dies. 5-Fluorouracil can only be given parenterally 500 mg–1000 mg/m^2 administered on two occasions in a 28-day cycle.

Side effects include a high risk of teratogenicity. As there is a risk of severe damage to kidneys and stomach, monitoring of gastrointestinal function and urinary excretion are important aspects of nursing care. More rarely, angina may result some time after drug administration, and the patient should be advised to report any chest discomfort.

Like 5-fluorouracil, **methotrexate** is also an anti-metabolite, but one that acts as a folic acid antagonist. It mimics folic acid but is inactive, so that it prevents the cell converting folic acid to reduced folate, an essential part of the metabolic pathway needed for the synthesis of DNA. The cell is then unable to replicate. Methotrexate can be given orally or parenterally usually 50 mg/m^2 i.v. on days one and eight of a 28-day cycle of therapy. Severe side effects include liver, kidney and stomach toxicity, as well as risk of teratogenicity. More rarely, impaired respiratory function may also result.

Doxorubicin is a cytotoxic antibiotic, that is, it belongs to a group of antibiotics either derived from the mould *Streptomyces* or with similar characteristics but produced synthetically. They are all too toxic for general anti-infection use. Doxorubicin is not cell cycle specific but is particularly potent in phase S. It works by intercalation, whereby the drug is inserted between nucleotide pairs of the two strands of DNA. As a result the shape of DNA becomes unstable and it cannot be used to produce RNA or proteins and nor can it replicate. Doxorubicin can only be administered parenterally usually i.v. 30 mg/m^2, on two occasions in a 28-day cycle. Side effects include the risk of severe myelosuppression, and some risk of teratogenesis and hypersensitivity reaction.

Dexamethasone is a corticosteroid hormone that has anti-inflammatory effects. It therefore reduces oedema and minimises symptoms such as pain associated with the pressure of oedema. It also has an antiemetic effect although the mechanisms through which it operates are not well understood. In the adult, dosage range is 5–20 mg, given once daily. It can be given orally or parenterally. Long-term therapy may produce toxic effects associated with excess hormone levels (see Chapter 10 *Drugs and endocrine disorders*).

Currently, in metastatic breast cancer, **paclitaxel** and a related drug **docetaxel** are being used. They are mitotic inhibitors produced originally from extracts taken from needles of the Pacific Yew Tree. Several drug trials have demonstrated a significant anti-tumour effect in second-line therapy, and further work continues to determine the optimum dosage and regime (D'Andrea and Seidman, 1997). Paclitaxel and docetaxel work in G2 and M phases by causing an overproliferation of microtubules. Normally these form the spindle along which chromatids move during cell replication. When there are too many microtubules the spindle cannot form and the cell cannot divide. These drugs are given intravenously, in doses of 135–250 mg/m^2 infused over periods of 3 or 24 hours

for paclitaxel, and 75–100 mg/m^2 infused over 1 hour for docetaxel, both in 3-week cycles.

Patients receiving paclitaxel and docetaxel are at high risk of dose-limiting neutropenia as a result of bone marrow suppression. Various severe hypersensitivity responses are also likely and because of this a corticosteroid, an antihistamine and an H$_2$ antagonist are given before treatment begins (see Chapter 5 *Drugs and immunological disorders* and Chapter 14 *Drugs and gastrointestinal disorders*). Significant risk of fluid retention associated with docetaxel can be reduced by administration of dexamethasone 8 mg twice daily for 5 days starting 24 hours before docetaxel therapy begins (D'Andrea and Seidman, 1997). Alopecia and peripheral sensory nerve damage may also result.

Tamoxifen is an example of a hormone antagonist. It is not cell cycle specific and acts by binding to oestrogen receptors in the cytoplasm. In cancer cells that need an oestrogen stimulus in their metabolic pathways, this will inhibit DNA synthesis. Many breast tumours are influenced by circulating oestrogens, which are produced from the ovaries in premenopausal women. Currently tamoxifen is undergoing drug trials to judge its effectiveness in prevention of breast cancer (Leonard, 1996), though its main use is in treatment of advanced breast cancer. The dosage is 10–20 mg orally twice daily. The main side effects are teratogenesis and infertility, but other symptoms associated with the menopause may occur such as hot flushes and menstrual irregularities although these are generally well tolerated.

In postmenopausal women oestrogens are produced in lesser quantities by tumour cells themselves as well as fat, muscle and liver cells in which the enzyme aromatase converts adrenal androgens to oestrogens. Aromatase inhibitors such as **aminoglutethimide** and **formestane** suppress the female sex hormones that stimulate tumour growth and are used for patients in whom cancer progresses or recurs after tamoxifen treatment. Both are associated with limiting side effects. For example, aminoglutethimide affects other cellular enzyme-dependent adrenocorticoid pathways as well as oestrogen ones. It also causes skin rashes and lethargy. Formestane has limited bioavailability and must be given by intramuscular injection fortnightly, leading to possible inflammatory reactions at the injection sites. A new aromatase inhibitor, **anastrozole**, is in clinical trial at present and may prove more effective than tamoxifen alone or may have an increased anti-tumour effect in conjunction with tamoxifen (Howell, 1996).

Megestrol acetate, administered orally 40 mg four times daily, is the commonest progestin and is used in advanced cancer for progestin-sensitive tumours. Its adverse effects include teratogenesis, fluid retention, thromboembolic disease and decreased glucose tolerance. The patient's fluid balance should therefore be monitored and checks made for the onset of deep vein thrombosis and diabetes mellitus.

CERVICAL CANCER

Cervical cancer is defined as a neoplasm of the uterine cervix. It can be detected in the early, curable stage by the pap tests.

Pathophysiology

The incidence of early neoplastic cervical change peaks between the ages of 20 and 40 years, whereas invasive cancer peaks at 45–65 years. Human papilloma virus (HPV) infection of the cervix is a sexually transmitted disease (see Chapter 16 *Drugs and reproductive disorders*). A small number of women with this type of infection will develop invasive cervical carcinoma. It is associated with sexual behaviour, the risk increasing with coitus at an early age and multiple sexual partners. There is also a high incidence in those societies in which female sexual behaviour is restricted but promiscuous male sexual behaviour is tolerated, such as Latin America. Cervical cancer is also associated with conditions producing immunosuppression, such as HIV infection (see Chapter 5 *Drugs and immunological disorders*). This may explain its association with smoking (Nowak and Handford, 1994).

Benign tumours of the cervix are uncommon. Invasive malignant change occurs after abnormal progressive cytological precursor states, together termed cervical intraepithelial neoplasia or CIN (**Table 6.1**). In this process, normal cells can be replaced with increasingly abnormal ones (dysplasia). However, 50% of individuals with CIN I have spontaneous regression of the change. The area of cervix particularly prone to neoplastic change is the junction between the part of the cervix covered in squamous cell epithelium and that with a mucus-secreting columnar cell surface, the squamocolumnar junction. At CIN III stage, the change is localised to the epithelial layer of cells and is equivalent to a preliminary stage of carcinogenesis termed carcinoma-in-situ (see **Table 6.1**). Twenty per cent of patients with CIN III develop invasive carcinoma within

Classification of cervical dysplasia	
Grade	Criteria
CIN I	Mild dysplasia
CIN II	Moderate dysplasia: less than two-thirds of the cells of the epithelium are dysplasic
CIN III	Carcinoma-in-situ: severe dysplasia in more than two-thirds of the cells of the epithelium

10 years (Stevens and Lowe, 1995). The invasive tumour may be an adenocarcinoma or squamous cell carcinoma. Various types of HPV have been discovered in tumour biopsies, and it is known that HPV proteins can inactivate tumour suppressor gene products so enabling the development of cancerous change. Immunosuppression prevents recognition and destruction of neoplastic cells allowing them to grow, replicate and mutate further. The commonest symptom is vaginal bleeding, and later invasion of tumour into the bladder or urethra may cause urinary obstruction.

Pharmacological management

Laser therapy is curative for CIN lesions. Surgery is the primary treatment for invasive tumour stage 1 and radiotherapy for stages 2 and 3. Chemotherapy may be useful as palliative treatment in case of distal metastasis. **Cisplatin** is an alkylating type of chemotherapeutic agent containing platinum and is administered i.v., 25 mg/m^2 twice during a 28-day cytotoxic regime. It acts by forming DNA interstrand links and thus restricts DNA synthesis. It is distributed widely in all body tissues but does not easily cross the blood–brain barrier. There is a risk of long-term accumulation of the drug. It is teratogenic and there is high risk of severe damage from extravasation, hypersensitivity reaction and ear and kidney damage. Synergistic side effects occur with several other cytotoxic agents and with radiotherapy. For detail of methotrexate and fluorouracil see the section on breast cancer above. Folinic acid is given not only to rescue normal cells (see earlier section *Bone marrow suppression*) but also to potentiate the action of 5-fluorouracil.

ENDOMETRIAL CANCER

Endometrial cancer is defined as a malignant neoplastic disease of the endometrium of the uterus that most often occurs in the fifth or sixth decade of life.

Pathophysiology

This is the commonest invasive cancer of the female genital tract and accounts for approximately 7% of all malignancies in women, although the mortality is lower than that of cervical cancer. Incidence peaks during and after the menopause, and obese nulliparous women who are at risk of diabetes and cardiovascular disease are typically at risk of endometrial cancer. There is more rarely a hereditary component seen in those families who also have increased risk of breast cancer (Nowak and Handford, 1994).

Cancers of the endometrium are generally types of adenocarcinoma. Perimenopausal endometrial cancer is associated with hyperplasia and is oestrogen dependent whereas postmenopausal cancer is not. The link with obesity can be explained in terms of the oestrogen production of fatty tissue. As the tumour grows it spreads to myometrium and cervix or to the uterine tubes and ovaries. Occasionally the tumour invades the bladder or rectum. Spread is via local pelvic lymph nodes and through small lymphatic channels in the uterine and vaginal wall. Distal metastasis most commonly occurs in lung and bone. Perimenopausal heavy and or irregular periods or post-menopausal vaginal bleeding may be the only symptom (Stevens and Lowe, 1995).

Pharmacological management

Most tumours are stage 1 at diagnosis and this accounts for the good prognosis. Total hysterectomy and bilateral oosalpingectomy is the primary treatment with radiotherapy. As endometrial cancer is hormone dependent, in metastatic disease progestins such as **megestrol** (see *Breast cancer* section) may produce a response.

OVARIAN CANCER

Ovarian cancer is defined as a malignant neoplastic disease of the ovary that occurs most frequently in women between 40 and 60 years of age and occasionally in young adult women.

Pathophysiology

This accounts for approximately 5% of female cancers in the United Kingdom but has a high mortality. Environmental influences on causation are suggested by the low incidence in Japanese women in Japan but an incidence approaching that of US women among Japanese immigrants. Ovarian cancer occurs most commonly in women over the age of 40 years who are nulliparous, which suggests that hormones are involved in its cause.

Ovarian tumours may be benign or malignant. This cancer can derive from several different cell types. The commoner types of ovarian cancer are cystic epithelial tumours, containing either mucoid or serous fluid. More rarely, solid tumours or malignant germ cell tumours such as choriocarcinoma occur, the latter being highly malignant. Overall, the high mortality associated with ovarian cancer, with a 5-year survival of only 20%, is attributable to the lack of symptoms in early disease and metastatic spread by the time of diagnosis. Spread is via the peritoneum as well as by blood and lymphatics to the bowel, liver and lungs. The ovary is also a common site of metastatic growth from primary tumours of breast and gastrointestinal tract. Symptoms can be ignored initially as they are nonspecific. They include vague abdominal discomfort and bloating, anorexia, dyspepsia and flatulence (Nowak and Handford, 1994).

Pharmacological management

Bilateral oophorectomy and total hysterectomy with omentectomy is performed. In stage 2 or in more advanced disease, regimes, including **cisplatin** and **cyclophosphamide** (see *Breast cancer* and *Cervical cancer* sections for further detail) are used. Concurrent intravenous mannitol is usually infused in order to prevent drug precipitation in the kidney (see also Chapter 15 *Drugs and urological*

disorders). **Paclitaxel** may be used for metastatic disease that has not responded to previous chemotherapy (see *Breast cancer* section).

The rare choriocarcinoma, a type of germ cell cancer, although highly malignant is very susceptible to chemotherapy. After evacuation of the uterine contents, **methotrexate** alone may effect a cure. If central nervous system involvement is suspected, intrathecal methotrexate may be given. Metastases in other systems are treated with a more aggressive combination regime, for example cyclophosphamide (see *Breast cancer* section), dactinomycin and vincristine. **Dactinomycin** is a cytotoxic antibiotic given i.v. 0.3 mg–0.4 mg/m² twice during a 28-day cytotoxic cycle that acts by an alkylating effect and is not cell cycle specific. It is associated with severe bone marrow depression, liver damage and risk of tissue destruction on extravasation. **Vincristine** is a mitotic inhibitor given i.v. 1.2 mg–1.5 mg/m² once per week in a 28-day cycle associated with a high risk of liver damage and with convulsions. It acts in mitosis by binding to tuberlin, thus preventing formation of the microtubules that make up the spindle along which chromatids organise themselves. As a result, DNA and RNA synthesis is prevented and cell division cannot take place.

PROSTATIC CANCER

Prostatic cancer is defined as a malignant neoplastic disease of the prostate gland.

Pathophysiology

Worldwide, prostatic cancer accounts for 5–20% of all male cancers. In the United Kingdom it is the second most common cancer and it is more common in the United Kingdom and USA than in Eastern Europe or the Far East. Men who migrate from an area of low incidence to an area of high incidence become at high risk of prostatic cancer, which suggests that environmental elements are involved in the causation. There is a genetic component suggested by the increased incidence in families in which other members have prostate, testicular or, possibly, breast cancer. It is commoner in men living in urban rather than rural areas. Incidence increases with advancing age, rarely occurring in men under 40 years old. Eighty per cent of prostate cancer is diagnosed in men over the age of 65 years.

Most neoplasia affecting the prostate is a benign hyperplasia, affecting men from the age of 45 years and causing symptoms in most men over the age of 70 years. The commonest malignant tumour is an adenocarcinoma, and many tumours are stimulated by testosterone. It arises from cells at the periphery of the prostate gland. As a result, invasion occurs first through the surface of the prostate and metastasises to the bones of the lower spine and pelvis, the gastrointestinal tract, the liver and lung through blood and lymphatic circulations. It is later that the tumour mass spreads medially to the urethra and base of the bladder, eventually producing urinary symptoms. These include frequency of micturition, poor stream and nocturia. Lower back pain may result from spinal metastases. Five-year survival relates to the stage of tumour at diagnosis, ranging from 90% to 10% (Price and Wilson, 1992).

In the life cycle of this type of tumour, there is often a long refractory period, with malignant cells in a dormant state corresponding to the G0 phase of the cell cycle before it progresses to an actively invasive stage. Occasionally, therefore, treatment decisions are difficult, given the usually advanced age at diagnosis, as without treatment the individual may live many years before dying of an unrelated condition.

Pharmacological management

Prostatectomy and radiotherapy are the first-line treatments. As prostatic cancer is hormone dependent, in relapse or metastatic disease, anti-androgens such as **flutamide** are useful. Flutamide acts by blocking androgen receptors on cells in the target tissues. Dosage is 250 mg 3 times daily taken orally. Therapy usually involves a combination of anti-androgen with a gonadotrophin-releasing hormone analogue such as **goserelin**. The latter decreases luteinizing hormone secretion and so inhibits production of testosterone at the luteinizing hormone target tissues (see Chapter 16 *Drugs and reproductive disorders*). It is given in depot formulation of 3.6 mg, implanted in the anterior abdominal wall and renewed monthly for 6 months. If patients have an initial response then they may

be offered bilateral orchidectomy as an alternative to further drug therapy, as resistance is common to second-line or continuing drug therapy and prognosis is consequently limited. However, both forms of treatment are associated with unpleasant feminization effects, which patients may find difficult to tolerate.

CANCER OF THE TESTIS

Cancer of the testis is a malignant neoplastic disease of the testis. An undescended testicle is often involved.

Pathophysiology

Unlike prostatic cancer, cancer of the testis is a disease that affects generally young men, aged between 20 and 40 years. It is more prevalent in UK and US men than in Japanese men and the incidence is increasing in the United Kingdom and USA. It is believed that many of these tumours arise from developmental abnormalities and that the risk is increased by up to 40-fold in those who have incomplete descent of a testis. A link with high scrotal temperature has been suggested. More recently, exposure to increased levels of environmental oestrogen *in utero* or after birth have been recognised as potential influences in causation (Nowak and Handford, 1994).

Ninety-seven per cent of testicular tumours arise from germ cells and are either seminomas or teratomas. Seminomas are formed from primitive germ cells that would normally differentiate to spermatocytic tissue and they account for 50% of germ cell tumours. Other germ cell tumours can be categorised as teratomas (Stevens and Lowe, 1995).

Spread from seminomas is generally to the regional lymph nodes, whereas spread from other tumours is via the bloodstream to the lungs and liver. Symptoms are generally few and include unilateral testicular swelling and discomfort. This has implications for the nurse as health promoter. Informing men about testicular self-examination is likely to increase early diagnosis and improve prospects for cure.

Pharmacological management

Recent improvements in treatment have led to a high cure rate. Unilateral orchidectomy is the central treatment feature with radiotherapy and/or chemotherapy as adjuvant options. If, after excision, there is no evidence of tumour then the patient has a 90% chance of complete cure. Prognosis worsens for more advanced tumours, with a 20% cure rate for stage 4 tumours. Tumours at stage 2 may respond to combination chemotherapy involving **cisplatin** with **etoposide**. For stage 3 and 4 tumours **bleomycin** and **vinblastine** may be added to the regime. Etoposide, given i.v. 100 mg/m^2 on 2 occasions in a 21-day cytotoxic cycle and vinblastine, given i.v. 7.5 mg/m^2 once during each 21-day cytotoxic cycle, are mitotic inhibitors, with etoposide acting in S and G2 phases and vinblastine active in M phase. Side effects include bone marrow suppression, liver, lung and kidney damage and convulsions. Bleomycin, given i.v. 30 i.u. weekly during each 21-day cytotoxic cycle is a highly toxic cytotoxic antibiotic associated with pneumonitis, pulmonary fibrosis, infertility and teratogenesis. It acts by preventing the inclusion of thymidine into DNA so that DNA cannot be produced.

BLOOD AND LYMPHOID CANCERS

LYMPHOMAS

Lymphomas are neoplasms arising from lymph tissue and are classified broadly as Hodgkin's disease and non-Hodgkin's lymphomas. Many classification systems exist that further subdivide these two main categories in various complex ways.

HODGKIN'S DISEASE

Hodgkin's disease is a malignant disorder characterised by painless, progressive enlargement of lymphoid tissue, usually first evident in cervical lymph nodes.

Pathophysiology

There is a peak of incidence of Hodgkin's disease at 20–30 years and another at 60–70 years. It is commoner in men than women. In children it occurs almost exclusively in boys less than 10 years of age. Incidence is particularly high in Jewish people in the United Kingdom and USA (Souhami and Moxham, 1990).

It arises from abnormal lymphoid cells with two nuclei, the Reed–Sternberg cells, affecting lymph nodes, spleen or liver. More rarely bone marrow, central nervous system or lungs may be involved. How Reed–Sternberg cells are formed is unclear and has been the focus of research for many years. Other features of Hodgkin's disease include infiltration of the affected nodes and organs by other cells such as lymphocytes, plasma cells, histiocytes and fibroblasts (Stevens and Lowe, 1995). Biopsy allows histological classification of the tumour. The overall 10-year survival figure is over 80% in the lymphocyte-predominant cases but only 5% for the lymphocyte-depleted category.

Any lymph node may be involved, but Hodgkin's disease commonly affects those in the neck. Spread progresses to neighbouring and then more distant nodes. The main symptom is a rubbery painless swelling of the affected node, which usually enlarges slowly over several months. Later generalised symptoms include pyrexia and night sweats, weight loss, pruritus and pain in the nodes associated with alcohol use.

Pharmacological management

It is frequently curable as the tumour is sensitive to radiotherapy and chemotherapy. In early disease, radiotherapy is the treatment of choice. In more advanced stages, chemotherapy is given with allopurinol to prevent acute tumour lysis syndrome. There are many schedules, often given in alternating regimes. Details of doxorubicin can be found in the *Breast cancer* section. Bleomycin and vinblastine are found in the testicular cancer section. **Dacarbazine** is an alkylating agent that inhibits DNA and RNA synthesis and also interrupts the purine production metabolic pathway. It is given i.v., 375 mg/m² twice in each 28-day cycle and it is associated with bone marrow depression, vomiting and eye and nervous system damage. Because of the risk of sterility in young sufferers, the nurse should ensure that sperm or oocyte banking is discussed with patients before therapy begins.

NON-HODGKIN'S LYMPHOMA

Non-Hodgkin's lymphoma describes any kind of malignant lymphoma except Hodgkin's disease.

Pathophysiology

In the United Kingdom this occurs more frequently than Hodgkin's disease and accounts for approximately 2% of all malignancies. It is rare below the age of 50 years and thereafter incidence increases steadily. It affects men and women equally but incidence is high in Black Americans. Geographical variation is evident, with a low incidence in Japan.

Non-Hodgkin's lymphomas can be classified in many ways based on differences in cell site, shape and size. Most lymphomas derive from B cells, some from T cells and some from other cell types; they cover a range of malignancy, from low grade to high grade. Low-grade tumours may have a long period of initial dormancy before entering an aggressively growing phase whereas high-grade tumours tend to maintain a higher level of malignancy throughout their life cycle

Often the disease affects several lymph glands in different parts of the body. It is generally asymptomatic although advanced disease is associated with systemic symptoms, as in Hodgkin's disease, and anaemia may also result. The tumours can cause pressure or obstruction symptoms as they enlarge. Lymphomas can also arise from lymph tissue in the gastrointestinal tract, skin, brain, thyroid, bone and testis (Neal and Hoskin, 1997). Five-year survival depends on histological grade and stage but 10-year survival of low- and high-grade tumours is similar, at approximately 45%.

Pharmacological management

Low-grade and localised non-Hodgkin's lymphoma is treated with radiotherapy and cure can be expected. Non-localised tumour cannot be cured, but long remissions can be achieved and symptoms controlled with chemotherapy, including use of cyclophosphamide, doxorubicin, vincristine and **prednisolone**. High-grade tumour is treated with chemotherapy and radiotherapy to locally affected areas.

In this regime, prednisolone is given for its anti-cancer effect as it produces a change in the hormonal cellular environment that adversely influences the activities of the cells. It is also an anti-inflammatory agent and can be given in various chemotherapeutic regimes to reduce swelling and pain resulting from pressure (see Chapter 3 *Classes of drugs*). It also has an antiemetic effect although this is not a recognised use of such steroid therapy.

MULTIPLE MYELOMA

Multiple myeloma is defined as a malignant neoplasm of the bone marrow.

Pathophysiology

This disease is one of many, usually rare, malignancies that affect plasma cells, and occurs mainly in those aged over 60 years. The cause is unknown, although there is some familial association. It occurs equally in men and women in the United Kingdom, with an incidence of approximately 3 per 100 000 (Neal and Hoskin, 1997).

Large numbers of mainly plasma cells are derived from malignant B cells in the bone marrow. These abnormal plasma cells usually produce a specific type of antibody (monoclonal antibody) called a paraprotein, which is similarly abnormal. As the plasma cells proliferate in bone marrow they destroy skeletal tissue, probably by secretion of osteoclast-activating factors such as interleukins-1 and -6 and tumour necrosis factor. The result is calcium depletion and other metabolic disturbances and osteoporosis. As a result patients may present with crush fractures of the skull or spine. Anaemia may result from replacement of erythropoiesis space by tumour in the marrow, though thrombocytopenia and neutropenia are less common initially. It is associated with suppression of normal immune cell production (hypogammaglobulinaemia), leading to risk of death from overwhelming infection. The abnormal immunoglobulins often separate into sections and become deposited in the kidney tubules (light chain section) or glomeruli (amyloid), where they cause damage (Stevens and Lowe, 1995).

Pharmacological management

The average survival for patients with stage 1 multiple myeloma is 4 years and cure is rarely possible; treatment is aimed at reducing the number of malignant plasma cells and controlling symptoms. In patients under the age of 50 years, high-dose **melphelan** followed by bone marrow transplant may increase survival time. Alternatively, combination regimes may be used, sometimes in conjunction with melphelan. Melphelan is given orally, as an induction dose of up to 10 mg daily for 7–10 days. Maintenance therapy is 0.15–2 mg daily depending on leucocyte and platelet counts. It is associated with some risk of bone marrow suppression, alopecia and infertility. **Carmustine** (BCNU), given i.v. 30 mg/m^2, once during a 21-day cycle, is a nitrosurea type of alkylator-like agent that is not cell cycle specific. Its side effects include severe bone marrow suppression, infertility and teratogenesis. Radiotherapy is used to provide symptomatic treatment for bone pain.

LEUKAEMIAS

Leukaemia is a malignant neoplasm of blood-forming organs.

Pathophysiology

In the majority of leukaemia patients the cause cannot be identified. It is suggested that exposure to ionising radiation may be responsible for approximately 20% of all childhood leukaemias and 10% of adult ones. Rarely, leukaemia is linked with a congenital disease, for example Down's syndrome. There is current research interest in the influences of prenatal and infant environmental factors. In adults occupational exposure to benzene or other chemicals may be a cause. A virus common to southern Japan and the Caribbean has been linked with types of leukaemia. Chemotherapy earlier in life is also a known risk factor (Price and Wilson, 1992).

The leukaemias are the most common type of neoplastic disease of leucocytes. They are a group of related malignancies derived from primitive blood-forming cells in the bone marrow. Acute leukaemias are characterised by proliferation of immature or blast cells. Chronic leukaemias involve proliferation of more mature cells. In both types, the white cell production zone in bone marrow is overwhelmed by abnormal cells, leaving the individual affected open to infection. Bone marrow enlargement is accompanied by varying degrees of anaemia and thrombocytopenia (Darby and Roman, 1995).

Pharmacological management

Prospective randomised trials have determined UK protocols for treatment of acute lymphoblastic leukaemia in children (UKALL). The results are reviewed 5 yearly and revised protocols published. Chemotherapeutic treatment for leukaemias involves inductive or initial regimes started on diagnosis that aim to achieve remission. In childhood acute lymphoblastic leukaemia intensification regimes follow the induction therapy. Intrathecal **methotrexate** is given at both these stages of the programme to treat abnormal leucocytes in the central nervous system. In children and adults consolidation treatment may be given when remission is achieved and stem cells harvested from the bone marrow; it involves radiotherapy to the brain and further intrathecal methotrexate. A maintenance regime will usually continue for up to 2 years.

The following are used in **all** inductive and intensification schedules for children. **Asparaginase** is classed as a miscellaneous type of agent. It can be given s.c., i.m. or i.v. in paediatric inductive therapy; it is given s.c. 6000 i.u. on day four of the schedule, then 3 times weekly for 9 doses. It is an enzyme that breaks down asparagine so the cell cannot use it to synthesise vital cell proteins. Adverse effects include liver, lung, kidney and central nervous system damage. The use of daunorubicin, thioguanine and cytabarine is discussed in the acute myeloid leukaemia (AML) section below. Oral allopurinol 100 mg/m^2 thrice daily commences 24 hours before chemotherapy and continues for 14 days. Because of the high risk of infection, antibiotic therapy is given during the chemotherapy programme.

For adults and children with relapsing acute leukaemias high-dose chemotherapy with bone marrow transplantation is increasingly used. Monoclonal antibodies can also be used to recognise and help to destroy abnormal bone marrow cells before bone marrow transplant.

The following are used in induction regimes for adults with AML. **Daunorubicin** (60 mg/m^2 i.v. given twice), is a cytotoxic antibiotic particularly associated with risk of hair loss, bone marrow suppression, congestive heart failure, liver damage and tissue destruction on extravasation. It is active in all phases of the cell cycle but is particularly effective in the S phase. **Cytarabine** is an antimetabolite acting as a pyrimidine antagonist, which can be administered intravenously, intrathecally or subcutaneously (for example 200 mg/m^2 given i.v. (twice). Adverse effects include a high risk of severe bone marrow suppression and liver, kidney, stomach, lung and heart damage. **Thioguanine** (for example, 100 mg/m^2 orally twice daily on two days in the regime) is also an antimetabolite, but is a purine inhibitor and is associated with liver and kidney toxicity.

In chronic myeloid leukaemia (CML) **busulphan** given orally 4 mg/m^2 daily is used to reduce the peripheral leucocyte count to below 15×10^9/L. Lower, maintenance doses of busulphan may continue although resistance usually develops, at which time an alternative combination therapeutic regime is commenced. An alkylating agent, busulphan is effective in all phases of the cell cycle and is associated with moderate bone marrow suppression and pulmonary fibrosis. Bone marrow transplant achieves prolonged remission in some cases (Neal and Hoskin, 1997).

Chronic lymphatic leukaemia (CLL) is usually treated with non-aggressive chemotherapy to match the generally slow progression of the disease. **Cyclophosphamide**, a DNA and RNA alkylating agent, may be used in conjunction with allopurinol. Low-dose radiation treatment may be used to reduce splenomegaly. Prolonged remissions can be expected.

RESPIRATORY SYSTEM CANCER

LUNG CANCER

Lung cancer is a pulmonary malignancy attributable to a number of factors, including cigarette smoking and asbestos.

Pathophysiology

Lung cancer is the commonest cause of death from malignant disease in the United Kingdom. It affects men more frequently than women, although the incidence in men is falling more sharply than that in women. Incidence rises with age reaching a peak at over 55 years of age. Inhaled carcinogens cause this type of cancer. Approximately 90% can be linked to tobacco smoke inhalation, either directly or from passive inhalation. The increasing incidence in developing countries can be attributed to more people smoking. Other carcinogenic agents implicated include asbestos, particularly blue asbestos, and long-term exposure in the home to radon gas emitted from granite rocks on which the house is built. More rarely, occupational exposure to various hydrocarbons or metals such as nickel is involved (Rees *et al.*, 1993).

Lung cancers can develop anywhere in the airways, but most commonly arise from the larger bronchi. All are derived from parts of the bronchial epithelium. Overall they can be categorised as small cell lung carcinomas (SCLC) or non-small cell lung carcinomas (NSCLC). There are several types of small cell carcinomas, which together account for a quarter of all lung cancers. They are an ectopic source of hormone or peptide secretion, for example antidiuretic hormone. Small cell carcinomas metastasise early in their life cycle and are therefore associated with a poor prognosis.

Non-small cell carcinomas include squamous carcinoma, responsible for 50% of all lung cancers, and adenocarcinoma (15%), a particularly slow growing cancer which usually develops in the periphery of the lung, and anaplastic tumour, which is so poorly differentiated that the cell origin cannot be determined. The tumour spreads around and along the length of the airways, producing symptoms of irritation or obstruction to airflow, generally late in the disease. These symptoms include cough, often unproductive, weight loss, haemoptysis, dyspnoea, wheeze and chest pain. Later dysphagia caused by compression of the oesophagus can occur, or hoarseness caused by invasion of a recurrent laryngeal nerve.

Metastatic spread in lung cancer is to bone, brain, kidney, liver, bone marrow, meninges, adrenal glands and skin via the bloodstream. Tumour cells can also spread across the surface of the pleural cavity. Via lymphatic nodes the disease can spread to the previously unaffected lung, spinal cord and superior vena cava. In approximately 70% of patients, metastasis is present on diagnosis and accounts for the poor prognosis. Small cell carcinoma has a 1-year survival of 45%. Of the few operable non-small cell carcinomas, 5-year survival figures range from 5 to 50%, depending upon the tumour stage (Donnellan and Crown, 1997).

Pharmacological management

Primary treatment in small cell lung cancer is with chemotherapy rather than surgery or radiotherapy.

Treatment of non-small cell lung cancer in early stage disease involves surgical excision. Palliative treatment may involve a mix of radiotherapy and chemotherapy to reduce symptoms. Cyclophosphamide, cisplatin, etoposide and vincristine are commonly used.

GASTROINTESTINAL TRACT CANCERS

OESOPHAGEAL CANCER

Oesophageal cancer is a malignant neoplastic disease of the oesophagus.

Pathophysiology

In China, Japan, South Russia, Iran, India and the Middle East, oesophageal cancer is the commonest cause of death. In Europe the incidence is highest in northwest France. It occurs most commonly in men aged 50 years or more. Predisposing factors include alcohol and tobacco use, and individuals who combine the two have a much greater risk. It is also linked with gastro-oesophageal reflux, nutritional deficiency such as low levels of vitamin A, B or C or of trace elements such as zinc, magnesium or iron (Stevens and Lowe, 1995).

Benign tumours of the oesophagus are rare. The majority of oesophageal cancers are squamous cell carcinomas and arise from the middle and lower part of the oesophagus. Approximately 20% are adenocarcinomas and occur low down in the oesophagus. Ten per cent are of various rare histological types. Prognosis is generally poor; 5-year survival is less than 10%. This is because of early metastasis via local lymphatics and the late onset of symptoms, which occur only when the tumour is compromising the lumen. Dysphagia eventually results and the patient may also report an unexplained weight loss (Price and Wilson, 1992).

Pharmacological management

Options for the treatment of oesophageal cancer include surgical excision, but surgery with the aim of cure is rarely undertaken as it is effective only in early stage disease and 5-year survival after radical resection is less than 20%. Radiotherapy, chemotherapy, repeated dilatation treatment and laser treatment to vaporise the part of tumour obstructing the lumen are other alternatives, used alone or in combination (Jaskiewicz, 1994). Palliative chemotherapy may include **cisplatin** and/or **mitomycin**. Mitomycin is a cytotoxic antibiotic associated with risk of tissue destruction on extravasation. It is given intravenously 5–20 mg/m^2 every 3–8 weeks.

STOMACH CANCER

Stomach cancer is defined as a malignant neoplastic disease of the stomach.

Pathophysiology

It occurs more commonly in men than women, and worldwide the incidence is slowly falling. However, there are great variations in incidence, with highest rates occurring in the Far East particularly Korea and Japan, and a low incidence in some parts of North America (Park et al., 1997). It is linked with social class, the highest incidence occurring in social class 5, and incidence rises with increasing age. Individuals with pernicious anaemia, those who have previously had partial gastrectomy, people with blood group A and those with a family history of stomach cancer have a higher incidence.

The commonest stomach cancer is an adenocarcinoma, which spreads through the stomach wall and ulcerates through the mucosal surface. It may result from a fall in gastric acid production, which predisposes to bacterial overgrowth of the stomach. This bacterial overgrowth in turn may convert food components to carcinogens. The worldwide variation in incidence also suggests a dietary link. As the tumour grows it invades local lymphatics and blood supply, metastasising to liver, bone and lungs. It may also spread through the abdominal cavity, causing ascites to form because of obstruction to venous and lymphatic drainage from the abdominal cavity. Overall prognosis for stomach cancer is poor, with less than 15% surviving for 5 years, although treatment in early disease can produce a 90% survival. Unfortunately the poor prognosis is the result of symptoms that tend to occur only late in the disease and initially are easy to ignore. They include epigastric discomfort and anorexia; dysphagia, vomiting (possibly haematemesis), malaena, weight loss and jaundice occur as later features.

Pharmacological management

Stomach cancer may be cured by partial or total gastrectomy. Survival depends upon the stage at operation. Fifty-five per cent survive for 5 years if the tumour is limited to mucosa or submucosa, but only 2.5% of tumours are limited to this stage at operation. Overall, 20% of patients who have had surgical excision survive for 5 years. Chemotherapy and radiotherapy are adjuvant and palliative options. In advanced stomach cancer **5-fluorouracil** in combination with other drugs such as **doxorubicin** and **etoposide** may be given to reduce the adverse effects of metastasis, particularly in lung and liver.

COLORECTAL CANCER

Colorectal cancer is defined as a malignant neoplastic disease of the colon.

Pathophysiology

Colorectal cancer is the second most common cancer in the West, causing 15% of all malignancies in men and women. The incidence increases with age; it starts at 20 years of age and peaks in the 60–80 age group. A diet high in saturated fat and low in fibre is implicated in causation. It may alter bacterial flora and bile acids, which in turn may influence the pathogenesis of malignant change. Rarely, genetic predisposition may be involved as in the autosomal dominant condition familial polyposis in which individuals develop multiple colonies of polyps in the colon, which undergo malignant transformation usually before the age of 40 years. Long-standing Crohn's disease of the colon or ulcerative colitis may also rarely predispose to cancerous change, as may the presence of non-familial adenomata (Knowles and Jodrell, 1997).

In the United Kingdom, approximately one-half of colorectal cancers occur in the rectum followed, in frequency of occurrence, by the sigmoid colon and then more proximal areas of the colon. The commonest type of colorectal cancer is adenocarcinoma arising from the glandular epithelium of the mucosa. The tumour spreads locally through the bowel wall, invading adjacent organs such as the bladder or nearby loops of bowel. It metastasises to liver and lungs via the blood supply and lymphatics. Prognosis and treatment is related to the stage of the disease process.

It may be asymptomatic until late in the disease and symptoms are easy to ignore at first, causing delay in diagnosis. Symptoms include change in bowel habit, which may be constipation or diarrhoea, or both in an alternating pattern. Rectal bleeding of fresh blood from the surface of a tumour in the rectum or of altered blood from more proximal colonic tumour sites may also be present. Later symptoms of anaemia (see Chapter 12 *Drugs and cardiovascular disorders*) and intestinal obstruction may cause the patient to seek medical help.

Pharmacological management

Of the 80% of patients who have operable tumours, surgical excision is the main treatment. Cure rates, particularly for rectal cancer, differ widely but overall approximately 50% of patients develop local or metastatic recurrence. This has stimulated various continuing trials worldwide to determine the best combination of surgery with preoperative or postoperative radiotherapy and chemotherapy. For example the UK Quasar I trial is testing the value of different adjuvant chemotherapy regimes and it will be followed up by a Quasar II trial. Trials of more advanced disease suggest certain regimes, including **5-fluorouracil** with folinic acid, increase disease-free survival. In future a more specific modulator of the enzymatic effects of 5-fluorouracil than folinic acid, such as **raltitrexed**, may be shown to improve treatment response in clinical trials. Recently, adjuvant chemotherapy given by hepatic portal infusion has produced promising results (Laffer *et al.*, 1995).

SKIN CANCER

Skin cancer is defined as a malignant neoplastic disease of the skin

PATHOPHYSIOLOGY

A major stimulus to malignant change in the skin is exposure to ultraviolet radiation from the sun, so it generally occurs on areas of skin exposed to sunlight. Incidence of skin cancer in the United Kingdom has increased by over 50% in the past decade. More rarely, chronic irritation and previous exposure to radiotherapy and various chemical agents may lead to cancerous change in the skin.

There are various types of skin neoplasms and most are very rare. Common tumour types are melanocytic naevi (moles), which can arise from cells in the basal level of the epidermis or from the dermis. Some occur in childhood whereas others are more common in adults and most people have some. A few people have large numbers as a familial characteristic. The great majority of naevi are benign, but occasionally they may undergo malignant change. This has health promotional implications for nurses who should inform patients about the importance of inspecting their moles regularly, checking for any change in size, colour or surface texture. Suspicious 'moles' should be excised and biopsied (Stevens and Lowe, 1995).

Malignant melanomas arise from melanocytes and are rare in dark-skinned people; however, the incidence is rising sharply in the United Kingdom among white-skinned individuals, particularly in those subjected to ultraviolet radiation from childhood (Autier *et al.*, 1997). They occur mainly in young and middle-aged adults. Anywhere on the skin may be affected, but they appear most commonly on the trunk in men and the lower part of the legs in women. Nose, mouth, vagina and anus are rarer sites. Metastasis to any tissue is possible and can happen early in the life cycle of the tumour. Tumours are infiltrated by lymphocytes and occasionally complete regression of tumour occurs. This suggests an immune response may influence growth of the tumour.

Pharmacological management

Melanomas are relatively resistant to radiotherapy and chemotherapy, though surgery may be curative in the early stages. Various drugs may be combined to combat metastatic disease, for example **dacarbazine** with **dactinomycin**, or **vinblastine** with **bleomycin** and **cisplatin**.

Increasingly, **colony-stimulating factors** and **interferons** (α, β and γ) are being used in various trials to augment the body's immune system and increase its destruction of the tumour while protecting the bone marrow from the suppressive effects of chemotherapy (Lilley *et al.*, 1996).

Basal cell carcinoma (BCC) is more common than squamous carcinoma, although both arise from skin keratinocytes. The former occurs generally on the face, neck and hands and the incidence increases after the age of 40 years, to a peak in the elderly. Metastasis is rare.

Treatment of BCC skin cancer involves surgical excision or radiotherapy and cure is expected in 95% of patients. Rarely, cytotoxic therapy may be given as palliation in metastatic disease.

CANCER IN THE YOUNG

Although the incidence of cancer increases with advancing age, when it occurs in the young it can have particularly

6.1 CHILDHOOD CANCERS AND PARENTAL SMOKING

- There is increasing evidence that parental smoking, particularly cigarette smoking, is associated with increased risk of childhood cancers of various types. Approximately 13% of these cancers might be attributable to parental smoking.
- Hypotheses concerning mechanisms by which sperm might be affected by constituents of cigarette smoke have been suggested, but have not yet been proved (Sorahan et al., 1997).

devastating outcomes. These may adversely effect the individual's psycho-socio-physical development. There is increasing evidence that parental smoking habits are a causative feature in childhood cancer. This has implications for the health promotion work of nurses, who should encourage young men and women to give up smoking using appropriate supportive programmes.

Malignant disease in adolescence

The life-threatening nature of cancer and prolonged treatment schedules with their unpleasant adverse effects can cause profound difficulties for individuals at this vulnerable stage in their lives. Developmental achievement of the following may be incomplete or delayed:

- Positive adult self-image because of alopecia and other adverse effects of therapy.
- Ability to adopt adult intimate relationships because of alopecia and other adverse effects and social isolation.
- Independence from family because of therapy-induced continuing dependency.
- Physical sexual maturation because of chemotherapy or radiotherapy damage to gonads.
- Emotional control because of all of the above (may be expressed in depression and anxiety).

Nurses can help by recognising these difficulties and by ensuring that health professionals actively inspire hope and encourage the patient to identify his or her own coping strategies (Whyte and Smith, 1997).

KEY POINTS

- People have differing abilities to withstand the effects of carcinogens.
- Cytotoxic chemotherapy produces a high risk of teratogenic change so its use is contraindicated in the pregnant woman with a malignancy.
- Cytotoxic chemotherapeutic agents should be given intravenously with great care to avoid local tissue destruction.
- Malignant tumours that are initially asymptomatic and that metastasise early are generally associated with a poor prognosis.
- People should observe their skin moles regularly to detect changes in colour, size and surface texture; they should seek early help if changes occur.
- Evidence exists to link parental smoking with the incidence of childhood cancers.

MULTIPLE CHOICE QUESTIONS

Any or none of the following answers may be correct.

1. Malignant change in cells is associated with
   a. return of the cell to a more primitive state
   b. a series of changes affecting the DNA of the cells
   c. abnormal stimulation of proto-oncogenes and anti-oncogenes
   d. the effects of initiators and promoters
   e. the ability to spread through invasion and metastasis

2. Chemotherapeutic agents
   a. act by interrupting one or more phases of the cell cycle
   b. are usually given in combined regimes
   c. are used primarily in treatment of benign neoplasms
   d. are used in adjuvant or palliative treatment schedules
   e. generally destroy cells that are in the G0 phase of the cell cycle

3. Commonly occurring adverse effects of cytotoxic drug therapy include
   a. development of resistance to the drug's actions
   b. damage to the fetus in early pregnancy
   c. increased feeling of wellbeing
   d. maintenance of bone marrow function
   e. nausea and vomiting

4. Alkylating agents are used in chemotherapeutic regimes
   a. to modify DNA and/or RNA
   b. although they are used rarely
   c. because they form cross-linkages between strands of nucleic acids
   d. despite adverse effects such as pulmonary fibrosis and kidney damage
   e. as they can affect many types of cancers because their action is not cell cycle specific

5. The antibiotics used in chemotherapy
   a. may be used to treat infection caused by myelosuppression
   b. are too toxic to be used in the treatment of infections
   c. act by converting malignant neoplasms to benign ones
   d. cause tissue destruction on extravasation
   e. include streptomycin and amoxycillin

6. Folinic acid may be given as part of a chemotherapeutic regime because it
   a. can be given orally
   b. inhibits an enzyme necessary for the production of DNA
   c. helps to prevent cancer cells from replicating
   d. aids recovery of purine and pyrimidine synthesis in non-malignant cells treated with high-dose methotrexate
   e. can enhance the effect of 5-fluorouracil

7. Biological response modifiers may be used in one or more of the following ways:
   a. to counteract damage to erythropoiesis centres
   b. as an alternate repair mechanism for mutated DNA in malignant cells
   c. increasingly in future, in ways that increase the specificity of their action
   d. to stimulate production of killer T cells, which recognise and destroy cancer cells
   e. to stimulate production of white blood cells, so increasing the body's resistance to infection

8. Malignant tumours of the testis
   a. are generally associated with a good prognosis
   b. commonly arise from germ cells
   c. may be associated with non-descent of the testis
   d. must be treated with chemotherapy as surgery is ineffective
   e. usually respond to orchidectomy with radiotherapy or chemotherapy

9. Breast cancer
   a. is the commonest cancer in women in the West
   b. may be oestrogen-dependent
   c. is not sensitive to chemotherapy
   d. can be treated with adjuvant chemotherapy
   e. has a poor prognosis if treated in stage 1 of the disease

10. Tamoxifen
    a. is a type of hormone antagonist
    b. increases the response of cells to oestrogen
    c. acts by blocking the response of cells to oestrogen
    d. can be used in palliative treatment of some breast cancers
    e. may cause menopause-like symptoms

REFERENCES

Autier P, Dore J, Gefeller O, Cesarini J, Lejeune F, Koelmel K, Lienard D, Kleesberg U, for the EORTC Melanoma Cooperative Group. Melanoma risk and residence in sunny areas *Br J Cancer* 1997; **76**:1521-1524.

Bleiberg H. Antiemetic treatment: what have we achieved? *Top Support Care Oncol* 1996; **20**:9-10.

Bodmer W. The somatic evolution of cancer. *J R Coll Phys London* 1997; **31**:82-89

Chang H-T, Mok K-T, Tzeng W-S. Induction of intraarterial chemotherapy for T4 breast cancer through an implantable port-catheter system. *Am J Clin Oncol* 1997; **20**:493-499.

D'Andrea G, Seidman A. Docetaxel and paclitaxel in breast cancer therapy: present status and future prospects. *Semin Oncol* 1997; **24(suppl)**:27-43.

Darby S, Roman E. Leukaemia and ionising radiation. *Biol Sci Rev* 1995; **7**:11-13.

Darling D, Tarin D. The spread of cancer in the human body. *New Sci* 1990; **127**:50-53.

Donnellan P, Crown J. The development of docetaxel in non-small cell lung cancer – docetaxel in new combinations and new schedules. *Semin Oncol* 1997; **24(suppl 14)**:14-18.

Espat NJ, Moldawar LL, Copeland EM. Cytokine-mediated alterations in host metabolism prevents nutritional repletion in cachectic cancer patients. *J Surg Oncol* 1995; **58**:77-81.

Hollinger M. *Introduction to pharmacology.* Washington: Taylor and Francis, 1997.

Holmes S. *Cancer chemotherapy, 2nd ed.* Dorking: Asset Books, 1997.

Hortobagyi G. Introduction: taxoids and the management of breast cancer. *Semin Oncol* 1997; **24(suppl 13)**:1-2.

Howell A. New endocrine treatment strategies. *Eur J Cancer Care* 1996; **5(suppl)**:2-3.

Jaskiewicz J. Quick recall: oesophageal cancer. *Eur Cancer News* 1994; **7**:1-5.

Jatoi I. Breast cancer: a systemic or local disease? *Am J Clin Oncol* 1997; **20**:536-539.

Klopvitch PM, Clancy BJ. Sexuality and the adolescent with cancer. *Semin Oncol* 1985; **1**:42-48.

Knowles G, Jodrell D. Recent developments in adjuvant chemotherapy for colorectal cancer. *Eur J Cancer Care* 1997; **6**:18-22.

Laffer U, Metzger U, Aberhard P. Long term results of single course of adjuvant intraportal chemotherapy for colorectal cancer. *Lancet* 1995; **345**:349-353.

Leonard R. The endocrine environment. *Eur J Cancer Care* 1996; **5(suppl)**:1-2.

Lilley L, Aucker R, Albanese J. *Pharmacology and the nursing process.* St. Louis: Mosby, 1996.

Lind J. Tumour cell growth and cell kinetics. *Semin Oncol Nurs* 1992; **8**:3-9.

McMillan S. Carcinogenesis. *Semin Oncol Nurs* 1992; **8**:10-19.

Neal A, Hoskin P. *Clinical oncology – a textbook for students.* London: Edward Arnold, 1997.

Nowak T, Handford A. *Essentials of pathophysiology.* Dubuque: Brown, 1994.

Park JO, Chung HC, Cho JY, Rha SY, You NC, Kim JH, Noh SH, Kim CB, Min JS, Kim BS, Roh JK. Retrospective comparison of infusional 5-fluoruracil, doxirubicin, and mitomycin-C combination chemotherapy versus palliative therapy in treatment of advanced gastric cancer. *Am J Clin Oncol* 1997; **20**:484-489.

Price S, Wilson L. *Pathophysiology – clinical concepts of disease processes, 4th ed.* St. Louis: Mosby, 1992.

Rees G, Goodman S, Bullimore J. *Cancer in practice.* Oxford: Butterworth Heinemann, 1993.

Risch HA, Jain M, Marrett LD, Howe CR. Dietary fat intake and risk of epithelial ovarian cancer. *J Natl Cancer Inst* 1994; **86**:1409-1415.

Skeel RT, Lachant NA, eds. *Handbook of cancer chemotherapy, 4th ed.* Boston: Little, Brown and Co, 1995.

Sorahan T, Prior P, Lancashire R, Faux S, Hulten M, Peck I, Stewart A. Childhood cancer and parental use of tobacco: deaths from 1971-1976. *Br J Cancer* 1997; **76**:1525-1531.

Souhami R, Moxham J. *Textbook of medicine.* Edinburgh: Churchill Livingstone, 1990.

Stevens A, Lowe J. *Pathology.* London: Mosby, 1995.

The Health of the Nation. *Key Area Handbook: Cancers.* London: Department of Health, 1995.

Van de Velde C. Preoperative chemotherapy in operable breast cancer: the influence of timing FEC in relation to surgery. *Drugs* 1993; **45(suppl)**:31-37.

Whyte F, Smith L. A literature review of adolescence and cancer. *Eur J Cancer Care* 1997, **6**:137-146.

7 Sylvia Prosser
DRUGS AND PSYCHOLOGICAL DISORDERS

INTRODUCTION

A person's mood may be altered pathologically in two main ways, elation or depression, each of which are extremes of states of mind experienced in everyday life. During the course of normal living, the individual experiences feelings of satisfaction or being positive when life goes well. At such times, problems seem less, energy abounds and people often seem pleasant and cooperative. At other, less happy times, energy levels seem low and the individual feels negative about life. The neurotransmitters that have been found to be of key importance in influencing mood are collectively termed biogenic amines, and influence the pattern of production of action potentials in the central nervous system neurons that produce them. Examples of these amines are dopamine and the monoamines serotonin and noradrenaline.

DISORDERS OF MOOD

Mood disorders may be subdivided into those involving one state, either elation or depression, which are termed unipolar mood disorders, and those involving oscillation between two opposite mood states, the so-called bipolar disorders. The external evidence of how a person feels is termed the affect, so mood disorders may manifest with the sufferer having either a flattened affect (depression), or appearing 'high', with an exalted mood state (mania). Specific neuroanatomical changes are associated with unipolar and bipolar mood disorders, respectively (Soares and Mann, 1997). Unipolar depression is described as being associated with decreased size of the frontal lobe, cerebellum, caudate and putamen. Bipolar disease has been associated with enlargement of the third ventricle, and reduced size of the cerebellum and possibly also of the temporal lobe.

DEPRESSION

The commonest unipolar mood disorder is depression. This may have no specific cause (endogenous depression) or may develop as a direct result of emotional trauma (reactive depression). It has been suggested that 6–10% of the Western population will experience a depressive illness at some time in their lives, and of these, 15–20% of sufferers will attempt suicide (Bennett, 1994). Mental illness was initially not well understood but, as biomedical knowledge increased, it became evident that depression involved disruption of a range of central nervous system monoamine receptors, and that the state also involved structures within the endocrine system that modulated the stress response: the hypothalamus and adrenal gland. The hypothalamic–pituitary pathway is responsible for mental arousal as a response to physical challenge and is maintained by mobilisation of the endocrine system. Increased secretion of cortisol enables the response to be sustained. The neurons in the hypothalamus that initiate this chain reaction are controlled by structures in the locus coeruleus that secrete noradrenaline. It therefore seems that depression may be an abnormal response to the stress reaction.

The effects of a severe disruption of the neurotransmitter system produces the state of clinical depression, in which the sufferer has an overall feeling of hopelessness and an inability to feel happiness or a sense of self-worth. Thought processes slow, producing 'poverty of thought', and sleep may be disturbed, with characteristic patterns of early waking and inability to return to sleep. Appetite may be reduced and the individual may exhibit psychomotor retardation, a pattern of slow physical movement and response. Constipation may be present and the sex drive is frequently diminished. Some depressed people have different behaviour patterns and may eat and sleep to excess. A patient may suffer depression in association with anxiety, in which case the medication needs to incorporate an anxiolytic to produce a calming effect as well as having antidepressant properties.

Pathophysiology

In the 1930s, it was discovered that the use of amphetamines raised the mood in sufferers of mild endogenous depression. Amphetamines lengthen the time that noradrenaline remains in the nerve synapses. This happens because noradrenaline stored at the nerve endings is released in increased amounts, and its re-uptake into the nerve endings is inhibited by impeding the chemical monoamine pump (**Fig. 7.1**).

Doctors treating hypertensive patients with reserpine in the 1950s inadvertently found another of the keys to understanding the neurobiological state that produces depression. Reserpine was known to deplete monoamine transmitters in the brain (Kolb and Whishaw, 1996) and it was noticed that patients receiving reserpine for hypertension became depressed. This suggested that the monoamine transmitters were responsible for maintaining mood.

Also in the 1950s, some patients being treated with iproniazid for tuberculosis were noted to be relieved of pre-existing depressive symptoms. Iproniazid was known to inactivate monoamine oxidase, an enzyme that enhances the breakdown of noradrenaline and serotonin. It was logical to suggest that depression was associated with depletion of noradrenaline and serotonin at the nerve endings in the brain.

Pharmacological management

Pharmacological treatment of depression involves the use of medication that affects the availability of amines within the brain synapses; specifically, the drugs prevent the breakdown of monoamines such as serotonin or noradrenaline so that their concentrations at nerve endings is increased. If the monoamines are allowed to accumulate at the nerve endings, then the sensations of depression diminish.

Some monoamine oxidase inhibitors maintain the levels of noradrenaline and serotonin by stopping the breakdown of these transmitter substances when they have re-entered the nerve endings. Thus, more amines are available for release to the synapses. Others forms of monoamine oxidase inhibitors (MAOIs) affect the ratio of noradrenaline to serotonin taken up into the nerve endings. Some agents inhibit only the uptake of serotonin (such as clomipramine) or noradrenaline (such as viloxazine). Some MAOIs such as mianserin do not work in this way at all, but seem to influence the feedback mechanism to the nerve ending; they cause secretion of the neurotransmitter to increase by inhibiting the negative feedback communication system that would otherwise suppress secretion of the neurotransmitter.

Antidepressants commonly have a delayed therapeutic onset of 1–2 weeks, which may be caused by the time taken to override the feedback mechanisms at the nerve endings (Laurence and Bennett, 1992). This poses a problem when caring for people with depression, because during this 'lag phase', they will think they are getting no benefit from their medication. Because this comes on top of the existing feelings of hopelessness, such patients may discontinue their medication before it has a chance to improve their feelings. As volition increases, there may be an increased risk of a suicide attempt, as a measure of energy has returned although the sufferer's mood remains bleak for a further period. Because of their effect in stimulating cerebral function, antidepressants may provoke epilepsy in people with organic brain damage, those with a familial tendency to epilepsy or those who have had electroconvulsive therapy in the past.

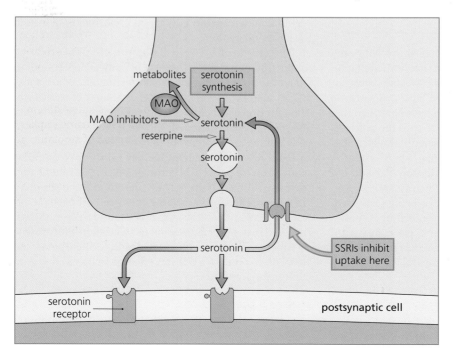

Fig 7.1 Site of action of specific serotonin reuptake inhibitors and monoamine oxidase inhibitors. SSRIs: specific serotonin reuptake inhibitors; MAO, monoamine oxidase. (From Page 1997, with permission.)

Tricyclic antidepressants

Tricyclic antidepressants (which inhibit the amine pumps returning the neurotransmitters to storage in the nerve endings) are well absorbed into body tissues, may become concentrated in the myocardium and are metabolised in the liver.

Drugs that inhibit the amine pumps tend to produce side effects; these are described as antimuscarinic. Muscarine is a substance that enters certain nerve endings when some types of poisonous fungi are ingested. Antimuscarinic effects are those of blockade of these particular receptors, notably the acetylcholine receptors, in the body. This gives rise to symptoms such as dry mouth, blurred vision, raised intraocular pressure and obstruction of the bladder neck, with subsequent difficulty in initiating micturition. Additionally, tricyclic antidepressants can cause postural hypotension, impotence in men and tremors and alterations of cardiac rhythm, so patients need to receive careful advice before they commence medication. Because of their toxic effects, these drugs may be lethal if the patient takes them in overdose. Tricyclic antidepressants tend to have varying degrees of sedative effect, which makes them useful for the patient with anxiety and depression. An example of a tricyclic antidepressant is dothiepin hydrochloride, given in doses commencing at 75 mg/day and increasing to 150 mg/day. If taken at night, the sedative agent has a beneficial effect upon the patient's sleep pattern.

Clomipramine hydrochloride is an example of a tricyclic antidepressant that has less marked sedative effects and that more selectively blocks serotonin re-uptake. A daily dose of 10 mg is given initially; this is increased to between 30 and 150 mg/day. Like dothiepin, clomipramine can be given in a single dose at bedtime to promote a better sleep pattern (Walker, 1996). Similar side effects to those of dothiepin may be experienced, and in both cases, patients should be warned against taking these agents in conjunction with alcohol. The patient should not drive or operate machinery as vigilance is reduced.

Monoamine oxidase inhibitors

Monoamine oxidases are a group of enzymes that play a role in the metabolism of serotonin, noradrenaline, dopamine and adrenaline. Correspondingly, they take their effect at adrenergic and dopaminergic nerve endings. The enzymes are found in brain cells and in peripheral nerve endings that use adrenaline, noradrenaline or dopamine as transmitters. Because this group of drugs inhibits breakdown of the neurotransmitters concerned with maintenance of mood, they produce an antidepressant effect. However, because additionally they influence a range of nerve endings within the sympathetic nervous system, numerous potentially dangerous side effects may occur. The sympathomimetic effect can involve promotion of a feeling of wellbeing and increased energy, which is helpful

for the depressed patient, but psychosis may result from overadministration or in a susceptible individual. Because this class of drugs enhances the effects of the sympathetic nervous system, a potentially lethal hypertensive crisis may occur if any concurrent sympathomimetics (such as amphetamines, which liberate stored noradrenaline) are taken. In addition, if the patient has a diet that is rich in amines, a hypertensive crisis can be provoked. For this reason, people taking MAOIs are warned to avoid a variety of foods, including pickles; cheese, which is converted into tyramine; broad beans, which contain the adrenaline precursor dopa; and wine, which contains tyramine (Laurence and Bennett, 1992). Severe headache, hypertension and bradycardia are experienced in hypertensive crisis. Convulsions in people with a family history of epilepsy may occur in those taking MAOIs. If taken in overdose, MAOIs can induce hypomanic states, extreme fluctuations of blood pressure and unconsciousness.

An example of an MAOI is phenelzine, which may be prescribed for patients who have failed to respond to other antidepressants for reactive depression (Walker, 1996). A dose of 15–30 mg three times daily may be given. Once the depressive symptoms have been controlled, the patient may be prescribed a maintenance dose of 15 mg on alternate days. Because of the risk of postural hypotension, phenelzine is not suitable for elderly patients, and the preparation is also not suitable for children. Phenelzine potentiates the effects of pethidine, morphine, adrenaline and amphetamine. The interaction with dopamine and levodopa make it unsuitable for patients being treated for Parkinson's disease (Walker, 1996).

Tranylcypromine is an MAOI that is sometimes prescribed for adult patients with depression complicated by phobic symptoms. A dose of 10 mg is given twice daily, in the morning and afternoon. Once the symptoms are stable, a maintenance dose of 10 mg daily is given. Sleep disturbances may trouble patients receiving this medication.

Selective serotonin re-uptake inhibitors

This group of antidepressants constitutes a new development in the treatment of depression. As the name implies, the drugs work by potentiating the action of serotonin at the nerve endings. Because of the distribution of the serotonin transmitting nerve endings, selective serotonin re-uptake inhibitors (SSRIs) seem to have fewer unwanted side effects, and are safer than tricyclics and MAOIs when taken in overdose. Sedation is not produced, and so SSRIs are helpful for patients suffering depression without symptoms of anxiety. A popular medication at present is fluoxetine, which is prescribed as a dose of 20 mg daily for depression. In the same dosage, fluoxetine is useful in the treatment of obsessive compulsive disorders, as the drug seems to produce insouciance (a 'carefree' mood). Eating disorders have been associated with disruption of adrenergic, serotonergic and opioid transmitter systems in the central nervous system. In larger doses (60 mg daily), fluoxetine is used for the treatment of patients with bulimia nervosa. The use of this preparation in children has not yet been sufficiently documented to allow its use for this age group. Fluoxetine is metabolised by the liver and excreted by the kidneys. Its removal from the body is a lengthy process, which has to be taken into account if medication is changed to another family of antidepressants; when administered over a prolonged period, the active drug will still be present for weeks (Walker, 1996). Patients need to be advised that, should hypersensitivity reactions (rash, urticaria, bronchospasm) occur, they need to discontinue the medication and seek medical help. Some patients develop headaches caused by the effects of serotonin as a vasodilator and, in some patients, gastrointestinal disturbances may occur.

MANIA: A DISORDER OF HEIGHTENED AFFECT

Mania is characterised by marked elevation of mood, resulting in inappropriate elation and impaired judgement. There may be a perception of being invincible, or of being in possession of special powers, coupled with extreme over-excitability. It is thought that mania results from overstimulation of the noradrenaline transmitter system, so treatment is aimed at reducing this stimulation. Mania may develop in patients who have been taking antidepressants such as MAOIs or tricyclics, or as a result of levodopa therapy for Parkinson's disease. Patients with severe episodes of mania require neuroleptic therapy (see below). Promazine may be given orally, or haloperidol intramuscularly.

Pathophysiology

The exact pathophysiology of mania and the mode of action of the neuroleptics used are not well understood, but it is known that haloperidol is a strong and specific blocker of the dopamine receptor sites in the brain. Study of manic patients in the 1940s showed that their urine contained elevated levels of urea. Experimental use of lithium, initially to correct the urinary abnormality, was found to quieten the mental state. Lithium appears to work via nerve transmitters in a mechanism mediated by cyclic AMP. This compound acts as a metabolic building block for ATP and also acts as a biochemical messenger within cells.

Pharmacological management

Lithium is administered in doses of between 0.2 and 2.0 g daily, and it is readily absorbed via the gastrointestinal tract. The dose is monitored carefully and adjusted to provide a therapeutic plasma level of between 0.6 and 1.2 mmol/l, 12 hours after the most recent dose taken. Because of the small size of the molecule and its solubility in water, lithium rapidly diffuses throughout body tissues, but it is taken up more readily in the brain, bones and thyroid. Patients should keep to the same brand of the drug to maintain maximal control of the plasma levels. Lithium moves within the body compartments in a manner similar to sodium, and its excretion is related to sodium levels: if sodium is depleted, lithium is retained. In order to obtain a therapeutic effect, the dose of lithium has to approach levels at which it is toxic, so patients receiving this preparation require close monitoring for toxic effects, and care is needed in situations in which body sodium is depleted, such as dehydration from excessive diuretic therapy or gastrointestinal disorder.

The toxic plasma level of lithium is reached at 2.0 mmol/l. At this level, the patient may experience slight nausea and diarrhoea. Lithium is slow to leave the body and, as the plasma levels increase, central nervous system dysfunction becomes evident, with tremor, dizziness, tinnitus, unsteadiness, blurred vision, impaired speech and deteriorating consciousness levels. Fatal hypotension, disordered cardiac rhythm and renal failure may develop.

Patients who have been taking lithium as long-term therapy (over 3–5 years) risk damage to the metabolically active cells of the nephron, and may also develop hypothyroidism. Those caring for patients receiving long-term lithium must realise the need for regular screening of thyroid and renal function, and patients need to be alert to the early signs of lithium toxicity. Lithium may be stopped rapidly, although manic symptoms may recur around a fortnight later. There is a risk of potentiating the effects of any neuroleptic therapy taken concurrently. If a patient takes non-steroidal anti-inflammatory drugs, the effect of lithium is enhanced because excretion of lithium is reduced. Administration of lithium during pregnancy can cause cardiac abnormalities and goitre in the fetus. Because of the sodium and water shifts that take place in pregnancy, the lithium levels of the mother may become unstable.

ANXIETY AND AGITATION

Anxiety is part of the natural arousal response, involving activation of the sympathetic nervous system to prepare the body for 'fright, fight or flight'. Activation of the sympathetic nervous system causes tachycardia; bronchodilatation; increase of transmission of nerve action potentials and therefore tremor; constriction of the vasculature to the alimentary tract and sensations of faintness, nausea, sweating and skin pallor caused by diversion of blood flow to the brain, heart and skeletal muscles at the expense of skin capillaries. Because of the increase in cerebral blood flow, the individual feels ill at ease. Secretion of adrenaline reinforces the vasopressor effect of the arousal response; if the stimulus persists, cortisol will be produced in increased amounts by the adrenal cortex, and the blood sugar and free lipid levels will be elevated to provide sufficient muscle fuel for possible rapid flight. In addition, the immune response may be diminished because of the raised cortisol levels in those experiencing a sustained stress response (see **Fig. 7.2**).

Pathophysiology

Anxiety disorders occur when the individual experiences extreme anxiety for no rational reason. Panic disorder affects 1–2% of the population (Carlson, 1991). The sufferer feels extreme anxiety and, between attacks, feels anxious lest the panic state return. This anxiety may develop into a phobic state, for example claustrophobia. The tendency to panic disorder may be genetically transmitted and appears to have a biochemical basis, in that panic disorder can be precipitated by raised levels of lactic acid or carbon dioxide. Positron emission tomography has been used to examine brain activity during panic attacks. Before the attack, the activity of the parahippocampal gyrus increases, and during a panic attack, the anterior portion of the temporal lobe shows increased activity.

Pharmacological management

Pharmacological treatment of anxiety disorders involves the use of anxiolytic preparations. The 'fright–flight' symptoms can be treated by giving preparations that block the sympathetic β-adrenergic response, for example propanolol capsules 40 mg 1–3 times daily. The benzodiazepines are effective in reducing anxiety symptoms at doses that do not cause sedation. This group of preparations bind to γ-aminobutyric acid (GABA) receptors on nerve cell membranes and inhibit cerebral function. Benzodiazepines may work as anxiolytics by altering dopamine and noradrenaline transmission in addition to modifying the effect of cerebral serotonin (Bennett, 1994). The benzodiazepines are lipid soluble and therefore well absorbed into the brain when taken orally. There is evidence to suggest that people who have personalities that are particularly timid may have a decreased number of benzodiazepine-sensitive receptors in their brains. If benzodiazepine-sensitive receptors are present in the brain, then it is likely that some naturally occurring substance, which normally binds to these receptors, is insufficiently produced in people with anxious personalities. Treatment of anxiety-related disorders frequently involves psychotherapy in addition to drug treatment. Panic attacks are often treated with tricyclic or monoamine oxidase antidepressants rather than the benzodiazepines, which are not particularly effective in such conditions.

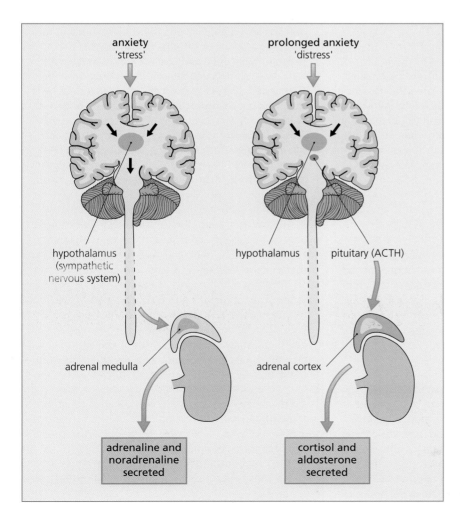

Fig 7.2 Acute and chronic anxiety. ACTH, adrenocorticotrophic hormone.

OBSESSIVE–COMPULSIVE DISORDERS

These are disabling states in which the sufferer is unable to stop thinking certain thoughts and undertaking particular ritualised actions. The person with obsessive–compulsive disorder (OCD) has insight into the uselessness of the thoughts and actions, but remains unable to break from the cycle of completing them. Obsessive–compulsive disorder often starts in young adults and affects about 2% of the population. Obsessions may centre around cleanliness, counting, checking that an action has been done or avoiding a particular activity (such as not looking in mirrors). Obsessive–compulsive disorder appears to be associated with Tourette's syndrome, which causes the sufferer to repeat involuntary actions such as a movement or an exclamation, and appears to have a genetic component (Carlson, 1991).

Pathophysiology

Positron emission tomography scanning studies have indicated that the frontal lobes, caudate nucleus and cingulate gyri of people with OCD have increased glucose metabolism levels. The neurotransmitter serotonin has been found to mediate washing, cleaning and danger-avoidance behaviours.

Pharmacological management

Obsessive–compulsive disorder is associated with alteration in cerebral serotonin metabolism, and the pharmacological treatment of OCD therefore involves the use of the antidepressant agents clomipramine, 100–150 mg daily (a larger dose than for depression), fluoxetine, 20–60 mg daily, or fluvoxamine, 100–200 mg daily. These drugs act by blocking serotonin re-uptake at synapses, and thus diminish the repetitive behaviours.

BIPOLAR DISEASE: MANIC DEPRESSIVE DISORDER

In these conditions, the individual experiences oscillation between the two opposing mood states of mania and depression. The mood swings occur in regular cycles, commonly lasting several months each. Since the development of noninvasive imaging of the brain, a range of suggestions has been made related to the pathophysiological changes that occur in manic depressive illnesses.

Pathophysiology

Nuclear magnetic resonance spectroscopy has been used to identify increased levels of choline in the basal ganglia of patients with mood disorders. Patients with mood disorders may have altered metabolism of phospholipids and abnormal energy production in the frontal and temporal lobes (Soares and Mann, 1996). It has been suggested that there may be localised abnormalities of the metabolism of high-energy phosphates in the frontal lobes of the brains of patients with bipolar disorder (Kato et al., 1995). Others have associated the characteristic fluctuations in mood states with disorders of ion pump mechanisms within the neurons and have suggested that people with bipolar mood states have slower nerve conduction rates (El Mallakh et

PERSON CENTRED STUDY 1

Marjorie, a woman in her late thirties, held a job that she found challenging and rewarding. She had been subject intermittently to sudden lowering of mood, which she described as the mental equivalent of being let down rapidly in a lift, after which she felt anxious and inadequate. She had always tended to be a 'worrier'.

Marjorie was having a difficult time at work, and began to find that she was thinking about her job even when she was at home at the weekend, and that she tended to have unpleasant sensations in the pit of her stomach when this happened. She then began to wake quite early on work days, and would lie in bed feeling more and more anxious about the forthcoming day. One day when the alarm clock rang, she felt so afraid that she was unable to get out of bed. Being able to do nothing but cry, she was obviously unable to go to work. Her partner made an urgent appointment for her to visit the general practitioner who prescribed dothiepin. For about 2 weeks, Marjorie continued to feel extremely anxious and unable to cope. She felt lost and empty, the medication made her head feel 'muzzy' and her mouth was dry. It was difficult to read for any length of time because of blurring of vision and impaired concentration. After about a fortnight, she realised that a change had taken place.

It took several months before Marjorie was able to return to work, and it took considerable courage to do so. Gradually, her medication dose was reduced and then finally discontinued. Marjorie continued to receive counselling for some months after returning to work.

1. How might you explain Marjorie's abdominal symptoms?
2. Why did Marjorie's family doctor prescribe dothiepin, rather than fluoxetine?
3. What advice would Marjorie have been given when she was first prescribed her medication?

al., 1996). Although the precise biological basis of bipolar disorders remains obscure, there may be changes in the nerve communication pathways that regulate groups of neurotransmitter systems (Lachman and Papalos, 1995). As the groups affected control two opposing types of nerve activity, the result is a series of swings from one mood extreme to the other.

Pharmacological management

Lithium carbonate is prescribed to contain the symptoms of mania, and also to prevent the recurrence of depressive episodes. For treatment of the initial condition, one 450 mg tablet is usually given twice a day, and the dose is titrated to maintain a serum level of 0.5–1.5 mmol/l. Once the condition is brought under control, a maintenance dosage is given to achieve plasma levels of 0.5–1.0 mmol/l. For a discussion of the hazards of lithium therapy, see the section explaining the pharmacological management of mania (page 100).

For those patients who are unable to respond to lithium, carbamazepine may be given in an initial divided dose of 400 mg daily. The normal dosage range is up to 600 mg daily in divided doses, although as much as 1600 mg daily may be needed. Patients with bipolar disease should not receive antidepressants on any sustained basis as their use will provoke a recurrence of the manic state (Gelder *et al.,* 1994).

DISORDERS OF THINKING

In these conditions, neural dysfunction causes disordered thought processes. If the disease state advances, disorganisation of the personality may develop in addition to alteration of the mood.

SCHIZOPHRENIA AND ANTIPSYCHOTIC THERAPY

Schizophrenia produces a syndrome of disabling effects upon the sufferer. The condition may run a fluctuating course and is characterised by 'positive' and 'negative' symptoms. Positive symptoms include aggression, over-activity, delusions (misguided beliefs) and hallucinations (perceptions having no basis in reality). Negative symptoms encompass apathy and flattened affect (depression). The schizophrenic syndrome describes bizarre patterns of thought and perceptions for which no tangible predisposing causes can be found.

Emotions and mood are modulated within the limbic system, a series of structures that developed from the brainstem and spinal cord at the time when amphibians and reptiles were evolving. These areas therefore represent relatively ancient parts of the central nervous system. A triple-layered covering developed around and above the brainstem, and was originally named the 'limbic lobe' by anatomists. Interest in these structures grew and, because

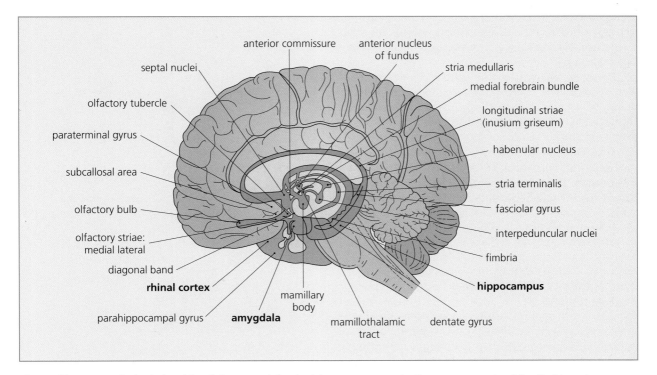

Fig 7.3 The anatomical relationship of the amygdala, the hippocampus and other components of the limbic system. (From Page 1997, with permission.)

of the proximity of the olfactory apparatus, the structures that make up the limbic system (**Fig. 7.3**) were named the rhinencephalon, literally 'smell-brain' (Kolb and Whishaw, 1996). The role of the limbic system remained obscure until 1937 when Papaz became interested in the origins of the emotions. In 1994, the role of structures within the limbic system related to the processing of memories was described (Petri and Mishkin, 1994). The rhinal cortex was found to process memory of objects, the hippocampus, spatial memory and the amygdala, emotional memory.

Pathophysiology

Study of the brains of schizophrenia sufferers using magnetic resonance imaging (MRI) and computerised tomography (CT scanning) in addition to post-mortem dissection and histological analysis have demonstrated the presence of a range of structural abnormalities. Post-mortem examinations indicated that the brains of people who had been schizophrenic weighed less than normal, and that the intracerebral ventricles tended to be enlarged. The tissue of the prefrontal cortex and the parahippocampal gyri were thinner than usual. Kolb and Whishaw (1996) found disorganisation of the arrangement of the neurons of the brains of schizophrenic people, with loss of parallel alignment of the nerve cells (**Fig. 7.4**). These structural anomalies were described in people of all ages past the stages of embryonic development. Studies of twins, one of each pair of whom suffered from schizophrenia, showed different patterns of activation of the prefrontal cortex during card-sorting activities, but not during other psychological tests. It appears, therefore, that there is an alteration of the structure and the function of the prefrontal cortex of people with schizophrenia.

The nerve cells of the prefrontal cortex use dopamine as a neurotransmitter. Interestingly, drugs such as cocaine, levodopa and amphetamines, which enhance transmission at the dopamine synapses, are capable of producing psychotic symptoms similar to those of paranoid schizophrenia.

Theories as to the cause of schizophrenia are associated with the functioning of the dopamine transmitters. The presence of increased numbers of dopamine D_2 receptors in the brains of schizophrenic patients has led to a range of theories of how schizophrenia is caused.

Two subtypes of schizophrenia appear to exist. Type 1 or 'acute' schizophrenia is characterised by delusions, hallucinations and thought disorder, so-called 'positive' symptoms, which could be associated with abnormal dopamine neuron activity. Type 2 or 'chronic' schizophrenia has 'negative' features such as flattened affect and poverty of thought, which could be associated with alteration to the architecture of the cerebral tissue. These theories are strengthened by the condition of chronic amphetamine abusers, who tend to display type 1 symptoms, but to have no structural change demonstrable within their cerebral tissue.

Pharmacological management

Pharmacological treatment for schizophrenia consists of two main approaches: treatment of the acute episode (the 'positive' symptoms) and maintenance therapy to keep the patient in a stable state of remission. Neuroleptics, also called antipsychotic drugs, are drugs that help to control the symptoms of schizophrenia by quietening mood and emotions. They therefore tend to flatten the affect, producing feelings of indifference and slowing psychomotor activity.

The preparations that help in the treatment of acute schizophrenia tend to be those that antagonise the

7.1 POSSIBLE CAUSES OF SCHIZOPHRENIA

Too much dopamine being produced by the nerve cell. The dopamine receptors are hypersensitive, with normal or excessive amounts of dopamine being secreted at the synapses.

Dopamine at the synapses is not being properly antagonised (inactivated).

Some malfunction of the controlling feedback mechanism.

An imbalance between the activity of the dopamine neurons and their cortical antagonists, which secrete the neurotransmitter glutamate.

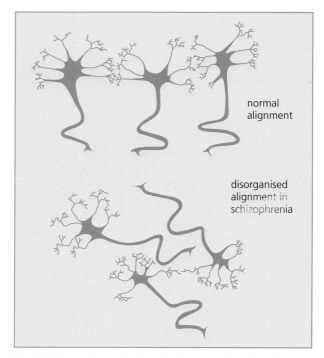

normal alignment

disorganised alignment in schizophrenia

Fig 7.4 Alteration to brain cell alignment in schizophrenia.

dopamine receptors in the frontal and temporal lobes of the brain. The main groups of drugs include pheno-thiazines such as chlorpromazine, 50–1000 mg daily; promazine 40–800 mg daily and thioridazine 75–200 mg in divided doses, which are useful for patients with 'positive' symptoms. Thioxanthines such as flupenthixol may be given as an oil-based depot injection of 20 mg/ml or as tablets in divided doses of 1–3 mg daily. Flupenthixol has additional antidepressive properties, which make it useful for 'negative' symptoms of schizophrenia. Butyrophenones such as haloperidol may be given orally or intramuscularly in variable doses according to the severity of the mental symptoms. The oral dose ranges from 1.5 to 20 mg daily. Emergency treatment of severely ill patients normally ranges from 5 to 10 mg haloperidol intramuscularly, although grossly disturbed patients may need doses of 100–120 mg daily. The 'active' or positive symptoms are easier to remedy than the 'negative' lethargic ones. The aim is to stabilise and maintain the patient on the lowest continuing dose that produces effective results; this is preferably an oral dose and is usually around 3–10 mg haloperidol daily.

Haloperidol is used for a range of mental disorders: as treatment for psychoses in schizophrenic patients and also for the treatment of behavioural problems such as aggression and hyperactivity in people with learning difficulties; for agitation states in elderly patients and to control restlessness and impulsive behaviour in Gilles de la Tourette's syndrome. Haloperidol may also be prescribed for children with hyperactivity or aggressive states. The dosage of haloperidol varies according to the individual's symptoms, but ranges from 1.5 to 3 mg twice or three times daily for adults with moderate disorder. Severely disturbed patients may receive 3–5 mg twice or three times daily. Children may receive a maintenance dose of 0.025–0.05 mg/kg body weight per day. The preparation may be given orally as tablets or syrup, or by intramuscular or intravenous injection. In doses of 0.5–1 mg daily, haloperidol is used to treat nausea and vomiting, and in parenteral doses of 3–15 mg daily, it is helpful in the control of persistent hiccoughs.

Because the symptoms of schizophrenia include deluded thought processes, sometimes complicated by the fixation that a third party is intent on harming the patient, it is difficult to obtain the cooperation of the patient in taking neuroleptic medication. Approximately 40% of schizophrenic patients do not take the tablets they are prescribed (Laurence and Bennett, 1992). For these reasons, the preparations may be administered within oil-based depot preparations that require intermittent injection every 1–4 weeks, often given by the community psychiatric nurse. The agents commonly given include fluphenazine, haloperidol and flupenthixol.

Newer drugs used in the treatment of schizophrenia include antipsychotics that selectively influence dopamine or serotonin transmission. Clozapine blocks D_1 and D_2

dopamine and serotonin$_2$ receptors and has been found to be useful in the treatment of patients with schizophrenia that had been previously unresponsive to treatment. The drug is expensive and has unpleasant side effects such as sedation, postural hypotension, excessive salivation and fever. Weight gain and agranulocytosis may also occur. Because of the risk of side effects, the patient is initially prescribed small doses and these are then gradually adjusted upwards, usually to within the range of 200–450 mg daily.

Risperidone is another of the newer antipsychotic agents that may be used for its strong serotonin$_2$ blockade and antagonism of dopamine D_2 receptors. It is effective for the control of positive and negative schizophrenic symptoms, and also for the symptoms of depression, guilt and anxiety that may accompany schizophrenia. It produces blockade of α-adrenergic receptors, so can produce postural hypotension. Additionally, sleep disturbances, anxiety and headaches may occur in association with risperidone therapy (Larsen and Ashleigh, 1996).

Pharmacological treatment to maintain remission may include the use of haloperidol or fluphenazine, which can be given as a depot preparation 2–4 times per week. The drug dosage selected is the lowest that will achieve effective symptom control. The usual maintenance dose of fluphenazine is 12.5–100 mg, given every 2–5 weeks.

There are two types of dopamine receptor in the central nervous system: D_1 and D_2 receptors. In addition to existing in the limbic system, these are present in the vicinity of the hypothalamus, where endocrine releasing factors are secreted, and in the extrapyramidal motor tracts. When non-specific dopamine antagonists are used, the D_1 and D_2 receptors are affected indiscriminately, and endocrine dysfunction and extrapyramidal motor symptoms are produced.

Because of the problem of causing side effects by blocking the dopaminergic receptors, neuroleptic therapy, particularly chlorpromazine, tends to produce a spectrum of side effects. In the central nervous system, by its action upon the hypothalamus and reticular formation, where awareness states are modulated, chlorpromazine causes emotional quietening and a general state of indifference. Pain perception is reduced (Laurence and Bennett, 1992), and lethargy and sleepiness commonly occur. Chlorpromazine has a range of effects upon muscle functioning: in cases of pre-existing neurological damage, muscle spasticity may be reduced, but in large doses dystonia (excessive muscle contractility) is produced. Chlorpromazine has antiemetic properties and can be used within a symptom control regime to reduce hiccoughs or pruritus in palliative care contexts. Chlorpromazine blocks α-adrenoreceptors and the resulting loss of muscle tone in the vascular walls can produce postural hypotension. (This vasodilator property also makes chlorpromazine useful in promoting heat loss in cases of hyperthermia, as in malignant hyperpyrexia after anaesthesia; see Chapter 3 *Classes of drugs*.)

Extrapyramidal effects caused by the unwanted blockade of motor tracts include parkinsonism and tardive dyskinesia, which produces involuntary movements of the face, limbs and trunk. The altered mobility is thought to be associated with loss of the neurotransmitter GABA, the secretion of which is inhibited in patients receiving chronic neuroleptic therapy.

ALZHEIMER'S DISEASE: A DEGENERATIVE DISORDER OF MEMORY AND COGNITION

This condition, which is the commonest cause of dementia (Fujimoto and Shimomura, 1996), is not currently curable by pharmacological or other means. However, medication may be used to limit the symptoms of the disease, and clinical trials continue to search for ways of preventing or halting the progress of the dementia.

Alzheimer's disease is characterised by an insidious onset followed by a variable rate of deterioration of cognitive function. The earliest sign is short-term memory loss. This is caused by the impaired function of neurons in the cerebral cortex and hippocampus. The decrement in function is associated with a decrease in the production of acetylcholine in the brain, which is caused by a lack of the enzyme acetyltransferase. There appears to be a direct relationship between the extent of depletion of acetyltransferase and the loss of intellectual function. The reduction of other neurotransmitters such as somatostatin, noradrenaline, serotonin and the enzyme dopamine β-hydroxylase have been suggested as possible causes of the disease, but currently the major focus of investigation for pharmacological treatment of Alzheimer's disease is centred upon correcting the acetylcholine transmitter system (Drachman & Leber, 1997).

Pathophysiology

Post-mortem specimens from the brains of patients with Alzheimer's disease show the presence of abnormal proteins deposited in the cerebral tissues; β-amyloid plaques and neurofibrillary tangles produced by abnormal neurons alter the normal architecture of the brain. The presence of helical tau proteins impede the normal transmission pathways between neurons. There appears to be a correlation between the extent of the abnormal deposits and the degree of disability shown by the patient when alive (Fujimoto and Shimomura, 1996). A familial form of Alzheimer's disease has been identified in which the amyloid precursor gene on chromosomes 21 and 14 has mutated. The β-amyloid plaque formation appears to be accelerated by the presence of apolipoprotein E, which binds to the lesions. The likely pathological processes associated with Alzheimer's disease are summarised in **Figure 7.5**.

Patients with Alzheimer's disease tend to follow a slow and unremitting path of deterioration, commencing with short-term memory lapses (see **Case Study 7.2**), and finishing with virtually complete disability and death from infections such as stasis pneumonia. It is important to differentiate early Alzheimer's disease from treatable conditions such as depression. The prognosis for a patient with established Alzheimer's disease is variable, ranging between 2 and 20 years. The average life span from the commencement of the disease is around 8 years (Fujimoto and Shimomura, 1996). Medication must be given with caution to sufferers with Alzheimer's disease as they are susceptible to adverse influences upon the central nervous system.

Pharmacological management

Therapeutic treatment to slow or halt brain failure is at present experimental in nature. Trials are being conducted using metabolic enhancers to improve cerebral metabolism of oxygen and glucose; to increase metabolic enzyme efficiency in the brain; to potentiate dopamine and serotonin and to block α-adrenoceptors. The theory that depletion of acetylcholine is important in the pathogenesis of Alzheimer's disease has led to the development of substances that increase the concentration of acetylcholine at the synapses and increase the sensitivity of the acetylcholine receptors. Choline and lecithin (acetylcholine precursors) have been administered in an attempt to

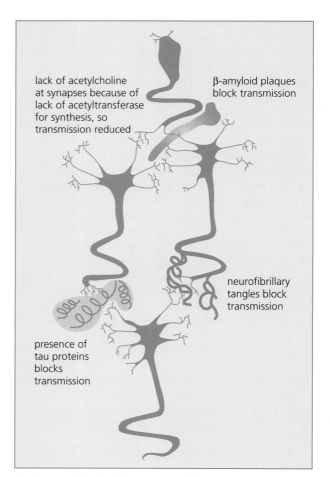

lack of acetylcholine at synapses because of lack of acetyltransferase for synthesis, so transmission reduced

β-amyloid plaques block transmission

neurofibrillary tangles block transmission

presence of tau proteins blocks transmission

Fig 7.5 Pathological changes in Alzheimer's disease.

increase intracerebral acetylcholine levels. Cholinesterase inhibitors such as physostigmine and tetrahydroaminoacridine (TCA or tacrine, 10 mg four times daily for 6 weeks) have been used to lengthen the dwell time of acetylcholine in the synapses, and they appear to produce some improvement in cognitive function. Unfortunately, TCA carries a risk of hepatic toxicity. The best results have been obtained by intracranial infusion, which carries its own specific risks.

Symptomatic treatment of Alzheimer's disease is more widely established than treatment to slow the disease progression. Antidepressants are prescribed for lowered mood states, and sedative antidepressants may help agitation and insomnia. If the patient is not agitated, SSRIs may be prescribed. Benzodiazepine hypnotics such as temazepam, 7.5 mg, are given for sleep disorders. Long-acting hypnotics

PERSON CENTRED STUDY 2

Edward was in his early fifties when those who knew him began to notice that he was becoming increasingly absent minded. At this point, Edward himself realised that he was forgetful, but attributed it to mental stress as the business he ran was in difficulties because of the financial recession. However, neither the business nor Edward's memory improved. The seriousness of the situation became clear when Edward made a series of judgmental errors that took his business to the verge of bankruptcy. Edward's family could no longer simply attribute his lapses to pressure of work. He now forgot what he was saying in the middle of sentences and sometimes forgot where he was trying to get to. Edward loved golf, but after he tried to play a shot with the club held upside down, his wife made him visit their family doctor. The doctor sent him to the nearest neurological centre for investigation to exclude organic brain disease. A computerised tomography scan demonstrated changes consistent with Alzheimer's disease, with atrophy of the cerebral cortex and dilatation of the intracerebral ventricles. He received some relief from his agitation from haloperidol 0.5 mg twice daily; temazepam 7.5 mg at night and his depression was helped by fluoxetine 20 mg daily.

1. How could you explain Edward's early symptoms of absent mindedness to his wife?
2. What pharmacological treatment may Edward have been prescribed in an attempt to halt the progress of the disease?
3. What information would Edward's wife be given about his prognosis?

are avoided as the medication has a tendency to accumulate and increase the risk of falls. Anxiolytics are helpful in controlling agitation, although the effects of excessive medication may mimic an exacerbation of the dementia. If the patient suffers from hallucinations, delusions or paranoia, antipsychotic therapy such as haloperidol, 0.5–1.0 mg, or fluphenazine may be prescribed. These may help the agitation and confusion that develops during the evening if they are given during the late afternoon or early evening. The progressive nature of Alzheimer's disease means that the lowest dose of medication that obtains the desired effect should always be given. Relatives need to be kept realistically aware that the aim of palliative treatment is to minimise the symptoms, but that symptom reduction does not mean that the condition has been halted or cured.

ATTENTION DEFICIT HYPERACTIVITY DISORDER (ADHD)

ADHD has a prevalence of 0.5–1.0% in the United Kingdom using the International Classification of Diseases criteria for hyperkinetic disorder (Taylor et al., 1991). It is a neurodevelopmental disorder that impacts upon the key areas of children's development. There are three areas of dysfunction: overactivity and restlessness, inattentiveness and distractibility, and impulsiveness and social disinhibition. Most cases of ADHD occur in otherwise normal, non-abusive families that are neither materially nor socially deprived.

Pathophysiology

The motor hyperactivity and decreased attention spans are probably attributable to no single cause. The following have been suggested as causes of ADHD: brain damage, genetic predisposition, dopamine deficiency, encephalitis, high levels of environmental lead and food hypersensitivity.

Pharmacological management

Treatment should always be multifaceted and individually tailored; drug treatment should never be used alone. Psychostimulants have become the mainstay of treatment in the United Kingdom and the USA; 75–85% of children benefit from their use. The most commonly used agent is methylphenidate, a controlled drug. The protocol starts with a dose of 5 mg per day and this is increased by 5 mg every 2 days until the usual effective dose of 20–40 mg per day is achieved. The maximum daily dose should not be more than 60–80 mg. The last dose should be given 4 hours before bedtime (Bramble and Pearch, 1997). Side effects are usually transient, involving appetite suppression, nausea, abdominal pain, nervousness, irritability and insomnia. Headaches and dizziness require blood pressure to be checked. Long-term effects on height and weight need to be regularly reviewed and, as the child moves into the peripubertal growth spurt, the effectiveness of the medication needs to be reassessed.

Contraindications to pharmacological treatment include psychosis, epilepsy, Gilles de la Tourette's syndrome and the child being a member of a chaotic, drug-abusing family. Other drugs in the psychostimulant class are **dexamphetamine** (at double the starting dose of methylphenidate) and **pemoline** (at four times the starting dose of methylphenidate). The action of all the drugs is to increase the release of noradrenaline and dopamine from neurons.

DRUGS USED TO CHANGE BEHAVIOUR RELATED TO EATING

Weight gain as a result of stored fat occurs when the energy store is enlarged because the intake of energy as food exceeds the output of energy as bodily work. Preparations that increase bodily work and in consequence the physiological energy needed and/or decrease the drive to eat are likely to produce catabolism of the energy stores and reduction of body mass. Therefore, preparations enhancing the effect of the sympathetic nervous system are likely to reduce body weight, although there are likely to be side effects of stimulation of the sympathetic nervous system. People suffering from eating disorders may be helped by taking pharmaceutical preparations to alter their drive to consume food.

APPETITE SUPPRESSION

Interest in appetite suppression by the use of medication was raised in the 1930s when it was noted that people taking amphetamines lost the desire to eat, although this effect, which originated from direct stimulus of the sympathetic nervous system, was lost after a few days. A range of preparations was developed in order to control appetite in those who had a strong medical need, but not the will power, to lose weight. It became evident that some of the preparations used to treat depression by raising mood and energy levels could also be used to influence eating in those who reduce their intake of energy.

Drugs used in the treatment of obesity tend to be short-lived in effectiveness and to produce a risk of abuse. Appetite suppressants may act centrally, by affecting catecholamine or serotonin neurotransmitters. They boost energy expenditure and reduce the drive to eat, thus putting the subject into a negative energy balance. There is interest in the possibility of identifying and developing the use of peptides such as leptin and satietin (Frederich *et al.*, 1995); these peptides are thought to control the body's fat content by a biofeedback system in which, once the 'ideal' fat content of the body is reached, fat is no longer deposited in the adipose tissues, but is removed from the body.

Peripheral agents used to produce weight loss act by impeding absorption from the gastrointestinal tract by inhibiting parts of the digestive enzyme cascade (see Chapter 14 *Drugs and gastrointestinal disorders*).

MIND-ALTERING DRUGS AND SUBSTANCE ABUSE

For generations, humans have been using chemicals that influence the way the mind works. Sometimes the aim of this use was medicinal, at other times it was to obtain interesting mental and physical sensations. The chemicals may be obtained from plants or fungi, or may be artificially synthesised; the active chemicals have been found to bind to specific nerve cell receptors, suggesting that similar substances must occur naturally in the body (**Fig. 7.6**).

One of the oldest of these substance groups are the opiates, which are obtained from the dried exudate of the unripe seed heads of certain poppies. The synthetic substitute, diamorphine (heroin), has been taken to obtain a feeling of euphoria and unreality. Diamorphine is used under the Misuse of Drugs Act (1971) as a legitimate analgesic (see Chapter 18 *Pharmacological management of pain*).

'Designer drugs' such as α-methyl fentanyl ('China White') are taken for their central nervous system stimulant properties, but, because of erratic processing methods, they may be of unpredictable strength. Amphetamine ('Speed'), used to gain the effects of prolonged central nervous system stimulation, works by potentiating the effects of noradrenaline at the nerve synapses.

Withdrawal from habitual use of opiates produces a range of symptoms associated with overstimulation of the central nervous or musculoskeletal systems.

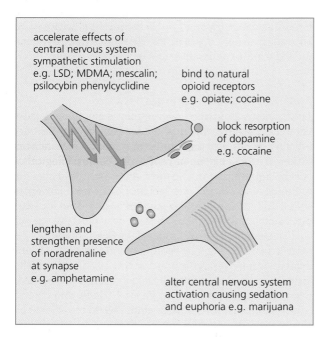

accelerate effects of central nervous system sympathetic stimulation e.g. LSD; MDMA; mescalin; psilocybin phenylcyclidine

bind to natural opioid receptors e.g. opiate; cocaine

block resorption of dopamine e.g. cocaine

lengthen and strengthen presence of noradrenaline at synapse e.g. amphetamine

alter central nervous system activation causing sedation and euphoria e.g. marijuana

Fig 7.6 Modes of action of 'mind-altering' drugs. LSD, lysergic acid diethylamide; MDMA, methylenedioxymetamphetamine.

Withdrawal from any regularly used narcotic substance produces unpleasant symptoms. Because the effects of withdrawal from methadone are less intense, this substance is used to rehabilitate opiate abusers.

CENTRAL NERVOUS SYSTEM STIMULANTS

Cocaine is derived from the leaves of the coca plant, which are chewed or sucked to obtain a feeling of physical power and energy and hunger reduction. Cocaine produces a sympathomimetic effect because it blocks the reabsorption of dopamine from the synapses into the synaptic clefts. When taken in easily absorbed forms, a 'rush' of intense wellbeing is experienced.

PSYCHEDELIC SUBSTANCES

Various naturally occurring and synthetic substances have been taken to alter sensory perception. Lysergic acid diethylamide (LSD) was first produced in laboratories in the 1930s and was heavily used during the 1970s. It mimics sympathetic nervous system stimulation in addition to provoking visual hallucinations and a sense of altered sensory input. For example, sounds may be 'seen', colours 'heard' or inanimate objects may appear to take on life. A 'bad trip' may produce a sense of panic. Some long-term users develop permanent changes in thought and actions that are similar to those of schizophrenia.

Mescaline (3,4,5-trimethoxyphenylethamine) is structurally similar to dopamine and noradrenaline. This substance is produced by the flowering heads of certain cacti. When taken, it alters sight, smell, touch and hearing sensations. A synthetic chemical that is similar in structure and effects is methylenedioxymetamphetamine (known as MDMA or Ecstasy). This produces an initial sympathomimetic effect, followed by the development of a tranquil, reflective mood. Use of MDMA can cause destruction of neurons using tryptamine transmitters in the cerebral cortex and hypothalamus, and withdrawal from prolonged use can produce states of deep depression. Deaths of young people at clubs and parties have occurred, probably caused by the heat stress and dehydration that develop as a result of the tireless dancing that is possible after taking this preparation.

Psilocybin is a mind-altering compound that is found in the Liberty Cap ('Magic') mushroom. Psilocybin is structurally similar to LSD and serotonin. When the chemical is taken, the temperature, pulse and respiratory rates become raised, the pupils are dilated and the user experiences hallucinations.

Phenylcyclidine (PCP) was initially developed in the 1950s as an anaesthetic agent. The substance is known by the street names of 'Angel Dust' or 'PeaCe Pill'. It is used as a substitute for mescaline or psilocybin. Phenylcyclidine produces a sense of intoxication and dissociation in users, and the effects last for between 4 and 6 hours. Nystagmus is a noticeable feature, along with muscular rigidity, sweating and apathy. Users of PCP feel themselves to be superhuman and their behaviour may become hostile and aggressive. When under the effects of this chemical, users experience a diminished sense of physical pain. Heavy usage may produce respiratory depression, convulsions, hypoglycaemia and rhabdomyolysis – breakdown of skeletal muscle fibres – with the consequent risk of renal failure. 'Bad trips' or PCP overdosage may cause psychotic behaviour; this can be treated with haloperidol. Long-term use may cause the development of personality disorders and confusional states (Eoff and Bates, 1996).

Marijuana has received attention as a useful analgesic substance for patients in intractable pain. However, at present it remains an illegal substance in the United Kingdom. The psychoactive chemicals are concentrated in the flowering tips of the hemp plant. The main psychotropic substance is δ-9 tetrahydrocannabinol (THC). When the plant is burned in a 'joint', the process produces a range of additional chemicals. THC influences the central nervous system, producing relaxation, sedation and euphoria. Marijuana intoxication produces altered time and space perception, a sense of wellbeing and heightened sensory experiences. Dizziness, dry mouth, throat and eyes and tachycardia are less welcome effects. Small doses have little effect upon reaction times, but if one or two 'joints' are smoked, psychomotor performance is markedly impaired and it is unsafe to drive or undertake other tasks requiring fine judgement. First-time users may experience panic attacks, and short-term memory loss occurs in habitual users. The use of marijuana is associated with decreased testosterone levels and spermatogenesis and long-term heavy use of marijuana has been associated with loss of motivational drive and with the development of attention deficit disorder (Eoff and Bates, 1996).

DRUG DEPENDENCY AND TOLERANCE

Some drugs acting upon the central nervous system cause changes that impel the individual to continue to use them whether or not they are needed to remedy a specific condition. Dependence upon drugs may be physiological or psychological.

Physiological changes include tolerance and dependence, mechanisms that are not well understood. In **tolerance** states, a biochemical change occurs with the result that more of a given substance is needed to produce the same effect. This may be because of alterations to enzyme systems and changes in the secretion of transmitter substances such as endorphins, enkephalins or GABA. Physical **dependence** is a potential problem for those taking preparations that act upon the central nervous system, particularly depressants such as might be used as analgesics or sedatives. Drugs that cause excitability of the central nervous system tend not to produce symptoms of dependence to the same extent. Once the substance that produced the dependence is no longer taken, the bodily adaptive responses probably continue unmodified, hence the physical signs of drug dependency. These vary according to the drug that was used but may include anxiety, sweats, chills and tremors.

Any substance that alters consciousness, and a strange range of other substances such as laxatives, diuretics and non-opioid analgesics, may create **psychological dependence**. The dependence may be linked to the process of taking the agent or to the effects of the substance itself. The individual has beliefs related to the powers of the substance that influence their perception of the need to take the substance. An illustrative example is cigarette smoking. Many young women currently have an obsession with being thin and many believe that smoking prevents weight gain. The act of getting and lighting a cigarette, holding it, inhaling and exhaling the smoke and finally extinguishing the cigarette into an ash tray are clearly rituals that are savoured by many smokers. In addition to dependence on the ritual, there develops a physical dependence upon the chemicals contained within cigarette smoke. For a dedicated smoker trying to give up the habit, there may well be additional issues associated with giving up smoking that are not addressed by the application of a nicotine patch to the skin.

KEY POINTS

- The patient being treated for depression will not immediately feel any benefit from the medication.
- The antimuscarinic effects of tricyclic antidepressants may prove lethal if these drugs are taken in overdose.
- Patients taking MAOIs should avoid foods rich in tyramine because of the risk of hypertensive crisis.
- Lithium has a narrow therapeutic margin, and so regular monitoring of serum levels is necessary to avoid toxic accumulation of the drug.
- Sufferers from panic disorders may find it helpful to know that there is a preventable biochemical cause of their symptoms.
- Depot injections may help to counteract the problem of non-compliance in schizophrenia patients.
- Symptoms of Alzheimer's disease can be controlled; the disease process is at present incurable.
- Drugs used to treat obesity have a short-lived effect and are susceptible to abuse.

MULTIPLE CHOICE QUESTIONS

1. A patient with unipolar depression is likely to have which of the following alterations within the central nervous system?
   a. loss of normal neuronal alignment
   b. increased glucose metabolism in the frontal lobes
   c. abnormal metabolism of phospholipids
   d. premature breakdown of monoamines
   e. premature breakdown of acetylcholine

2. A patient receiving pharmacological treatment for unipolar depression may be prescribed
   a. reserpine
   b. serotonin
   c. dothiepin hydrochloride
   d. muscarine
   e. sodium valproate

3. Hazards of antidepressant medication include the development of
   a. postural hypotension
   b. excitability
   c. headaches
   d. convulsions
   e. all of the above

4. Mania is thought to be caused by
   a. an abnormality of the dopamine receptor sites
   b. accumulation of urea at the synapses
   c. reduced nerve conduction rates
   d. accumulation of tau proteins at the synapses
   e. increased glucose uptake in the frontal lobe

5. When a patient is prescribed lithium therapy, the patient must be observed for all of the following except
   a. hypothyroidism
   b. hypertension
   c. renal failure
   d. ataxia
   e. hyponatraemia

6. During a panic attack, which of the following abnormalities may be present?
   a. increased β-adrenergic response; and increased carbon dioxide levels
   b. increased activity in the temporal lobe; and increased acetylcholine at the synapses
   c. low arterial pH; and increased activity in the parahippocampal gyri
   d. increased temporal lobe activity; and increased cerebral γ-aminobutyric acid (GABA)
   e. dizziness and tingling of the extremities

7. Mrs Smith suffers from acute anxiety attacks for which her family doctor has prescribed a benzodiazepine preparation. She is worried that they will make her sleepy during the day. What facts would you have in mind when discussing this with her?
   a. that Mrs Smith's anxiety may be a learned response
   b. that anxious patients are thought to lack active benzodiazepine receptors and that benzodiazepine therapy therefore provides a replacement therapy
   c. that benzodiazepines are effective anxiolytics and do not tend to produce sedation
   d. that Mrs Smith may need to be referred for psychotherapy
   e. all of the above

8. Michael suffers from schizophrenia. At present he has feelings of persecution and his conversation hops from topic to topic. How could you help Michael and his family to ensure that he continues to receive appropriate medication?
   a. by explaining that his drugs will not harm him
   b. by arranging for his medication to be prescribed in liquid form
   c. by ensuring that the community psychiatric nurse is aware of his discharge from hospital
   d. by explaining that it may be helpful for his medication to be prescribed in depot formulation
   e. by arranging for Michael to have group therapy

9. Michael has been prescribed a neuroleptic drug for his schizophrenic episodes. Which of the following are adverse effects of neuroleptic therapy?
   a. agitation
   b. hesitancy of micturition
   c. indifference
   d. nausea
   e. dystonia

10. The degenerative changes of Alzheimer's disease may be slowed by treatment with drugs to change the concentration of neurotransmitters at the synapses to
    a. increase the concentration of acetylcholine
    b. inhibit the production of acetylcholine
    c. potentiate noradrenaline
    d. block serotonin
    e. potentiate dopamine

REFERENCES

Bennett JP. Drugs for the treatment of movement disorders. In Brody TM, Larner J, Minneman KP, Neu HC, eds. *Human pharmacology: molecular to clinical.* St Louis: Mosby; 1994:363-371.

Bramble D, Pearch J. Attention deficit hyperactivity disorder: a rational guide to paediatric assessment and treatment. *Curr Paediatr* 1997; **7:**26-41.

Carlson NR. *Physiology of behaviour.* Boston: Allyn and Bacon, 1991.

Drachman DA, Leber P. Treatment of Alzheimer's disease – searching for a breakthrough, settling for less. *N Engl J Med* 1997; **336:**1245-1247.

El Mallakh RS, Pant B, Looney SW. Nerve conduction velocity and H-reflex recovery in bipolar illness *J Neuropsychiatr Clin Neurosci* 1996; **8:**412-416.

Eoff JC, Bates RG. Drug abuse. In Herfindel ET, Gourley DR, eds. *Textbook of therapeutics.* Baltimore: Williams and Wilkins, 1996. 1203-1226

Frederich RC, Hamann A, Anderson S, Löllman B, Lowell BB, Flier JS. Leptin levels reflect body lipid content in mice: evidence for diet-induced resistance to leptin action. *Nature Med* 1995; **1:**1311-1314.

Fujimoto D, Shimomura SK. Alzheimer's disease. In Herfindel ET, Gourley DR, eds. *Textbook of therapeutics.* Baltimore: Williams and Wilkins, 1996. 1797-1822

Gelder M, Gath D, Mayou R. *Concise Oxford textbook of psychiatry.* Oxford: Oxford University Press, 1994.

Kato T, Shioni T, Murashita J, Hamakawa H, Takahashi Y, Innubushi T, Takahashi S. Lateralised abnormality of high energy phosphate metabolism in the frontal lobes of patients with bipolar disorder detected by phase-encoded 31P-MRS. *Psychol Med* 1995; **25:**557-566.

Kolb B, Whishaw IQ. *Fundamentals of human neuropsychology.* New York: WH Freeman, 1996.

Lachman HM, Papalos DF. A molecular model for bipolar affective disorder. *Med Hypothesis* 1995; **45:**255-261.

Larsen PD, Ashleigh EA. Response to risperidone: a two edges sword? *J Californian Alliance Mentally Ill* 1996; **7/2:**17-18.

Laurence DR, Bennett PN. *Clinical pharmacology.* Edinburgh: Churchill Livingstone, 1992.

Page C. *Integrated Pharmacology.* London: Mosby, 1997.

Petri HL, Mishkin M. Behaviourism, cognitivism, and the neuropsychology of memory. *Am Sci* 1994; **82:**30-37.

Soares JC, Mann JJ. The anatomy of mood disorders: a review of structural neuroimaging studies. *Biol Psychiatr* 1997; **41:**86-106.

Taylor E, Sandberg S, Thorley G, Giles S. *The epidemiology of childhood hyperactivity.* (Maudsley Monographs No 33.) Oxford: Oxford University Press, 1991.

Walker G. *ABPI data sheet compendium.* London: Walker Publications, 1996.

8 Pauline Runyard
DRUGS AND NEUROLOGICAL DISORDERS

INTRODUCTION

The nervous system is affected by the general pathological processes of inflammation and infarction, and is the site of specific diseases that affect its specialised tissues, resulting in neurodegeneration and demyelination. Because of the compact anatomy of the nervous system even small lesions result in severe disturbances of function. This is made worse by the fact that neurons, because they lack the capacity for cell division, cannot be replaced once they are lost.

The cells in the nervous system that are of pathological significance are: **neurons**; **astrocytes**, which act as specialised supporting cells; **oligodendrocytes**, which form myelin; and **microglia**, which are similar to monocytes/macrophages both in type and function.

SPECIFIC DISORDERS OF THE CENTRAL NERVOUS SYSTEM

RAISED INTRACRANIAL PRESSURE

Because of the enclosed nature of the brain, any increase in its size as a result of lesions (as occurs with tumour growth), increased cerebrospinal fluid (CSF) volume (as a result of infection or malformation or obstruction of the CSF tract) or an increase in blood volume (e.g. head injury or stroke) results in raised intracranial pressure. Cerebral oedema, which occurs as a direct result of trauma, infection, haemorrhage, tumour, ischaemia, infarct or hypoxia, also leads to raised intracranial pressure. Cerebral oedema causes an increase in the fluid content of brain tissue and a further increase in brain size, resulting in movement within the brain and compression of its structures, which may then lead to tearing of associated blood vessels and thus further damage.

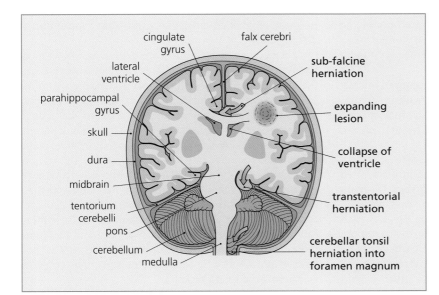

Fig 8.1 Cerebral herniation. (From Stevens & Lowe 1995, with permission.)

Pathophysiology

Compression of the brain may result in the displacement of CSF and an alteration in cerebral blood volume in an attempt to offset increasing intracranial pressure. A small increase in intracranial pressure may give rise to episodes of confusion and drowsiness, accompanied by slight pupillary changes and alteration in the respiratory rate. When a rapidly expanding lesion occurs, such as an extradural haemorrhage, there may be vomiting caused by medullary movement and stimulation of the vomiting centres, headache caused by stimulation of pain-sensitive nerve endings associated with stretched vessels, and papilloedema caused by the increased pressure on the CSF in the optic nerve sheath leading to its impaired flow. There is also the danger of cerebral herniation when one area of the brain shifts from one brain compartment to another (**Fig. 8.1**). Careful and regular observation of the patient who has suffered head trauma will allow the detection of the earliest signs of an enlarging brain lesion.

Should the intracranial pressure continue to rise there is a resultant reduction in neuronal oxygenation; this leads to systemic arterial vasoconstriction in an attempt to overcome the increased intracranial pressure. When intracranial pressure approaches arterial pressure, the brain tissues begin to experience hypoxia and hypercapnia and there is a rapid deterioration in the patient's condition. The patient shows the following signs and symptoms: a decreasing level of arousal, Cheyne–Stokes respirations and/or central neurogenic hyperventilation, pupils that become sluggish and dilated, a widened pulse pressure and bradycardia.

Pharmacological management

When cerebral oedema is present and there is the need for emergency measures to be undertaken, an intravenous infusion of **20% mannitol** is given. Mannitol is an osmotic diuretic and when it enters the extracellular fluid, it draws water from the cells to increase the extracellular fluid volume. When mannitol enters the glomerulus of the nephron its osmotic effect prevents reabsorption of water from the tubules back into the blood, thereby increasing urinary output.

Parenteral **dexamethasone 10 mg may be given initially** for the treatment of cerebral oedema. It has minimal mineralocorticoid activity and maximal anti-inflammatory activity (Margioros *et al.*, 1994) (see Chapter 3 *Classes of drugs*).

STROKE

Stroke is the third leading cause of death in the United Kingdom and affects 120 000 people each year. It occurs more frequently in men and those over 55 years of age.

Stroke is defined as rapidly developing signs of focal (or global) disturbance of cerebral function that last more than 24 hours and have a vascular cause. Stroke may be the result of a cerebral infarction (80% of strokes) or primary intracerebral haemorrhage and/or subarachnoid haemorrhage (20%). The consequent rise in intracranial pressure is caused by ischaemia and necrosis leading to cerebral oedema or by cerebral tissue haemorrhage.

Pathophysiology

Signs and symptoms will vary according to the area of brain affected. After an infarct there is often disturbance in motor and/or sensory function of one side of the body resulting in hemiparesis and/or hemiplegia. Dysphasia and dysphagia may also occur, in addition to other sensory losses; there may also be an accompanying change in personality.

Intracerebral haemorrhage is often the result of hypertension and clinical signs will depend on the location and size of the bleed. Subarachnoid haemorrhage caused by a ruptured or leaking aneurysm will often manifest as a severe sudden headache that may be followed by a loss of consciousness.

During the first year after a stroke approximately 50% of those affected will die, either as a direct result of the initial stroke or because of a secondary stroke. Nearly one-third of those surviving will need help in caring for themselves (Bonita, 1992).

Pharmacological management

A major trial undertaken in 1996 on the most effective treatment during the acute post-stroke phase has confirmed that **aspirin** and **dipyridamole** taken in combination reduce the risk of secondary stroke after 24 months by 38% (International Stroke Trial Collaborative Group, 1997). The critical time for treatment to commence is up to 3 hours after the stroke (Taylor, 1998).

Aspirin is given orally as an anti-platelet drug; it acts by decreasing platelet aggregation and may inhibit thrombus formation on the arterial side of the circulation, where anticoagulants have little effect. When given in combination with **dipyridamole**, another anti-platelet drug, **aspirin** can be given in doses as low as **25 mg twice daily**; if necessary, higher doses may be given, up to a **maximum of 300 mg daily**.

Aspirin may cause bronchospasm and gastrointestinal haemorrhaging. Although it does more good than harm there are a significant number of people who are allergic or intolerant to aspirin. It is essential to confirm by computerised tomography scan whether there is any doubt as to the cause of the stroke, as anti-platelet treatment, if administered when the cause is a cerebral haemorrhage, could prove fatal.

Dipyridamole is a vasodilator that, in combination with warfarin, reduces thrombus formation. Its action is to interfere with platelet function by increasing the cellular concentration of cyclic AMP. The European Stroke Prevention Study 2 has reported that low-dose **aspirin** and **modified-release dipyridamole** when combined prevent ischaemic strokes in patients who have suffered a previous stroke or transient ischaemic attacks.

Side effects include gastrointestinal effects, myalgia, dizziness, headache, hypotension, hot flushes and tachycardia.

New drugs undergoing evaluation

New areas of treatment for stroke that are undergoing trials are thrombolytics such as **streptokinase** and **alteplase**; trials have shown a higher mortality rate within the first 4 weeks, but improved results after 3–6 months (with less residual physical disability). The best results were obtained when treatment was commenced within 3 hours of the stroke. However, ischaemic stroke **must** be confirmed before the treatment commences.

Neuroprotective agents are also being studied; their action is to protect against cell damage and minimise nerve degeneration within the brain. **Chlormethiazole** is the drug under trial but so far results have been disappointing (Taylor, 1998).

ENCEPHALITIS

This is an acute viral infection with central nervous system involvement, the most common causative agents are herpes simplex type 1 and arthropod-borne (mosquito-borne) viruses that have a seasonal incidence, for example Eastern equine encephalitis or St. Louis encephalitis. The latter is more common and less serious. Japanese encephalitis occurring in Asia and the Pacific area is transmitted accidentally to humans by mosquitoes whose main host is birds or pigs. A vaccine is available for travellers to these areas if an epidemic is in progress (Meers *et al.*, 1995).

Encephalitis may also occur as a secondary complication of systemic viral diseases such as poliomyelitis and mononucleosis (glandular fever) or as a result of a viral illness such as rubella. Encephalitis has on rare occasions resulted from vaccination with a live attenuated virus vaccine (e.g. measles, mumps and rubella) (Paradiso, 1995).

Pathophysiology

The pathological changes vary according to the causative agent. Herpes simplex type 1 mainly causes haemorrhage and necrosis of the temporal and frontal lobes. Arthropod-borne encephalitis causes widespread nerve cell degeneration, with a secondary inflammatory process producing oedema and necrosis of tissue, with or without haemorrhage. The overall result is an increase in intracranial pressure that can lead to herniation. Clinical signs and symptoms of encephalitis are fever and delirium or confusion progressing to unconsciousness; seizures may occur as the disease progresses, as may cranial nerve palsies, paraesthesia and paresis, involuntary movement and abnormal reflexes. Signs of marked raised intracranial pressure may also be present.

Pharmacological management

The antiviral agent **aciclovir is administered intravenously** for adults with encephalitis simplex at 10 mg/kg over 1 hour, repeated every 8 hours. For a child up to 3 months old 10 mg/kg is given every 8 hours for 10 days. For children between 3 months and 12 years of age 250 mg/m^2 is given every 8 hours for 10 days (BNF, 1998). **Aciclovir** acts effectively on the herpes simplex virus because the effective encoding mechanism of the virus makes it more sensitive to aciclovir than the unaffected host cells. Aciclovir accumulates and becomes trapped within the viral cell, leading to inactivation of the virus. Measures are also needed to recognise and manage increased intracranial pressure.

MENINGITIS

The causative organism may be viral or bacterial in origin. Viral meningitis, often referred to as aseptic meningitis, occurs only in the meninges and is caused by many different viruses. Its spread is by coughing and sneezing microbe-laden droplets from the mucosa of the respiratory tract. The infection is usually self-limiting but headaches and tiredness may persist for 1 year or more.

Bacterial meningitis is caused by an infection affecting the pia mater and arachnoid, the subarachnoid space, the ventricular system and the CSF. Access to the CSF is gained when the organism invades the bloodstream, usually from the oropharynx, and crosses the meninges that surround the brain and spinal cord. Cerebral spinal fluid acts as a culture medium for the rapid growth of bacteria, which subsequently initiate an inflammatory response of the meningeal lining. This inflammatory response leads to vascular oedema and increased permeability of vessel walls. Neutrophils are delivered to the subarachnoid space, and these lead to the formation of a purulent exudate, which is distributed to the cranial and spinal nerves and into the perivascular spaces of the cortex. Within the cortex the number of microglia and astrocytes increase (Paradiso, 1995).

The major bacteria responsible for the occurrence of meningitis are *Streptococcus pneumoniae*, *Haemophilus influenzae* and *Neisseria meningitidis*. They are usually spread by coughing, sneezing or kissing, and are responsible for more than 200 deaths per year in the United Kingdom. Of these deaths 150 are caused by *Neisseria meningitidis* group B (Day, 1996).

Streptococcus pneumoniae affects older adults and young children and is carried in the upper respiratory tract of 30% of the population. It causes 10% of all meningitis cases and is often referred to as pneumococcal meningitis. It has a higher mortality rate (approximately 20%) than other forms of meningitis. No vaccination is yet available.

Haemophilus influenzae type b (Hib) meningitis is usually preceded by bacteraemia; it has a sudden onset and commonly progresses to unconsciousness. It used to account for approximately 40% of bacterial infections in children, but in 1992 the immunisation of infants with **Hib conjugate vaccination** began and by 1994 the coverage of infants aged 12 months or under was 93%; records of Hib meningitis in 1997 were at an all time low, but over the last two years, outbreaks of the infection have been given prominence in the national UK news. The vaccine was originally made from a polysaccharide present in the capsule of the bacteria but it was poorly antigenic in children under 2 years of age, who are most at risk. Its antigenicity has now been much improved by attaching the antigen to another larger molecule. **Hib vaccine** is given for primary immunisation in a course of three doses of 0.5 ml given by deep subcutaneous or intramuscular injection at monthly intervals in a different limb from other vaccines.

Neisseria meningitidis (**meningococcus**) is highly pathogenic and is the causative organism for meningococcal meningitis and meningococcal septicaemia. The meningococci are subdivided into eight serological groups (A–D, W135, X, Y, Z) according to the antigenic structure of their capsule. Serogroups A–D and W135 cause most cases of meningococcal infection, with one or other of these predominating in a particular geographical location. In the United Kingdom 70% of meningeal infections are attributable to serogroup B and 26% to serogroup C. Fifty per cent of meningococcal infection occurs in children under 5 years of age, but a second peak has been observed in 15–19 year olds. There are three common syndromes of meningococcal disease: meningitis alone, septicaemia alone, which is life threatening and often manifests with a rash, and meningitis with septicaemia. The mortality is less than 5% with meningococcal meningitis but is increased tenfold in the presence of septicaemia. Active immunisation is available by **vaccination for serogroup A and C meningococcus** for the control of local outbreaks of meningococcal meningitis, and for those travelling abroad to high-risk areas for longer than 1 month; a single dose of 0.5 ml is given by deep subcutaneous or intramuscular injection. A vaccination for serogroup B is currently undergoing trials.

Pathophysiology

With meningococcal meningitis the signs and symptoms have a quick onset and rapidly progress to being very severe. A vasculitic rash may be present (petechiae), which necessitates urgent treatment. The rash is caused by sludging of the circulation, which produces microclots in the skin capillaries that are seen as purple lesions. These microclots occur throughout capillary networks and use up the clotting factors inappropriately, so there is a paradoxical situation in which bleeding occurs, but multiple microclots are present. This condition is called disseminated intravascular coagulopathy and is responsible for some of the deaths from meningococcal meningitis.

General symptoms occur as a result of the meningeal inflammatory process causing headache, vomiting, irritability, photophobia and drowsiness possibly leading to coma. These are accompanied by fever, neck stiffness and 'focal' neurological deficits, for example hemiparesis caused by inflammation and occlusion of a cerebral artery supplying a particular area of brain. Intracranial pressure can also cause dilated, unresponsive pupils, and lid and eye movement weakness as a result of third cranial nerve damage. Brudzinski's sign or Kernig's sign may prove positive because inflamed nerves are stretched as they pass through inflamed meninges close to the spinal cord. Complications can occur as a sequelae of the initial infection and can be acute or chronic: hydrocephalus caused by persistent obstruction to CSF flow through narrowed channels or by pus blocking reabsorption through the arachnoid granulations; encephalitis; deafness as a result of damage to the eighth cranial nerve, which occurs in 5–40% of sufferers; and some degree of mental handicap, particularly after Hib meningitis.

Pharmacological management
Meningitis caused by meningococci

- Parenteral **benzyl penicillin** is administered (**intravenous benzyl penicillin** may be preferable) in order to halt the rapid progression of the disease.
- If there is a known penicillin allergy then the broad-spectrum antibiotic **cefotaxime** is recommended.
- Should the development of cerebral oedema be suspected then **intravenous dexamethasone** should be given immediately.
- **Rifampicin** is given for 2 days before hospital discharge.
- **Anticonvulsants** may be necessary if a fit or convulsion occurs.

If disseminated intravascular coagulopathy is present, medication is required to restore the normal clotting or fibrinolytic balance; this would probably be undertaken in an intensive care unit and is not discussed further here.

Meningitis caused by pneumococci

- Parenteral **benzyl penicillin** unless the organism is resistant.
- **Cefotaxime** is given if the organism is resistant. If organism remains highly resistant then **vancomycin** is added.

Meningitis caused by *Haemophilus influenzae* group B

- **Chloramphenicol** or **cefotaxime** is administered.
- **Rifampicin** is given for 4 days before discharge from hospital.

PERSON CENTRED STUDY 1

Mary explained that her 4-year-old daughter Lana had been 'whinging' during the early evening after her tea. She had given her some analgesic, popped her on the sofa in front of the TV with her father and older brother and told her she could sit with them until bedtime. When she undressed her two hours later she had seen one dark coloured spot under her knickers and Lana had been reluctant to have the light on in the bathroom. Mary said she felt devastated that she had not brought her to the hospital more quickly.

1. Why did Lana have photophobia and neck stiffness?
2. What was happening in the blood to produce the spot?
3. What medication would the hospital team commence – what route would they be given and why?

group (Mathewson-Kuhn, 1994). Secondary causes include poisoning, for example from carbon monoxide and heavy metals. Parkinsonism may be caused by drugs, most commonly phenothiazines, in which case the effect may be reversible [MPTP (1-methyl-4-phenyl-1,2,5,6-tetra-hydropyridine) – found in illegal designer drugs – has focused attention on toxins being a causative factor (McCance & Huether, 1994); Parkinsonism can also be produced by post-traumatic and metabolic events (repeated hypoglycaemic attacks).

Atrophy of the cerebral cortex and neuronal loss has been seen to occur in over 50% of people with Parkinson's disease. The principal pathological feature of Parkinson's disease is the degeneration of the dopaminergic nigrostriatal pathway, which is composed of the substantia nigra, with fibres synapsing in the caudate and putamen basal ganglia. Parkinson's disease may occur because of a fundamental defect in mitochondrial oxidative function. Restoration of this function may be possible through brain grafting of normal fetal brain cells and of genetically modified carrier cells, both of which have shown preliminary success (Bennett, 1994).

NEURODEGENERATIVE DISEASES OF THE SPECIALISED TISSUES OF THE NERVOUS SYSTEM

PARKINSON'S DISEASE

Parkinson's disease is a chronic progressive movement disorder affecting people over the age of 45 years. Symptoms do not appear until approximately 80% of the capacity to produce dopamine has been lost. The progression of the disease may vary in rate and character from one person to another. The disorder is characterised by disturbance of movement with rigidity, slowness of voluntary movement (bradykinesia), akinesia and tremor, which often first manifests in the fingers and thumb, producing the characteristic pill rolling movement. The tremor disappears during voluntary movement and sleep. There is a disturbance of posture, and the normal arm swing associated with walking is absent (**Fig. 8.2**). Speech develops a characteristic monotone. Severity of the disease is related to the degree of loss of the dopaminergic neurons in the substantia nigra and also loss of the dopaminergic receptors in the striatum, which further reduces the dopaminergic action. Dopamine has an inhibitory effect on movement by opposing the excitatory effect of acetylcholine. This imbalance results in the enhancement of cholinergic activity and the signs and symptoms of Parkinson's disease.

Pathophysiology

Parkinson's disease usually appears in later life and is found to affect 1 person in every 100 in the 60–70 year age

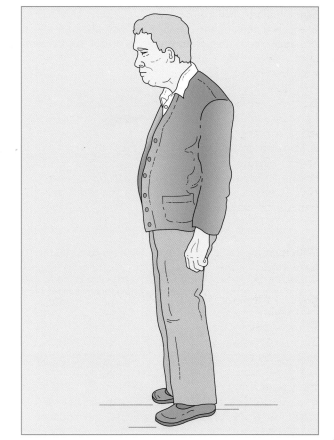

Fig 8.2 Parkinson's disease. (From Stokes 1998, with permission.)

Pharmacological management

Drug therapy is aimed at balancing the dopaminergic and cholinergic activity by reducing cholinergic activity or enhancing dopaminergic function (**Fig. 8.3**). Medication will provide relief from symptoms but is not curative and aims to maintain maximum independence of movement for as long as possible.

This can be achieved by:
- Replacing dopamine.
- Use of dopamine agonists to stimulate surviving dopamine receptors.
- Prolonging action of dopamine by inhibiting metabolism.
- Use of anticholinergic (muscarinic) drugs (Downie *et al.*, 1995).

Replacing dopamine

Dopamine is unable to cross the blood–brain barrier so **levodopa** is given instead. **Levodopa** is the precursor of dopamine and acts by replenishing depleted striatal dopamine by its ability to cross the blood–brain barrier. It is broken down to dopamine in the central nervous system. Once converted it acts as a neurotransmitter that facilitates movement and postural reflexes. Only 10% of **levodopa** is able to cross into the central nervous system as the majority is decarboxylated in the peripheral tissues of the liver and gut; this results in the possible side effects of nausea, vomiting, anorexia and postural hypotension.

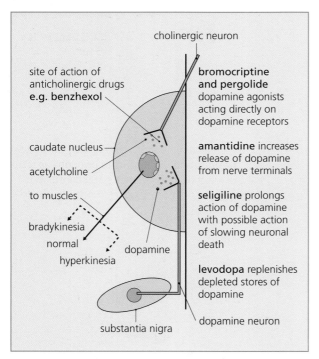

Fig 8.3 Action of drugs given in Parkinson's disease to balance dopaminergic and cholinergic activity.

To overcome this an extracerebral dopa-decarboxylase inhibitor is administered, such as **benserazide** or **carbidopa**, which prevents the peripheral degradation of levodopa to dopamine, and thereby increases the concentration of levodopa within the central nervous system. Effective brain concentrations of levodopa are thus achieved without the administration of such high doses. There is also less delay in onset of therapeutic effect and earlier reduction of bradykinesia and rigidity.

Dosage of levodopa is initially 50–100 mg twice daily given with carbidopa. This is gradually increased until a compromise is reached between increased mobility and degree of side effects. **Levodopa** and **carbidopa** administered in combination has resulted in a 75% reduction in the dose of levodopa required to maintain maximum effectiveness. This combination has also achieved less variation in the daily control of symptoms and a greater degree of clinical improvement (Mathewson-Kuhn, 1994). Levodopa with carbidopa is very effective for a number of years, then there is a slowing of response, which is probably attributable to further degeneration of the nigrostriatal neurons because of progression of the disease. It is important to note that caution is needed when giving levodopa to patients with open-angle glaucoma.

Side effects of levodopa are varied:
- Nausea and vomiting occur as a result of stimulation of the chemoreceptors in the medulla by the newly formed dopamine and are reduced by giving levodopa in divided doses with meals or by the administration of an antiemetic e.g. cyclizine. When given with food absorption rate is slowed and therefore peak absorption is lower.
- Constipation can also occur but can be avoided by increasing fluids and adding fibre to the diet.
- Cardiovascular effects result in postural hypotension and cardiac arrhythmias. Dopamine is thought to collect in noradrenaline nerve terminals, where it serves as a false transmitter.

Adverse effects of long-term levodopa therapy can include:
- Restlessness.
- Abnormal involuntary movements, which may be facial or effect the trunk, resulting in rocking movements. The hypersensitivity of the dopamine receptors is believed to increase. Akinetic spells, which are part of the on–off phenomenon, may occur, interspersed with abnormal involuntary movements. These effects often occur at the peak of drug action or at the end of the period of drug action.
- These side effects can be decreased by the addition of **amantadine** or **bromocriptine** to treatment as well as by adjusting the diet and times of meals (Matthewson-Kuhn, 1994).
- A drug-induced psychosis can cause behavioural disturbances, which may result in depression, dreams and confusion, delusions and insomnia. The drug will need to be reduced or withdrawn.

8.1 DRUG INTERACTIONS

- Monoamine oxidase inhibitors should be stopped 14 days before levodopa commenced as it interferes with central monoamines, leading to an accumulation of dopamine. If given simultaneously they can give rise to the dangerous effects of hypertension and hyperthermia.
- Antipsychotic drugs e.g. phenothiazines should not be administered concurrently with levodopa as they exacerbate the disease.
- Pyridoxine is present in multivitamin preparations in amounts greater than 5 mg and acts as a cofactor in the decarboxylation of levodopa to dopamine thus promoting its rapid conversion in the periphery. The result is a decreased amount of levodopa transported to the brain.

Chinese medicine, when integrated with the administration of levodopa, may help to reduce its side effects (Li-G, 1995).

Dopamine agonists

Amantadine is an antiviral agent that has been found to relieve the symptoms associated with parkinsonism. It can be used alone during the early stages of Parkinson's disease when tremor is not the major symptom. When a patient is in the advanced stages, it is administered with **levodopa**. It is not as effective as levodopa but it produces a more rapid response with fewer side effects. **Amantadine** has also been shown to be an effective prophylactic treatment for influenza A (see Chapter 5 *Drugs and immunological disorders*). Its action is to increase the activity of dopamine in the periphery and central nervous system by increasing synthesis, facilitating release and inhibiting cellular dopamine re-uptake. It is believed also to have anticholinergic effects in that it increases the peripheral and central adverse effects of anticholinergic drugs.

Amantadine, which is given orally, is well absorbed from the gastrointestinal tract and is quickly distributed to tissues and body fluids. Onset of action occurs after 15 minutes, reaches its peak in 1–4 hours, and has a duration of action from 12 to 24 hours and a half-life of 24 hours. Amantadine crosses the blood–brain barrier and 90% of amantadine is excreted unchanged in the urine. If the urine is acidic the rate of excretion is increased.

Amantadine is usually well tolerated and the reactions that do occur are transient and reversible. Side effects include:

- Gastrointestinal disturbances (anorexia, nausea, vomiting and constipation).
- Psychic disturbances (hallucinations, confusion, nightmares, anxiety, difficulty with concentration); these are probably related to the increased dopaminergic activity.
- Dermatological effects (mottling, peripheral oedema, rash). The purplish mottling is caused, in women, by the vasoconstriction that results from the local release of catecholamines.
- Anticholinergic effects of dry mouth, blurred vision, urinary retention, slurred speech, mood changes, dizziness and ataxia.

Contraindications to use of amantadine include:
- Hypersensitivity to the drug.
- A history of seizures, liver disease, cardiac disease or psychiatric problems as amantadine increases dopaminergic and catecholamine activity, which can trigger seizures and psychic side effects and increase cardiac stimulation.
- Pregnancy or lactation.

Bromocriptine and **pergolide** are ergot derivatives and are used clinically for the treatment of Parkinson's disease. Their action is on the postsynaptic dopamine receptors in the basal ganglia. These receptors are different to those acted upon by levodopa. These receptors are seen in the central nervous system, cardiovascular system, pituitary–hypothalamic axis (see Chapter 10 *Drugs and endocrine disorders* for the action of bromocriptine) and in the gastrointestinal tract. They are more effective than the anticholinergic drugs and amantadine in treating parkinsonism. They are very useful as an adjunct to levodopa or levodopa–carbidopa when fluctuations to treatment are occurring. This is probably because they have a longer duration of action, particularly **bromocriptine**, which is biphasic: the initial phase is about 4.5 hours and the second phase is 45–50 hours. **Pergolide** is for oral administration only and is commenced at a starting dosage of 50 μg for 2 days, then gradually increased by 100–150 μg every 3 days until optimal therapeutic dosage is achieved of **3 mg/day in three divided doses**.

Pergolide **must not** be stopped abruptly in patients receiving it chronically as an adjunct to levodopa as it may precipitate the onset of hallucinations and confusion.

Bromocriptine and **pergolide** are partially absorbed from the gastrointestinal tract and metabolised in the liver. Their systemic bioavailability is only a small fraction of the administered dose.

Adverse reactions associated with bromocriptine and pergolide are generally related to their activity as dopaminergic agonists, and can be divided into those that occur initially and those that occur after long-term treatment:
- Initial effects include nausea, vomiting and postural hypotension. Gastrointestinal effects are reduced if the drugs are taken with food or if the dose is reduced.
- It is important to be aware of the possibility of sudden cardiovascular collapse after the administration of the **first dose**.

⚠ 8.2 DRUG INTERACTIONS

- When bromocriptine and antihypertensives are given simultaneously the patient must be observed for the occurrence of hypotension.
- The effectiveness of bromocriptine and pergolide are reduced when given with phenothiazines, metoclopramide and haloperidol as the latter antagonise the effects of dopamine.
- Bromocriptine, when given with antihistamines, alcohol and sedative hypnotics, increases their sedative effects.
- Bromocriptine and pergolide are contraindicated in persons who are sensitive to ergot derivatives.
- Because of their dopaminergic effect on the heart and brain, bromocriptine and pergolide are used cautiously in patients prone to cardiac dysrhythmias or who have a history of psychic disturbances.
- Dosage of bromocriptine and pergolide is reduced if there is impairment of the liver because of their poor metabolism
- Bromocriptine and pergolide are not recommended for use during pregnancy or in children aged under 15 years.

• Long-term effects are constipation, mental disturbances (confusion, hallucinations etc.), dyskinesia, alcohol intolerance with bromocriptine and somnolence and rhinitis with pergolide.

Cabergoline is a newer dopamine agonist given orally once daily at a dosage ranging from **2 to 6 mg/day**. It is effective when given to patients affected by 'on–off' mobility problems with daily fluctuation in motor performance. It is given in addition to levodopa–carbidopa therapy, and has enabled a gradual reduction in the dose of the latter by substantial amounts, thereby reducing their adverse effects.

Adverse effects of cabergoline include:
• Nervous system: dyskinesia, hyperkinesia, hallucinations or confusion.
• Gastrointestinal system: nausea, vomiting, dyspepsia and gastritis.
• Cardiovascular system: dizziness and hypotension.
• Respiratory system: symptomatic pleural effusion/fibrosis.

For patients on long-term treatment with cabergoline it is not recommended that other ergot alkaloids are administered until further information is available. It is recommended that cabergoline is not administered simultaneously with drugs that have dopamine antagonist activity (e.g. phenothiazines, butyrophenones, thioxanthenes and metoclopramide) as these might reduce the therapeutic effect of cabergoline.

Prolongation of dopamine action

Selegiline hydrochloride is a monoamine oxidase-B inhibitor but if the dose does not exceed 10 mg per day then food and drug interactions do not occur. It is given in addition to levodopa or levodopa–carbidopa when the patients exhibits a decreased response. It inhibits the action of the enzyme monoamine oxidase, resulting in a reduction of dopamine catabolism and an increase in the concentration of dopamine in the brain synapses. **Selegiline** has also been shown to delay the onset of disability in early Parkinson's disease.

Adverse reactions are very similar to those of levodopa. Additional neurological reactions are loss of balance, anxiety, mood changes and headaches. There may also be an exacerbation of the adverse effects of levodopa, necessitating a reduction in the dose of levodopa by 15–40%.

Selegiline has been shown to increase the effects of levodopa, pethidine and tricyclic antidepressants. Richard *et al.* (1997) have discussed how they found minimal toxicity when selegiline was combined with an antidepressant and how there was an absence of the **serotonin syndrome**, which is thought to cause changes in mental status and motor and autonomic function.

Tolcapone is an orally active specific inhibitor of peripheral catechol-O-methyltransferase (COMT). The use of tolcapone leads to an increase in the transport of levodopa into the brain. It has therapeutic potential when given in addition to levodopa in the treatment of patients with Parkinson's disease. It is particularly effective in stabilising patients with end-of-dose phenomena, leading to an increased duration of 'on' time. The initial dose is **100 mg three times daily up to 200 mg**, and should lead to a reduction in the daily dosage of levodopa (Spencer and Benfield, 1996).

Side effects include dyskinesia, nausea, sleep disorders, anorexia and diarrhoea.

Anticholinergic/antimuscarinic drugs

The drugs most commonly used are **benzhexol 5–15 mg, benztropine 1–4 mg, orphenadrine 150–300 mg, procyclidine 10–20 mg** and **trihexyphenidyl**. These drugs are particularly useful for treating young patients or those who have minimal symptoms or who cannot tolerate levodopa or levodopa–carbidopa.

Cholinergic neurons in the basal ganglia possess dopamine receptors which, when activated, inhibit their production of acetylcholine. In Parkinson's disease with the loss of dopamine there is an increased synthesis and release of acetylcholine, and an intensified excitatory effect. Anticholinergic drugs block the effects of elevated acetylcholine in the peripheral tissues of the body (particularly

PERSON CENTRED STUDY 2

Mr Simons is a very fit 78-year-old married man. He has had Parkinson's disease for a number of years, which is successfully treated with levodopa and carbidopa combined. One morning he had an important meeting to attend at his local club and in his rush not to be late he could not remember whether he had taken his normal medication of levodopa and carbidopa. Being aware of the benefits he obtains from taking the drug, he took another dose before he went out just to be sure and drove to the club in his car.

When he arrived he went to leave his car but felt dizzy and had to sit down again (postural hypotension), when he finally entered the club he had to dash to the toilet to be sick (gastric irritation). Mr Simons continued to feel dizzy and a colleague telephoned his wife to inform her of the situation. She suggested telephoning the doctor. On hearing this Mr Simons angrily knocked the telephone to the floor (aggression).

1. Why do you think Mr Simons showed the symptoms of postural hypotension, gastric irritation and aggression?
2. What future advice would you give Mr Simons about his medication?

the smooth muscle) and within the central nervous system, leading to a reduction in the tremor, rigidity and excessive salivation. Anticholinergic drugs have been found to be beneficial in drug-induced parkinsonism (Mathewson-Kuhn, 1994). These drugs are well absorbed from the gastrointestinal tract and can cross the blood–brain barrier.

The most common adverse reactions are dry mouth, constipation, blurred vision, tachycardia and dizziness. These drugs are contraindicated in urinary retention and glaucoma, and reactions can occur when they are given alongside antihistamines and tricyclic antidepressants.

Drugs that may also be given because of their anticholinergic effects but are not considered to be anticholinergics are **amitriptyline**, an antidepressant; **diphenhydramine**, an antihistamine; and **ethopropazine**, a phenothiazine.

Other drugs that may be given to treat specific aspects of parkinsonism

Baclofen and **benzodiazepines** are given to relieve the spasticity that occurs and act by reducing the afferent input to

ventral motor neurons, thereby reducing the efferent outflow to the muscles.

'On–off' effects of movement, when there are sudden fluctuations in disability, have been greatly reduced by the administration of **apomorphine**. It has also been noted that changes in diet such as a reduction in protein intake may also play a part, as there is competition between levodopa and amino acids for transport across the blood–brain barrier.

MOTOR NEURON DISEASE (AMYOTROPHIC LATERAL SCLEROSIS)

Little is known about the aetiology of motor neuron disease, but it is now believed to be inherited in 5–10% of patients. It is an autosomal dominant trait and is age related. Motor neuron disease occurs in 1 in 50 000 people, with an overall incidence of 6000 people in the United Kingdom (Rose, 1992).

Pathophysiology

The pathological changes that take place in motor neuron disease are caused by the death and degeneration of motor neurons in the motor cortex, brainstem and anterior horn cells of the spinal cord, resulting in death of either upper or lower nerve cells. Physiological effects are muscle weakness, atrophy and flaccidity when the lower anterior horn cells are affected and weakness and hyper-reflexia with upper neuron involvement. When certain motor nuclei of the brainstem are involved the resulting bulbar palsy causes slurred speech, difficulties with swallowing and a risk of choking.

Pharmacological management

Hyoscine is effective in reducing the excess salivation that occurs in motor neuron disease; it is a muscarinic blocking agent and acts on the vomiting centre in the medulla. It can be given sublingually, 0.3 mg 6 hourly, or as 4-hourly intramuscular injections of 0.4–0.6 mg or subcutaneously using a syringe driver with the dose varying between 0.8–2.4 mg. It is administered until the excess salivation diminishes.

DEMYELINATING DISEASES

MULTIPLE SCLEROSIS

The peak incidence of multiple sclerosis is between the ages of 20 and 40 years, with a slight female predominance. Multiple sclerosis is thought to be the result of a genetic susceptibility to mounting an inappropriate immune response to viral infections (Stevens and Lowe, 1995).

Pathophysiology

The pathogenesis of multiple sclerosis is an immune response of unknown origin, causing areas of demyelination, termed plaques, within the brain and spinal cord. In the areas of recent demyelination there are to be seen small vessels encircled by lymphocytes. Macrophages enter the lesion where they phagocytose damaged myelin, accumulate lipid and form foam cells. There is also seen an infiltration of T cells and B cells, emphasising immune activation. Astrocytes, which are seen around the margins of the plaque, are enlarged. The plaques are often seen at the angles of the lateral ventricles, in the cerebellar peduncles and in the brainstem. In an old lesion a small proportion of axons spanning the plaque may be seen to be lost. The early common clinical signs are limb weakness, blurring of vision, lack of coordination and abnormal sensation. There is a great variation in outcome.

Pharmacological management

The goal of pharmacology is to modulate the immune response.

Interferons are named after their ability to interfere with viral RNA and protein synthesis. **Interferon β-1b** is primarily synthesised in macrophages and fibroblasts, and has a potent antiviral action. The inhibition of viral replication by interferon may result from the induction of an enzyme that inhibits viral replication by catalysing the breakdown of viral RNA. Side effects of interferon β-1b in multiple sclerosis patients include skin reactions, flu-like symptoms, fatigue, leucopenia, new or worsened depression and new or worsened headache (Neilley *et al.*, 1996).

Immunoglobulin was administered to the relapsing–remitting form of multiple sclerosis and was found to be effective and well tolerated. This was undertaken in a randomised placebo-controlled trial of 1 month during which immunoglobulin therapy was administered intravenously (Fazekas *et al.*, 1997).

Baclofen (maximum dosage 80 mg/day) is a skeletal muscle relaxant and is effective in relieving spinal spasticity in patients with multiple sclerosis. Baclofen is a chemical analogue of the inhibitory neurotransmitter, γ-aminobutyric acid (GABA), and acts by inhibiting the release of excitatory transmitters at the spinal level. It is well tolerated with few side effects.

Dantrolene sodium is a direct-acting skeletal muscle relaxant, which acts on the muscle by interfering with the release of calcium ions from the sarcoplasmic reticulum, thus weakening the force of contraction. It does not interfere with nerve impulse transmission as the centrally acting muscle relaxants do. It is not as effective at treating spasticity of the spinal cord as **baclofen** but it is particularly useful in treating patients with spasms that cause pain. Dantrolene does produce muscle weakness and is therefore used with caution in patients with borderline strength. As dantrolene has the potential for causing drug-induced hepatitis, patients should undergo baseline liver studies and need to be made aware of the symptoms that occur with hepatitis. The drug is stopped after 45 days if no benefits are observed.

NEUROMUSCULAR JUNCTION DISORDER

MYASTHENIA GRAVIS

Myasthenia gravis is characterised by muscle weakness arising from defective neuromuscular transmission. It occurs predominantly in women. The disease is caused by an autoimmune process in which antibodies are formed against the acetylcholine receptors in muscles. These antibodies are present in 80% of people with active myasthenia gravis (**Fig. 8.4**) (Paradiso, 1995).

Pathophysiology

The antibodies attach to the acetylcholine receptors at the neuromuscular junction and make them unable to bind to acetylcholine. This leads to muscle weakness, which more commonly affects the muscles of the eye, lips, tongue, throat, neck and shoulders. Limb muscles may be affected and movement restricted. These symptoms may be exacerbated by emotional disturbances, strenuous exercise and pregnancy. Sufferers of this disease may experience temporary or permanent remissions.

Pharmacological management

The treatment of myasthenia gravis falls into two main areas: anticholinesterase drug therapy and immunosuppressive drug therapy.

Anticholinesterase drug therapy

Acetylcholine is broken down by the enzyme cholinesterase. If the action of cholinesterase is inhibited, the concentration of acetylcholine at the motor end plates rises and its action is potentiated to enhance neuromuscular transmission and neuromuscular strength. Pyridostigmine is usually the drug of choice. Patients usually experience improvement in muscle strength 30 minutes after taking the medication, and the duration of its action is 3–4 hours. The dose, which is usually between 10 and 12, 60 mg tablets daily, is determined by the patient's response. Anticholinesterase drugs should be used with caution. Too much medication can increase weakness, potentially leading to a life-threatening cholinergic crisis, and some drugs may be contraindicated because they affect the action of anticholinesterase drugs.

Also, anticholinesterase agents produce muscarinic side effects, which include increased salivation, sweating, increased gastric secretion and gastrointestinal upsets, motility and diarrhoea, an increase in bronchial secretions and muscle twitching. A concurrent administration of an antimuscarinic such as oral atropine (0.5 mg) or propantheline (15–30 mg) may be required to counteract these side effects. These drugs, however, must be used with caution in order not to make secretions thick and sticky. Although anticholinesterases are of value in treating the weakness, they do not alter the natural history of the disease.

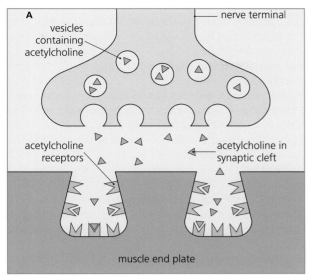

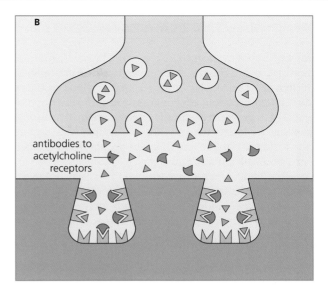

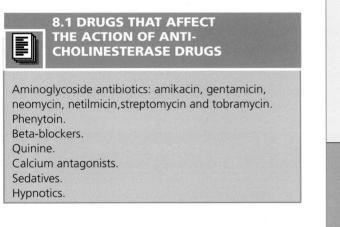

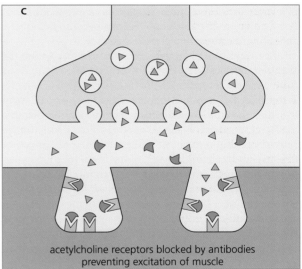

Fig 8.4 The pathogenesis of myasthenia gravis.

8.1 DRUGS THAT AFFECT THE ACTION OF ANTI-CHOLINESTERASE DRUGS

Aminoglycoside antibiotics: amikacin, gentamicin, neomycin, netilmicin, streptomycin and tobramycin.
Phenytoin.
Beta-blockers.
Quinine.
Calcium antagonists.
Sedatives.
Hypnotics.

Immunosuppressive drug therapy

The aim of immunosuppressive drugs such as corticosteroids, azathioprine, cyclosporin and cyclophosphamide is to inhibit the production of antibodies, thereby reducing the number of circulating acetylcholine-receptor antibodies that are specific to the disease process in myasthenia gravis. This form of treatment may be beneficial in patients with a limited response to pyridostigmine.

Characteristically there is a 'lag' between the start of treatment and the first signs of sustained improvement. Initially, steroid therapy can increase weakness and cause an exacerbation of symptoms (Kernich and Kaminski, 1995).

Azathioprine is often used when steroids are contraindicated. It can also be used in combination with prednisolone in patients who respond slowly to steroids. The action of azathioprine is much slower than that of steroids and some patients are unable to tolerate the drug because of the side effects.

Cyclosporin and cyclophosphamide, the actions of which are discussed in detail in Chapter 6, are not used routinely and are reserved for those unable to tolerate steroids or azathioprine or those who have been unresponsive to other forms of immunosuppressive drugs.

Plasma exchange involves the removal of plasma from the serum and the replacement of albumin. The aim is to remove or reduce to a minimum those constituents that aggravate the disease, thereby reducing the amount of circulating acetylcholine-receptor antibodies. The effects of plasma exchange are short lived, approximately 4–12 weeks, with a maximum improvement usually after 2–3 weeks. Effective treatment by immunosuppression further reduces the production of acetylcholine receptor antibodies (Pundare, 1994).

ABNORMAL ELECTRICAL BRAIN ACTIVITY

EPILEPSY

Epilepsy is a symptom that shows itself in the form of **recurrent** seizures. It is estimated that 1 person in 200 in the United Kingdom experiences recurrent seizures, but not all will progress to chronic epilepsy, defined as having seizures for longer than 5 years. It is estimated that there are between 150 000 and 350 000 people in the United Kingdom with chronic epilepsy.

Pathophysiology

A seizure is a sudden uncontrolled burst of abnormal neuronal activity within the brain. The possible cause of the abnormal neuronal activity is a dysfunction of the inhibitory action of the GABA neuron. These neurons have been found so far only within the central nervous system (Marieb, 1994) in the grey matter of the brain and spinal cord. A seizure commences with the high-frequency firing of a group of neurons; if the firing continues and inhibition does not occur, then normal neurons become involved in spreading the abnormal electrical activity.

The signs and symptoms of a seizure vary, as no two seizures are alike (Matthewson-Kuhn, 1994), and can result from a variety of causes. The basic classification of seizures is based on aetiology and they are either idiopathic or symptomatic. The cause of idiopathic seizures is unknown and they tend to start in childhood or adolescence. Symptomatic seizures have a predetermined cause such as congenital defects, hypoxia at birth, head injury, brain tumours, infection of the central nervous system, vascular insufficiency, substance abuse and chemical poisoning with alcohol, amphetamines, lead and some insecticides. Metabolic causes include electrolyte and glucose imbalances, hypoxia, vitamin deficiencies and drug interactions. Epilepsy is further classified into two broad groups: partial seizures and generalised seizures. Partial (focal) seizures are localised to one area of the brain, whereas generalised seizures involve both cerebral hemispheres of the brain.

Signs and symptoms of seizures

Partial (focal) seizures can occur as:
- **Simple partial seizures**, which arise from a localised area of the brain and may involve motor neurones (abnormal movement of one limb) or sensory neurones (abnormal sensation) or both. Consciousness is not lost and duration is short.
- **Complex partial seizures** in which consciousness is impaired or lost and motor activity is often seen in the form of non-reflex actions, resulting in bizarre inappropriate behaviour.

Generalised seizures are seen in:
- **Absence seizures (petit mal)**, which occur most commonly in children; they do not have motor involvement and result in a brief loss of consciousness (see **Box 8.1 on epilepsy in childhood**). These seizures usually disappear during adolescence.
- **Myoclonic seizures** consist of sudden single or multiple uncontrollable jerks.
- **Tonic or clonic seizures (grand mal)** are the most common form of seizure and are characterised by a sudden loss of consciousness, followed by muscle rigidity (tonic phase) and then a period of jerking of the limbs (clonic phase). Full consciousness is usually regained within 1 hour.

Pharmacological management

The management of epilepsy is by drug therapy or surgical intervention. Drug therapy is by the administration of anti-convulsant or anti-epileptic drugs. These drugs act in two ways; first, they prevent the spread of neuronal excitation, which is caused by excessive depolarisation, by exerting a stabilising effect on excitable cell membranes. This is brought about by reducing the transport of sodium ions across the neuronal cell membrane, leading to its stabilisation. Drugs that act here are **carbamazepine** and **phenytoin**. The second mode of action is by suppressing the focus of neuronal discharge by enhancing the activity of neurotransmitters such as GABA, which act by blocking the synaptic transmission, resulting in the reduction or abolishment of excessive discharge. This is a prime focal point

---

8.1 CHILDHOOD EPILEPSY

Children are not diagnosed as epileptic until they have been observed to have had three fits not caused by hyperpyrexia and have distinctive changes as screened by electroencephalogram (EEG).

Two drugs are commonly available for treatment: sodium valproate, usually reserved for children suffering petit mal; carbamazepine for grand mal. These drugs are used singly in the first instance, titrated against weight and symptom control.

When the maximum dose is reached with poor symptom control (max daily dose for sodium valproate is 35 mg/kg and for carbamazepine: under 1 year, 200 mg; 1–5 years, 400 mg; 5–10 years, 600 mg; 10–15 years, 1 g) a second drug is added.

Liver function tests are carried out routinely every 3 months and also blood tests for those on carbamazepine.

For those children entering their teens, night-time fits are particularly monitored as epilepsy sufferers cannot apply for a licence to drive a motor vehicle if they are unstable.

for certain anti-epileptic drugs. The goal of pharmacology is to reduce or eliminate seizures without impairing mental or motor function and with minimal side effects.

The choice of anticonvulsant will depend on the particular type of seizure the patient experiences and the patient's age and sex. Knowledge of occupation and whether the patient suffers from fatigue and stress are important as these factors can trigger an attack. Other factors that may be considered are the cost of the medication, and whether the patient ingests large quantities of alcohol and/or caffeine, as these interfere with the action of some anticonvulsants. Another important consideration is the patient's acceptance of the treatment plan. The trend in medication is towards monotherapy as anti-epileptic drugs may interact with each other in two ways:

- Alteration in the metabolism of the other drug.
- Change in their ability to bind to plasma proteins, leading to toxicity e.g. valproate may increase the toxicity of phenytoin by displacing it from its plasma binding sites.

The recommended drugs used are carbamazepine, **sodium valproate**, phenytoin, **lamotrigine** and **vigabatrin**.

Carbamazepine is commenced at a low dose of 200 mg/day orally, which is increased as necessary by 100 mg per day weekly until control is established or toxicity occurs. The slow introduction of this drug helps to reduce the side effects of nausea and visual disturbances. Other side effects are sedation, dizziness, headache, skin rashes (5%), granulocyte suppression and hyponatraemia.

Carbamazepine is metabolised in the liver to epoxide. This compound is believed to contribute to the neurotoxicity that often develops in patients taking this drug. Carbamazepine is a powerful inducer of liver enzymes that increase its clearance rate. This results in a significant reduction in its half-life over the first few weeks of treatment, necessitating increasing doses during the first 4–6 weeks.

Carbamazepine reduces the effectiveness of other anti-epileptic drugs and the oral contraceptive pill by increasing their metabolism.

Conversely ciprofloxacin, verapamil and diltiazem inhibit the metabolism of carbamazepine and may lead to toxicity. Antibiotics increase the serum concentration of carbamazepine, phenobarbitone and phenytoin.

Carbamazepine is now selected as the drug of choice for women and children over 5 years of age because it does not cause coarsening of facial features, hirsutism or gingival hyperplasia.

Sodium valproate is an analogue of the inhibitory neurotransmitter GABA, which results in an increase in the concentration of GABA at the synapses. Sodium valproate is effective against a variety of seizures, especially myoclonic seizures. The initial dose is 100–200 mg once or twice daily up to 0.8–1.2 g in divided doses, given orally.

⚠ 8.3 SODIUM VALPROATE

Elevation of liver enzymes and blood ammonia is common in patients receiving sodium valproate therefore caution is needed if it is to be given to children and those with liver disease. Lethargy may be a problem in early therapy. Other common side effects are tremor, alopecia and weight gain. Less common side effects are coagulation disorders secondary to depletion of fibrinogen, and hepatitis, which is rare.

Sodium valproate displaces phenytoin from its plasma protein, which interferes with its metabolism and thereby increases the metabolism of sodium valproate.

Therapy should be introduced slowly and taken with food, to overcome the gastrointestinal disturbances associated with this drug. Enteric-coated tablets are also available to overcome this problem.

Phenytoin is suitable for the treatment of generalised and complex partial seizures. It is administered orally with an initial dose of 150–300 mg in one or two divided doses, up to 300–400 mg daily. Although a very effective anti-epileptic drug, it is unsuitable for many patients because of its many side effects. Gastrointestinal irritation is minimised when the drug is administered with or immediately after meals.

Phenytoin limits seizure propagation by altering the transport of ions. It is almost wholly metabolised by the liver, which may become saturated at or around the therapeutic range. The result of this is that a small increase in dosage may lead to a large increase in the plasma level, leading to the dose-related adverse effects of nystagmus, diplopia and ataxia. To overcome these adverse effects phenytoin plasma levels should be maintained between the therapeutic range of 10–20 mg/l. The dose at which this transition occurs varies from patient to patient, therefore all doses of phenytoin must be individualised.

Gingival hyperplasia, hirsutism, acne and coarsening of facial features make phenytoin unsuitable for women and children. The side effects in some people include skin rash, blood dyscrasias and immunological reactions. Phenytoin is found to be associated with deficiencies of calcium, vitamin D and folic acid, which in turn lead to hypocalcaemia and osteomalacia.

Alcohol and warfarin may stimulate phenytoin metabolism and decrease blood levels. Isoniazid, chloramphenicol and cimetidine may decrease phenytoin metabolism and increase blood levels. Phenytoin may decrease the effectiveness of digoxin and oral contraceptives.

Lamotrigine is a newer anti-epileptic drug for the adjunctive treatment of partial seizures and secondary generalised tonic or clonic seizures, which are not controlled by other anti-epileptic drugs.

Side effects include diplopia, blurred vision, dizziness, drowsiness, headache and rashes.

Vigabatrin is used for the treatment of chronic epilepsy that has not been treated satisfactorily by other anti-epileptics.

Side effects are similar to those of lamotrigine.

STATUS EPILEPTICUS

Status epilepticus occurs when there are repeated seizures without the patient regaining consciousness. This may be caused by non-compliance, abrupt stoppage of anti-epileptic medication, withdrawal of alcohol or other drugs, metabolic-induced deficiencies and events of neurological origin (stroke, meningitis or head injury).

Pathophysiology

Status epilepticus exists when there is no recovery between three episodes of seizures or when seizure activity lasts more that 30 minutes. If termination of status epilepticus is not achieved there is a 15% or less risk of mortality as a result of severe cerebral hypoxia and hyperthermia caused by excessive muscle activity. Acidaemia, cardiovascular collapse and renal shutdown may also occur.

Pharmacological management

Airway and patient safety should be maintained. The intravenous administration of **diazepam** emulsion 10–20 mg is given over 3–6 minutes and is repeated every 30 minutes if necessary. **Lorazepam** may be given as it has a longer rate of duration. Intravenous **phenytoin** 15–20 mg/kg is the second drug of choice and repeated doses of 100–150 mg are given every 30 minutes.

CHANGES IN CEREBRAL BLOOD FLOW

MIGRAINE

Migraine affects 1 in 10 of the population; the incidence in women is double that in men. The first attack usually occurs between childhood and early adulthood. During the reproductive period about 20% of women suffer migraine, particularly those aged in their early 40s.

Migraine produces a recurrent throbbing headache with neurological symptoms lasting between 2 and 72 hours. It is accompanied by visual and gastrointestinal disturbances in the form of photophobia, nausea and vomiting. Migraine is classified into two main types:
- Migraine without aura (common migraine, affecting about 80% of sufferers).
- Migraine with aura (classic migraine, affecting about 20% of sufferers).

8.4 ANTI-EPILEPTIC DRUGS DURING PREGNANCY

There may be a change in the frequency of seizures during pregnancy. The occurrence of a seizure during pregnancy puts both the mother and baby at risk, because of hypoxia and other metabolic changes. There is an increased risk of neural tube and other defects in women who are on anti-epileptic drugs: 7% compared with 2–3% for the general population (Matthewson-Kuhn, 1994). These malformations are particularly associated with carbamazepine, phenytoin and valproate. Women who become pregnant while on these medications should be counselled and offered antenatal screening and a second trimester ultrasound scan. Children of mothers who have epilepsy have an increased risk of malformations even if anti-epileptic drugs are not used during pregnancy (Stringer, 1994). Single drug therapy and a decrease in the level of medication is recommended.

The aura can be either visual, in the form of blind spots, or sensory disturbances such as 'pins and needles' moving up one arm to the face. The period of aura may last from 10 to 60 minutes. Other early premonitory signs and symptoms are:
- Mood swings.
- Hyperactivity.
- A feeling of hunger or thirst, or a craving for sweet foods.
- Fluid retention may occur accompanied by oliguria.
- Onset of headache followed by diuresis.

Causes of migraine are known as trigger factors; of these, dietary and stress factors are the most common. Dietary factors most frequently associated with migraine are foods and drinks that contain tyramine, which is believed to act on neurotransmitter pathways in the brain. These are cheeses, especially blue cheeses, chocolate and wine, particularly red wine. Other food triggers are caffeine, alcohol, tea, citrus fruits, eggs and fried and spicy foods. Stress-causing factors are anxiety, tension, sleeplessness and a change in the normal daily routine. Other triggers are environmental: particularly loud noise, flashing lights, fluorescent lighting and television or computer screens. Women are also affected by hormonal triggers such as pregnancy, oral contraception, hormone replacement therapy and menstruation, all of which are associated with a change in the hormonal levels of oestrogen and progesterone.

Pathophysiology

The accepted but unproven theory is that there is spasm and constriction of the cerebral arteries, causing transient ischaemia, followed by dilatation of the meningeal vessels and sterile inflammation of their walls, producing the throbbing nature of the headache. Accompanying the vasodilatation is a change in nerve activity and neurotransmitter levels. One of these is serotonin, a hormone and a neurotransmitter; one of its actions is to cause vasoconstriction. Serum levels of serotonin have been found to be increased just before a migraine attack and then fall sharply at the onset of the headache. Studies of cerebral blood flow have shown a reduction during the early and aura phases, with a greater increase in blood flow during the headache phase.

Pharmacological management

Drug treatment of migraine tends to be acute or prophylactic.

Acute treatment

This usually commences at the beginning of an attack and can be directed at reducing cranial pressure by constriction of cranial blood vessels. Some migraine headaches respond to analgesics such as **aspirin** or **paracetamol** but as peristalsis is often reduced during migraine attacks their absorption may be poor. It is recommended that dispersible or effervescent preparations should preferably be used. **Ergotamine** is used in patients who do not respond to analgesics. It is a natural amino acid alkaloid of ergot that is derived from a fungus grown on rye, which has α-adrenergic blocking properties. It is available in oral, sublingual, suppository and inhaler form. Doses of 6–8 mg per attack and 10–12 mg per week should not be exceeded. It can be used alone or in conjunction with 'over the counter' migraine preparations. These preparations contain simple analgesics with or without an antiemetic. Administration of **ergotamine** should be limited to no more than twice a month. If vomiting is made worse by ergotamine or as a result of the migraine then an antiemetic can be given such as **metoclopramide 10 mg** orally. It promotes gastric emptying and normal peristalsis, so other drugs taken orally are better absorbed. **Prochlorperazine 5 mg** and **domperidone 30 mg** are also useful as they can be given rectally as suppositories if the patient is vomiting persistently.

Ergotamine should not be administered to persons with known hypersensitivity, sepsis, vascular disease, hepatic or renal disease, marked atherosclerosis, hypertension and anaemia. All of these conditions may be worsened because of its vasoconstrictor properties. Ergotamine is contraindicated in pregnancy as it is a powerful uterine stimulant.

Nausea is a common side effect; other adverse reactions include tingling and numbness, cold peripheries and general malaise. Ergotamine should not be given in intervals of less than 4 days as regular use of ergot can result in limb pains, venous thrombosis, gangrene and ergotism. Ergotism is the most common side effect, signs of which include nausea, vomiting and abdominal cramps.

Concomitant administration of nitroglycerine increases the availability of ergot, resulting in increased vasoconstriction and a danger of severe hypertension.

Sumatriptan is a serotonin$_1$ agonist that reverses the cerebral vasodilatation believed to cause migraine headache. The dose is 50–100 mg orally as soon as possible after the onset of the headache; the dose should not be repeated for same attack, but may be repeated if migraine recurs; maximum 300 mg in 24 hours. By subcutaneous injection using auto injector, the dose is 6 mg as soon as possible after onset; the dose should not be repeated for the same attack, but may be repeated after not less than 1 hour if symptoms recur, not exceeding 12 mg in 24 hours. It is not recommended for those aged over 65 years or for children.

Transient pain may be experienced at the injection site. Feelings of pressure, heaviness and tingling in various parts of the body, particularly the face, neck and upper chest, flushing, dizziness and drowsiness may also occur. These feelings can be very alarming to the patient and he or she needs to be forewarned and reassured that the feelings will be short lived. Chest pain and tightness that mimic angina may occur as a result of vasospasm. This may lead to arrhythmia, ischaemia or myocardial infarction; if so, the sumatriptan will need to be discontinued and a doctor alerted.

Contraindications include ischaemic heart disease, previous myocardial infarction and uncontrolled hypertension.

Non-steroidal anti-inflammatory drugs (NSAIDs) such as **ibuprofen** and **naproxen**, 500 mg given orally, or **diclofenac sodium**, 100 mg suppositories or 75 mg intramuscularly, have also been found to be effective in the acute treatment of migraine. Their effectiveness is thought to be because of direct action on the meningeal artery inflammation. They also appear to have prophylactic properties when taken continuously. For side effects and contraindications see Chapter 5 *Drugs and immunological disorders*.

Prophylactic treatment

Some patients require prophylactic medication taken daily to prevent migraine, usually if they have more than two migraine headaches per month. The main groups of drugs given are **beta-blockers**, **serotonin antagonists** and **tricyclic antidepressants**.

Beta-blockers such as **propranolol**, **metoprolol**, **nadolol** and **timolol** are all effective in the prevention of migraine. Their exact mode of action is unknown, but it may result from the effect of beta-blockers on peripheral resistance. The most common drug used is **propranolol**; its effective dose is **10–40 mg** three times daily. Side effects include insomnia, nightmares, fatigue and depression. Propranolol should never be given to patients with asthma, cardiac failure, peripheral vascular disease or depression. These contraindications tend to limit the use of beta-blockers, as does their interaction with **ergotamine**.

Pizotifen, 0.5–3 mg daily, given orally, is an antihistamine and serotonin antagonist structurally related to the tricyclic antidepressants. It acts by blocking the serotonin receptors in the smooth muscle of some cranial arteries, resulting in a reduction in the frequency and severity of migraine attacks. **Cyproheptadine**, 4 mg at night, is also an antihistamine with serotonin-antagonist and calcium-channel blocking properties. It may also be tried in refractory cases.

Tricyclic antidepressants such as **amitriptyline**, 10–50 mg at night, may be administered.

There is some evidence that the calcium-channel blockers **verapamil** and **nifedipine** may be useful in migraine prophylaxis.

SLEEP DISORDERS

The two major disorders concerning sleep are narcolepsy and insomnia.

NARCOLEPSY

People with narcolepsy lapse into sleep during waking hours. These episodes last for about 15 minutes and may often be triggered by a pleasurable event. This condition can be extremely hazardous as there is no prior warning of an attack. The person is advised not to operate or go near machinery or drive a car and to refrain from such pleasures as swimming or having a bath. Narcolepsy occurs as a result of abnormal timing of rapid eye movement (REM) sleep, with frequent episodes of REM sleep during the day and less REM sleep during the night.

Pathophysiology

The cause of narcolepsy has not been established but there is believed to be a link between the class II antigen DR2, a part of the major histocompatability complex. Most people with narcolepsy are found to carry this antigen.

Pharmacological management

Dexamphetamine is given, 10 mg daily in divided doses for adults, and 5 mg daily in divided doses for the elderly. It is increased by 10 mg daily at intervals of 1 week to a maximum of 60 mg for adults and increased by 5 mg daily at intervals of 1 week to a maximum of 30 mg for the elderly. Driving and other hazardous activities can resume once the patient is stabilised. **Dexamphetamine** is a central nervous system stimulant and has a direct action on α and β receptor sites in the body.

Its use is contraindicated in those with cardiovascular disease, moderate to severe hypertension, hyperthyroidism, glaucoma, those taking monoamine oxidase inhibitors and those in whom there is a known hypersensitivity to amphetamines.

Side effects are varied. In the nervous system they include insomnia, restlessness, irritability and excitability and talkativeness. In the cardiovascular system they include dizziness, headaches and convulsions, hypertension, tachycardia, palpitation and cardiac arrhythmias; and in the gastrointestinal system they include nausea, vomiting, anorexia, abdominal cramp, diarrhoea, dry mouth and metallic taste.

INSOMNIA

Insomnia is a disorder not a specific disease; it is a symptom of many diseases. Insomnia may be transient, short-term or chronic and is characterised by:
- Difficulty in falling asleep.
- Difficulty in staying asleep.
- Short unrefreshing sleep.

Transient insomnia is a condition that affects most people at some time, particularly when they are anxious or upset. It may also be caused by disturbances in the normal awake–sleep cycle, which leads to desynchronisation of the circadian rhythm and is seen to occur in shift workers and as a result of jet lag. Short-term insomnia is often the result of an emotional problem such as bereavement, or marital and work-related problems. Long-term insomnia is associated with chronic depression, drug or alcohol abuse and chronic pain disorders. Insomnia can also have an iatrogenic cause and is associated with the following drugs: amphetamines, steroids, central adrenergic blockers, bronchodilating agents and caffeine, which is also contained in many over-the-counter prescriptions.

Elderly people have true insomnia caused by age-related changes. Their total sleep time is decreased quite markedly and they take longer to fall asleep. They awaken earlier in the morning and more frequently during the night (**Fig. 8.5**). These changes in their sleep pattern may be associated with changes in lifestyle, lack of daily routine, physical ailments (e.g. sleep apnoea, nocturnal myoclonus, 'restless legs', dyspnoea and cerebral degeneration), desynchronisation of their circadian rhythm and incorrect use of sedatives. **It should be noted that**, with regard to sedatives in the terminally ill in relation to insomnia, these should not be omitted when a patient is receiving opiate medication as an opiate is not a sedative.

Insomnia is frequently seen in psychiatric illness, particularly in anxiety states and depressive illness (see Chapter 7 *Drugs and psychological disorders*). Choosing a medication with a secondary hypnotic effect to treat the illness can assist in relieving the insomnia.

Chronic insomnia is an inability to obtain the amount or quality of sleep needed to function adequately during the daytime, causing tiredness during the day and associated mood disturbance. Insomnia and daytime sleepiness are symptoms and not specific diseases. Insomnia is the symptom of many diseases. Treating insomnia with drugs relieves the symptoms only; if used for an extended period

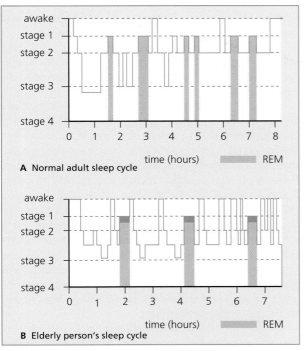

A Normal adult sleep cycle

B Elderly person's sleep cycle

Fig 8.5 Sleep cycles. REM, rapid eye movement.

such drugs bring about changes in the normal sleep cycle, which in itself leads to sleep disturbances. It is recommended that before medication commences the underlying cause should be determined and treated and, where required, advice and information given to assist and promote sleep.

Sleep occurs when there is a reduction in the activity of the reticular formation centre and hypothalamus in the brainstem. The neurotransmitters that play an important part in REM sleep are acetylcholine and noradrenaline, whereas those that play an important part in non-REM sleep are serotonin and GABA. Peptides are also known to be involved with non-REM sleep but their role is not clearly understood and further research is being undertaken into these sleep-promoting peptides (Domino, 1994).

Pathophysiology

Insomnia is a consequence of increasing age, when stages III and IV (non-REM) sleep become less prominent and the elderly spend much less time in these stages. Patients with serious mental diseases such as depression and schizophrenia also have severe sleep disturbances during these stages, as well as an earlier onset of REM sleep than other people. The neurotransmitters implicated in wakefulness are acetylcholine, catecholamines (including dopamine and noradrenaline), histamine and glutamic acid. Because such a large variety of neurotransmitters are implicated, drugs acting on them affect wakefulness as well as the different stages of sleep.

Pharmacological management

Sleep promoting drugs act as central nervous system depressants and include the following groups of drugs:

- **Benzodiazepines:** these are hypnotic drugs that produce drowsiness and induce sleep.
- **Barbiturates:** usage is not recommended; these drugs act as a sedative (calms the patient and reduces their activity) and as a hypnotic.
- **Antihistamines:** act as a hypnotic and as a sedative and are occasionally used for children.
- **Miscellaneous sedative–hypnotic drugs**.

Benzodiazepines act by enhancing the inhibitory presynaptic or postsynaptic actions of GABA. When benzodiazepines are taken orally they reach peak blood and brain concentrations within 1–2 hours. Their action is to reduce the latent period and prolong the duration of sleep. Approximately 25% of normal sleep is REM sleep. When taking benzodiazepines this can be reduced by as much as 75%. When the benzodiazepine is stopped, there is a rebound effect on REM sleep as the body tries to make up for what has been lost. Nightmares occur with severe rebound, causing the patient to resort to retaking their medication. It is for this reason, and because of the danger of drug dependence, that the medication should not be prescribed for periods longer than 2–3 weeks.

In the elderly, who have a reduced amount of REM sleep normally, the effects are greater; the patient appears 'groggy', depressed, unstable, shaky and agitated, and periods of amnesia are seen. It is recommended that elderly people should be prescribed short-acting benzodiazepines, which have a hypnotic action. These are **loprazolam**, 1 mg at bedtime, elderly 0.5–1.0 mg; **lormetazepam**, 0.5–1.5 mg at bedtime, elderly 500 µg; **temazepam**, 10–20 mg at bedtime, elderly 10 mg. The action of the drug can be greatly extended if the patient has a deteriorating renal or liver function. In such patients the dosage should be reduced accordingly. **Nitrazepam**, 5–10 mg at bedtime, elderly 2.5–5 mg, is a long-acting hypnotic and is used less frequently for treatment, especially in the elderly.

Contraindications include respiratory depression, acute pulmonary insufficiency; severe hepatic impairment, myesthenia gravis and sleep apnoea syndrome. Side effects include drowsiness and light-headedness the next day; confusion and ataxia (especially in the elderly); amnesia may occur, as may dependence.

Alcohol and benzodiazepines when taken together can result in a greater loss of coordination than when taken singularly. There is also an increase in the sedative effects of the benzodiazepine. Benzodiazepines are also known to decrease the elimination of digoxin, leading to increased risk of toxicity.

Benzodiazepines and their metabolites are widely distributed in body tissues. They cross the blood–brain barrier and the placenta, and are distributed into breast milk.

They are believed to cause fetal abnormalities and are therefore not recommended during pregnancy. Long-term use in late pregnancy may cause dependence in the neonate, resulting in withdrawal symptoms.

The use of barbiturates is not now recommended, but they may still be used for the treatment of intractable insomnia in patients already taking barbiturates. They should be avoided in the elderly. Long-acting barbiturates such as phenobarbitone are still used as previously discussed in the section on epilepsy.

Sedative antihistamines such as **diphenhydramine** are available as over-the-counter medication for adults; they aid relief of temporary sleep disturbance, and can be combined with paracetamol for the relief of temporary sleeplessness and night-time pain.

The antihistamine **promethazine**, 25 mg at bedtime, is available over the counter for adults and may be taken as a night sedation and for insomnia. **Promethazine** is also available for children aged 2–5 years, dose 15–20 mg, and for 5–10 year olds, 20–25 mg, but the use of hypnotics for children is not recommended.

Because of their prolonged duration of action, these medications may lead to drowsiness the following day.

Miscellaneous sedative-hypnotic drugs

Zolpidem and **zopiclone** are not benzodiazepines but act on the same receptors. They have a short duration of action with little or no hangover effect, but should not be used for long-term treatment. Side effects include nausea and vomiting and those seen with the benzodiazepines.

Chloral hydrate now has limited use as a hypnotic although previously it was given frequently to the elderly. Dependence occurred with prolonged usage. Gastric irritation was a common side effect.

Triclofos, 10–20 ml, is given orally in solution; it is a chloral derivative, but causes less gastric irritation. It can be used for insomnia but only in the short term, because of the danger of dependence. Contraindications include cardiac disease, hepatic or renal impairment, pregnancy and breast feeding. Side effects include abdominal distension, flatulence, vertigo, rashes, headache, malaise delirium (especially in the elderly), ketonuria, excitement and nightmares.

Chlormethiazole, 1–2 capsules or 5–10 ml syrup, is given for severe insomnia in the elderly. It is a useful hypnotic as it does not cause a hangover effect, but should not be administered for long-term use as dependency occurs. It is given for very short-term use in younger adults to relieve alcohol withdrawal symptoms. It may also be used for the treatment of status epilepticus.

In the presence of cardiac and respiratory disease, confusion can occur due to hypoxia. If hepatic and renal impairment are present, excessive sedation can result.

Contraindications include acute pulmonary insufficiency and alcohol-dependent patients who continue to drink. Side effects include nasal congestion and irritation, increased bronchial secretions, conjunctival irritation and headache.

KEY POINTS

- Raised intracranial pressure causes cerebral compression; nursing vigilance is required to detect the early signs, which may indicate a need for surgical decompression.
- Low-dose aspirin is prescribed as prophylaxis against future thrombosis after a stroke caused by a thrombotic episode.
- Severe meningococcal meningitis can lead rapidly to collapse and death, therefore a combination of broad-spectrum antibiotics should be commenced immediately.
- Medication for Parkinson's disease is given to control symptoms; patients should be observed for signs of diminishing response to the drugs.
- Patients with Parkinson's disease and motor neuron disease may lose their ability to swallow; if this occurs there is a risk of inhalation pneumonia.
- The progress of multiple sclerosis is variable and characterised by remissions and exacerbations; symptoms are made worse by fatigue.
- Epileptic women receiving carbemazepine may need particular advice related to family planning as the drug inactivates oral contraceptives.
- A migraine attack may be provoked by the consumption of foods containing tyramine.
- Insomnia is a symptom not a disease. Long-term treatment with hypnotics may cause further disturbances to the sleep cycle.

MULTIPLE CHOICE QUESTIONS

Choose the correct answers.

1. Raised intracranial pressure is detected by
a. epistaxis
b. alteration in pupil size
c. confusion
d. leakage of cerebral spinal fluid
e. vomiting

2. The effective treatment for stroke is
a. aspirin
b. dexamethasone
c. heparin
d. dipyridamole
e. mannitol

3. Meningitis vaccination is available for
a. *Haemophilus influenzae* type B
b. *Streptococcus pneumoniae*
c. *Neisseria meningitidis* group A
d. *Neisseria meningitidis* group B
e. *Neisseria meningitidis* group C

4. Bacterial meningitis results in the formation of a
a. granuloma
b. purulent exudate
c. partial loss of hearing
d. slowly occurring dementia
e. thrombosis

5. Postural alterations in Parkinson's disease are characterised by all of the following except
a. difficulty with writing
b. orthostatic hypotension
c. short, accelerated steps
d. festinating gait
e. tremor

6. Drug therapy in Parkinson's disease is aimed at
a. increasing cholinergic activity
b. decreasing dopaminergic function
c. decreasing cholinergic activity
d. increasing dopaminergic function
e. balancing the dopaminergic and cholinergic activity

7. The drugs given to maximise the effects of levodopa are
a. benserazide
b. cyclizine
c. amantadine
d. carbidopa
e. bromocriptine

8. The side effects of the administration of anticholinesterase agents may include all of the following except
a. a decrease in bronchial secretions
b. sweating
c. diarrhoea
d. increased salivation
e. gastrointestinal upsets

9. Which of the following statements about phenytoin is false?
a. it commonly causes hiccups, stomachache and vomiting
b. it causes dose-related ataxia and nystagmus
c. it is the safest drug used in the treatment of epilepsy
d. it is associated with hirsutism and gingival hyperplasia
e. it is used to treat generalised tonic or clonic seizures

10. Prophylactic treatment for migraine is
a. pizotifen
b. sumatriptan
c. aspirin
d. verapamil
e. propranolol

REFERENCES

Bennett JP. Drugs for the treatment of movement disorders. In: Brody TM, Larner J, Minneman KP, Neu HC, eds. *Human pharmacology molecular to clinical*. St Louis: Mosby, 1994:363-371.

Bonita R. Epidemiology of stroke. *Lancet* 1992; **339**:342-344.

Bramble D, Pearce J. Attention deficit hyperactivity disorder: a rational guide to paediatric assessment and treatment. *Curr Paediatr* 1997; **7**:26-41.

British Medical Association. *British National Formulary*. London: Royal Pharmaceutical Society of Great Britain, 1998

Day M. Meningitis – case notes. *Nurs Times* 1996; **92**:19.

Domino EF. Drugs for sleep disorders. In: Brody TM, Larner J, Minneman KP, Neu HC, eds. *Human pharmacology molecular to clinical*. St Louis: Mosby, 1994:449-455.

Downie G, MacKenzie J, Williams A. *Pharmacology and drug management for nurses*. Edinburgh: Churchill Livingstone, 1995.

Fazekas F, Deisenhammer F, Strasser Fuchs S, Nahler G, Marroli B. Immunoglobin in relapsing-remitting multiple sclerosis is effective and well tolerated. *Lancet* 1997; **349**:589-593.

International Stroke Trial Collaborative Group. The international stroke trial: a randomised trial of aspiring, subcutaneous heparin, both or neither among 19 435 patients with acute ischaemic stroke. *Lancet* 1997; **349**:1569-1581.

Kernich CC, Kaminski HJ. Myasthenia gravis: pathophysiology, diagnosis and collaborative care. *J Neurosci Nurs* 1995; **27**:207-215.

Li-G. Atropine, levodopa or methyldopa: serious side effects. *J Tradit Chin Med* 1995; **15**:163-169.

Mathewson-Kuhn M. *Pharmaco-therapeutics*. Philadelphia: FA Davis, 1994.

Margioros AN, Gravanis A, Chrousos GP. Glucocorticoids and mineralocorticoids. In: Brody TM, Larner J, Minneman KP, Neu HC, eds. *Human pharmacology molecular to clinical*. St Louis: Mosby, 1994:473-481.

Marieb EN. *Human anatomy and physiology, 3rd ed.* Redwood City, CA: Benjamin Cummings, 1994.

McCance LK, Huether SE. *Pathophysiology the biologic basis for disease in adults and children*. St. Louis: Mosby,1994.

Meers P, Sedgwick J, Worsley M. *The microbiology and epidemiology of infection for health science students*. London: Chapman and Hall, 1995.

Neilley LK, Goodwin DS, Goodkin DE, Hauser SL. Side-effect profile of interferon beta-1b in multiple sclerosis 'results of an open label trial'. *Neurology* 1996; **46**:452-454.

Paradiso C. *Pathophysiology*. Philadelphia: JB Lippincott, 1995.

Pundare L. Therapeutic apheresis. *Professional Nurse* 1994; **9**:626-631.

Richard IH, Kurlan R, Tanner C, Factor S, Hubble J, Suchowersky O, Waters C. Deprenyl (selegiline) eldepryl and antidepressants. *Neurology* 1997; **48**:1070-1077.

Rose V. Understanding motor neurone disease. *Professional Nurse* 1992; **9**:784-786.

Spencer CM, Benfield P. Talcapone. In: *CNS Drugs*. Auckland: Adis International, 1996.

Stevens A, Lowe J. *Pathology*. London: Mosby, 1995.

Stokes M. *Neurological Physiotherapy*. London: Mosby, 1998

Stringer JL. Drugs for seizure disorders (epilepsy's). In: Brody TM, Larner J, Minneman KP, Neu HC, eds. *Human pharmacology molecular to clinical*. St Louis: Mosby, 1994:351-361.

Taylor D. Issues in stroke. *Pharm J* 1998; **60**:489-491.

Taylor E, Sandberg S, Thorley G, Giles S. *The epidemiology of childhood hyperactivity*. (Maudsley Monographs No 33.) Oxford: Oxford University Press, 1991.

9 Julie Fegan
DRUGS AND HEAD AND NECK DISORDERS

INTRODUCTION

The eyes, ears, nose and throat include the special senses that help people to communicate. The loss of these special senses can sometimes damage an individual life more than the loss of a limb. Many disorders of the eyes, ears, nose and throat will involve changes over a lifetime, attributable to ageing and degeneration of sight, hearing, smell, taste and the efficiency of swallowing. These cannot be reversed by pharmacological means but the acute conditions may. Some degenerative functions can be reversed by surgical techniques such as cataract extraction, implantation of lenses or cochlear implants. Damage to nervous tissue is irreversible, but there are devices that boost function, hearing aids for example. Contact lenses and spectacles may restore near normal accommodation and refraction in the eye. More difficult can be the problems of balance that are associated with disease in the vestibular apparatus of the ear. The nose and throat are prone to infections and hypersensitivities such as acute or chronic rhinitis; infection and inflammation can impair smell, breathing and speech.

The internal and external structures of the eye and ear are intimately connected with neurological function. Therefore, drugs that can affect the nervous system may have some effect on the nervous supply innervating these important sensory organs. Drugs can be ototoxic and may affect hearing or balance, or both. Many systemic diseases can cause temporary or permanent damage to the eye and/or ear. Sensorineural loss from disease or trauma can lead to the loss of any of the special senses, depending on the nerve supply affected. Many of these problems can be dealt with surgically; many can be modified by pharmacological means.

ADMINISTRATION OF DRUGS TO THE EYE

When administered as eye drops, drugs penetrate the globe, probably through the cornea (**Fig. 9.1**). However, undesirable systemic effects can occur because of absorption via conjunctival vessels or from the nasal mucosa after the excess fluid from the eye drops has drained into the nose via the tear ducts. For example, **timolol** (a beta-blocker) given as eye drops may induce bronchospasm or bradycardia in susceptible people. This systemic absorption is highly variable. When two different eye drops are used at the same time of day, for instance **pilocarpine** and **timolol** in glaucoma, dilution and overflow can occur when one immediately follows the other so the patient should be advised to allow a 5-minute interval between the different drops.

In general, it is not advisable for patients to continue wearing contact lenses, particularly soft contact lenses, when receiving eye drops. Some drugs and preservatives can accumulate in hydrogel lenses and may induce toxic reactions. Ointments should never be used in conjunction with contact lens wear. Many drugs given systemically can also have an effect on contact lens use (**Table 9.1**). Contact lenses require scrupulous care. Complications of poor compliance can lead to ulcerative keratitis and conjunctival problems such as purulent or papillary conjunctivitis.

DRUGS FOR TEAR DEFICIENCY

Artificial tears, sterile water and normal saline can be used to keep the cornea moist and avoid ulceration. Carbomer 940 (polyacrylic acid) 0.2% – one drop – can be instilled 3–4 times a day. This will relieve symptoms in keratoconjunctivitis often seen in patients with rheumatoid arthritis. Patients need to be reminded that their vision will be blurred and their eyes sticky with this medication. They should put other eye drops in before these and wait 30 minutes before applying contact lenses. Under anaesthetic or heavy sedation, eyes may be protected from drying with Vaseline gauze pads if surgery is prolonged. For the newborn undergoing ultraviolet light treatment, the eyes may be protected with shields or eye masks.

DRUGS FOR LOCAL ANAESTHESIA

Oxybuprocaine hydrochloride, **proxymetacaine hydrochloride**, **lignocaine hydrochloride** and **amethocaine**

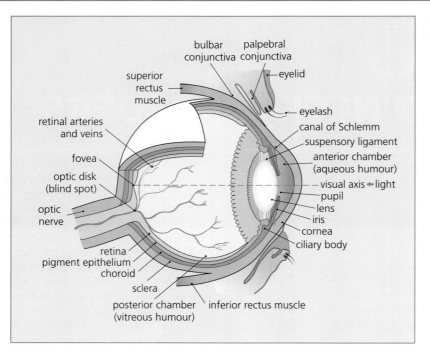

Fig 9.1 Anatomy of the eye.
(From Page 1997, with permission.)

Drugs and contact lenses	
Drugs that reduce blink rate	Anxiolytics, hypnotics, antihistamines and muscle relaxants
Drugs that reduce tear production	Antihistamines, antimuscarinics, phenothiazines and related drugs, some beta-blockers, diuretics and tricyclic antidepressants
Drugs that increase lacrimation	Ephedrine and hydralazine
Drugs that cause conjunctival inflammation	Isotretinoin
Drugs that may cause ocular or eyelid oedema	Primidone
Drugs that may cause irritation	Aspirin (appears in tears and may be absorbed by the lens) and high-dose oestrogen contraceptives
Drugs that may discolour lenses	Rifampicin and sulphasalazine

Table 9.1 Adverse effects of systemic drugs on contact lens wear

hydrochloride are used for topical desensitisation in minor surgical procedures (for action see Chapter 3 *Classes of drugs*). Care must be taken with patients receiving these medications as they will not be aware of particles touching the cornea and thus are at risk of accidental injury. A pad should be kept over the eye until the drug effect has worn off.

DRUGS THAT CAN DAMAGE THE EYE
As the eye is controlled by the somatic nervous system and the autonomic nervous system, drugs that affect the function of any of these systems may in some way affect the function of the eye. CS gas and Mace used in civil disorders or for personal protection contain **capsaicin**, which activates sensory nerve receptors causing pain,

inflammation and lacrimation. The same chemical is found in chilli peppers so the eyes should never be touched after cutting up chillies.

Long-term glucocorticosteroids applied topically and systemic drugs such as **phenothiazines** used in schizophrenia can cause cataracts. **Chloroquine**, an early malarial drug now used for rheumatoid conditions, can cause reversible cataracts and also irreversible retinopathy if the dose is not kept below 250 mg per day. Long-term topical or systemic glucocorticosteroids can cause 'steroid glaucoma'.

Taking as little as 10 g of methanol, found in 'moonshine' and poteen, damages the retinal ganglion cells that form the optic nerve and can cause blindness. Hepatic enzymes convert the methanol to formaldehyde, which rapidly reacts with the proteins; this is the reason it is used as a tissue fixative in the laboratory. **Indomethacin**, **ethambutol**, **tamoxifen** and **phenothiazines** have adverse effects on the retina, which seem to be dose dependent.

9.1 OXYGEN DAMAGES THE EYE

A specific problem with premature infants placed in a high-oxygen environment is retrolental fibroplasia produced by the inappropriate growth of blood vessels into the vitreous humour; it is triggered by abrupt removal of the infant from the high-oxygen environment.

DISORDERS OF THE EYE

INFLAMMATION, INFECTION AND HYPERSENSITIVITY

Local intraocular inflammation and uveitis can be treated with a short course of glucocorticosteroids applied topically to the eye. Glucocorticosteroids have marked anti-inflammatory actions, but they also produce many side effects, including excessive suppression of the immune system and exacerbation of infections. Most of these side effects can be avoided if smaller doses are applied locally, although this can be associated with a local suppression of the immune system. They work by suppressing the inflammatory response (see Chapter 3 *Classes of drugs*). Systemic glucocorticosteroids may be appropriate for severe eye diseases such as scleritis, episcleritis and blinding uveitis. Correct diagnosis is vital as glucocorticosteroids can worsen an inflamed eye produced by a dendritic ulcer caused by herpes simplex, and can lead to blindness or loss of the eye.

CONJUNCTIVITIS

Conjunctivitis is an inflammatory condition that affects the conjunctivae and is usually caused by viral or bacterial infection, chemical irritation or allergy. It can be caused by a variety of microorganisms (**Table 9.2**). Diagnosis of acute or chronic bacterial conjunctivitis involves isolating the causative organism, which may involve Gram-staining for bacterial type and/or Giemsa stain for the histological examination of cells. Treatment involves testing for antibiotic sensitivity and administration of the appropriate antibiotic eye drops or ointment.

Pathophysiology

The eye is normally protected by immunoglobulin A in the tears, which constantly wash the eye. In all cases of conjunctivitis, the inflammatory process that occurs by the

	Acute bacterial	Chronic bacterial	Viral	Trachoma	Allergy
Types of conjunctivitis					
Examples	Staphylococcal, streptococcal	*Moraxella* sp. tuberculous	Herpetic, adenoviral	*Chlamydia trachomatis*	Pollen allergy, cosmetic allergy
Incidence	Common	Uncommon	Very common	Uncommon	Very common
Appearance	Suppuration, diffuse redness	Extreme redness, little secretion	Redness, lacrimation, chemosis	Papillation, follicle formation	Redness, lacrimation, chemosis
(Vardaxis, 1995)					

Table 9.2 Types of conjunctivitis

insult of infection, chemical or allergy causes the signs and symptoms, namely redness, oedema, pain and lacrimation. **Acute bacterial conjunctivitis** ('pinkeye') is highly contagious and often caused by Gram-positive organisms (see **Table 9.2**). The onset is acute, with mucopurulent drainage from one or both eyes. Preventing spread of the organism with meticulous hand washing and separate towels is important. The disease is frequently self-limiting and resolves spontaneously within 10–14 days, although antibiotic eye drops are usually effective. **Viral** conjunctivitis is caused by an adenovirus, with mild to severe symptoms. Some strains cause a pharyngitis or it may manifest as keratoconjunctivitis. Both diseases are contagious, with watering redness and photophobia. If the conjunctivitis is **allergic** it will be the result of a type I hypersensitivity reaction, producing itching associated with photophobia, burning and gritty sensations in the eye. Chronic conjunctivitis is a persistent condition that requires identification of the cause for effective treatment. Trachoma (chlamydial conjunctivitis) is caused by *Chlamydia trachomatis* and is often associated with poor hygiene. It is the leading cause of preventable blindness in the world. The severity may vary but inflammation and vascularisation of the cornea with scarring of the conjunctiva and eyelids leads to blindness.

Pharmacological management

Drugs such as antibiotics may be given systemically to treat an eye condition but infections are usually treated with eye drops or ointments. Antibacterial drugs used for eye infections include broad-spectrum antibiotics such as **chloramphenicol**, **ciprofloxacin**, **framycetin sulphate**, **gentamicin**, **neomycin sulphate** or **ofloxacin**. Gentamicin is specifically used for *Pseudomonas aeruginosa* infections, **ciprofloxacin** for corneal ulcers, **chlortetracycline** for chlamydial (trachoma) infections, **fusidic acid** for staphylococcal infections and **propamidine isethionate** for *Acanthamoeba* keratitis. Side effects with antibacterial drugs used topically in the eye are minimal and may include stinging and itching. Chloramphenicol, the most widely used, has been associated with aplastic anaemia, although rarely, and ciprofloxacin is best avoided in children as it is particularly likely to cause local burning and itching. Chlamydial organisms are sensitive to local or systemic antibiotics. The action of antibiotics is discussed in Chapter 5 *Drugs and immunological disorders* and Chapter 3 *Classes of drugs*.

The treatment of allergic conjunctivitis may include antihistamines, steroids and vasoconstrictors. Systemic corticosteroids can be given to treat the eye. Topical corticosteroids should only be used in the short term because they can cause 'steroid glaucoma' and should never be used in undiagnosed red eye in which the cause may be herpes simplex; their use can produce a dendritic ulcer, leading to loss of vision or of the eye. **Antazoline** is useful but is a sympathomimetic, which should be avoided in angle-closure glaucoma. **Levocabastine** can be used in seasonal allergic conjunctivitis but may cause local irritation, blurred vision, local oedema, urticaria, dyspnoea, headache and drowsiness. **Lodoxamide**, **nedocromil sodium** and **sodium cromoglycate** are antiinflammatory and are used for the topical treatment of inflammation and allergic conjunctivitis but may cause transient burning and stinging. There are few antiviral drugs available. Aciclovir is used to treat corneal ulcers caused by herpes simplex and ganciclovir is used to treat cytomegalovirus infection of the eye, which occurs in patients with AIDS.

Fungal infections are rare but may occur in agricultural workers after injuries to the eye, especially in hot and humid climates. Orbital mycosis is rare and usually is spread from the paranasal sinuses. Increasing age, debility or immunosuppression may encourage fungal proliferation. The spread of infection via the bloodstream occasionally produces a metastatic endophthalmitis. Many different fungi are capable of producing ocular infection and can be identified in the laboratory. Antifungal preparations for the eye are not generally available so treatment will be carried out at specialist centres. Information can be obtained from the nearest hospital ophthalmology unit or from Moorfields Eye Hospital, City Road, London EC1V 2PD or telephone 0171 253-3411.

KERATITIS AND CORNEAL ULCERATION

Keratitis is an infection or inflammation of the cornea, either from outside (exogenous) from infective causes or inside the cornea (endogenous) from allergic or toxic states.

Pathophysiology

A common manifestation of keratitis is corneal ulceration. Corneal ulcers may be bacterial or viral infections or be secondary to long-standing inflammation caused, for example, by trauma. Viral corneal infections are caused by herpes zoster virus and by adenoviruses; the latter cause epidemic outbreaks because of their contagious nature. In most cases the ulcer will heal but in some cases it can cause scarring or have the following serious complications:

- Scarring leading to opacities.
- Corneal perforation followed by prolapse of the iris.
- Descemetocoele, an outpouching of Descemet's membrane through the ulcerated outer layers of the cornea.
- Hypopyon, a collection of pus within the anterior chamber.
- Staphyloma, a nodule of darkly coloured tissue caused by the bulging of the cornea or sclera.
- Uveitis, endophthalmitis, cataract or secondary glaucoma.

Pharmacological management

Corneal ulcer and keratitis require specialist treatment and may call for subconjunctival or systemic administration of antibiotics. **Endophthalmitis** is a medical emergency that also calls for specialist management and often requires parenteral, subconjunctival or intraocular administration of antibiotics. Dendritic ulcers are a common form of ulcerative keratitis caused by herpes virus infection of the cornea, so called because of the tree-like structure. After debridement of the ulcer the eye is treated with **aciclovir** plus a broad-spectrum antibiotic to prevent secondary bacterial infections.

GLAUCOMA

Glaucoma includes several conditions that cause a rise in intraocular pressure and thus may cause ischaemia and degeneration of the optic nerve. The aqueous humour is formed by the ciliary epithelium in the posterior chamber and flows through the pupil to the angle formed by the cornea and iris. Here it filters through the trabecular meshwork and enters the canal of Schlemm for return to the venous circulation. Glaucoma results from the impeded outflow of aqueous humour from the anterior chamber of the eye and contributes to the incidence of blindness each year. The condition may be asymptomatic and a considerable loss of peripheral vision may occur before medical attention is sought. Routine screening of people aged over 40 years and those with a family history of glaucoma is important.

Pathophysiology

Three main types of glaucoma exist: congenital (infantile) glaucoma, closed-angle glaucoma and open-angle glaucoma. Congenital glaucoma is caused by the anterior chamber retaining its fetal configuration, with the trabecular network attached to the root of the iris or with a membrane across the anterior chamber. Early surgical treatment is necessary to prevent blindness.

Primary open-angle glaucoma (**Fig. 9.3A**) is an abnormal increase in intraocular pressure in the absence of an obstruction between the trabecular meshwork and the anterior chamber. It is usually, however, an abnormality of the trabecular meshwork impairing the flow from the meshwork to the canal of Schlemm. It tends to manifest in patients over the age of 35 years, may be an inherited condition and is the most common form of glaucoma – accounting for about 90% of cases. Free testing is available after the age of 35 years for those whose parents suffer the condition. Primary open-angle glaucoma is usually asymptomatic and chronic, causing progressive loss of visual field unless appropriately treated. In some patients the cause may be iatrogenic as topical corticosteroids can cause a rise in intraocular pressure and in some sensitive people, systemic corticosteroids can also do so.

In primary closed-angle glaucoma (**Fig. 9.3B**) the anterior chamber is narrow and outflow becomes impaired when the iris thickens as a result of pupil dilatation. As the iris thickens it reduces or eliminates the access to the angle between the base of the iris and sclera, where aqueous reabsorption occurs. Primary closed-angle glaucoma usually occurs as the result of an inherited anatomic defect; it is usually bilateral but may not be symmetrical in development and occurs in about 5–10% of cases. Treatment is primarily surgical by removal of part of the iris (iridectomy).

Secondary glaucoma is caused by diseases that obstruct aqueous flow. Secondary open-angle glaucoma may be caused by particles in the aqueous humour that block the trabecular meshwork, for example degenerate lens

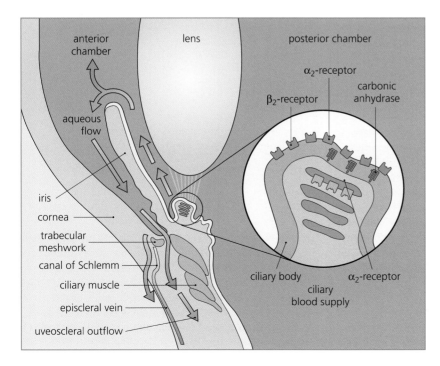

Fig 9.2 Production and drainage of the aqueous humour.

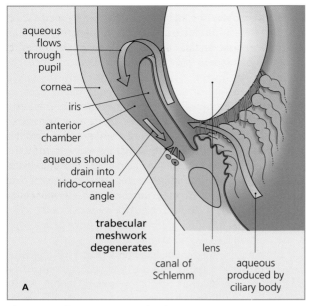

Fig 9.3A Primary open-angle glaucoma.
(From Stevens & Lowe 1995, with permission.)

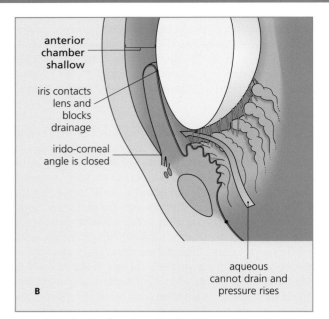

Fig 9.3B Primary closed-angle glaucoma.
(From Stevens & Lowe 1995, with permission.)

material, pigment from melanocyte lesions or macrophages that accumulate in response to haemorrhage or inflammation (**Fig. 9.3C**). Adhesions between the iris and cornea that are caused by uveitis or that are secondary to vascular proliferation of retinal vessels may result in secondary closed-angle glaucoma.

Pharmacological management

Treatment is usually pharmacological and involves five classes of drugs: β-adrenergic blockers, adrenergic agonists, parasympathomimetics, carbonic anhydrase inhibitors and hyperosmolar agents. All but the carbonic anhydrase inhibitors and hyperosmolar agents are given topically, that is they are instilled as eye drops.

β-adrenergic blockers

Topical beta-blockers (**betaxolol hydrochloride**, **carteolol hydrochloride**, **levobunolol hydrochloride**, **metipranolol** and **timilol maleate**) reduce intraocular pressure by reducing the rate of production of the aqueous humour (see **Fig. 9.2**). Beta-blockers also reduce intraocular pressure if given by mouth but this route is not used. These drugs administered as eye drops may be systemically absorbed and are therefore contraindicated in patients with bradycardia, heart block or heart failure. They should also not be used in any patient with asthma or obstructive airways disease.

Adrenergic agonists

The adrenergic agonists (adrenaline, dipivefrine hydrochloride and guanethidine monosulphate) produce mydriasis

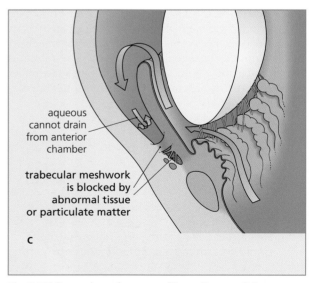

Fig 9.3C Secondary glaucoma. (From Stevens & Lowe 1995, with permission.)

(pupillary dilatation) (**Fig. 9.4**). Adrenaline probably works by reducing the rate of production of aqueous humour and by increasing the outflow through the trabecular meshwork. It is contraindicated in closed-angle glaucoma because it is a mydriatic unless an iridectomy has been carried out. Many people become sensitive to these drugs over time, developing a red eye that persists until treatment is discontinued.

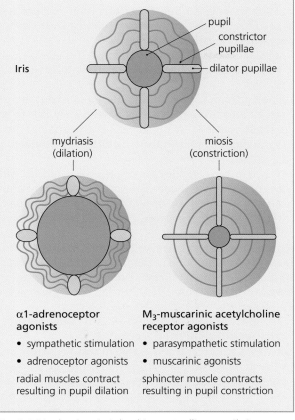

α1-adrenoceptor agonists
- sympathetic stimulation
- adrenoceptor agonists

radial muscles contract resulting in pupil dilation

M₃-muscarinic acetylcholine receptor agonists
- parasympathetic stimulation
- muscarinic agonists

sphincter muscle contracts resulting in pupil constriction

Fig 9.4 Mechanism involved in controlling pupil size.

Parasympathomimetics

Physostigmine sulphate increases concentration of acetylcholine at cholinergic transmission sites causing prolonged miosis and a fall in intraocular pressure by opening up drainage channels. Drops are available in 0.25 and 0.5% solutions and should be instilled 2–6 times per day according to response. They can cause blurred vision, irritation of the conjunctiva and lid twitching. They are often used in conjunction with **pilocarpine hydrochloride** or **pilocarpine nitrate**, which acts directly on cholinergic receptor sites. These solutions are available in 0.5, 1, 2, 3 and 4% strengths and may be instilled 2–6 times per day according to response. Nurses must advise the patient to keep these medications in the fridge, to renew them each week, not to touch the dropper and that visual acuity will be reduced in dim light.

Carbonic anhydrase inhibitors

Acetazolamide and **dichlorphenamide** are systemic drugs that are useful when beta-blockers cannot be used. Acetazolamide inhibits carbonic anhydrase, thus bicarbonate is reduced in aqueous humour and the water is therefore secreted. Dichlorphenamide has a similar but more prolonged action and both drugs have a diuretic effect and a moderate incidence of side effects, particularly in the elderly, of paraesthesia, hypokalaemia, lack of appetite, drowsiness and depression.

Hyperosmolar agents

Mannitol acts by increasing the osmolarity of the glomerular filtrate, which raises the osmotic pressure of the fluid in the renal tubules. This decreases the reabsorption of water and increases the urinary output. An intravenous infusion of 1.5–2 g/kg of a 15–25% solution of mannitol is given over 0.5–1 hour. Blood pressure should be monitored and signs of dehydration must be watched for. **Glycerol** acts by

---

PERSON CENTRED STUDY 1

Leslie went to the optician to have the prescription for his reading glasses checked. To his surprise he was referred to his local ophthalmology department because the optician had found that his intraocular pressures were raised. In the Outpatient's Department the ophthalmologist explained that he had glaucoma and asked if anyone in his family had ever had this condition. Leslie was also puzzled when the doctor asked him if he had asthma or chronic obstructive airways disease as he could not see a connection between those conditions and his newly diagnosed eye condition. He came home with timolol eye drops and strict instructions to store these in the fridge, not to touch the applicator tip and to discard any of the drug that remained after the date mark on the container. As he expected that the drops would 'cure' his condition he was surprised when told he would have to have a new prescription as soon as the old drops were discarded and would have to return to the ophthalmologist for regular check-ups.

1. How would you explain to Leslie why he will always need some kind of treatment for glaucoma?
2. What is the connection if Leslie has another family member with glaucoma?
3. Why might the doctor ask about asthma and chronic obstructive airways disease before prescribing treatment?
4. Why is it important to store the drops in the fridge, not to touch the applicator tip and to discard any of the drug that remained after the date mark on the container?

drawing fluid into the colon; it is given by 4 g suppository. It is a laxative so patients should be advised to expect increased bowel action.

EYE DISEASES CAUSED BY SYSTEMIC PROBLEMS

Cataracts and a characteristic **retinopathy** are features of diabetes mellitus; some newly diagnosed diabetics experience transient blurred vision when they begin insulin treatment until their body water has stabilised. Hypertension, sickle cell anaemia and AIDS can affect the retinal blood vessels or the retina itself. Multiple sclerosis patients may experience visual disturbances by demyelination of the optic nerves. **Uveitis** can be found in some patients with tuberculosis. **Conjunctivitis** is a symptom of exophthalmos in those with hyperthyroidism. Babies born to mothers with active sexually transmitted diseases may have inflammation of the conjunctiva and cornea.

DISORDERS OF THE EAR

HEARING LOSS

Hearing loss may be classified as conductive (usually caused by some abnormality in the external or middle ear), sensorineural (usually caused by some abnormality in the inner ear, auditory nerve or brain), or mixed (i.e. with features of conductive and sensorineural hearing loss). The structure of the ear is illustrated diagrammatically in **Figure 9.5**.

Pathophysiology

Conductive hearing loss occurs when a change in the outer or middle ear impairs sound from being conducted to the inner ear by interference in air conduction. In most cases temporary hearing loss is caused by occlusion of the external ear canal by wax. Careful removal of the wax restores hearing. Other conditions that may cause conductive hearing loss include foreign bodies lodged in the ear canal, benign tumours of the middle ear, carcinoma of the ear canal or middle ear and Eustachian tube dysfunction. These must be dealt with symptomatically. The following are causes of conductive hearing loss:

- Acute otitis externa (see below).
- Acute and chronic otitis media and its complications (see below).
- Barotrauma (e.g. after blast injuries) may lead to temporary hearing loss or permanent if there is damage to the auditory ossicles.
- Perforation of the tympanic membrane by trauma or infection.
- Otosclerosis (a rare disease involving the ossicles with formation of new bone of a vascular, spongy nature caused by a genetic predisposition, twice as common in women, with onset between 15 and 30 years of age).

Barotrauma and perforation will require symptomatic treatment of symptoms until healing takes place. Treatment of the underlying cause generally eliminates the hearing loss but a hearing aid is used if the hearing loss is greater than 40–50 decibels.

Pharmacological management

Ear wax is a normal bodily secretion that provides a protective film on the meatal skin and only needs to be removed if it causes deafness or interferes with a proper view of the eardrum during a clinical examination. Wax can be softened with simple remedies such as warm **almond oil** or **olive oil**, **sodium bicarbonate** ear drops or mixtures of **urea hydrogen peroxide** or **docusate sodium**. Some preparations contain organic solvents, for example **paradichlorparabenzene**, which can cause irritation of the meatal skin. The warm solution is introduced into the ear canal with the affected ear uppermost and left for 5–10 minutes. Several treatments may be needed over several days. After softening the wax, the ears may be syringed very gently with warm water. **Caution:** A person who has hearing in only one ear should not have the other ear syringed

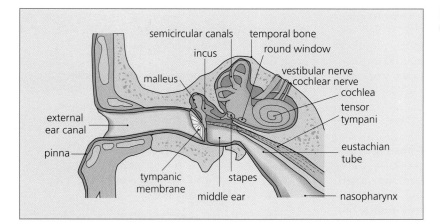

Fig 9.5 Structure of the ear.
(From Page 1997, with permission.)

because even a slight risk of damage is unacceptable. The ear should not be syringed if the patient has a history of recurring otitis externa (see below), a perforated eardrum or has had previous ear surgery (George, 1999).

SENSORINEURAL HEARING LOSS

The most common type of permanent hearing loss is **presbycusis**, a pattern of sensorineural hearing loss in the elderly, with loss of high tones combined with distortion. There is no pharmacological treatment for this degenerative condition, but treatment of an accompanying conductive hearing loss may improve acuity. Congenital or neonatal sensorineural hearing loss may be caused by maternal rubella, ototoxic drugs, prematurity, traumatic delivery, erythroblastosis fetalis and congenital hereditary malformation; there are no pharmacological treatments. **Tinnitus** is a complaint of buzzing, ringing, pulsating or hissing noises heard by the patient in the ears or head region. It may be caused by Ménières disease, labyrinthitis, ear wax, alcohol abuse, ototoxic drugs, neoplasms, vascular diseases, presbycusis and otosclerosis. It does not occur in vestibular neuronitis, and benign positional vertigo. Distinguishing between vertigo and tinnitus can help in making a differential diagnosis of Ménières disease. Important causes of acquired sensorineural deafness include:

- **Excessive noise** (formerly industrial exposure, now usually caused by the use of personal stereos at high volumes by young people (Stevens and Lowe 1995)).
- **Ototoxic drugs** (see below).
- **Post-infective** (non-inherited congenital deafness caused by maternal rubella, now rare; cytomegalovirus, toxoplasmosis and post-meningitis – the most common cause in children).
- **Acoustic neuroma** and **head injury** (important causes in adults).

Pathophysiology

Presbycusis is most common in the elderly. It may be caused by atrophy of the basal end of the organ of Corti (**Fig. 9.6**), a decrease in the number of auditory receptors, vascular changes or stiffening of the basilar membranes with slowly progressive hearing loss.

Pharmacological management

Treatment of the primary cause of hearing loss may improve but not reverse the hearing loss. Degeneration of the organs of hearing cannot be reversed by drug treatment. Early treatment of cytomegalovirus infection with **ganciclovir**, a relative of aciclovir, may help prevent hearing loss but should not be used with zidovudine because of myelosuppression. **Foscarnet** is also active against cytomegalovirus but is nephrotoxic. Ganciclovir and foscarnet are usually only used for cytomegalovirus when sight is threatened. Toxoplasmosis is generally self-limiting but

treatment is necessary if there is eye involvement or for those who are immunosuppressed. Treatment of choice is **pyrimethamine** and **sulphadiazine** given for several weeks under the care of a specialist. Pyrimethamine is a folate antagonist so weekly blood tests and folinic acid supplements are needed. Alternative regimens may use pyrimethamine with **clindamycin**, **clarithromycin** or **azithromycin**. Long-term secondary prophylaxis is required after treatment of toxoplasmosis in AIDS. For the treatment of meningitis see Chapter 8 *Drugs and neurological disorders*.

OTOTOXICITY

Four clinically important classes of drugs cause inner ear toxicity: antibiotics, diuretics, some chemicals and tobacco and alcohol. Most drug ototoxicity is associated with antibiotics, particularly aminoglycosides (**neomycin**, **kanamycin** and **streptomycin**) but also **erythromycin**, **minocycline**, **vancomycin** and diuretics (**ethacrynic acid** and **frusemide**). The chemicals that cause inner ear toxicity include salicylate, quinine, carbon monoxide, nitrogen mustard, arsenic, mercury and gold.

Pathophysiology

The cells of the cristae and maculae in the inner ear or the cells of the organ of Corti are damaged by increased concentrations of **antibiotics** in the endolymph. This increased concentration of drugs in the endolymph is toxic to cells of the organ of Corti. **Diuretics** alter the sodium–potassium balance, causing extracellular fluid accumulation and changes in the microstructure of secretory cells. Quinine, mercury and lead affect the neural pathways of hearing, including the spinal ganglia, the eighth cranial nerve and the cochlear nucleus. The site of action for the other

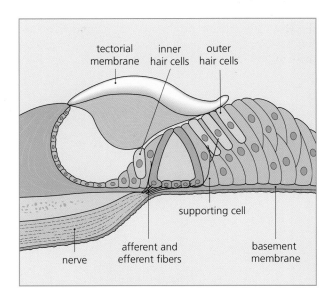

Fig 9.6 The organ of Corti. (From Page 1997, with permission.)

chemicals, including alcohol and tobacco, is unclear but most produce tinnitus followed by a high-tone sensorineural hearing loss (McCance and Huether, 1998).

Pharmacological management

Concurrent administration of aminoglycosides with diuretics should be avoided. Damage is often dose related and the elderly are most at risk of ototoxicity. Care is aimed at preventing further hearing loss because the loss is usually permanent. When there is already sensorineural hearing loss, ototoxic drugs should be avoided if at all possible. Topical ototoxic antibiotics should not be used when there is a perforation, although some specialists have used the polymyxins or aminoglycosides (e.g. neomycin) because it is considered that the pus in the middle ear associated with otitis media carries a higher risk of ototoxicity than the drops themselves (George, 1999).

VERTIGO

Dizziness is a word used for a wide variety of symptoms and can range from a vague feeling of unsteadiness to the light-headedness associated with anxiety. The site of the symptom must be determined: whether it is in the limbs, the chest or the head. Vertigo is usually described by patients as the sensation of rotation in which the person feels that their surroundings are spinning or moving. Vertigo often causes loss of balance.

Pathophysiology

Vertigo usually occurs with inflammation of the semicircular canals in the ear and may be caused by disease of the labyrinth, vestibular pathways or their central connections

(**Fig. 9.7**). Motion sickness is one kind of vestibular disorder. Vertigo may be associated with Ménières disease, labryrinthitis, ear wax, alcohol abuse, ototoxic drugs, neoplasms, vascular diseases, vestibular neuronitis and benign positional vertigo. It does not occur in presbycusis and otosclerosis.

Pharmacological management

The most effective drug for motion sickness is **hyoscine**, which can cause drowsiness, blurred vision, dry mouth and, in adult men, possible urinary retention, so caution should be exercised in administering this to elderly men. Hyoscine is contraindicated in closed-angle glaucoma. **Antihistamines** are slightly less effective, but are generally better tolerated (George, 1999). There is no evidence that one is better than another but their duration and side effects differ (drowsiness and antimuscarinic effects). If sedation is desirable then **promethazine** and **dimenhydrate** can be useful. In general, a less sedating antihistamine such as **cyclizine** or **cinnarizine** is preferred. **Metoclopramide** and the phenothiazines (except promethazine) act selectively on the chemoreceptor trigger zone and are therefore ineffective. Treatment of vertigo in its chronic form is seldom fully effective but antihistamines such as dimenhydrate or a phenothiazine such as prochlorperazine may help.

OTITIS EXTERNA

Inflammation of the external ear involving the skin and meatus as a result of infection is fairly common. Otitis externa may also be allergic in origin, often from antibiotic drops used to treat an infection. If severe, infection can progress down to the level of cartilage – this occurs with

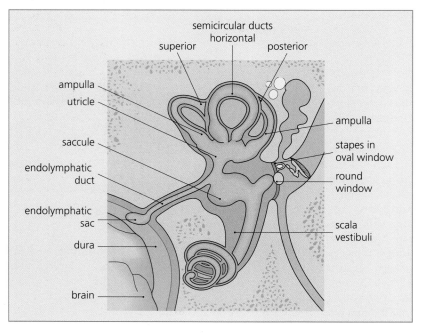

Fig 9.7 The peripheral vestibular system. (From Page 1997, with permission.)

furunculosis of the ear, a boil on the auricle. Most cases of otitis externa manifest as 'swimmer's ear', so called because of the regularity with which swimmers have this kind of infection from poorly disinfected pools.

Pathophysiology

The organisms are usually bacterial or fungal and rarely viral:

• *Pseudomonas* spp., *Staphylococcus* spp. and diphtheroids.
• *Streptococcus* spp.
• *Aspergillus niger* and *Candida albicans* (otomycoses).
• Herpes viruses (viral cause).

Symptoms are a result of the inflammatory process caused by the infection and immune response, and are either localised as in the furunculosis or are diffuse. The most common fungus is *Aspergillus niger*, black threads of which can be identified in the inflammatory exudate and may even be visible in the ear canal. The patient may have exquisite pain, redness, swelling and the production of pus, with hearing loss on the affected side. The pain is exacerbated by moving the jaw as in chewing. If it is left untreated, the fever and pain disappear but the discharge persists. Itching of the ear becomes chronic, resulting in scratching of the ear with the finger or an object, thereby aggravating the condition. The ear should be cleaned of all debris and a swab taken for microbiological investigation. Medicated dressings may be applied.

Pharmacological management

Medications include topical antibiotics such as **chloramphenicol**, **framycetin**, **gentamicin** and **neomycin** for bacterial infections, **clioquinol** for bacterial and fungal infections and **clotrimazole** for fungal infections. Topical steroid preparations (**betamethasone sodium phosphate**, **dexamethasone**, **flumethasone pivalate**, **hydrocortisone**, **prednisolone sodium phosphate** and **triamcinolone acetonide** may be used, especially if there is marked oedema (see Chapter 3 *Classes of drugs*). Dressings are changed daily and the laboratory report for sensitivity is taken into consideration. Systemic antibiotics are only given if the patient presents with pyrexia. Once treated the patient should be taught not to scratch their ears, to keep water out and to dry them thoroughly with clean cotton wool after swimming or bathing.

OTITIS MEDIA

Otitis media is inflammation of the middle ear caused by infection with viruses or bacteria or by allergy. Although normally mild, acute otitis media can produce serious complications with long-lasting effects such as deafness.

Pathophysiology

Upper respiratory tract viral infections are frequently accompanied by acute inflammation in the middle ear and the inner lining of the eardrum. Secondary bacterial infection may occur, increasing the risk of perforation of the eardrum. Children are particularly susceptible because the narrow Eustachian tube can become obstructed by the adenoids at the lower end (Stevens and Lowe, 1995). The main complications are persistent perforation of the eardrum, otitis media with effusion ('glue ear') and acute mastoiditis, which is now rare since the introduction of antibiotics. It is believed that adequate treatment for allergic rhinitis could prevent otitis media from occurring. Acute otitis media in children has a multifactorial aetiology and economic and antimicrobial implications (Boccazzi and Careddu, 1997). Because it is difficult to distinguish between bacterial and viral infections on clinical examination, nasal swabs are taken as they are relatively noninvasive and can exclude a bacterial cause. Local epidemiology will also give the doctor information, as the choice of antibiotic must take into account the antibiotic-resistant strains prevalent at the time.

Pharmacological management

As the middle ear is inaccessible to ear drops an infection must be treated with systemic antibiotics. High levels of antibiotic resistance are now being seen in the three principal pathogens: *Streptococcus pneumoniae*, *Haemophilus influenzae* and *Moraxella catarrhalis* (Cohen, 1997). Both *H. influenzae* and *M. catarrhalis* are efficient producers of β-lactamases; more recently pneumococci have become more resistant through altered penicillin binding proteins. Some antimicrobials have remained effective against the majority of these three bacterial species, for example **amoxicillin** and **clavulanic acid** (Jones, 1997). The newer macrolides, **azithromycin** and **clarithromycin**, provide good coverage in penicillin-resistant *S. pneumoniae* and β-lactamase-producing *H. influenzae*. Both drugs achieve higher, sustained concentrations in middle ear fluid than do the β-lactam antibiotics (Block, 1997, Arguedas *et al.*, 1997). However, it is now suggested that early treatment with antibiotics may not be necessary. In six studies of children with otitis media, 60% of children were pain free after 24 hours without antibiotics, and 2–7 days after presentation only 14% still had pain. Early use of antibiotics reduced the risk of pain by 41% and contralateral otitis media by 43% (Del Mar *et al.*, 1997). Antibiotics were associated with vomiting, diarrhoea or rashes. From the studies it is apparent that only 1 in 17 children needs antibiotics early to prevent pain. The other 16 would have been able to wait until nasal swabs were taken and cultured for antibiotic sensitivity so that the appropriate antibiotic could be given for the specific microbe.

OTITIS INTERNA

Labyrinthitis is an inflammation of the inner ear that involves the labyrinth. The most common cause is an extension of infection and inflammation from acute or chronic otitis media. Less commonly it may occur from meningitis extending into the inner ear.

Pathophysiology

The organisms involved include β-haemolytic *Strepto-coccus*, *S. pneumoniae*, *Staphylococcus* spp., *H. influenzae*, coliforms, *Pseudomonas* spp. and *Neisseria meningitidis*, in any combination. There is usually a purulent exudate, loss of labyrinthine function and loss of hearing. Regardless of whether severe disease develops, the most severe symptoms are experienced with diffuse inflammation. The patient usually presents with vertigo (see above), vomiting, nausea and nystagmus (involuntary rapid movement of the eyeball).

Pharmacological management

Systemic antibiotics are used against the causative organism (see Chapter 5 *Drugs and immunological disorders*). Beta-haemolytic *Streptococcus* is sensitive to **penicillin**, but it is important to discover the causative organism and a broad-spectrum antibiotic may be used initially.

MÉNIÈRES DISEASE

This vestibular disorder causes proprioceptor dysfunction so that standing or walking is impossible in an acute attack. The disease usually first affects people between the ages of 40 and 60 years, one ear being affected initially and in 25% of patients the other ear is involved later (Vardaxis, 1995). The symptoms include **vertigo**, which is often preceded by a feeling of pressure in the ear and followed by malaise for several days. **Nausea** and **vomiting** are almost always associated with attacks and may be very difficult to control. The patient will also complain of **hearing loss**, which is particularly pronounced before and after an attack. This hearing loss is progressive, with distortion of any sound still perceived. **Tinnitus** is also present and worse before the attacks, preceding all other symptoms by a period of months or years.

Pathophysiology

Ménières disease is an idiopathic condition associated with increased pressure within the endolymphatic system in the inner ear. The raised endolymph pressure distends the membranous labyrinth, and the hair cells of the organ of Corti show a progressive degeneration. The cause of Ménières disease is unknown but there is marked distension of the cochlear duct by excess fluid, such that the vestibular membrane of Reissner, which separates two fluids of different composition, bulges into the scala vestibuli (see **Fig. 9.8**). This membrane may rupture, allowing the two fluids to mix. Histological study has been difficult (Stevens and Lowe, 1995).

Pharmacological management

Attacks of Ménières disease occur in bouts, becoming more frequent and more severe over time, and eventually causing deafness in the affected ear (Vardaxis, 1995). Advice may be for the patient to stay on a low-fluid, low-salt diet. Medical treatment with vestibular sedatives (e.g. **cinnarizine** or **prochlorperazine**) is unsatisfactory but **betahistine hydrochloride** (16 mg three times a day initially, with 24–48 mg daily as a maintenance dose), promoted as a specific treatment for Ménières disease, may be helpful (Kumar and Clark, 1994).

Diuretics (**hydrochlorothiazide** and **frusemide** with potassium replacement) are used to limit endolymph production. **Meclozine hydrochloride** and **cinnarizine** are antihistamines that may help the vertigo, tinnitus, nausea and vomiting. **Aminoglycosides** induce a stable decrease in vestibular function. Vestibular suppressants (sedatives, antihistamines, anticholinergics and narcotics) may be used for severe attacks. A benzodiazepine such as diazepam or lorazepam not only provides sedation but also acts on the medial and lateral vestibular nuclei to suppress otolithic and semicircular canal activity (Page *et al.*, 1997).

DISORDERS OF THE NOSE AND THROAT

INFECTION AND INFLAMMATION

Rhinitis, acute or chronic inflammation of the nasal mucosa, and rhinorrhoea manifest with excessive watery secretions from the nasal mucosa. Both may occur as a result of viral infections or an interaction between antigens and tissue-bound IgE antibodies within the nasal mucosa.

PERSON CENTRED STUDY 2

Dean is 3 years old. He is at present flushed and miserable and insists on holding his blanket to the left side of his head. His mother Danielle, realising that once again he has earache, takes his temperature and finds that he has a fever of 38.7°C. She takes him to the family doctor who examines his ears with some difficulty, as Dean is very uncooperative. The doctor prescribes a broad-spectrum antibiotic and some paracetamol syrup. Later at home Dean's grandmother says he will 'grow out of' this problem and he does not need antibiotics, but Danielle wonders whether he should be put onto the waiting list for insertion of grommets.

1. How would you explain the recurrent earache to Danielle?
2. Why might grommets not be appropriate for Dean at this time?
3. Why is a broad-spectrum antibiotic appropriate for this earache?
4. Why is Dean's grandmother partly right?

Sympathetic activity reduces rhinitis and rhinorrhoea, clears the nasal passages and facilitates breathing. Sympatholytic drugs (adrenergic neuron blockers and α-adrenoceptor antagonists) can cause nasal congestion. Unfortunately, no treatment is effective against the most common viral infection to cause rhinitis and rhinorrhoea, the common cold (Page *et al.*, 1997). **Interferon** was once suggested, but as one dose was so expensive, it was not thought reasonable to use it for colds.

ALLERGIC RHINITIS

Perennial and seasonal allergic rhinitis affects millions of people and can lead to serious complications such as chronic sinusitis and otitis media. The symptoms include sneezing, rhinorrhoea, nasal congestion and pruritus, which can lead to irritability, insomnia and fatigue. The cause is usually pollens, dusts and moulds.

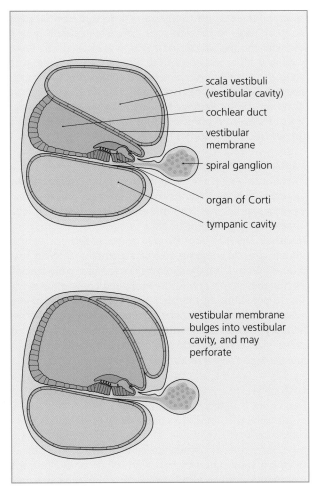

Fig 9.8 Changes in Ménière's disease. (Top) Normal cochlea and (below) affected cochlea. (From Stevens & Lowe 1995, with permission.)

Pathophysiology

The pathophysiology of allergic rhinitis results from a type 1 hypersensitivity reaction (see Chapter 5 *Drugs and immunological disorders*). The symptoms are attributable to the biological effects of mast cell degranulation. The nasal passages contain a large number of mast cells and are sensitive to the effects of histamine released from them, causing inflammation of the mucous membranes of the nose. The inflammation is caused by vasodilatation, hypersecretion of mucus, oedema and swelling. Because the mucous membranes of the respiratory tract are continuous with those of the nose (accessory sinuses, nasopharynx, and upper and lower respiratory tract), they too are adversely affected by the allergic reaction.

Pharmacological management

Sufferers may find antihistamines and H_1 receptor antagonists useful in relieving the symptoms of allergic rhinitis. Nonsedating products such as **acrivastine**, **astemizole**, **cetirizine hydrochloride**, **fexofenadine hydrochloride**, **loratadine**, and **terfenadine**, sometimes in combination with a decongestant, may be used. These newer drugs, although not causing sedation and psychomotor impairment because they cross the blood–brain barrier only to a small extent, cannot alleviate pruritus of non-allergic origin.

Older antihistamines still used for hay fever and urticaria include azatadine maleate, brompheniramine maleate, **chlorpheniramine maleate** (used for emergency treatment of anaphylactic shock – see Chapter 19 *Pharmacological management of medical emergencies*), clemastine, diphenhydramine hydrochloride (also a drug available over the counter, used for temporary sleep disturbances in adults), phenindamine maleate, **promethazine hydrochloride** (also used for emergency treatment of anaphylactic shock) and trimeprazine tartrate (also used as a premedication).

Topical intranasal corticosteroids are another important component of management of allergic rhinitis (see Chapter 3 *Classes of drugs*). **Beclomethasone, betamethasone, budesonide, flunisolide, fluticasone, mometasone** and **triamcinolone** are used prophylactically for the treatment of allergic rhinitis when started 2–3 weeks before the season commences, although they may have to be continued for several months. Perennial rhinitis may require their use for years. Side effects include dryness, irritation of the nose and throat, epistaxis and rarely ulceration, nasal septal perforation (usually following surgery) and raised intraocular pressure. Taste may also be disturbed if the nasal spray is swallowed. Hypersensitivity reactions, including bronchospasm, have also occurred.

Very disabling symptoms occasionally justify the use of **systemic corticosteroids**, for students taking important examinations for example. **Cromoglycate**, **nedocromil** and topical antihistamines (**azelastine** and **levocabastine**) are also used in allergic rhinitis.

Allergen immunotherapy (hyposensitisation) is used in patients not managed adequately with pharmacotherapy. Except for bee and wasp stings, allergy-specific hyposensitisation is not very effective in asthma but can be effective in allergic rhinitis if sensitivity to a particular allergen can be proved.

Rare hazardous arrhythmias are associated with **astemizole** and **terfenadine**, particularly when concentrations of these drugs are raised in the blood or when they are taken together. The dose should not be exceeded (astemizole 10 mg only daily and terfenadine 120 mg only daily) and must be avoided in liver impairment. They should not be given with ketoconazole, itraconazole, or other **imidazole antifungals**, nor with **erythromycin** and **clarithromycin**. Electrolyte imbalances such as hypokalaemia may occur if they are taken with **diuretics**. Other potentially arrhythmogenic drugs such as **anti-arrhythmics**, **antipsychotics**, **tricyclic antidepressants** should not be taken at the same time as astemizole and terfenadine.

THROAT INFECTIONS

As many infections of the respiratory tract are self-limiting and leave little residual damage, the use of antibiotics in bacterial infections carries a unique risk of development of resistant organisms. In the absence of life-threatening infection the choice of antibiotic should be based on culture and sensitivity tests of the causative organism. Some organisms, however, produce such a characteristic pattern that clinical diagnosis and prescription of antibiotic can be based on presentation alone.

EPIGLOTTITIS

Epiglottitis is a life-threatening inflammation of the epiglottis usually caused by *H. influenzae* type B. The oedema of inflammation can obstruct the airway and spread above and below to the trachea and bronchi. If this occurs respiratory distress is more severe and the outcome less favourable.

Pathophysiology

Patients present with inspiratory stridor, fever and severe respiratory distress. The child or adult will be unable to swallow because of the swelling and oedema of inflammation. Examination of the throat may cause laryngospasm and respiratory collapse. Nasotracheal intubation or tracheotomy is necessary in rapidly increasing obstruction. Pneumonia, cervical lymph node inflammation, otitis and rarely meningitis or septic arthritis may occur during the course of epiglottitis.

Pharmacological management

The cephalosporin derivatives (**cefuroxime**, **cefotaxime** and **ceftriaxone**) are used to treat epiglottitis, with **chloramphenicol** as a second-line drug. Chloramphenicol is effective but can cause a lethal aplastic anaemia (see Chapter 5

Drugs and immunological disorders). The incidence of epiglottitis is diminishing as increasing numbers of children receive *H. influenzae* type B immunisation. The disease is now more common in adults.

PHARYNGITIS

Pharyngitis is a sore throat most likely to be caused by viruses, but allergy or bacteria can also be the cause. A sore throat is an initial symptom in colds and flu. Antihistamines that relieve rhinitis and earache usually work as well on the sore throat. It may be important to control the allergy to avoid a secondary bacterial infection in inflamed tissues. Viral sore throats generally resolve except in immunosuppressed or immunodeficient patients. Bacterial sore throats do not resolve readily so if a sore throat persists it will need to be treated with systemic antibiotics.

Pathophysiology

Streptococcus pyogenes, a β-haemolytic Gram-positive cocci, produces most troublesome infection by producing streptokinase to dissolve clots, which explains how it spreads. It is an acute throat infection associated with fever, pain and inflammation of the pharynx and tonsils, with white patches of pus on pharyngeal epithelium. Rheumatic fever and glomerulonephritis complications may result in heart and kidney damage because of hypersensitivity reactions. One strain produces an erythrogenic toxin, which causes the rash of scarlet fever.

Pharmacological management

There are no effective drugs to treat throat inflammation caused by viruses. Over-the-counter lozenges or sprays may cause a sore tongue and lips, and those containing local anaesthetics may relieve pain but lead to sensitisation (George, 1999). Warm or cold water gargles or syrupy liquids may be soothing and **paracetamol** or **aspirin** may reduce the pain, but the soreness does resolve fairly quickly. Fortunately *S. pyogenes* has remained completely sensitive to penicillin, but there is no effective vaccine to prevent the infection. Therefore **phenoxymethylpenicillin** or **benzyl penicillin** are the first-line antibiotics for this group of bacteria. **Erythromycin** and **cephalexin** would be second and third choices of treatment, respectively.

LARYNGITIS

Laryngitis is usually caused by the common cold and is only treated with antibiotics in the event of secondary infection. The larynx may also be affected by 'croup'; this is called laryngotracheobronchitis and is an acute viral inflammation of the respiratory tract with subglottic swelling and respiratory distress accompanied by a high-pitched sound during inspiration. Croup is usually caused by parainfluenza virus, less often RSV (respiratory syncytial virus), influenza A or B and the bacterium *Mycoplasma pneumoniae*. Laryngitis has also been caused by the diphtheria organism, now fortunately very rare in the United Kingdom because of immunisation.

Pathophysiology

Viruses called rhinoviruses cause colds and thus laryngitis. They are RNA viruses with an envelope that is composed of fats and polysaccharides. The virus works by injecting the RNA into a host cell or by the cell phagocytosing the virus particle. The virus then breaks up the cell's own DNA, produces viral protein capsids and assembles new virus particles until the cell bursts (lyses). The body's phagocytes and the antiviral protein interferon, produced by the virus-infected cells, soon limit the infection.

In bacterial croup caused by *Corynebacterium diphtheriae*, inflammation and infection of the upper airways, including pharyngitis and rhinitis, proceeds to laryngeal inflammation. Diphtheria causes the mucosa of the larynx to become coated with a fibrous exudate, which closes the airway.

Pharmacological management

Bacterial infections are often secondary to viral infections and may be treated in the usual way with systemic antibiotics, the choice of which is determined by the causative organism. There are no effective pharmacological treatments for the common cold virus. For *M. pneumoniae* infection tetracyclines are effective but are deposited in growing bones and teeth bound to calcium, causing staining and occasional dental hypoplasia, so they should not be given to pregnant or breastfeeding women or children under 12 years of age. Immunisation against diphtheria has made this serious disease rare; however, **benzylpenicillin** is effective for diphtheria infection. It must be given by injection as it is inactivated by gastric acid. Benzylpenicillin may cause convulsions in high doses after being given intravenously or in renal failure.

'OVER-THE-COUNTER' DRUGS

Many over-the-counter preparations are bought by the public for dealing with the common coughs and colds suffered by children and adults. They usually consist of expectorant and soothing substances, but the drawbacks of suppressing a cough are rarely outweighed by the benefits. If sleep is disturbed such preparations can be useful, but may cause sputum retention and this can be harmful in patients with chronic bronchitis and bronchiectasis.

EXPECTORANTS

These are claimed to promote expulsion of bronchial secretions but there is no evidence that any drug can facilitate expectoration. It is a myth that subemetic doses of ammonium chloride, ipecacuanha and squill act as expectorants (George, 1999). However, a simple expectorant mixture may serve a useful placebo function (see Chapter 2 *Introduction to pharmacology*).

SOOTHING COUGH PREPARATIONS

Soothing cough preparations with syrup or glycerol are believed by some patients to soothe a dry irritating cough. Simple linctus has the advantage of being cheap and harmless. Paediatric simple linctus is particularly useful in children and sugar-free versions are available.

COMPOUND COUGH PREPARATIONS

Compound cough preparations are on sale to the public but the rationale is sometimes dubious (George, 1999). In the event of overdosage the Poisons Information Services should be contacted for full details of the ingredients. Many of these commercial products contain **paracetamol**, systemic nasal decongestants (see below), **antihistamines**, expectorants (see above), menthol and eucalyptus, and sweet syrups. Because many of these preparations contain antihistamines, which may cause drowsiness, they may affect the ability to drive or operate machinery.

NASAL DECONGESTION

The nasal mucosa is sensitive to changes in atmospheric temperature and humidity and these alone may cause slight nasal congestion. The nose and nasal sinuses produce a litre of mucus in 24 hours (George, 1999) and much of this finds its way silently into the stomach via the nasopharynx. Being aware of this passage of mucus may lead some to believe they have sinusitis.

In rhinitis and the common cold, short-term use of **decongestant** nasal sprays or drops may give symptomatic relief. As these contain sympathomimetics they cause vasoconstriction of mucosal blood vessels, which in turn reduces the thickness of the nasal mucosa. They can cause rebound congestion as they wear off by a secondary vasodilatation. The safest, **ephedrine hydrochloride**, can work for several hours. The stronger sympathomimetics (**oxymetazoline**, **phenylephrine** and **xylometazoline**) are more likely to cause a rebound reaction. All of these preparations may cause a **hypertensive crisis** in patients taking monoamine oxidase inhibitors.

Non-allergic watery rhinorrhoea associated with perennial rhinitis responds well to **ipratropium bromide**, an antimuscarinic that can cause dryness, irritation and epistaxis. Antimuscarinics (also called anticholinergics) inhibit the stimulation of the postganglionic parasympathetic receptors. **Vasodilatation** is a feature of parasympathomimetics just as **vasoconstriction** is a feature of sympathomimetics. Thus the congestion is reduced more centrally than locally. The same drug is very useful in asthma as a bronchodilator for the same reason (see Chapter 11 *Drugs and respiratory disorders*).

The systemic nasal decongestant **pseudoephedrine hydrochloride**, unlike the local application in nasal sprays, does not cause rebound nasal congestion, but may interact with other sympathomimetics. Pseudoephedrine hydrochloride should therefore be **avoided** in patients with hypertension, hyperthyroidism, coronary heart disease, diabetes mellitus and in patients taking monoamine oxidase inhibitors. Side effects can include dry mouth, urinary retention and constipation, although this is unlikely with inhalation (McKenry and Salerno, 1995).

KEY POINTS

- Medications applied topically as eye drops will penetrate the eyeball but may also have systemic effects.
- Infection and inflammation of the eye should be promptly and adequately treated to prevent permanent damage to the eye.
- Screening for glaucoma is important because the increased intraocular pressure which occurs may produce considerable loss of peripheral vision before symptoms are noticed.
- Hearing loss needs good assessment to deal with problems such as earwax and to rule out sensorineural hearing loss which may be a result of other pharmacological management.
- Ear infections may not be treated with antibiotics until nasal swabs are cultured to select an appropriate antibiotic.
- Infection and inflammation of the nose and throat may be caused by viruses, bacteria or allergy.
- Over-the-counter drugs bought by the public for coughs and colds may have other systemic effects which nurses need to know in order to advise patients.

MULTIPLE CHOICE QUESTIONS

Choose all that are correct

1. Eye drops can be absorbed via the
   a. conjunctiva
   b. eye lids
   c. nasal mucosa
   d. pharynx
   e. stomach

2. Contact lenses can be damaged by
   a. tears
   b. oestrogen
   c. diuretics
   d. aspirin
   e. ampicillin

3. The following medications can be used for eye infections:
   a. Augmentin
   b. carbamazepine
   c. gentamicin
   d. aciclovir
   e. nystatin

4. Glaucoma is when
   a. the vitreous humour grows
   b. the ciliary processes do not function
   c. the canal of Schlemm is obstructed
   d. the anterior chamber pressure rises
   e. a patient loses their vision

5. Eye abnormality can occur as a result of
   a. swimming
   b. diabetes
   c. hypertension
   d. pregnancy
   e. ageing

6. Drugs taken systemically that affect the eye are
   a. alcohol
   b. coffee
   c. steroids
   d. phenothiazines
   e. antibiotics

7. Hearing loss is caused by
   a. otitis externa
   b. otitis interna
   c. ototoxicity
   d. systemic disease
   e. diabetes mellitus

8. Side effects of topical nasal corticosteroids include
   a. irritation of nose and throat
   b. dryness
   c. nosebleed
   d. glaucoma
   e. bronchospasm

9. Otitis media should be treated with
   a. benzyl penicillin as a first-choice drug
   b. an antibiotic chosen after a throat swab for culture and sensitivity
   c. chloramphenicol given as ear drops
   d. an antibiotic chosen after a nasal swab for culture and sensitivity
   e. azithromycin or clarithromycin

10. Rhinitis and rhinorrhoea
    a. are always allergic in origin
    b. require sympatholytic drugs
    c. are treated with H_1 receptor antagonists
    d. if left untreated can cause serious complications
    e. should have antibiotics to control secondary infections

REFERENCES

Arguedas A, Loaiza C, Rodriguez F, Herrera ML, Mohs E. Comparative trial of 3 days of azithromycin versus 10 days of clarithromycin in the treatment of children with acute otitis media with effusion. *J Chemother* 1997; **9**:44-50.

Block SL. Causative pathogens, antibiotic resistance and therapeutic considerations in acute otitis media. *Pediatr Infect Dis J* 1997; **16**:449-456.

Boccazzi A, Careddu P. Acute otitis media in pediatrics: are there rational issue in empiric therapy? *Pediatr Infect Dis J* 1997; **16(3 Suppl):**65-69.

Cohen R. The antibiotic treatment of acute otitis media and sinusitis in children. *Diagn Microbiol Infect Dis* 1997; **27**:35-39.

Del Mar C, Glasziou P, Hayem M. Are antibiotics indicated as initial treatment for children with otitis media? A meta-analysis. *Br Med J* 1997; **314**:1526-1529.

George CF. *British National Formulary, no. 37*. London: British Medical Association and Pharmaceutical Press, 1999.

Jones RN. Can antimicrobial activity be sustained? An appraisal of orally administered drugs used for respiratory tract infections. *Diagn Microbiol Infect Dis* 1997; **27**:21-28.

McKenry L, Salerno E. *Pharmacology in Nursing*. London: Mosby, 1995.

Page CP, Curtis MJ, Sutter MC, Walker MJA, Hoffman BB. *Integrated pharmacology*. London: Mosby; 1997.

Stevens A, Lowe J. *Pathology*. London: Mosby, 1995.

Vardaxis NJ. *Pathology for the health sciences*. Edinburgh: Churchill Livingstone, 1995.

10 Pauline Runyard
DRUGS AND ENDOCRINE DISORDERS

INTRODUCTION

The endocrine and nervous systems are very closely linked and complement each other. The hypothalamus regulates the activity of the endocrine system and is itself closely linked to the nervous system, which responds rapidly to information received.

The endocrine, or hormonal, system is responsible for the regulation of cell activity and maintains the homeostasis within the body by responding to a changing internal and external environment. Most hormones are secreted by endocrine cells, others are secreted by nerves or are formed in plasma and interstitial fluid from products released by cells.

The endocrine system can be organised as follows:
• The hypothalamic–pituitary system.
• Discrete endocrine glands (adrenals, thyroid).
• Endocrine cells lodged in other organs (pancreas, digestive system, heart and kidneys).

THE HYPOTHALAMIC–PITUITARY SYSTEM

The hypothalamus has connections with the limbic system, which is particularly involved with the development and expression of emotions and is in turn influenced by the cerebral cortex. It is this connection between the limbic system and the hypothalamus that plays an active part in the modulation of the endocrine system.

Lying below and joining the hypothalamus is the pituitary gland, formed from two separate structures. The posterior pituitary gland (neurohypophysis) stores two hormones that are released in response to excitation from the hypothalamus. These hormones are antidiuretic hormone (ADH) and oxytocin. The anterior pituitary gland (adenohypophysis) secretes hormones in response to stimulation by 'releasing hormones' secreted by the hypothalamus; hormones secreted by the anterior pituitary stimulate or inhibit the secretion of hormones by target endocrine cells; in turn, the levels of these hormones circulating in the blood affect the secretion of the appropriate 'releasing hormones' by the hypothalamus (**Fig. 10.1**). This is known as a negative feedback loop (**Fig. 10.2**). Hormones secreted from the anterior pituitary gland are of two types: somatotrophic hormones and glycoprotein hormones. The somatotrophic hormones are adrenocorticotrophic hormone (ACTH), melanocyte-stimulating hormone (MSH), growth hormone (GH) and prolactin, and the glycoprotein hormones are thyroid-stimulating hormone (TSH), follicle-stimulating hormone (FSH) and luteinizing hormone (LH), the male equivalent of which is interstitial cell stimulating hormone (McCance and Huether, 1994).

The hypothalamus contains neurosecretory cells that are able to synthesise and secrete the 'releasing hormones' that regulate the anterior pituitary; these neurosecretory cells also synthesise and package other hormones along with their binding proteins for delivery and storage in the posterior pituitary gland. The most common consequence of a disorder occurring within the hypothalamus or pituitary is an excess or deficiency of one or more hormones.

DISORDERS OF THE ANTERIOR PITUITARY GLAND

HYPOPITUITARISM

Hypofunction of the anterior pituitary gland known as hypopituitarism is caused by infarction of the gland, as seen in Sheehan's syndrome (see Chapter 16 *Drugs and reproductive disorders*); by removal or destruction of the gland as a result of disease, trauma or infection; or by the presence of an adenoma, which is the most common cause of disease in the pituitary and acts by compression.

Hormonal alterations in glandular tissues may result from the following:
• Change within the structure of the glandular tissue.
• Dysfunction of regulating mechanisms.
• Decrease in excretion of hormones or their inactivation.
• Peripheral resistance to the action of the hormones.

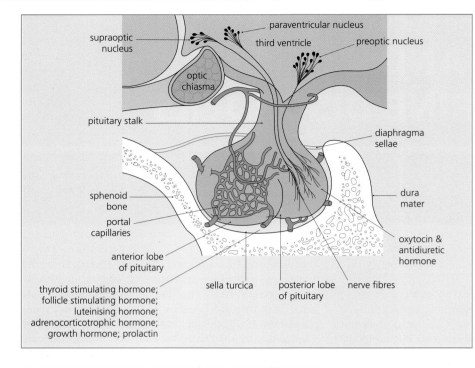

Fig 10.1 Pituitary and hypothalamus and their hormones. (From Stevens & Lowe 1995, with permission.)

Figure labels: paraventricular nucleus, supraoptic nucleus, third ventricle, preoptic nucleus, optic chiasma, pituitary stalk, diaphragma sellae, sphenoid bone, dura mater, portal capillaries, anterior lobe of pituitary, oxytocin & antidiuretic hormone, thyroid stimulating hormone; follicle stimulating hormone; luteinising hormone; adrenocorticotrophic hormone; growth hormone; prolactin, sella turcica, posterior lobe of pituitary, nerve fibres

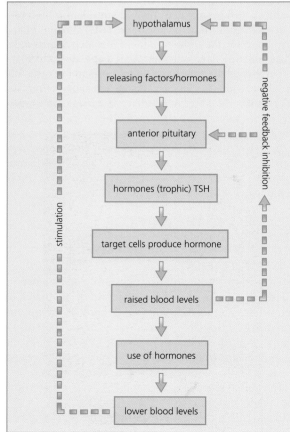

Figure labels: hypothalamus, releasing factors/hormones, anterior pituitary, hormones (trophic) TSH, target cells produce hormone, raised blood levels, use of hormones, lower blood levels, stimulation, negative feedback inhibition

Fig 10.2 Hormone production: negative feedback. TSH: thyroid stimulating hormone.

The aetiology of endocrine gland disorders can be classified as primary (disease within the pituitary), secondary (the result of a hypothalamic disorder) or functional.

Pathophysiology

Growth hormone is the first to be affected by compression of the secretory cells, and is readily seen in the young child of short stature (dwarfism). Children's growth may be affected by their genetic inheritance, the food they eat, the amount of love they receive, the time of year, the extent of their activity and the activity of their endocrine glands (Tanner, 1989). The hypothalamus produces growth hormone releasing hormone (GHRH), which acts on the anterior pituitary. This is stimulated by sleep, exercise, physical and emotional stress, increased protein intake and hypoglycaemia.

Short stature may be caused by having 'short genes', congenital conditions such as skeletal dysplasia, chronic organ or emotional disorders and endocrine deficiency.

Alterations in sexual and reproductive functioning in the young are caused by the lack of follicle-stimulating hormone (FSH) and luteinizing hormone (LH). In adult men and women hyposecretion of FSH and LH causes infertility and amenorrhoea, respectively.

The other four trophic hormones are prolactin, melanocyte-stimulating hormone, adrenocorticotrophic hormone and thyrotrophin. The effects of the last two are discussed further on in the chapter when the adrenal and thyroid glands are examined.

Panhypopituitarism is when all the anterior pituitary hormones are deficient as is antidiuretic hormone from the posterior pituitary gland.

Pharmacological management

Before 1985 GH was harvested from human cadavers and appeared to transfer Creutzfeld–Jakob disease. Today genetically engineered hormone is given by daily injection, sometimes with anabolic and sex steroids (Wardhaugh, 1992). **Somatotrophin** is biosynthetically identical to natural GH and the daily dose given in the evening by subcutaneous injection is calculated according to weight. Thus the dose increases as the child grows. The normal level of hormone in the blood is 15–20 mU/l; somatotrophin treatment is indicated in children whose GH blood levels are 7 mU/l or below.

Of the children who present for treatment, 50% have some hormonal deficiency that affects sexual development. **Gonadotrophins** are given when children are aged 11–12 years to initiate puberty. Thirty per cent of these children are also overweight; their energy expenditure is below normal. These children need to be encouraged to be more active. The follow-up is 3 monthly to check blood pressure and to look for symptoms of diabetes, as these are known to develop in adults who produce excess GH.

Luteinizing hormone and follicle-stimulating hormone are discussed in Chapter 16 *Drugs and reproductive disorders.*

HYPERPITUITARISM

An adenoma within the pituitary may contain secretory pituitary cells, leading to an oversecretion of pituitary hormones or to a combination of oversecretion and undersecretion of pituitary hormones. In 60–80% of functioning adenomata, excess prolactin is produced (see Chapter 16 *Drugs and reproductive disorders*), 15% of the remainder produce GH, and a few produce ACTH.

Pathophysiology

The major disease resulting from a hypersecretion of GH is **gigantism,** which occurs before closure of the epiphyseal plate, or **acromegaly** in adults (**Fig. 10.3**). Acromegaly is a slowly progressive disease more often seen in men aged in their 40s and 50s. The physical changes seen are caused by the proliferation of connective tissue, an increase in the cytoplasmic matrix and an increase in bony proliferation. Acromegaly is recognised by the enlargement of the head, showing forward projection of the jaw and protrusion of the frontal bone. Hands and feet will also be enlarged. There is a change in body posture caused by the proliferation of cartilage; this results from the increased somatomedin produced by the liver, which occurs as a result of the change in the secretory pattern of GH. Because of the excessive cartilaginous and bony overgrowth, there is a degenerative arthritis of the major synovial joints. Diabetes mellitus occurs in 15% of patients with acromegaly because of inhibition of peripheral glucose uptake, which leads to hyperinsulinaemia and the resistance to insulin at the cellular level. Hypertension and left heart failure occur in 30–50% of patients with acromegaly, but pathophysiological changes are not understood (McCance and Huether, 1994). Headaches occur in 50–87% of patients but appear unrelated to size or extension of the tumour or the presence of hypertension. Because it is a space-occupying lesion, it is associated with symptoms of headache and seizures; as it is close to the optic nerve, it is also associated with visual disturbances.

Pharmacological management

This can be by removal of the tumour to relieve pressure within the brain, irradiation to reduce tumour size or medication to suppress GH production.

Bromocriptine mesylate is available as 1 mg and 2.5 mg tablets or 5 mg and 10 mg capsules. It acts as a potent dopaminergic receptor agonist. These receptors can be found in the pituitary–hypothalamic axis, cardiovascular system, gastrointestinal system and central nervous system. It is metabolised by the liver and has a biphasic half-life of 45–50 hours (Mathewson-Kuhn, 1994). It must be used cautiously if patients have a history of cardiac disease or psychiatric disturbances. Initial adverse reactions include nausea, vomiting, dry mouth, leg cramps, cardiac arrhythmias and orthostatic hypotension. It is also known to cause peptic ulceration in acromegaly patients (Downie *et al.,* 1995). Effects are minimised if low doses are administered initially and if they are given with food and at bedtime.

It is important that bromocriptine is not given with other dopamine receptor blocking agents such as the phenothiazines (e.g. chlorpromazine) and butyrophenones

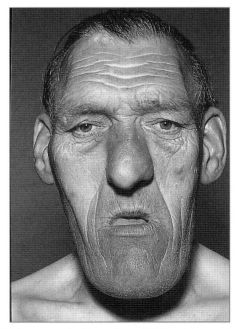

Fig 10.3 Acromegaly. (From Page 1997, with permission.)

(e.g. haloperidol) as these may negate its clinical effect (Evans *et al.*, 1994). **Bromocriptine** is also used in the treatment of idiopathic Parkinson's disease (see Chapter 8 *Drugs and neurological disorders*) and has the additional side effects of confusion, visual or auditory hallucinations and limb pain.

Octreotide is an analogue of somatostatin, and is being developed further for the future treatment of acromegaly. There are hopes that it may be possible to administer it orally rather than by subcutaneous injection. At present octreotide is being given for the treatment of carcinoid and vasoactive intestinal polypeptide tumours. It acts on specific receptor sites in the pituitary plasma membranes, brain synaptic membranes and cellular membranes of pancreatic islet cells. Octreotide appears to decrease intracellular calcium levels, thus influencing the communication mechanisms inside the cell.

DISORDERS OF THE POSTERIOR PITUITARY GLAND

Diseases of the posterior pituitary are rare and, if they occur, are seen in association with abnormal ADH (also known as vasopressin) secretion.

SYNDROME OF INAPPROPRIATE ANTIDIURETIC HORMONE SECRETION

Syndrome of inappropriate ADH secretion (SIADH) is mainly caused by the ectopic secretion of ADH by tumour cells. The tumours that this syndrome has been associated with are oat cell adenocarcinoma of the lung, carcinoma of duodenum and pancreas, leukaemia, lymphoma, Hodgkin's disease, sarcoma and squamous cell carcinoma of the tongue.

Pathophysiology
Transient SIADH may occur after any type of surgery because of the postoperative fluid volume shifts within the body. It may also be caused by pulmonary infection: infected lung tissue may produce ectopic ADH. Inappropriate ADH secretion occurs in some psychiatric patients as a result of their drug regimes, and has also occurred after the administration of the following medications: hypoglycaemic medications, barbiturates, general anaesthesia, vincristine, nicotine, morphine, diuretics and synthetic hormones. These drugs act by stimulating ADH release or by potentiating circulating ADH.

Pharmacological management
Treatment for SIADH is to correct the hyponatraemia, which occurs in various degrees of severity, by the administration of **hypertonic saline** alongside a fluid restriction of below 800 ml/day until sodium levels are normal. Normal urine output occurs within 3 days along with a 2–3 kg weight loss. Excessive release of ADH by the pituitary has been shown to respond to the administration of **phenytoin**.

DIABETES INSIPIDUS: HYPOSECRETION OF ANTIDIURETIC HORMONE

Diabetes insipidus may be a permanent or transient deficiency in ADH synthesis or release, osmoreceptor dysfunction or a decrease in kidney responsiveness to ADH. The end result is the excretion of large volumes of dilute urine (polyuria) and extreme thirst (polydipsia). According to severity urine output can range from 4 to 12 litres per day.

Pathophysiology
The presenting symptoms occur as a result of the following:
- Interference of ADH synthesis, transport, or release from the posterior pituitary caused by primary brain tumours, infections and trauma.
- Insensitivity of the renal collecting tubules to ADH as a result of irreversible disorders such as polynephritis, amyloidosis and polycystic disease. Drugs, for example lithium carbonate and general anaesthetics, may also induce a reversible form of diabetes insipidus by inhibiting the production of cyclic AMP, leading to a reduction in the metabolic pathway necessary for ADH to be effective.

Pharmacological management
Water replacement is essential for neurogenic diabetes insipidus along with the administration of the synthetic ADH analogue **desmopressin**. Desmopressin is preferred because of its effective antidiuretic effect without the vasopressor effect of ADH, which causes an increase in cardiac rate and output. The dosage is 1–2 µg given once daily by intramuscular or subcutaneous injection or, by nasal spray, 10 µg per metered dose with a maintenance dose of 10–20 µg once or twice a day. Desmopressin is also effective in the treatment of primary nocturnal enuresis in adults and children.

 10.1 NASAL PREPARATIONS

Patients on nasal preparations must be instructed carefully in the proper use of the device, as it may cause nasal congestion and local ulceration.

Antidiuretic hormone (vasopressin) may be used for diabetes insipidus, but must be given with extreme caution to patients with cardiovascular problems because of its additional vasoconstrictor effects. However, because of these vasoconstrictor effects, it is very useful for the initial treatment of bleeding **oesophageal varices**, as is **terlipressin**.

The following drugs interact with ADH by potentiating its effects: carbamazepine, chlorpropamide, clofibrate, urea, fludrocortisone and tricyclic antidepressants. Those drugs that inhibit the effects of ADH include demeclocycline, noradrenaline, lithium carbonate, heparin and alcohol.

 10.2 VASOPRESSINS

All ADH analogues may cause water intoxication, indicated by drowsiness, listlessness, weakness, headaches, seizures and coma. Extreme care must be taken when administering these drugs.

DISCRETE ENDOCRINE GLANDS

Two hormones released from the anterior pituitary gland that have a specific and direct effect on two further endocrine glands are TSH and ACTH. When released into the circulatory system, they are recognised by their specific target cell hormone receptors, and bind with them in order to initiate appropriate intracellular activities. Thyroid-stimulating hormone and ACTH are both lipid soluble and are classified as steroid hormones. They are relatively small molecules and cross the plasma membrane by simple diffusion. When entering the cell, TSH first binds to receptor molecules in the cytoplasm and then diffuses into the nucleus. Adrenocorticotrophic hormone diffuses directly into the nucleus. Once activated by either hormone, the receptor binds to specific sites on the chromatin of the target cell DNA, bringing about an increase in RNA transcription with a corresponding increase in the synthesis of specific proteins.

THE THYROID GLAND

The thyroid gland is composed of two cell types, which secrete two different types of hormones. The bulk of the gland is made up of thyroid follicle cells, which synthesise two hormones: thyroxin (T4), which is the major hormone secreted, and tri-iodothyronine (T3). The majority of T3 is formed at the target tissue receptors where T4 is converted to T3 by the enzymatic removal of one iodine group. Both hormones are constructed of two tyrosine amino acids bound to either three or four iodine atoms. (Iodine enters the thyroid epithelial cells by active transport; phospholipids possibly act as the carrier.) (Dunn and Dunn, 1994). This binding of iodine takes place in the lumen of the follicle, which contains thyroglobulin colloid, and is then stored. Under the influence of TSH, thyroglobulin colloid plus iodinated tyrosines are removed from storage. Lysosomal action then splits the protein, which is converted to active T4 and T3 and by diffusion T4 and T3 pass to the capillaries and into the circulation.

The second cell type within the thyroid gland is the parafollicular or 'C' cell, found in clusters between the follicles. Parafollicular cells produce the hormone calcitonin, which acts by inhibiting the action of osteoclasts in bone, thereby helping to maintain calcium homeostasis.

With the exception of tumours and Hashimoto's disease, most forms of thyroid enlargement are caused by hyperplasia of the cells that form the thyroid follicle. The structural hyperplasia responsible for enlargement of the organ may be associated with normal (euthyroid), increased (hyperthyroid) or reduced (hypothyroid) secretion of thyroid hormones, according to the stimulus producing the hyperplasia.

EUTHYROID HYPERPLASIA

Hyperplasia of the thyroid is present on post mortem of many elderly people and is associated with a multinodular goitre. The nodules contain very little colloid and are seen to be mainly composed of thyroid follicle cells. The cause is unknown but thought to be associated with fluctuating levels of TSH.

HYPERTHYROIDISM

Hyperplasia of the thyroid follicles and their cells can be seen as an enlargement of the thyroid gland. The increase in cell numbers is often accompanied by an increase in cell function, with excessive production and secretion of T4 and T3, leading to the clinical features that are associated with hyperthyroidism. Most of the clinical features are known collectively as **thyrotoxicosis** and are the result of a permanently raised metabolic rate (**Fig. 10.4**).

The second and most important cause of hyperthyroidism is Graves' disease, which manifests with diffuse enlargement of the thyroid gland and exophthalmos (protuberant, staring eyes) caused by the expansion of adipose tissue behind the eye orbit. Graves' disease is the result of diffuse thyroid hyperactivity caused by the presence of an IgG antibody called long-acting thyroid stimulator (LATS). These are autoantibodies that are directed to thyroid membrane receptors where they stimulate the thyroid to synthesise and secrete thyroid hormone continuously, irrespective of requirements. The secretion of thyroid hormone is no longer under the control of TSH from the pituitary. There is an increase in the number of lymphoid cells, with hyperplasia of the thyroid acini and an enlargement of their nuclei. The thyroid shows diffuse fleshy enlargement although the follicle lumen contains virtually no stored

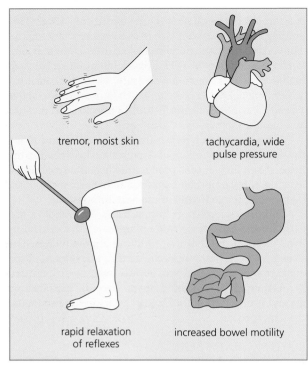

tremor, moist skin

tachycardia, wide
pulse pressure

rapid relaxation
of reflexes

increased bowel motility

Fig 10.4 Signs and symptoms of hyperthyroidism.

collagen. Patients with Graves' disease have a high incidence of the human lymphocytic antigen (HLA) (Stevens and Lowe, 1995).

The production of excess thyroid hormone can also occur as a result of an autonomous nodule of hyperactive thyroid tissue that is not under the control of TSH and may be caused by a thyroid adenoma or by a multinodular goitre.

Pathophysiology

The pathological changes seen are loss of subcutaneous fat, reduction of skeletal muscle bulk and, occasionally, cardiomyopathy. These changes are a direct result of the effect that circulating thyroid hormone has on the body's cellular activities, leading to an increase in oxygen consumption; this results in heat intolerance, rapid heart rate, diarrhoea, anxiety and restless hyperactivity.

Pharmacological management

Radioactive iodine or **surgery** is used to block the synthesis or effects of excess thyroid hormone and, if undertaken with care, can lead to the complete control of hyperthyroidism. There are several **antithyroid drugs** whose actions are to inhibit the synthesis or release of thyroid hormones. All are used to treat hyperthyroidism, though some may be used in conjunction with certain iodides to bring about a euthyroid state before surgery, or may be used in conjunction with radioactive iodine therapy to hasten recovery and to bring symptoms under control.

Carbimazole and **propylthiouracil** are available as tablets and can be used in the long-term treatment of hyperthyroidism or in preparation for thyroidectomy. Carbimazole and propylthiouracil have a greater affinity for iodide than thyroglobulin. This prevents iodination of the tyrosine residue in thyroglobulin and thus the synthesis of T4 and T3 in the colloid of the follicle. Propylthiouracil affects the processing of T4 to T3 in the peripheral tissues. This effect on processing has a marked physiological effect because T3 is 10 times more active than T4.

Both drugs can cause the serious side effect of bone marrow depression, which may lead to agranulocytosis. The patient should immediately report a sore throat, mouth ulcers, fever or rashes as these can be an early sign of bone marrow depression. Other common side effects are skin rashes and pruritus, which should disappear spontaneously without withdrawal of the drug. It can be taken in carefully monitored doses during pregnancy. As both drugs are secreted in breast milk it is important that breast feeding is not undertaken. The medication should be taken with food to reduce gastric irritation.

Carbimazole and propylthiouracil both enhance the effects of anticoagulants, leading to bleeding or the presence of bruising.

Carbimazole

Carbimazole is given in an initial daily dosage of 20–60 mg in two or three divided doses. It is not effective for 10–14 days, as the thyroid continues releasing its existing reserves of hormones. The patient gradually becomes euthyroid over subsequent weeks. The dose is then progressively reduced until a maintenance dosage of 5–15 mg as a single dose is achieved. The dose may be determined by clinical status and continues for 12–18 months. If relapse occurs when the medication is stopped, then further measures may need to be considered.

Propylthiouracil

Propylthiouracil is given 300–600 mg daily. The dose is divided in the same way as carbimazole and is reduced gradually until a maintenance dose of 50–150 mg is reached. It has a rapid onset compared with carbimazole and is used in the management of hyperthyroidism before surgery and to treat thyrotoxic crisis.

Iodine and iodides

These come in solution and are given as 2–6 drops twice daily, preferably diluted in milk and taken after meals. Iodides are usually given before surgery as the benefits are only sustained for a short period. Iodine and iodides act by inhibiting the release of T3 and T4 from the thyroid into the plasma. This reduces thyroid function very rapidly and simultaneously reduces the vascularity of the thyroid gland.

The use of over-the-counter cough and cold remedies containing iodides should be avoided during treatment with iodine or iodides.

Radioactive iodine (sodium iodide I-131)

This means of treatment is recommended for patients with large thyroids and moderately severe hyperthyroidism (Dunn and Dunn, 1994). It is administered orally in doses of 4–10 µCi for hyperthyroidism and 50 µCi for malignancies. It passes quickly into the circulation and concentrates in the thyroid. It destroys follicular cells through the ionising effects of β radiation. **Propranolol** may be administered after this therapy to counteract the cardiac stimulation that is brought about by the temporary increase in circulating thyroid hormones. Radioactive iodine has a half-life of 8 days and is excreted in the urine.

HYPOTHYROIDISM

Hyperplasia of the thyroid leading to hypothyroidism can occur as a result of Hashimoto's disease and Graves' disease. In such cases, the balance has been reversed and the patient has passed from a hyperthyroid state, to a euthyroid state and then to a hypothyroid state through the gradual destruction of thyroid follicles by autoantibodies.

Hypothyroidism can also occur in response to surgical removal of the thyroid for malignancy or Graves' disease. Effects of thyroid hormone deficiency will not be revealed for several months until the store of T3 and T4 in the thyroid is depleted. It can also occur in areas of the world where dietary iodine is deficient. Hypothyroidism causes continuous stimulation of the thyroid follicles by TSH to produce thyroid hormone and leads to goitre formation.

Pathophysiology

When hypothyroidism is present in adults it is called **myxoedema** and manifests with non-pitting oedema (Fig. 10.5). This is caused by the accumulation of hydrophilic mucopolysaccharides and protein in the dermis and connective tissues throughout the body. The 'boggy' oedema is particularly noticeable around the eyes, hands, feet and in the supraclavicular fossa. There is also a thickening of the tongue, and laryngeal and pharyngeal mucous membranes. The effects of this is a slurring and hoarseness of speech, which are common in hypothyroidism. An inherited enzyme defect causes the failure of normal T3 and T4 synthesis leading to **cretinism** in children.

Pharmacological management

The normal daily production of thyroid hormones is T4, 70–90 µg and T3, 15–30 µg. The treatment of hypothyroidism is with replacement thyroid hormones, either natural or synthetic. Natural ones are derived from beef or pork. Synthetic forms of thyroid hormone have the same physiological effects as natural T3 and T4 but vary in their potency according to the ratio of each drug. Replacement medication is given orally before meals; it is absorbed by the gastrointestinal tract. When in the blood, the drugs are bound to thyroxin-binding globulin and two types of albumin made in the liver. This prevents them from being metabolised and excreted, giving them a longer half-life. It is the unbound portion that is pharmacologically active. Thyroxin does not reach its maximum effectiveness for several weeks, whereas T3 achieves full effectiveness in 4–8 days.

Tri-iodothyronine and T4 potentiate anticoagulants, enhance antidepressant effects and decrease the effectiveness of digitalis. They may increase the need for oral hypoglyaemic medications in type 2 diabetes.

Tri-iodothyronine

Because of its quick action, T3 is used in the treatment of severe and acute hypothyroid states. It can be given intravenously, often in conjunction with intravenous corticosteroids and fluids. The initial dose is 5 µg and it is increased weekly until a maximum dose of 60 µg is reached. In the treatment of myxoedema coma, 5–20 µg is given by slow intravenous injection.

Thyroxin

This is given for routine replacement therapy in hypothyroidism. The starting dose is 50 µg orally, slowly increased to 100–200 µg daily. To prevent irreversible brain damage (cretinism) occurring with congenital hypothyroidism, T4 must be given as soon as possible after birth. Thyroid hormones are also used to suppress the release of TSH from the pituitary gland in the treatment of Hashimoto's thyroiditis, thyroid cancer and active goitre, and in combination with antithyroid drugs to prevent the development of goitre in hyperthyroid patients.

Because they increase the metabolic activity of the body, they have particular effects on the:

- Neurological system, causing tremors, headache, nervousness, insomnia and irritability.
- Cardiovascular system, causing palpitations, increased blood pressure, tachycardia, arrhythmias, angina and fever.
- Gastrointestinal system, causing a change in appetite, weight loss, nausea and vomiting.
- Reproductive system, causing menstrual irregularities (Mathewson-Kuhn, 1994).

It is important to note that if the pulse rate is above 100 beats per minute a doctor should be consulted and it should be stressed to the patient the importance of carrying a medic alert card.

THE PARATHYROID GLANDS

The parathyroids produce a hormone, **parathyroid hormone** (PTH), that is important for calcium balance. There are usually four parathyroid glands, and these are situated

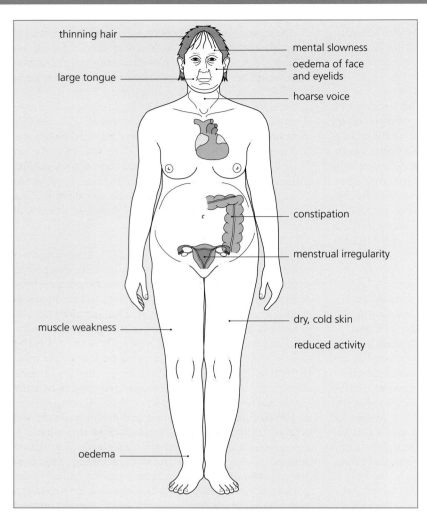

thinning hair

mental slowness

oedema of face
and eyelids

large tongue

hoarse voice

constipation

menstrual irregularity

muscle weakness

dry, cold skin

reduced activity

oedema

Fig 10.5 Changes associated with myxoedema.

behind the thyroid gland. When too much PTH is produced, **hypercalcaemia** (raised blood calcium) develops and when too little, **hypocalcaemia** occurs. Parathyroid hormone acts directly on the kidney by decreasing reabsorption of phosphate and increasing tubular reabsorption of calcium. It also acts on the bone by activating osteoclasts to break down the bony matrix and release calcium and phosphate into the blood. The third action is to increase intestinal absorption of calcium by the intestinal mucosal cells.

HYPERPARATHYROIDISM

Hyperparathyroidism is characterised by increased secretion of the PTH; the cause may be primary, secondary, or tertiary.

Primary hyperparathyroidism occurs when one or more hyperfunctioning glands do not respond to the normal feedback of serum calcium and secrete PTH autonomously. The most common cause is a benign parathyroid tumour in one of the glands; this accounts for approximately 80% of cases.

Secondary hyperparathyroidism is a parathyroid response to hypocalcaemia. Parathyroid hormone is secreted in excess, but the kidneys, which are the target organs, have failed and calcium levels remain low.

Tertiary hyperparathyroidism is when autonomous secretion of PTH occurs as hyperplastic parathyroid cells lose their sensitivity to circulating calcium levels; it is often seen to occur as a result of chronic renal failure.

Pathophysiology

Hyperparathyroidism results in **hypercalcaemia** and bone demineralisation. The consequences of hyperparathyroidism are:

- The overstimulation of bone to release calcium into the bloodstream. If this process continues, bone deformities can occur.
- An increase in the amount of calcium being delivered to the kidneys, which results in hypercalciuria and kidney stones. The renal tubules respond by producing an alkaline urine, which can lead to metabolic acidosis, as a result

of the elimination of bicarbonate to make the urine alkaline.
• Hypophosphataemia caused by hypercalcaemia.

Hypercalcaemia may also be caused by malignant disease, vitamin D intoxication and immobilisation – often as a result of paraplegia in the young and Paget's disease in the elderly. The major symptoms of hypercalcaemia are polydipsia and polyuria, caused by the decreased responsiveness of the renal tubules to ADH, and constipation along with anorexia, nausea and vomiting. Kidney stones and cardiac arrhythmias can also occur.

Pharmacological management
Disodium pamidronate is an anti-neoplastic agent that lowers the serum calcium levels in patients with malignancies who have resulting bone metastases. **Frusemide**, a diuretic, reduces serum calcium concentration by increasing calcium excretion. **Calcitonin** lowers the serum calcium by reducing the renal tubular reabsorption and increasing calcium deposition in the bone. This is available as a porcine derivative or is synthetically produced as **salcatonin** (salmon calcitonin), which is also used for postmenopausal osteoporosis. The route of administration is subcutaneous or intramuscular. As it is a peptide, it is destroyed in the stomach if taken orally. The dose ranges according to the condition treated from 50 IU salcatonin three times weekly to 100 IU daily for Paget's disease.

Side effects include nausea, vomiting, diarrhoea, flushing, paraesthesia and an unpleasant taste in the mouth.

HYPOPARATHYROIDISM
Hypoparathyroidism is a rare endocrine disorder and is brought about by deficient PTH secretion or the decreased effectiveness of PTH on target tissues. This primarily occurs as a result of damage to the parathyroid glands secondary to thyroid surgery. When hypoparathyroidism occurs with hypocalcaemia, it is considered a metabolic crisis.

Pathophysiology
A lack of PTH activity results in a decrease in serum calcium because of reduced reabsorption of calcium from the renal tubules and the bone. Simultaneously, serum phosphate levels are increased (hyperphosphataemia) as a result of the reabsorption of phosphates. Hypocalcaemia causes a lowering of the threshold for nerve and muscle excitation, so that a nerve impulse may be initiated by a slight stimulus anywhere along the length of a nerve or muscle fibre (Paradiso, 1995). The resulting symptoms are muscle spasms, hyper-reflexia, clonic–tonic convulsions and laryngeal spasm.

Hypocalcaemia and hyperphosphataemia in the absence of renal or gastrointestinal disease suggest hypoparathyroidism as the causative factor.

Hypoparathyroidism appears to result from hypomagnesaemia. Once magnesium levels are restored then the parathyroid glands return to normal. Hypomagnesaemia may be related to chronic alcoholism, malnutrition and malabsorption.

Pharmacological management
Vitamin D is not itself biologically active and needs the presence of bile salts to activate it. When activated, vitamin D promotes the absorption of calcium from the diet via the intestinal mucosa.

Excess consumption of vitamin D can cause calcification of the tissues, severe muscular weakness and abdominal pain.

THE ADRENAL GLANDS

Each adrenal gland consist of two distinct endocrine components: the cortex and the medulla. The adrenal cortex produces three main groups of hormones: mineralocorticoids, glucocorticoids and gonadocorticoids.

Aldosterone is the most abundantly produced (95%) and the most potent **mineralocorticoid**. It is responsible for maintaining sodium and water balance and comes under the direct influence of the kidneys (see Chapter 15 *Drugs and urological disorders*).

Glucocorticoids, which include cortisol, cortisone and corticosterone, are secreted from all three regions of the cortex. It is only cortisol that is secreted in significant amounts. The action of glucocorticoids on their target cells is to alter the DNA transcription process.

Gonadocorticoids are the sex hormones. The male hormones are androgens, of which testosterone is the most common. A small amount of female hormones (oestrogen and progesterone) are produced. Both sexes have male and female sex hormones in appropriate proportions for their gender. (For replacement therapy see Chapter 16 *Drugs and reproductive disorders*.)

Production of glucocorticoids and sex steroids is controlled by ACTH secreted by the anterior pituitary gland. Control of glucocorticoid secretion is by the negative feedback loop, whereas gonadocorticoids do not appear to exert feedback inhibition. Excessive production of these adrenocortical hormones is usually caused by an ACTH-producing adenoma of the pituitary or, more rarely, an adenoma of the adrenal cortex.

CUSHING'S SYNDROME
Cushing's syndrome is chronic hypercortisolism (excessive levels of circulating cortisol) caused by the hyperfunctioning of the adrenal cortex, with or without pituitary involvement. Cushing's syndrome that occurs in older adults, particularly men, usually results from ectopic ACTH secretion. Adrenal tumours are more common in

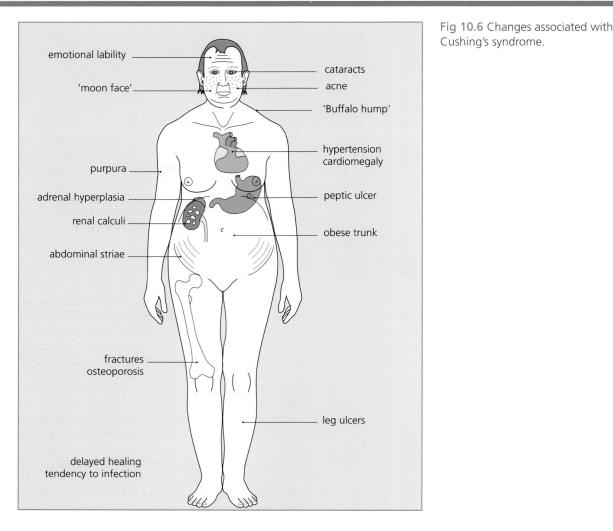

Fig 10.6 Changes associated with Cushing's syndrome.

children, especially girls. Cushing's syndrome usually occurs in those aged between 30 and 50 years of age. Causes of hypercortisolism may also include ectopic ACTH secretion by an oat cell carcinoma of the lung (McCance and Huether,1994).

The most common cause of cortisone excess is the administration of large doses of glucocorticoid drugs. The end result is that the patient develops a **Cushing-like syndrome** (Fig. 10.6).

Pathophysiology

Elevated levels of cortisol have exaggerated effects, causing symptoms in almost every body system:
- Adipose tissue accumulates in the abdomen and behind the shoulders (buffalo hump).
- Arms and legs become thinner because of the catabolic effects of cortisol on peripheral tissues. Accelerated protein catabolism leads to muscle wasting, which causes weakness and difficult movement.

- Protein loss also leads to:
  - Osteoporosis (which can lead to pathological fractures).
  - Loss of collagen, which leads to thinning skin through which capillaries are more visible. Capillaries are easily stretched by adipose deposits. These changes account for the purple striae frequently observed in the trunk area.
  - Weakened blood vessel support (making bruising easier as smaller vessels rupture).
- Glucocorticoids are thought to have an effect on mood, which may explain the mood changes that occur, from euphoria to depression.
- Amenorrhoea is believed to be caused by an increase in androgen levels.
- Long-term elevation of cortisol levels causes suppression of the immune system.
- Changes in skin pigmentation occur because of stimulation of melanocytes by ACTH.
- Steroids, e.g. cortisol, antagonise insulin and lead to an

increase in serum glucose levels and a possible diabetic state; polyuria is sometimes present (Paradiso, 1995).

Whatever the cause, two observations consistently apply to individuals with Cushing's syndrome: first, the diurnal or circadian secretion patterns of ACTH and cortisol is lost, and second, they do not increase their ACTH and cortisol secretion in response to a stressor.

Pharmacological management

Ketoconazole 200–400 mg may be given orally once daily with food. It is a broad-spectrum antimycotic agent and was used primarily for treatment of **fungal infections**. It acts by altering membrane permeability and, because it has been shown to inhibit cortisol biosynthesis, has been used as an additional therapy for patients with Cushing's syndrome. Gynaecomastia may develop in men. Ketoconazole, because of its properties of decreasing levels of testosterone in men, brings about a rise in serum LH and FSH. This has prompted investigations into its treatment for **prostatic cancer** (Winter, 1994). Other treatment is by radiation or surgery. If Cushing's syndrome is caused by administration of large doses of steroids, signs and symptoms will disappear when these are gradually withdrawn. Side effects include nausea, vomiting, abdominal pain, headache and rashes.

10.3 KETOCONAZOLE

Ketoconazole is not safe for patients with impaired liver function. If the treatment is to last for longer than 14 days then the patient needs liver function tests before treatment, after 14 days and then monthly.

Metyrapone acts by inhibiting the production of cortisol in the adrenal cortex, which leads to an increase in ACTH production, which in turn leads to increased synthesis and release of cortisol precursors. It is used to prepare patients with some forms of Cushing's syndrome for surgery, and has been found helpful in controlling the symptoms of the disease when it is caused by carcinoma of the bronchus that is not amenable to surgery. The dose is 750 mg every 4 hours for 6 doses for adults, and a minimum of 250 mg every 4 hours for 6 doses for children. Side effects include occasional nausea, vomiting, dizziness, headache, hypotension and sedation.

ADDISON'S DISEASE

The most common cause of primary adrenal hypofunction is the destruction of the cortex of both adrenals by autoimmune adrenalitis. It is often associated with autoimmune

PERSON CENTRED STUDY 1

Mary Evans aged 60 years is complaining of poor healing of a wound on her arm, which occurred 2 months ago. When examining the wound the nurse notices that there is bruising and discoloration of the skin. She asks whether this was caused by the injury, Mary answers 'No'. The nurse then asks whether there has been an increase in her weight over the past few months; Mary replies 'Yes'.

1. What do you think her problem could be?
2. What further questions do you need to ask Mary?

thyroid disease, autoimmune gastritis and other endocrine autoimmune diseases. Other causes include familial adrenal insufficiency, amyloidosis, metastatic destruction of the adrenal glands, adrenal haemorrhage and infections. Ninety per cent of the adrenal glands must be destroyed before the manifestations of hypocortisolism are evident.

Pathophysiology

Autoimmune adrenalitis causes atrophy and hypofunction of the adrenals. Autoantibodies are present in 50–70% of individuals with Addison's disease. The autoantibodies appear to be cell specific for the adrenal cortex. A combination of cell membrane and cytoplasmic antibodies and cell-mediated immune mechanisms contribute to the pathology of the disease. There appears to be a genetic defect in the immune surveillance mechanism of the cells, causing a deficiency of immune suppresser cells. This deficiency within the adrenocortical cells leads to a proliferation of immunocytes directed against specific antibodies (McCance and Huether, 1994). The result is a chronic deficiency in circulating levels of the hormones aldosterone and cortisol. Decreased levels of aldosterone lead to reduced sodium absorption and increased sodium excretion. Water is excreted along with sodium, leading rapidly to hypovolaemia and hypotension. Potassium moves in the opposite direction to sodium, resulting in hyperkalaemia. Other clinical manifestations are lethargy, weakness, anorexia, nausea and vomiting, for which the cause is not known. Vitiligo, white patchy areas of depigmented skin, occurs as a result of autoimmune destruction of melanocytes. If symptoms are untreated the individual may develop an Addisonian crisis, with severe hypotension and vascular collapse.

Pharmacological management

Fludrocortisone acetate, which is a mineralocorticoid, may be given daily with a dose range between 50 and 300 μg. If glucocorticoid activity is required then cortisone or hydrocortisone are given also. Unwanted side effects are oedema, weight gain, hypertension and electrolyte disturbances.

HYPERALDOSTERONISM

The primary cause of hyperaldosteronism (Conn's disease or primary aldosteronism) is a benign single adrenal adenoma, which causes excessive aldosterone secretion. Secondary hyperaldosteronism occurs in patients with renal artery stenosis, cirrhosis of the liver, nephrotic syndrome and severe heart failure.

Pathophysiology

Excessive aldosterone secretion, occurring as the result of primary hyperaldosteronism, leads to fluid and electrolyte imbalance through increased sodium reabsorption with corresponding hypervolaemia. Characteristically, the patient has an extracellular fluid volume overload and suppression of the normal feedback mechanism of renin secretion. Oedema does not occur under normal circumstances because of the renal tubular 'escape' mechanism, which allows the rate of sodium excretion to be reset, and thus prevents further sodium retention. This 'escape' mechanism operates in the proximal tubules and causes additional sodium to pass to the distal tubules, where the sodium is, to some extent, reabsorbed in exchange for potassium. This mechanism, although protecting the body from excessive sodium reabsorption and oedema, increases urinary losses of potassium. Patients present with hypertension caused by sodium and water retention, severe generalised muscular weakness caused by the hypokalaemia, cardiac arrhythmias and polyuria; patients may also be thirsty.

Pharmacological management

Spironolactone is the most effective drug in the treatment of primary aldosteronism. It is a potassium-sparing diuretic that is metabolised to canrenone, which antagonises the action of aldosterone on the distal tubule of the nephron. Aldosterone promotes the retention of sodium and the excretion of potassium by the kidneys. Canrenone reverses this effect, causing increased excretion of sodium and water, and retention of potassium. Spironolactone acts within 2–4 hours of oral administration (Downie et al., 1995). The normal oral dose of spironolactone is 100–200 mg daily, increasing to 400 mg when required. Surgical removal of the adenoma is undertaken when the patient is metabolically stable.

PANCREATIC ENDOCRINE TISSUE

The majority of pancreatic endocrine tissue is situated in the islets of Langerhans, found throughout the pancreas, with a few scattered endocrine cells situated in the ducts leading from the exocrine acini (Stevens and Lowe, 1995). There are five hormones secreted from these endocrine cells: insulin, glucagon, somatostatin, pancreatic poly-peptide and amylin, whose role is not fully understood. Somatostatin is also found in the stomach and the hypothalamus and is responsible in the pancreas for inhibiting the release of insulin and glucagon. Insulin is produced by 60% of the islet's β cells and is secreted in response to rising blood glucose levels. When insulin is released, its main metabolic effect is on muscle, adipose tissue and the liver. It also regulates the metabolism of glucose in the eye. Its action is to stimulate the transport of glucose and a number of other substances, including amino acids, phosphate, potassium and calcium, across the cell membrane into the cell (Hinchliff et al., 1996). This results in the reduction of blood glucose levels. Glucagon, which is produced by 20% of the cells in the islets, opposes the action of insulin and results in the increase of blood glucose levels. Failure to maintain adequate fasting blood glucose levels between 3.3 and 5.5 mmol/l is a possible indication of **diabetes mellitus**.

DIABETES MELLITUS

Diabetes mellitus is recognised clinically by the disturbance noted in carbohydrate, lipid and protein metabolism that results from an intracellular lack of glucose. There are two major types of diabetes mellitus: **type 1** insulin-dependent diabetes mellitus (IDDM) and **type 2** non-insulin-dependent diabetes mellitus (NIDDM). Both have different causes and respond to different lines of treatment and medication. There has recently been recognition of a type 3 diabetes, which affects people in midlife who are not overweight and who have an active lifestyle. These people do not respond to diet control and within a short time need insulin to maintain their blood glucose levels within a normal range. This third type of diabetes is as yet not well understood.

TYPE 1 INSULIN-DEPENDENT DIABETES MELLITUS

Type 1 IDDM most commonly occurs in youth and affects 25% of the diabetic population (Jacques, 1993). When 80–90% of the β cells have been destroyed, sufficient insulin can no longer be produced and the symptoms of polyuria, polydipsia and polyphagia result, followed by weight loss and fatigue. Insulin is necessary to allow the transport of glucose into most cells (the brain fortunately does not need insulin for glucose absorption). In the absence of insulin, protein synthesis ceases and wasting of muscle cells occurs. With the release of large amounts of amino acids into the plasma, combined with the fact that gluconeogenesis is no longer suppressed, hyperglycaemia occurs, resulting in glycosuria. Although blood glucose is elevated, the body produces gluconeogenic enzymes in an attempt to make more glucose available for cellular activity by activating glycogenolysis, lipolysis and gluconeogenesis. During the mobilisation of fats, excess acetyl CoA is produced, which forms cholesterol and ketone bodies, resulting in ketoacidosis. This leads to severe depression of the nervous system and results in a coma. Except for acetone, all the ketone bodies are organic acids and carry a negative charge. The ketones are excreted from the body in the urine. Because of their negative charge they remove the positive ions of sodium and potassium, which leads to an electrolyte imbalance and the person experiences abdominal pains and may vomit (Marieb, 1996). Acetone, which is more volatile, is excreted via the lungs and accounts for the 'fruity' breath in patients experiencing severe ketoacidosis. Additionally, there is an increase in the amount of stored triglycerides in the liver because of the lack of insulin. This excess of fatty acids within the liver leads to their conversion to phospholipids and cholesterol. These substances leave the liver and enter the blood as lipoproteins and can lead to the rapid development of atherosclerosis (Mathewson-Kuhn, 1994).

Pathophysiology

Type 1 IDDM has been thought to have an abrupt onset, but it is now believed that it has a distinctive natural history involving genetic susceptibility, a long preclinical period, immunologically mediated destruction of β cells and hyperglycaemia (McCance and Huether, 1994).

The exact nature of genetic susceptibility is not fully understood, but 10–13% of newly diagnosed diabetics have a parent or sibling with diabetes. There is also believed to be an increased susceptibility to environmental influences such as viral infections, resulting in cell-mediated destruction of β cells. Research findings support a genetic HLA link and if both HLA-DR4 and HLA-DR3 alleles are present, then the chances of that individual having IDDM are 20–40 times greater than that of the general population.

Research has demonstrated that islet cell antibodies exist for years before the occurrence of symptoms. Autoantibodies against insulin (IAA) have also been noted. These autoantibodies may form during the process of active islet cell and β cell destruction. Islet cell antibodies and IAA are believed to be the result of the autoimmune process rather than the cause.

The presence of islet cell antibodies provides a strong indication for an autoimmune origin and pathogenesis of IDDM. A local or organ-specific suppresser deficit may induce the autoimmune response. The exact sequence of events is unknown, but it is thought that environmental mechanisms play a role in the destruction of β cells by direct toxicity, by increasing the susceptibility of the β cells to another mechanism or by triggering an autoimmune response to β cells.

Hyperglycaemia occurs when 80–90% of the insulin-secreting β cells of the islets of Langerhans are destroyed. The initiating events of β cell destruction may be different from the final event that precipitates clinical symptoms. There is also considerable evidence to suggest that α and β cell functions are abnormal and that both a lack of insulin and a relative excess of glucagon exist in IDDM. Hyperglycaemia and hyperketonaemia cannot be caused by insulin deficiency alone; glucagon must be present in relative excess. This indicates that the metabolic abnormalities that occur are caused by both hormones. This could lead to an entirely new approach to the management of type 1 IDDM (McCance and Huether, 1994).

Pharmacological management

The correction of dehydration is of the utmost importance, along with the correction of sodium and potassium balance. Simultaneously, there may be a need for the administration of insulin on a sliding scale. All patients suffering from type 1 IDDM must be treated by injections of insulin. It cannot be given orally as it is destroyed by the gastric acid and enzymes.

Insulin was discovered in 1921 by Banting and Best *et al.* Originally it was extracted from the pancreas of an animal, usually beef (bovine) or pork (porcine), but as beef insulin was less like human insulin than pork, antibodies were formed, which limited its effectiveness. Porcine insulin was used primarily until 1983 when 'human insulin' was developed. Human insulin is slightly more soluble in an aqueous media, which accounts for its increased metabolic clearance rate. Biosynthetic human insulin was developed by recombinant DNA technology. Since then a semisynthetic insulin has been produced by replacing the amino acid alanine in pork with threonine, the amino acid necessary to change the pork insulin to the structure of human insulin.

There are now over thirty different insulin products available: rapid-acting, intermediate, long-acting and biphasic, which is a mixture of short-acting and intermediate-acting insulin. Apart from rapid-acting insulin, the others have been modified by using insulin as crystals (hence their cloudy appearance), which dissolve in the blood over a 24-hour period. Long-acting insulins are combined with zinc and can be active for up to 24 hours. Intermediate-acting insulins have the protein protamine or zinc added and are active for 8–12 hours. Biphasic insulins (which are gradually being withdrawn) are a mixture of 30% soluble human insulin and 70% isophane; this produces two main phases from a single injection and are usually given twice daily.

It is now widely recognised that an injection of animal insulin can, over time, cause the body to respond by forming insulin antibodies. Little is known of the effect of these antibodies on the body and, if large numbers form, whether these can lead to insulin resistance. Most new patients receiving insulin are given human insulin and some patients previously on animal insulin have been changed to human insulin to reduce the incidence of antibody formation. It has been noted that even human insulin does produce some antibodies.

Insulin works by binding to receptors on the cell membrane. A 'second messenger' is believed to be activated, enabling the metabolic processes of the cell to utilise glucose as a source of energy. All insulins have the same pharmacological action but their varying times of onset, peaks and duration of action allows individuals to select the insulin that best suits their own lifestyle.

Side effects for medium-acting and long-acting insulins affect various body systems:

- Central nervous system: headaches, lethargy, tremors, weakness, fatigue, delirium and sweating.
- Cardiovascular system: tachycardia and palpitations.
- Ears, eyes, nose and throat: blurred vision.
- Gastrointestinal system: hunger and nausea.
- Metabolism: hypoglycaemia.
- Skin: flushing, rash, urticaria, warmth, lipo-atrophy, erythema and pruritus.
- Systemic: anaphylaxis.

Insulin needs careful monitoring in hypersensitive patients and those with frequent hypoglycaemic attacks. The following increase hypoglycaemia: alcohol, beta-blockers, oral hypoglycaemics, monoamine oxidase inhibitors and octreotide. Other drugs interact with insulin to cause hyperglycaemia: thiazides, thyroid hormones, oral contraceptives, corticosteroids, lithium, diazoxide and loop diuretics.

The treatment for insulin overdose is glucose by mouth if the patient is conscious; if the patient is comatose the treatment is 50% glucose administered intravenously or 1 mg glucagon administered intramuscularly, intravenously or subcutaneously.

Types of insulin

Soluble insulin (human) 100 IU/ml is produced from a precursor synthesised by *Escherichia coli* or yeast using recombinant DNA technology. Soluble insulin can be given subcutaneously, intramuscularly or intravenously. It is particularly beneficial when treating a patient in a diabetic coma, newly diagnosed diabetes or unstable diabetes. When given intravenously, 50 IU/ml diluted in 50 ml normal saline is administered by an infusion pump. In the hospital it can be given intravenously on a sliding scale for diabetic ketoacidosis (DKA), coma, patients undergoing surgery or during labour.

Soluble insulins have a rapid rate of absorption; they begin to act within 15–60 minutes. The patient must eat within half an hour of administration. Peak activity is between 2 and 4 hours and duration is between 5 and 8 hours. These are also known as neutral insulins as they are the only insulins that can be given intravenously.

Rapid-acting **Insulin lispro** is an analogue of human insulin but is able to dissociate more readily into monomers than hexamers; this property allows its quicker absorption, more rapid onset and shorter duration of action when administered subcutaneously. It is administered immediately before a meal; absorption begins within 5 minutes and reaches its peak of activity within 1 hour. Plasma glucose levels can be expected to return to pre-meal values within 2 hours.

Insulin lispro may be given intramuscularly and intravenously. When given intramuscularly its half-life is 1 hour. Repeat injections are administered at hourly intervals (according to sliding scale regime) until glucose levels are settled. When given intravenously for the treatment of diabetic ketoacidosis it is given via a continuous infusion pump in normal saline; when blood glucose levels of 14 mmol/l are achieved, then the insulin is administered in 5% dextrose or dextrose saline to prevent too rapid a fall in blood glucose levels.

Studies undertaken on the rate of absorption of soluble insulin on various sites of the body have shown that it is more readily absorbed from the subcutaneous tissue of the abdomen than deltoid, femoral or gluteal sites. Because of this, it is recommended that the same area is used daily before a particular meal to maintain stability in glucose levels. It is also recommended that injection sites are rotated to prevent use of the same site within a month. There are relatively few side effects. The most common is localised fat accumulation or atrophy, allergic reactions and hypoglycaemia (Lawrence, 1994).

Intermediate-acting insulins may be mixed in the syringe with soluble insulin or may come already mixed. The insulin content may be bovine, porcine or human insulin and may be highly purified. These insulins are normally mixed with isophane or protamine. Onset of action for most mixtures is within 30–60 minutes because of the presence of soluble insulin. They have a peak activity after 4–8 hours, with a duration of 24 hours. Some mixtures come in the form of biphasic isophane insulin, but these are gradually being withdrawn. This is a sterile buffered suspension of porcine and human insulin, which is complexed with protamine sulphate. These are administered subcutaneously once or twice daily before breakfast and/or supper. If given twice daily there is a danger of the patient becoming hypoglycaemic around midnight. It is very important to ensure an adequate snack is taken before bedtime.

Isophane insulin is a suspension of bovine, porcine or human insulin to which protamine sulphate or another suitable protamine may be added. Their onset of activity is 2–4 hours, peaking between 4 and 12 hours, with a duration of 16–24 hours according to the particular suspension. Regular insulin will need to be given before each meal to prevent the post-prandial peaks in blood glucose levels.

Long-acting insulins tend to be insulin zinc suspension (mixed) in which bovine, porcine or human insulin is suspended. The larger particle complex formed leads to a longer period of action. The onset of action is after 4 hours, with a peak activity at 6–12 hours and a duration of action of 20–24 hours. These injections will need to be supported by the administration of regular short-acting insulin.

Eileen May has been admitted to the ward for stabilisation of her blood glucose levels. On assessing Eileen you established that she had been giving herself subcutaneous insulin injections for 6 years. When she was asked what insulin base she was using, she stated that she was originally using animal insulin, but is now taking 'human' insulin.

During the assessment Eileen talks about her last holiday and tells you that she felt very self-conscious about her appearance when wearing her swimming costume because of the 'lumpiness' of her skin on her thighs. You examine her legs and the lumpiness is evident. On further questioning, you discover that she has been injecting into her thighs, because it is less painful, particularly if she uses the same spot. Eileen also stated that she had first tried to give herself her insulin injection into her arm, but experienced hypoglycaemic symptoms.

1. Why has injecting into the same site caused poor control of her blood glucose levels?
2. Does it matter if sometimes she inadvertently gives herself an intramuscular injection?
3. What information could you give Eileen about rotating her injection sites?

TYPE 2 NON-INSULIN-DEPENDENT DIABETES MELLITUS

The cause of type 2 diabetes is unknown but is thought to be autosomal recessive. The people affected are usually aged over 40 years, and many are obese. Approximately 75% of the diabetic population are affected by type 2 diabetes, that is, about half a million people in the United Kingdom (Gill, 1991). Non-insulin-dependent diabetes mellitus is a long-term affliction and, although often asymptomatic, may manifest with classic hyperglycaemic symptoms; however, ketone bodies are present in only low concentrations in blood and urine and rarely lead to coma. Obesity is considered to be a precipitating factor for type 2, particularly in those individuals who are genetically at risk. Southern Asians have been shown to have a genetic predisposition to type 2.

Pathophysiology

In type 2 β cells have a decreased response to plasma glucose levels, and there is an increased secretion of glucagon. The decreased response of the β cells may be caused by the reduction in cell mass and their abnormal function. Amyloid deposits in the islets of the pancreas have been found in 10–40% of individuals with type 2, and their presence correlates positively with age of the individual and the duration and severity of the disease.

Obesity and subsequent insulin resistance are found to be present in 60–80% of people with type 2 in the West. Abnormalities of the insulin receptors in the cells of muscle and adipose tissues, and a reduction in the cells' glucose transporters are responsible for this insulin resistance (Hardie and Cohen, 1991). The abnormality in adipose tissues is particularly linked with central obesity.

Pharmacological management

Management of type 2 is by dietary modification of meals (which should be rich in fibre and complex carbohydrates), correction of hyperlipidaemia and hypertension, avoidance of smoking and sensible levels of exercise. The principle aim of treatment is to prevent long-term complications. Fifteen per cent of type 2 patients are able to attain a fasting blood glucose level of < 6 mmol/l with diet alone. A further 50% can attain this level of fasting blood glucose by the use of oral hypoglycaemic agents. Insulin is resorted to when these measures fail.

Sulphonylureas

The hypoglycaemic effect of antibacterial sulphonamides was first noticed in the 1940s. This led to the development of the 'first generation' sulphonylurea agents in the 1950s, of which **chlorpropamide** and **tolbutamide** are still used. The 'second generation' agents are more potent and include **glibenclamide**, **glipizide** and **gliclazide.**

The exact mechanism of sulphonylureas is not fully understood. Initially they stimulate the β cells of the pancreas to produce insulin by inhibition of the ATP-sensitive potassium channel, which leads to depolarisation of the cell membrane. Depolarisation allows extracellular calcium to flood into the cell, resulting in the stimulation of insulin secretion. It is believed that after a time, in some patients, sulphonylurea 'exhaustion' may occur (Holman and Turner, 1991). Sulphonylureas have been found to suppress hepatic glucose production and are thought to lower blood glucose by increasing the number of insulin receptors on the cell; they may also influence events within the cell once the glucose has been transferred inside.

The sulphonylureas are administered orally and are rapidly absorbed from the gastrointestinal tract. **Glipizide** is the only oral hypoglycaemic agent that must be taken on an empty stomach, as food delays absorption by approximately 40 minutes. **Chlorpropamide** is largely excreted unchanged in the urine. Most other sulphonylureas are metabolised primarily in the liver and excreted by the kidneys. Plasma concentrations of sulphonylureas show a poor correlation with dose given. This is believed to be because of the unexplained differences in the protein-bound or β-cell-bound components rather than the 'free' plasma fraction.

Side effects include nocturnal hypoglycaemia, which can occur with **chlorpropamide** if urinary elimination is impaired, leading to accumulation in the plasma. **Glibenclamide** given to patients with fasting blood glucose levels of 6–10 mmol/l can cause reactive hypoglycaemia after breakfast because it elicits a delayed β-cell response. It is recommended that the first dose of the day should be given at lunch time. Both these drugs should be used with caution in the elderly.

10.1 ENDOCRINE SYSTEM IN THE ELDERLY

With increasing age there is a decrease in hormone production but it does not appear to affect body structure and function. The major changes to occur are in the female endocrine system, with decline of the ovaries in the middle years of life. This has a major effect on calcium loss in the bones.

There is also a delayed and insufficient release of insulin by the beta cells of the pancreas in the elderly, and there is believed to be a decreased sensitivity to circulating insulin. During this period many people are diagnosed as pre-diabetics and should therefore be advised to attend diabetes-screening programmes, and encouraged to watch for the symptoms of this disease.

Chlorpropamide and **tolbutamide** have been found to be excreted in breast milk. All oral hypoglycaemic agents are highly bound to plasma proteins, which accounts for their differences in duration of action. Second generation agents have non-ionic binding compared with the ionic binding of the first generation. The result of this is that the second generation agents have less displacement reactions from other ionic-binding drugs, which should mean fewer drug interactions. Hypoglycaemic episodes may occur if a meal is omitted or there is an erratic pattern of exercise. Gastrointestinal disturbances may occur with any of the sulphonylureas at the beginning of treatment. **Chlorpropamide** and **tolbutamide** can have an antidiuretic effect and cause water retention, leading to headache, lethargy, swelling and low sodium levels. Chlorpropamide causes alcohol-flushing in 10% of patients, necessitating change to another sulphonylurea. Weight gain can occur with sulphonylurea therapy, but this is thought to be partly the result of patients being less strict with their diets.

Sulphonylureas can be affected by salicylates and other non-steroidal anti-inflammatory drugs, resulting in enhanced hypoglycaemic activity. Anabolic steroids inhibit the metabolism of the sulphonylureas as do allopurinol, chloramphenicol and warfarin; this leads to an increased sulphonylurea half-life. H$_2$ blockers such as cimetidine and ranitidine enhance the hypoglycaemic effect of sulphonylureas.

To avoid the effects of hypoglycaemia, the lowest dose possible of oral hypoglycaemic should be used when initiating therapy. **Chlorpropamide** is given in a single daily dose. The use of **tolbutamide** is discouraged by the size of the tablet and the need for three tablets daily. All other sulphonylureas can be given in single or divided doses.

Biguanides

Metformin hydrochloride is the only biguanide used to treat type 2 diabetes in the United Kingdom and is banned from use in the USA. It has the potentially dangerous side effect of lactic acidosis and hepatic damage. Its use should be avoided in elderly patients and those with cirrhosis, alcoholism, renal failure or heart failure as these conditions can contribute to fatal lactic acidosis.

Peripheral uptake of glucose is enhanced, possibly by increasing the sensitivity of insulin receptors, and brings about a reduction of gluconeogenesis in the liver, therefore lowering hepatic glucose output. These actions, when combined, slightly raise blood lactate levels in all patients. Metformin reduces blood glucose levels but does not cause hypoglycaemia.

Up to 20% of patients have gastrointestinal disturbances consisting of dyspepsia, anorexia, diarrhoea and occasionally an unpleasant metallic taste. Patients may also complain of a general malaise and fatigue. These effects can be minimised by starting the therapy at a low dose of 500 or 850 mg daily.

Cimetidine inhibits renal excretion of metformin, leading to increased plasma concentration.

Alpha-glucosidase inhibitors

Carbohydrates can only be absorbed after being broken down to monosaccharides by the presence of α-glucosidase enzymes in the brush border of the small intestine.

Acarbose is an inhibitor of intestinal α-glucosidase enzymes (maltase, isomaltase, sucrase and glucoamylase); it acts by binding to them and delaying the digestion and absorption of starch and sucrose. Because the binding is reversible it does not prevent the digestion and absorption of glucose after a meal, rather it reduces the rate at which these events occur. The clinical effect of α-glucosidase inhibition is a reduction in the post-prandial peaks of blood glucose levels. Acarbose does not cause weight gain (de Sonnaville and Heine, 1997).

Acarbose is administered orally, of which 1–2% is absorbed systemically. In addition, 35% is degraded to inactive metabolites by the intestinal or bacterial enzymes of the gastrointestinal tract. These metabolites are excreted in the faeces.

The condition of patients whose type 2 diabetes is inadequately controlled on a sulphonylurea or biguanide can be improved by the use of acarbose in addition to existing therapy. It has been seen to produce a reduction in the rate of rise and the peak levels of post-prandial blood glucose in such patients.

Side effects are predominantly gastrointestinal and are caused by an increase in gas formation from fermentation of unabsorbed carbohydrate in the bowel. This results in flatulence, abdominal distension and diarrhoea. This has been seen to abate or disappear in many patients with continued treatment. Hypoglycaemia does not occur when acarbose is administered as monotherapy.

The recommended dose of acarbose is 50 mg three times daily. This can be increased to 100 mg three times daily after several weeks, if clinical response is inadequate. A further increase to 200 mg three times daily may occasionally be necessary. In such pateints, liver enzymes must be carefully monitored. It is not clear whether any one therapy is better than others in preventing the development of long-term diabetic complications in type 2 diabetes.

Insulin action enhancer

Troglitazone is a new class of oral drug to counteract diabetes, which specifically targets insulin resistance by re-sensitising the body to the action of its own insulin. Insulin resistance is an underlying metabolic defect in type 2 diabetes, and there is increasing evidence that it is this that is central to the cardiovascular and microvascular consequences seen in this disease. Troglitazone has now had to be withdrawn because of unforeseen side effects on the liver. Research to find new drugs to counteract diabetes that have fewer side effects and the ability to reduce the morbidity associated with type 2 diabetes continues.

KEY POINTS

- The first indication of a pituitary tumour is often some form of visual disturbance.
- Patients with diabetes insipidus must have adequate monitoring and replacement of body water.
- Care is needed when antidiuretic hormone is taken by nasal spray as nasal congestion or ulceration may result.
- Antithyroid drugs may cause bone marrow depression. Patients should seek advice if they experience sore throats, rashes, fevers or other signs of infection.

- Patients being treated for hyperthyroidism may, over time, develop signs and symptoms of hypothyroidism and require revision of their management.
- Low circulating levels of PTH may lead to altered neuromuscular excitability and cardiac dysrhythmias.
- Patients with Cushing's syndrome tend to lose the flexible regulation of corticosteroids in response to stressors and circadian rhythms.
- Treatment for IDDM and NIDDM may become less effective over time and require adjustment of the treatment regime.

MULTIPLE CHOICE QUESTIONS

Choose the correct answers.

1. Which of the following systems or organs are closely linked with the endocrine system?
   a. hypothalamus
   b. pituitary
   c. pancreas
   d. heart
   e. kidneys

2. A disorder occurring within the endocrine system is likely to involve
   a. an excess production of a hormone because of excessive demand
   b. a decreased level of a hormone because of suppression by a circulating artificial hormone
   c. an increased inactivation of hormones
   d. peripheral resistance to the action of the hormones
   e. a decrease in excretion or inactivation of hormones

3. Precursor hormones that stimulate other hormones to be produced by their target organs include
   a. FSH and LH
   b. growth hormone
   c. TSH
   d. ACTH
   e. oxytocin

4. Thyroxin is essential for stimulating the proteins that act as enzymes within the cells of which of the following organs or tissues?
   a. spleen
   b. brain
   c. liver
   d. bone
   e. testes

5. The pathophysiological effects of hyperthyroidism are
   a. decreased bowel sounds
   b. increased heart rate
   c. weight gain
   d. decreased cardiac output
   e. increased vitamin metabolism

6. When hypercalcaemia develops, the normal physiological response of the body is to
   a. increase intestinal absorption of calcium
   b. increase in calcium absorption by the bones
   c. decrease PTH secretion by the parathyroid
   d. decrease release of calcium to the kidneys
   e. increase PTH secretion by the parathyroid

7. Which statement explains why increased skin pigmentation develops in untreated Addison's disease?
   a. the anterior pituitary gland, in attempting to increase the activity of the adrenal cortex by compensatory hypersecretion of ACTH, also hypersecretes MSH
   b. severe dehydration, a pronounced feature of this disease, causes cutaneous melanin to become greatly concentrated
   c. in this disease, accelerated protein catabolism results in the release of large amounts of melanin into the blood
   d. the prolonged, high serum potassium levels that characterise Addison's disease produce disintegration of melanin
   e. the loss of adipose tissue caused by vomiting and loss of appetite makes the melanocytes present in the skin more sensitive to the effects of ultraviolet light

8. Polyuria in diabetics is the result of
   a. increased glomerular permeability because of generalised vascular damage
   b. increased glomerular filtration in response to decreased serum albumin concentration
   c. increased volume of glomerular filtrate because of elevated blood pressure
   d. the amount of glucose filtered by the glomerulus being greater than that which can be reabsorbed, resulting in glycosuria accompanied by the loss of large amounts of water in the urine
   e. decreased water reabsorption caused by high tubular osmotic pressure

9. Ketosis in diabetes mellitus results from
   a. protein gain
   b. polyuria
   c. fat metabolism
   d. insufficient insulin secretion
   e. insufficient glucagon secretion

10. Diabetes insipidus involves a dysfunction of
    a. glucose metabolism
    b. ADH
    c. insulin production
    d. insulin resistance
    e. glucocorticoid insufficiency

REFERENCES

de Sonnaville HJJ, Heine RJ. Non-insulin dependent diabetes mellitus: presentation and treatment. *Medicine* 1997; **25**:23-26.

Dunn A, Dunn T. Thyroid and antithyroid drugs. In: Brody T, Larner J, Minneman K, Neu H. *Human Pharmacology: Molecular to Chemical, 2nd ed.* St Louis: Mosby, 1994, 515-522

Downie G, Mackenzie J, Williams A. *Pharmacology and drug management for nurses.* Edinburgh: Churchill Livingstone, 1995.

Evans W, Sollenberger H, Vance H. Hypothalamic-pituitary hormones. In: Brody T, Larner J, Minneman K, Neu H. *Human Pharmacology: Molecular to Chemical, 2nd ed.* St Louis: Mosby, 1994, 549-562, Chapter 41.

Gill GV. Non-insulin dependent diabetes mellitus. In: *Textbook of diabetes, vol 1.* London: Blackwell Scientific, 1991:24-29.

Hardie DG, Cohen P. Insulin action and responses: the biochemistry of post receptor events. In: *Textbook of diabetes, vol 1.* London: Blackwell Scientific, 1991:99-104.

Hinchliff SM, Montague S, Watson R. *Physiology for nursing practice, 2nd ed.* London: Baillière Tindall, 1996.

Holman R, Turner RC. Oral agents and insulin in the treatment of non-insulin-dependent diabetes mellitus. In: Pickup J, Williams G, eds. *Textbook of diabetes, vol 2.* London: Blackwell Scientific, 1991:462-476.

Jacques A. The use of insulin in diabetes mellitus. *Prof Nurs* 1993; **12**:190-192.

Lawrence JC. Insulin and oral hypoglycaemic agents. In: Brody T, Larner J, Minneman K, Neu H. *Human pharmacology molecular to clinical, 2nd ed.* St. Louis: Mosby, 1994:523-539.

Marieb EN: *Human anatomy and physiology, 4th ed.* Redwood City, California: Benjamin Cummings, 1996.

Mathewson-Kuhn M. *Pharmaco-therapeutics - a nursing process approach, 3rd ed.* Philadelphia: FA Davis, 1994.

McCance K, Huether S. *Pathophysiology, 2nd ed.* St. Louis: Mosby, 1994.

Page C. *Integrated Pharmacology.* London: Mosby, 1997.

Paradiso C. *Pathophysiology.* Philadelphia: J. B. Lippinocott, 1995.

Stevens A, Lowe J. *Pathology.* London: Mosby, 1995.

Tanner JM. *Foetus into man, 2nd ed.* Welwyn Garden City: Castlemead, 1989.

Wardhaugh B. Evaluating growth hormone treatment. *Nurs Stand* 1992; **6**:33-36.

Winter SJ. Androgens and antiandrogens. In: Brody T, Larner J, Minneman K, Neu H. *Human pharmacology molecular to clinical, 2nd ed.* St. Louis: Mosby, 1994:501-505.

11 Janet MacGregor
DRUGS AND RESPIRATORY DISORDERS

INTRODUCTION

The respiratory system consists of the airway passages, the lungs, the diaphragm and all the muscles that enable inspiration and expiration to occur. Its function is to ensure a constant and uninterrupted supply of oxygen to the body tissues in order that nutrients can be oxidised for energy release and carbon dioxide excreted, thus maintaining a dynamic physiological equilibrium. The three steps in this process are ventilation, diffusion and perfusion; perfusion is carried out by the cardiovascular system with which the respiratory system works in harmony (McCance and Huether, 1994). Respiration is controlled by spontaneous rhythmic discharges from the respiratory centre in the medulla, modulated by input from pontine and higher central nervous system centres and vagal effects from the lungs (Rang *et al.*, 1995). Voluntary breathing is possible by conscious control, which occurs by cortical impulses via the spinal tracts, for example when one is asked to hold one's breath. This conscious control is useful for the administration of inhaled medications as well as for talking, singing and laughing, the higher order abilities of *Homo sapiens*. All treatments for the respiratory system aim to ensure a constant oxygen flow by direct action on the tissues in the respiratory 'tree' or by action on other systems that coordinate respiratory function.

COMMON MANIFESTATIONS OF RESPIRATORY DISEASE AND THEIR TREATMENTS

SNEEZE

A sneeze is a way of forcefully expelling a foreign body or irritant from the upper airways and can be stimulated by the inflammation that a rhinovirus such as a 'cold' virus may cause. It is common in the early stages of a 'cold'. This symptom is usually self-limiting and requires no medication. However, it can be prolonged and debilitating in hay fever when the inflammation causes almost continuous sneezing. For this a steroidal nasal spray may be quite effective if used prophylactically. Beclomethasone dipropionate delivered in a metered spray of 50 µg per 'puff' can be used to reduce the inflammation and is not absorbed into the bloodstream. Sodium cromoglycate is also used prophylactically in the control of allergic rhinitis by topical inhalation administration (Hopkins, 1992).

SPUTUM

Sputum may be purulent, because of infection; frothy, as a result of pulmonary oedema; bloodstained, as in haemoptysis because of neoplastic effects on the blood vessels; or tenacious, as in cystic fibrosis or mucous plugging. Sputum changes, presence of blood (haemoptysis), dyspnoea and clubbing of fingers are all important indications in the patient suffering respiratory pathology and allow the practitioner to monitor the effect of medication.

Expectorants are said to liquefy mucus. Ammonia and ipecacuanha, however, are only useful as placebos (Downie *et al.*, 1995). Thick mucus is associated with the formation of polysaccharide fibres and acetylcysteine granules. Carbocisteine and methylcysteine act by splitting the disulphide bonds in mucus glycoprotein and are especially useful for the chronic respiratory disease sufferer (Hopkins, 1992).

NOISY BREATHING

Stridor is a rasping sound heard predominantly on inspiration. Croup consists of a cough that is caused by inflammation of the mucosa of the larynx, trachea, and bronchi, with narrowing of the subglottic area. Both of these conditions can be caused by viruses. Moist inhalations, nebulised steroids and adrenaline are all of uncertain benefit. Expiratory grunting is often found in infants with respiratory distress syndrome who are trying to create a positive airway, primarily during expiration, to maintain functional residual capacity.

11.1 'OVER-THE-COUNTER' PREPARATIONS

Many 'over-the-counter' preparations are a drug mixture, so caution is required in self-medication. Pregnant women and young children can be at risk.

In investigations of the throat and lung, amethocaine may be used as a spray onto the pharynx mucosa to suppress the cough reflex. This local anaesthetic acts by blocking the sodium channels of the small unmyelinated nerve fibres and thus blocking reception of sensory stimuli of foreign bodies, which could lead to aspiration. Local protocols are determined to ensure that patients are kept nil by mouth until the reflex recovers and danger of food or fluid aspiration is passed.

OTHER RESPIRATORY SYMPTOMS

Dyspnoea, shortness of breath and pain in breathing can lead to respiratory distress and may be treated with various respiratory drugs or with analgesics. The problem with some analgesics is that they may depress the respiratory system centrally or locally.

HYPOXIA

Hypoxia results from the decreased amount of oxygen in the air, loss of haemoglobin function, decreased production of red blood cells, disease of the respiratory and cardiovascular system and poisoning of the cytochromes in the cells (McCance and Huether, 1998). When pathological changes interfere with the vital activity of supplying tissues with oxygen, the resulting hypoxia (lack of oxygen in a cell in a tissue) and hypoxaemia (reduced oxygenation of arterial blood) upsets the homeostatic equilibrium of all body systems in a variety of ways. For example, kidneys produce erythropoietin to stimulate red blood cell production in the bone marrow, and brain cell membranes are unable to maintain the sodium–potassium pump and thus allow water to be retained, which causes oedema and convulsions.

Pathophysiology

When the oxygen supply to the cell is reduced, there is a rapid decrease in mitichondrial phosphorylation, which results in a lack of adenosine triphosphate (ATP) production. Anaerobic metabolism then generates ATP from glycogen until stores of the latter are depleted. As ATP levels drop, the plasma membrane's sodium–potassium pump and sodium–calcium exchange fails. Sodium and calcium build up in the cell and potassium leaks out. This leads to cell swelling as the sodium attracts water from the intersitial spaces. The endoplasmic reticulum dilates and ribosomes detach, thus reducing protein synthesis. If the hypoxia persists, vacuoles form in the cell cytoplasm and the cytosomes; damaged mitochondria and other cell structures swell and die.

Pharmacological management

Administration of oxygen is always a first-line treatment in hypoxia. There are many ways of delivering oxygen and local protocols of which to be aware for safe treatment. The nurse has a major responsibility in the safe administration of oxygen for her patient (Downie et al., 1995; Campbell and Glasper, 1995).

Oxygen is present as 21% of inspired air and can be administered therapeutically at concentrations from 21 to 90%. Face masks are a common method of delivery and are available to deliver oxygen concentrations up to 40%. Nasal cannula are excellent for low-flow requirements if tolerated by the patient, but care of the inside of the nares is important as the oxygen has a drying effect on the mucosa. Concentrations above 5% are not recommended via this route. Higher levels of oxygen, for example those used in paediatric treatments, can be achieved by the use of tents, adapted baby chairs and head boxes for very sick children. As they recover they do not tolerate the restriction or isolation, however.

Observation of safety precautions are vital. Oxygen is delivered in white-shouldered cylinders and is labelled oxygen. It is an inflammable gas; sparks and naked flames should be banned by clearly written and displayed labels. If the patient is receiving treatment at home, education is paramount for the family to maintain safe use. The immediate environment should be checked regularly, for example for kinked tubes, humidifying fluids and the patient's upright position. The respiratory rate and pulse should be regularly monitored, and if the patient is contained in a plastic hood, temperature should be monitored also (Downie et al., 1995).

OXYGEN DAMAGE TO HEALTH

The damage is caused by lipid peroxidation. Peroxisomes, small cell organelles that self-replicate by 'pinching' in half, contain one or more enzymes that use molecular oxygen to remove hydrogen atoms (oxidise) from various organic substances, producing hydrogen peroxide. One of the enzymes, catalase, uses the hydrogen peroxide generated by the other enzymes to oxidise a variety of substances, including phenol, formic acid, formaldehyde and alcohol. Another important function is to 'disarm' free radicals such as the superoxide radical by converting it to water. These peroxisomes are numerous in the kidneys and the liver where they detoxify harmful substances (Marieb, 1992).

OXYGEN AND THE PRETERM INFANT

Retinopathy of prematurity is caused in the preterm child if the latter is exposed to high concentrations, over 12 kPa, of oxygen (Carter, 1996). Vascularisation of the fetal retina is not complete until term, thus in preterm babies the peripheral retina is avascular. In those vessels that are present, if oxygen levels rise too high, constriction of the terminal branches occurs. If high oxygen therapy persists, new vessels proliferate from the sites of constriction into the vitreous and become covered in a fibrous material to form a fibrovascular membrane behind the lens, which contracts and pulls the neuroretina from the pigment epithelium at the vitreo-retinal interface (Coakes and Sellors, 1992). Thus, vision in these infants will be compromised. Treatment at present is under debate. Vitamin E, a lipid soluble antioxidant, is claimed to reduce platelet aggregation and lipid peroxidation in blood vessel walls (Muzulu, 1996). However, in premature babies, greater than 3 μmol/litre plasma of vitamin E causes haemolysis (see Chapter 12 *Drugs and cardiovascular disorders*). Current practice is to protect the cardiovascular system by preventing hypoxia – by the use of treatment with the lowest concentration of oxygen and weaning as soon as possible from oxygen therapy – and by preventing hypothermia, sepsis and hypoglycaemia. Oral preparations of vitamin E (there are no intramuscular preparations at present) are available and cause increased gastrointestinal osmolarity and may lead to necrotising enteritis.

Adrenocorticotrophic hormone may be given to produce an anti-inflammatory effect as it stimulates cortisone production. Cryotherapy (freezing) can be used to seal retinal holes by producing a local inflammation, resulting in the binding of the retinal and choroid layers; laser therapy (photocoagulation with xenon arc or argon laser) can be used for posterior lesions of grade III or IV to coagulate the pigment epithelium and the overlying neuroretina.

OXYGEN AND AGEING

Free radicals of oxygen that result from oxidative cellular metabolism can damage cell tissue. They are the normal products of cellular metabolism but are devastating to cells if they accumulate. The more you live the more you age. These oxygen atoms or molecules with unpaired electrons in their outermost orbit can combine with other nonradicals to form new free radicals, and, as a result, they can initiate or perpetuate reactions that affect cell membrane stability. They can also produce intracellular injury by damage to nucleic acids, and by destroying polysaccharides, oxidising proteins and peroxidising unsaturated fatty acids; they can kill and lyse cells and give rise to malignant transformations through DNA damage.

As human beings age, plasma constituents alter and, with the ravages of free radicals on cell structure, affect cardiovascular vessel integrity. Lipids, calcium and plasma proteins are deposited on vessel walls, further damaging basement membranes; this leads to atherosclerosis (McCance and Huether, 1998). It has been speculated that vitamin antioxidants, vitamin C (ascorbic acid) in combination with 100–400 IU/day vitamin E (α-tocopherol) and β-carotene (a precursor of vitamin A), may help to slow cardiovascular atherogenesis by inhibiting peroxidation of lipids and stimulating cell repair (Halliwell, 1993; Muzulu, 1996; Parfitt *et al.*, 1996), although optimal doses of supplementation have not been agreed. Vitamin C may also slow the loss of tissue plasticity associated with collagen cross-linking in ageing and diabetes mellitus (Seeley *et al.*, 1995; Pears, 1995) and detoxify inhaled oxidising pollutants.

However, excessive antioxidant intake may promote disease (Pears, 1995) and perhaps it is safer simply to consume a well balanced diet containing 500 g/day of fruit and vegetables.

DRUG ADMINISTRATION

Because the respiratory mucosa is very vascular, it can be used as a route for administration of drugs and in theory the lungs can be used for drug administration instead of giving injections. However, steroids are not absorbed and therefore their use in asthma is ideal in avoiding systemic effects of steroid use (see Chapter 3 *Classes of drugs*). Pharmacological preparations are prescribed for local application to the mucosa or for systemic effect on the blood and nervous supply. The respiratory system is lined with a moist mucosal surface protected by hairs in the nose and cilia throughout the system that waft debris towards the pharynx. A cough and sneeze reflex and microscopic macrophage activity complete the physical defences. Medications have to be administered in solutions or tiny particles in order to access the many passages of the 'tree', from which they can be absorbed. If the route is blocked, for example by a stricture or tumour, the medication cannot be taken up.

CHEMICAL CONTROL

Chemoreceptors monitor the acidity of arterial blood. Central receptors in the myelencephalon near the respiratory centre detect changes in the cerebrospinal fluid (CSF). Any change in arterial carbon dioxide level will be mirrored in the CSF across the blood–brain barrier. Respiratory alkalosis or metabolic alkalosis from the frequent ingestion of sodium bicarbonate, prolonged vomiting and diuretic therapy all result in a reduction of respiratory rate.

BEHAVIOURAL EFFECTS

The choices humans make in the air they breathe are not all under their control. Smoking tobacco irritates the fragile lining of the respiratory passages and kills the protective macrophage population in the mucosa, resulting in chronic bronchitis over time and cancer in susceptible individuals. Deep sea diving changes the pressure gradients in the alveoli, driving insoluble nitrogen bubbles into the blood, which causes the 'bends'; these bubbles can be fatal if they become lodged in the cranial blood vessels. Modern urban life, with its resultant traffic pollution (Soyseth *et al.*, 1995) and greater allergen load (Phelan, 1994; Day, 1995), has resulted in an increase in asthma in the young and a hastening of emphysema in the adult bronchitic population.

INTERACTION WITH OTHER SYSTEMS

Respiratory function is rapidly affected by some medication used in the treatment of cardiovascular conditions. Alveolar supply of oxygen responds automatically to blood supply at the interface between the alveoli and the pulmonary capillaries. When flow of blood is reduced, for example in heart failure or anaemia, the effects are immediate in the alveolar oxygen levels. Thus the medications for the cardiovascular system may well have an effect on respiratory rate and efficiency (Chapter 12 *Drugs and cardiovascular disorders*). Alveolar ventilation is closely related to the carbon dioxide excretion that can be measured in blood arteries. In chronic bronchitis and emphysema, alveolar underventilation leads to hypercapnia. This effect is also seen in central depression of respiration by narcotics and anaesthetics (McLeod, 1987).

MEDICATION ROUTES

It is important to understand the normal physiological function of individuals of all ages to assess differentiation in pathological function and preferred medication route. For example, a 4-week-old baby has a respiratory rate of 30–50 breaths per minute and is an obligatory nose breather (see **Box 11.1** for major differences that may affect treatments) so oral medications can be inhaled if the nose is not unblocked (Carter, 1996). At the other end of the age span, the elderly have loss of alveolar wall tissue and capillaries, which reduces gaseous exchange, and loss of elastic properties in chest wall tissue, which reduces chest compliance and thus reduces ventilatory reserve. Inhaled medication is more efficiently administered by mechanical nebuliser (see **Box 11.2**) in a fragile patient with bronchitis than a hand-held inhaler.

RESPIRATORY DISORDERS

COUGH

A dry hacking cough can be indicative of inhalation of irritant fumes, asthma, bronchitis, tumour or pneumonia. In young children stridor and croup can lead to an emergency situation.

Pathophysiology

The cough reflex (**Fig. 11.1**) maintains the open airway by forceful expiration of foreign matter that stimulates the irritant receptors. A cough may be dry or productive and require different medications.

11.1 PHYSIOLOGICAL REMINDERS ABOUT BABIES

- obligatory nose breathers
- narrow upper airway – air flow resistance
- the diaphragm is longer and cannot contract effectively
- glottis more cephalic and laryngeal reflexes more active
- epiglottis longer and extends further posteriorly
- areolar tissue present below the vocal cords – oedema risk
- trachea flexible due to very elastic cartilage
- respiratory tract short – susceptible to infection
- alveolar 'tree' not complete – small exchange surface
- ribs horizontal position – abdominal breathers
- high tracheal bifurcation – suctioning technique care (Carter, 1996, p. 88)

11.2 NEBULISER THERAPY

Effective therapy by nebuliser is achieved by selection of the appropriate system to deliver a specific drug to the specific target in the lungs. Conventional jet nebulisers deliver a flow related to the flow from the compressor that is less than the normal tidal volume breathing, thus 60–70% of the drug is wasted in expiration. Other systems can improve patient drug uptake by increasing flow, thus reducing drug particle size, or by the use of a breath assisted nebuliser, which will more nearly match an individual patient's inspiration flow rate. Good hygiene and care of the equipment must be addressed.

Correct technique is vital for the accurate delivery of drugs; a mouthpiece is more effective than a mask and will prevent irritation of the eyes, e.g. as with ipratropium bromide. However, masks are useful for small children and breathless/fragile clients.

Timing of drug delivery must be related to chest clearance. Bronchodilators should be given before chest physiotherapy; steroids and antibiotics afterwards. Tidal volumes should be measured before and 20 minutes after therapy. Observation is recommended of effectiveness of the drug, remembering that cold, non-isotonic, acidic or certain preservatives can cause broncho-constriction (Dodd, 1996).

Pharmacological management

Medication often only relieves the symptoms and can exacerbate the underlying pathology. Codeine linctus is effective because it acts on the 'cough centre' in the brainstem by inhibiting the release of excitatory neuropeptides through action on the μ receptors on sensory nerves in the bronchi (Rang *et al.*, 1995). However, it results in the thickening of secretions and inhibits ciliary activity; it also produces constipation in the gastrointestinal tract. The drug is presented in a sweet syrup, which is also soothing to the irritated airway.

CROUP

Viral croup accounts for 95% of childhood laryngeal infections. The incidence of croup is higher in boys and occurs more often in the winter months, in children aged between 3 months and 5 years (Lissauer and Clayden, 1997).

Pathophysiology

This is an upper respiratory obstruction caused by the inflammatory process. Children's tissues react with swelling in a larynx that is small and airways that are narrow. It is usually described according to the primary anatomical area affected, for example, epiglottitis. Croup is caused by a virus (respiratory syncytical virus, para-influenza virus) or more rarely, a bacterial (*Haemophilus influenzae*) infection. There is a mucosal inflammation and increased secretions, affecting the lungs, trachea and bronchi. The narrowing of an already small subglottic area compromises it: the negative pressure of inspiration is transmitted to the inflamed upper airway, causing it to collapse and obstruct airflow. Turbulent airflow across the swollen vocal cords causes inspiratory stridor and laryngeal spasm. The increasing obstruction leads to sternal and subcostal recession, increasing respiratory and heart rate and exhaustion (Lissauer and Clayden, 1997; McCance and Huether, 1998).

Pharmacological management

A common treatment for croup is with budesonide 1 mg/2 ml normal saline nebulised for two treatments 1 hour apart in the acute phase, reduced to 250 μg/ml twice daily for maintenance while the episode continues. This medication will reduce the inflammation in the mucosal lining

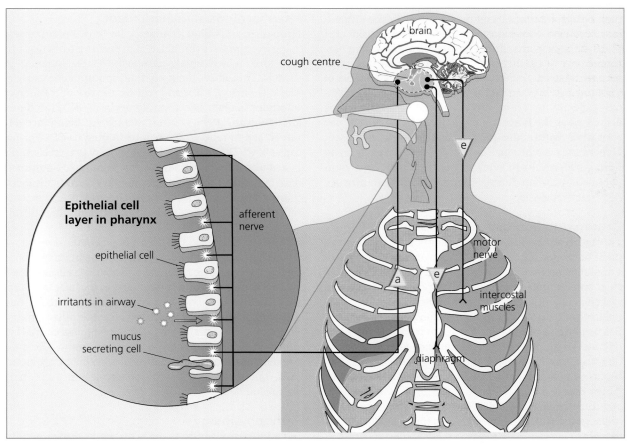

Fig 11.1 Cough reflex arc. (From Page 1997, with permission.)

of the upper respiratory tract. The child should be kept cool and older children respond well to sucking ice lollipops or drinking iced drinks. It is important to keep the family calm, watch for deterioration and have available emergency tracheal intubation equipment (Lissauer and Clayden, 1997). The respiration rate is monitored for a distressed state and children may have to be intubated until the swelling reduces.

BRONCHIOLITIS

This is the most common serious respiratory infection of infancy. It is rare after 1 year of age. Eighty per cent of cases are caused by the respiratory syncytial virus. It occurs in winter and spring. Half of the sufferers will have episodes of cough and wheeze until they are 3–5 years old. The babies present with tachypnoea, expiratory wheeze, subcostal and intercostal recession, mild fever, cyanosis and feeding difficulties. They may have a short history of coryzal symptoms.

Pathophysiology

In bronchiolitis there is infiltration with lymphocytes around the bronchioles. Cell-mediated hypersensitivity to viral antigens with release of lymphokines causes inflammation of the bronchiolar epithelium and activation of eosinophils, neutrophils and monocytes. As the submucosa becomes oedematous, cellular debris and fibrin form plugs within the bronchiolar lumen. Bronchospasm narrows many of the peripheral airways, which may also become blocked. Atelectasis occurs in some segments of the lung and hyperinflation in others. Functional residual capacity is often twice normal; compliance is decreased as the lungs are often overinflated and airway resistance within the lung is uneven and increased. Hypoxaemia can produce lactic acidosis; poor calorie and fluid intake results in ketoacidosis. This acidosis is compounded by carbon dioxide retention, which can produce respiratory acidosis.

Pharmacological management

Two hourly adrenaline nebulisers may be used for the treatment of bronchiolitis, although their use is controversial. Adrenaline acts on the sympathetic nerve endings of vascular smooth muscle to produce bronchial dilatation and vasoconstriction of the inflamed bronchiole linings, thus reducing mucus secretion. It is broken down in the liver. Babies must be carefully monitored for increased heart rate (Henney *et al.*, 1995), one of the many general effects of this drug. Another medication often used in high-risk babies is nebulised ribavirin, given for 12–16 hours or longer over 3–5 days (Henney *et al.*, 1995). It is expensive and must be given by small particle aerosol generator in order to reach the tiny bronchiole endings. Ribavirin is thought to interfere with the expression of messenger RNA, thereby inhibiting viral protein synthesis (Miller, 1992).

CYSTIC FIBROSIS

Cystic fibrosis is an inherited disease of the exocrine glands, particularly those involving the lungs and digestive systems. It is inherited in an autosomal recessive pattern and results from an abnormality of the **cystic fibrosis conductance regulator (CFTR)** on chromosome 7, which controls transport of salts and water across cell membranes (**Fig. 11.2**) (Hopkins, 1995).

Pathophysiology

In cystic fibrosis the mucus secretions in the lungs become thick and viscous and the mucociliary mechanism is impaired, causing mucus obstruction of the airways and respiratory tract infections. As progressive lung damage occurs, infections range from *Staphylococcus aureus*, *H. influenzae* and *Pseudomonas aeruginosa* to, more recently, a multidrug-resistant bacterium, *Pseudomonas cepasia*. Children are now supported with lifelong antibiotic cover, which has encouraged the development of more bacterial strains resistant to antibiotic assault (Hopkins, 1995) (see Chapter 3 *Classes of drugs*). The inflammatory response to infection leads to large numbers of leucocytes being present in the lungs; the byproduct of neutrophil breakdown is DNA, which forms viscous gels in the purulent sputum.

Pharmacological management

Human recombinant DNAse α can now be nebulised, using a compressor combination to ensure a particular particle size, which breaks down the extracellular DNA strands. This allows the more fluid sputum to be expectorated (Thomson, 1995) and reduces the risk of respiratory infections in cystic fibrosis sufferers by 28–37% (McKenry and Salerno, 1995). Gene therapy is being actively researched to replace the malfunctioning CFTR. Normal copies of CFTR can be transferred into airway epithelial cells by nebulised modified adenovirus or cationic liposomes; once there, their subsequent expression corrects the cystic fibrosis functional effect. In cell targeting it may be submucosal glands that are preferred (Stern and Alton, 1996).

RESPIRATORY DISTRESS SYNDROME

Respiratory distress syndrome may occur in infants born preterm who have no mature type 2 alveolar cells to secrete surfactant or adults who suffer injury to the lung from sepsis or multiple trauma. It is characterised by acute lung inflammation, leading to diffuse alveolocapillary injury. Postoperative respiratory failure can result in a clinical situation similar to respiratory distress syndrome. The most common problems that lead to respiratory failure are atelectasis, pneumonia, pulmonary oedema and pulmonary embolism.

Pathophysiology

In children and adults, damage occurs in respiratory distress syndrome because of the massive inflammatory

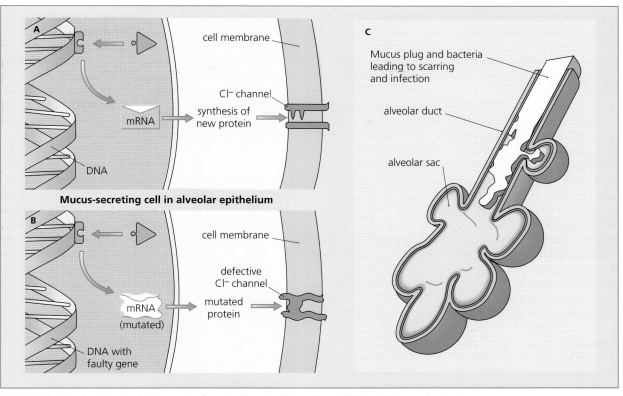

Fig 11.2 Pathophysiological elements of cystic fibrosis. (From Page 1997, with permission.)

response. The most important cell types and inflammatory mediators are the neutrophils, complement, endotoxins and tumour necrosis factor. The damaged pulmonary capillary endothelium stimulates platelet aggregation and intravascular thrombus formation. Neutrophils are then activated, often by endotoxins in sepsis. Neutrophils release proteolytic enzymes, oxygen free radicals, arachidonic acid metabolites and platelet-activating factors. They damage the alveolar cells and allow fluid, protein and blood cells to move from the capillary bed into the pulmonary interstitial cells and alveoli. This results in oedema and haemorrhage. The lung then becomes less compliant and less able to allow alveolar ventilation. The inflammatory response causes pulmonary vasoconstriction and thus hypertension and damage to the pulmonary vascular endothelium. Surfactant is inactivated in the adult as type 2 alveolar cells are impaired by the alveoli filling with fluid and collapsing. After 24–48 hours, a hyaline membrane forms and after 7 days, fibrosis obliterates the alveoli. This inflammatory response can ultimately cause a systemic response and multiple organ dysfunction syndrome.

Pharmacological management

In order to try and prevent respiratory distress syndrome in the infant born preterm, mothers who are expected to deliver premature infants are given **dexamethasone** or **betamethasone** 12 mg intramuscularly 12 hourly for 48 hours (four doses) to stimulate the maturation of the baby's lungs if there is time before delivery. Exogenous surfactant therapy can be given after the birth into the tracheal tube of the infant if the infant is ventilated with increased oxygen support. The active ingredients of surfactant are lecithin 60%, phosphatidyl glycerol and phosphatidyl inositol. 2.5 mg/kg curosurf with 2 minutes of manual ventilation are recommended (Sittlington *et al.*, 1991). **Beractant** (or **survanta**) are extracts of bovine lung and are given as 100 mg/kg birth weight (4 mg/kg). A minimum of four doses over 48 hours is given. Treatment shows a lower incidence of bronchopulmonary dysplasia and less damage caused by barotrauma as the lungs are ventilated. However, there is less consensus of opinion about immunogenicity, negative reaction with surfactant production, the doses and length of treatment and the optimal delivery procedures (Gardner, 1989). The partial pressure of oxygen is usually maintained at between 50 and 70 mmHg during treatments (Carter, 1993) and suctioning is usually delayed for 6 hours between treatments. Pulse oximetry should be maintained, transcutaneous oxygen and carbon dioxide levels monitored and care taken not to overinflate the lungs. Treatment for adults with respiratory distress syndrome include sedation to reduce oxygen need, support of cardiac function and steroids to reduce inflammation.

INFLAMMATORY AND INFECTIVE CONDITIONS OF THE RESPIRATORY TRACT

Inflammation of the respiratory system from allergy, trauma, drugs and infections causes pain, swelling and production of exudate. The airway passages are then narrowed and blocked, leading to the reduction of oxygen and carbon dioxide exchange. Constant blowing of the nose and sneezing irritates the mucosa lining of the upper airway passages.

INFECTIONS

Acute respiratory infections are usually caused by the invasion of tissues through the protective layer of mucus by viruses. Influenza, pneumonia and bronchitis are most often caused by viruses and may be followed by an opportunistic bacterium, for example *Streptococcus pneumoniae*, which will thrive in the damaged tissue.

INFLUENZA

This is caused by a virus that 'drifts' by changing its shape on a yearly basis. Immune responses that have developed against the strain of the previous year give no protection. For this reason, epidemics occur frequently across continents. Many elderly people have compromised immune responses and may have some damage to their lungs, thus they readily fall victim to this virus. Each winter, older people are offered vaccination in the United Kingdom, as are health professionals who may be in frequent contact with the disease.

Pathophysiology

Influenza viruses proliferate within cells by taking over the metabolic machinery of host cells and using it for survival and replication. They rapidly produce irreversible and lethal injury in the lungs of immunocompromised hosts.

Pharmacological management

Vaccines induce primary and secondary immune responses of a subclinical nature, so overt specific disease symptoms are not experienced. **Influenza virus vaccine, trivalent A and B (surface antigen/split virion)** are given intramuscularly in a dose of 0.5 ml. The vaccines need to be given annually to prevent infection with a new organism. Symptom relief such as aspirin 1 g every 6 hours is usually recommended to help relieve pyrexia and muscle and joint aches.

PNEUMONIA

Streptococcus pneumoniae infection probably affects 1 in 1000 people every year, with a mortality of 10–20% in adults (Payling, 1997).

A wide range of pathogens cause pneumonia in children, with different pathogens affecting different ages. Newborn babies are affected by β-haemolytic *Streptococcus*, and *E. coli* and *Chlamydia trachomatis* from the mother's genital tract. Older children are susceptible to respiratory synctial virus, *S. pneumoniae* and *H. influenzae*. *Mycoplasma pneumoniae* is common in the school-age child (Lissauer and Clayden, 1997). In all ages, pneumonia is often preceded by a viral infection.

Pathophysiology

Up to 60% of the population carries *S. pneumioniae* in the pharynx. It is spread by direct contact and oral expulsion. The bacterium reaches the lungs in susceptible individuals as it is not overcome by the normal respiratory defence mechanisms such as coughing and alveolar mast cell secretions. *Streptococcus pneumoniae* releases toxins that stimulate an inflammatory response, which, together with the toxins, damages alveoli and bronchi. Inflammation and oedema cause the alveoli to fill with dead cells and inflammatory exudate. Necrosis of the lung parenchyma may also occur. The lobe of the lung undergoes consolidation and the white blood count is usually elevated.

Pharmacological management

An effective vaccine against *S. pneumoniae* is available for high-risk patients. It s given as a single dose in the autumn (Payling, 1997). Currently, the best choice of antibiotic is a second generation cephalosporin, **cefuroxine**, 1–5 g 8 hourly intravenously. Oral **cefadroxil** 500 mg 12 hourly is useful for less severe conditions. If *M. pneumoniae* or *Chlamydia* infection is suspected, then erythromycin 500 mg 6 hourly is given (see Chapter 5 *Drugs and immunological disorders*).

ACUTE BRONCHITIS

This is an inflammation of the bronchi that often follows an upper respiratory tract infection. Cough and fever are the main symptoms. The patient often reports pain in the sternal area. The cause may be viral or bacterial in origin and may progress to pneumonia. The condition is common in patients who suffer from chronic bronchitis, in which case it may be termed acute-on-chronic bronchitis. Children may present with vomiting and have a wheeze with coarse crackles. There is a dispute about the term 'wheezy bronchitis' as many authorities define this as asthma (Lissauer and Clayden, 1997).

Pathophysiology

The causative organism invades the bronchial mucosa and produces an inflammatory response. Secretions may be purulent. The constant irritation leads to symptoms of a productive cough and substernal pain, together with all the symptoms of acute infection such as fever.

Pharmacological management

If the invading microorganism is a virus, the symptoms are self-limiting. Drugs such as **aspirin** are given to relieve the symptoms of fever and pain from coughing. Bacterial infections are treated with the appropriate antibiotics for the invading microorganism.

TUBERCULOSIS
(MYCOBACTERIUM TUBERCULOSIS)

Incidence of this chronic bacterial infection of the lung has increased in the inner cities of the United Kingdom by 12% from 1988 to 1992 (Thompson, 1993; Shaw, 1995). Worldwide, one-third of the population is infected (Peloquin and Berning, 1995). It is particularly active in the homeless, those infected with HIV and Southeast Asian immigrant communities in which many effects of poverty are compounded to facilitate the spread of infection (Smith, 1995). In maternity units catering for these populations, newborn babies are now vaccinated before discharge from the ward. In the tuberculous patient, the bacilli occur in three groups: metabolically active, metabolically inactive and necrotic (Spector, 1989). Three antibiotics are used initially to reduce the number of active bacilli quickly and prevent drug resistance. Long-term treatment is needed to cover the long periods of bacilli inactivity (Cooksey, 1995).

Tuberculosis presents particular challenges to those caring for patients with the disease. This is because of the characteristics of the causative organism, and because the disease process is associated with altered immune responses that influence the progress of the illness. Tuberculosis was one of the great killers of the nineteenth century. The development of vaccination, pasteurisation and the general improvement in social conditions has resulted in its reduced incidence. However, increased population migration, mutation of the *M. tuberculosis* bacillus and altered immune responses, particularly within vulnerable sections of society, have resulted in the current raised incidence of the condition (Porth, 1994; McCance and Huether, 1994).

The characteristics of the tubercle bacillus protect it against the humoral defences of the body and also make it resistant to some antibiotics. Tubercle bacilli are protected by a lipid capsule, which prevents hydrochloric acid from destroying the organism should it enter the stomach. The lipid capsule also protects the bacillus against breakdown in the body tissues, thus making tubercular lesions able to remain potentially active for a considerable time within the body. The lipid capsule also makes the broad-spectrum antibiotics commonly used for systemic infections ineffective against the tubercle bacilli, so an infected patient requires specific, prolonged treatment, which may prove problematic for some people. Tubercle bacilli are able to assume a semidormant state, within tissues and within cells such as macrophages after phagocytosis. In order to understand the principles of successful treatment of a patient with tuberculosis, it is important to consider the pathophysiology of the disease.

Pathophysiology

Tuberculosis in humans may be transmitted via bovine tuberculosis present in the milk of infected cows, which, if ingested, causes tubercular infection of the alimentary tract. In countries where milk is pasteurised and herds are vaccinated, bovine tuberculosis does not present much of a health problem. The human *M. tuberculosis* bacillus is an aerobic organism, and flourishes best in oxygen tensions of around 140 mmHg (Porth, 1994). For this reason, the apices of the lungs, which are particularly well ventilated, are likely to be a preferential site for tubercular infection. The organism is transmitted by minute droplets from respiratory secretions, so people living in close proximity have a greater risk of contracting the disease. The small size of the droplets allows mycobacteria to be inhaled directly into the alveoli.

Primary tuberculosis

If a person with no previous contact with the tubercle bacillus inhales the organism, specific immune responses are not immediately activated. A primary infection occurs, in which the organism becomes established in a terminal bronchiole or an alveolus, and the normal inflammatory response develops. The bacilli are ingested by macrophages, but, being protected by their lipid capsules, their destruction is not completely effective. The result is a localised area of necrotic tissue, macrophages, immune cells and tubercle bacilli. This lesion, called a Ghon's focus, becomes walled off from the surrounding tissues. At this stage, a tuberculin test will produce a positive result because the immune system has been stimulated and actively recognises the tubercle organism. If the person's immune system is healthy and the number of bacilli are small, the infection will be overcome, and the Ghon's focus will heal to produce a scar that may ultimately become calcified and be visible as a small spot on a routine chest X-ray. No pharmacological treatment will have been needed.

In some cases, the lesion may be dormant rather than healed, and becomes activated at a later time, progressing to the more advanced stages of the disease. This seems to be caused by a failure of the immune system to eradicate the disease initially or to keep it in check during the following months or years.

Progressive tuberculosis

In patients in whom the infection is substantial or the immune system is not fully effective, the tubercular infection is not arrested and the disease process continues. In this situation, the primary focus is inadequately isolated from the rest of the body and infective material is released locally. The lesion may open into one of the air passages, causing the lesion to be air-filled, and resulting in the release of bacilli and inflammatory material into the bronchiole, which produces a productive cough. If the lesion erodes into a blood vessel, haemoptysis occurs. The reactivated infection produces the signs of a low-grade infection: fever, sweats, especially at night, and in the more advanced cases, weight loss and malaise.

The bacilli may enter the bloodstream or the lymphatic circulation and produce infective lesions in lymph glands or distant organs or tissues. The bones, liver, kidneys, meninges or brain may be infected with multiple small lesions, a condition termed miliary tuberculosis.

Pharmacological management

Pharmacological preparations to treat tuberculosis must be effective against an organism that tends to remain dormant and that is becoming drug resistant; in its later stages, the disease may be characterised by large numbers of replicating microorganisms. For these reasons, the more commonly used antibiotics are not effective and specific antitubercular drugs are used in combination.

Rifampicin is rapidly absorbed in the stomach and stimulates hepatic function as much of the drug is reabsorbed by the entero-hepatic circulation system; thus it potentiates the effects of other drugs when used in combination. **Isoniazid** is a highly selective antibiotic for tuberculosis; in some patients it may cause a neuropathy if blood levels rise because of slow liver acetylation or liver damage. **Pyridoxine** must be given prophylactically to counteract the interference of isoniazid with pyridoxine metabolism (Hopkins, 1992). **Pyrazinamide** acts on inactivated bacilli and is effective in the first 3 months of treatment. It can raise serum uric acid levels and interfere with liver function. **Streptomycin** and **ethambutol** may be used for single-drug resistance, whereas multidrug resistance needs second-line drugs such as capreomycin or cycloserine (Cooksey, 1995).

Rifampicin is particularly useful as a treatment of mycobacteria that are in a semidormant state within cells. This preparation prevents the microorganisms from synthesising RNA, and therefore it acts as a bactericidal agent. Rifampicin is given orally in daily doses of between 450 and 600 mg. It is taken up well within the body tissues and crosses the blood–brain barrier when the meninges are inflamed, so it is an effective treatment when the tubercular infection has spread beyond the primary infection. Rifampicin potentiates the action of hepatic enzymes, and therefore it reduces the effectiveness of drugs that are degraded by the liver. For this reason, rifampicin causes inactivation of anticoagulants such as warfarin. It also reduces the effectiveness of corticosteroids, cyclosporin, digoxin, oral contraceptives, oral hypoglycaemics, narcotics and analgesics (Walker, 1995).

A striking but harmless effect of rifampicin therapy is that it may cause the urine, tears and sputum to turn a reddish colour. Wearers of soft contact lenses should be warned of this effect as their lenses may become permanently stained so that they are literally viewing the world through rose-coloured glasses.

Ethambutol is a bacteriostat and, by preventing division of the tubercle bacilli, slows the progress of the disease and inhibits the development of resistant forms of tuberculosis. Because, like rifampicin, it is absorbed readily from the alimentary tract and penetrates the body tissues easily, ethambutol is useful for the treatment of primary and progressive tuberculosis. The medication is given orally in doses of 15 mg/kg per day. In cases of tuberculous meningitis, the inflammation of the meninges enables the preparation to cross the blood–brain barrier (Laurence and Bennett, 1992). Ethambutol is excreted by the kidneys, so patients with impaired renal function must receive a reduced dose of the medication in order to avoid its toxic effects. There are relatively few side effects with ethambutol, although in some people it may cause optic neuritis, so it is important for the patient to report any difficulty that develops in reading small print with either eye. If this complication is not recognised, colour blindness, loss of part of the visual fields or more extensive blindness may result (Walker, 1995).

Isoniazid has a bactericidal effect upon *M. tuberculosis* regardless of whether the organism is multiplying within the tissues or inside macrophages. The preparation is given in doses of 5 mg/kg per day. It is particularly useful for patients with miliary tuberculosis. In elderly people, those who are poorly nourished or those who have liver disease or alcoholism, isoniazid can cause tingling and numbness of the hands or feet as a result of peripheral neuropathy. Some strains of tubercle bacilli are able to develop resistance to isoniazid. In order to reduce the likelihood of this occurring, patients may be prescribed isoniazid in combination with ethambutol.

Pyrazinamide is an effective agent against persistent, semidormant intracellular microorganisms. It is given orally in doses of between 20 and 30 mg/kg per day. It can cause joint pains and gout-like symptoms because pyrazinamide inhibits the excretion of urate from the kidney and thus produces hyperuricaemia.

Streptomycin may be used in combination with other antitubercular drugs. Because this substance is not easily absorbed from the intestine, it must be given intravenously or intramuscularly. Streptomycin is an aminoglycoside, that is, one of a group of substances that bind to bacterial ribosomes and cause the formation of abnormal amino acids that are lethal to the microorganism. Streptomycin has a toxic effect upon the vestibular branch of the auditory nerve and the hair cells of the vestibule, so patients receiving this treatment must be observed for nausea or dizziness, which could be permanently disabling if the toxicity is not detected quickly. For this reason, streptomycin therapy is discontinued if there is any suggestion of vestibular symptoms (see **Warning Box**). Streptomycin is now

11.2 ANTITUBERCULAR THERAPY

Antitubercular therapy is given in combinations of specific agents such as isoniazid, rifampicin, ethambutol and pyrazinamide for 2 months followed by a regime of rifampicin and isoniazid for a further 4 months (Brody *et al.*, 1994). Patients receiving treatment for this condition therefore have to comply with multiple therapy for a sustained period. Those in the community who are particularly susceptible to contracting tuberculosis include those with a diminished immune response as a result of pre-existing disease or poor social conditions. Such people may have difficulty accessing health advice. If, in addition, they suffer from alcoholism or malnutrition, there is a risk of problems caused by peripheral neuropathy. Health professionals therefore are faced with a dual challenge: to promote compliance to the therapeutic regime in a group who may be resistant to taking medication and to recognise the signs of adverse responses to the treatment in people who may tend to avoid contact with health professionals.

rarely used in the United Kingdom but it may be added if the organism is resistant to isoniazid.

CHRONIC BRONCHITIS

This is the most common chronic airway disease in the West. It is usually diagnosed when the patient has had a productive cough lasting for more than 3 months for 2 consecutive years (Nowak and Handford, 1994). The principal aetiological feature is chronic inhalation of irritating fumes such as cigarette smoke or industrial air pollutants such as sulphur dioxide. Ninety per cent of deaths from chronic obstructive pulmonary disease are connected to cigarette smoking (Whatling, 1995).

Pathophysiology

Inflammatory hyperaemia and exudate cause thickening of the bronchial mucosa. Hypertrophy and hyperplasia of the mucus-secreting glands produces excessive sticky mucus, which leads to a chronic cough. Metaplasia of the bronchial epithelium causes loss of cilia and their function in moving mucus from the lower airways to the pharynx for expectoration. Smaller airways become plugged and isolate inhaled organisms, which can then proliferate. When the airways are narrowed and occluded, hypoventilation produces hypoxia and hypercapnia. This triggers pulmonary vasoconstriction, which raises pulmonary pressure and the workload of the heart. Chronic hypoxia stimulates the kidney to secrete erythropoietin and thus encourage

production of red blood cells by the bone marrow. The viscosity of the blood increases and the haematocrit rises, which further increases the work of the heart (Nowak and Handford, 1994).

Pharmacological management

Management of the patient with chronic bronchitis includes preserving existing lung function. Cessation of smoking slows the decline in function. **Nicotine** replacement can be offered in the form of chewing gum – one 2 mg or 4 mg piece chewed for half an hour as desired to a maximum of 15, 4 mg pieces in 24 hours – and skin patches of 5, 10 or 15 mg over 16 hours or 7, 14 or 21 mg over 24 hours. Both routes give a maximum plasma concentration in 8–10 hours. They increase catecholamine release from the adrenal medulla by stimulating receptors in the central nervous system.

Bronchodilators are used: for example short-acting β agonists such as **salbutamol** by aerosol inhalation of 100–200 µg (one or two puffs) three or four times a day, and anticholinergics such as **ipratropium bromide** by inhalation of 20–49 µg three or four times a day. They can give an increased effect if they are given together, as salbutamol affects the nerves that dilate the bronchioles and ipratropium blocks the nerves that constrict them. In the older patient with chronic bronchitis, anticholinergics may be more effective as the sympathetic (dilatation effect) nerve endings tend to decline with age. The patient needs to receive bronchodilators regularly as permanent bronchoconstriction is usually present. **Oxygen** therapy should be given at a low concentration as these patients often have an altered respiratory drive mechanism. Antibiotics and steroids may be used as the disease progresses (Whatling, 1995).

EMPHYSEMA

Where destruction of the acini (end lobules) of the lungs occurs, gas exchange is compromised. Loss of small airway support allows the alveoli to collapse in exhalation and so the airflow is obstructed. There is decreased lung elasticity. Patients often appear thin and anxious, and have quiet breath sounds with pursed lips on expiration. The pursing of the lips is an unconscious attempt to keep the airways open during exhalation by producing a small positive airway pressure. There is a small sputum volume, respiratory distress on exertion of any sort and finger clubbing. In 1992 there were 25 172 deaths from emphysema in the United Kingdom. Although the condition is rare in nonsmokers, it can occur in patients with genetic conditions such as α_1-antitrypsin deficiency (**Fig. 11.3**).

Pathophysiology

Emphysema is characterised by loss of alveolar membranes and septa, which leads to abnormal enlargement of the terminal airspaces beyond the ends of the bronchioles. Bullae are formed when these sacs enlarge to diameters of over 1 cm. When the proximal and central parts of the lobules (acini) are distended, the condition is referred to as centrilobular emphysema. When the entire acinus is dilated, it is called panacinar emphysema. It has been suggested that the smoke particles inhaled by smokers stimulate macrophages to bring neutrophils to the area. These neutrophils secrete serine elastase, an enzyme that breaks down elastin. Excessive amounts of smoke particles encourage neutrophils and elastase secretion, which then damages alveolar tissue. Another view is that smokers have reduced levels of α_1-antitrypsin, an enzyme that removes elastase from the airways (Whatling, 1995).

Pharmacological management

Medication is the same as for chronic bronchitis.

ASTHMA

One in seven children in the United Kingdom suffers from asthma, and the numbers increase annually. Rising air pollution has been blamed, but one must not confuse factors that exacerbate asthma with those that cause the condition (Day, 1995). The link with cigarette smoking has been more thoroughly researched, as have the allergic effects of dust mites and pet hairs. The aim of treatment is to abolish symptoms, restore normal lung function, minimise the requirement for relief medication and enable normal growth in children.

Pathophysiology

Asthma is a common inflammatory reversible chronic obstructive airway disorder that occurs in children and adults and is divided into two kinds: extrinsic (implying a defined external cause) and intrinsic (in which no causative agent can be identified). Approximately 10–15% of the population are affected in their second decade and asthma is believed to be on the increase as a result of environmental factors (see **Fig. 11.4**). Stress and occupational exposure to sensitisers are also believed to play a part. For explanations of hypersensitivity, see Chapter 5 *Drugs and immunological disorders*.

Asthma is characterised by airflow limitation, which is reversible spontaneously or with treatment (although chronic inflammation may lead to irreversible airflow limitation), airway hyper-reactivity to a wide range of stimuli and infiltration of the bronchi with eosinophils, T lymphocytes and mast cells. The associated plasma exudation, oedema, smooth muscle hypertrophy, mucus plugging and epithelial changes lead to airway obstruction (**Figs. 11.5** and **11.6**).

Airway obstruction increases resistance to airflow, particularly during expiration, and causes hyperinflation of the respiratory structures distal to the obstruction. The

---

PERSON CENTRED STUDY 1

David Thresher is 55 years old and lives on the outskirts of a large industrial city, on a council estate with his wife and six children. He used to work as a quarryman until ill health forced him to give up work 5 years ago, and he has been unemployed ever since. There are few alternative employment opportunities locally, although most of his neighbours work in the local car factory.

He started having breathing difficulties 15 years ago, which were diagnosed as being caused by chronic bronchitis. In the past year his breathing has got steadily worse. His wife has complained about his smoking for years, trying to persuade him to give up, but Mr Thresher says smoking is one of his last pleasures in life.

Mrs Thresher says the family has 'got by' on unemployment and family benefits for the last 5 years, but she gets worried every winter by the mould that appears on the walls in the bedrooms, despite keeping the coal fire in the sitting room going all the time.

Usually Mr Thresher uses his salbutamol inhaler when he walks to the local shop and antibiotics when his sputum becomes green. However, he states that the antibiotics are not doing any good because he now coughs for 2 hours every morning on wakening.

1. Why is Mr Thresher experiencing breathlessness and a morning cough?
2. Why might ipratropium bromide by inhalation 20–40 µg three or four times per day be a more effective medication for Mr Thresher?

---

changes in resistance are not uniform throughout the lungs; regional differences exist, with a greater airflow to the less resistant areas. Hyperventilation is triggered by lung receptors responding to increased lung volume, and continued air trapping increases intrapleural and alveolar gas pressures, causing decreased perfusion of the alveoli.

Increased alveolar gas pressure, decreased ventilation and decreased perfusion lead to early hypoxaemia without carbon dioxide retention (hypercapnia). Hypoxaemia further increases hyperventilation by stimulating the respiratory centre. This causes the arterial carbon dioxide to decrease and pH to increase, which results in respiratory alkalosis. As the obstruction becomes worse, the number of

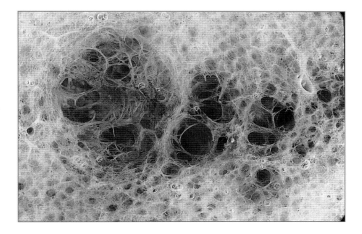

Fig 11.3 Emphysema. (From Stevens & Lowe 1995, with permission.)

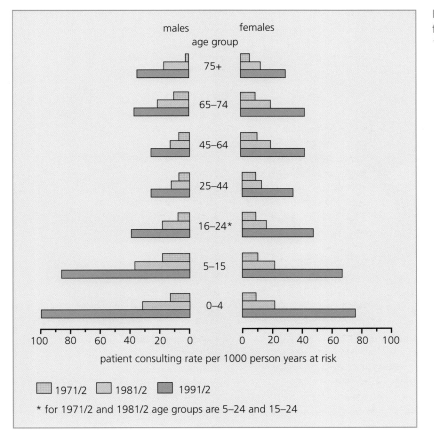

Fig 11.4 Patients consulting their GP for asthma. (From Stevens & Lowe 1995, with permission.)

alveoli being inadequately ventilated and perfused increases to the point where carbon dioxide retention and respiratory acidosis occurs. This signals respiratory failure.

The underlying pathophysiology in preschool children may be different in that they may not have appreciable bronchial hyper-reactivity. There is no evidence that chronic inflammation causes the episodic asthma that may accompany viral infections.

Pharmacological management

Drugs for asthma fall into two main categories: bronchodilators and prophylactic anti-inflammatory medications.

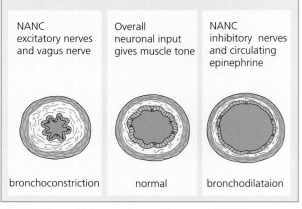

Fig 11.5 Bronchial smooth muscle tone. NANC: nonadrenergic, noncholinergic. (From Page 1997, with permission.)

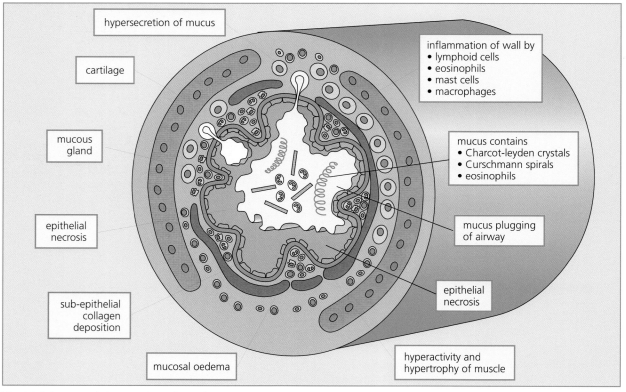

Fig 11.6 Structural changes in asthma. (From Stevens & Lowe 1995, with permission.)

Some bronchodilators, like salbutamol and terbutaline, can mimic adrenaline, which is naturally produced by stimulation of the adrenal medulla by the sympathetic nervous system. These bronchodilators selectively stimulate β_2 receptors in organs; in the bronchi they relax the smooth muscle so that the airway is opened. Other smooth muscle may be also affected; heart rate increases, blood vessels constrict, raising blood pressure, the iris muscles allow the pupils to dilate and a fine tremor may be evident. Salbutamol and **terbutaline** should be given 30 minutes before exercise as a prophylactic cover. Other bronchodilators, for example ipratropium bromide, work by blocking the vagal cholinergic receptors in the bronchioles to bring about bronchiolar dilatation and reduction of parasympathetically induced mucus secretion. These two types of drug are often given alternately to hospitalised children with good effect. It is recommended that if more than three doses per week are required, sodium cromoglycate is useful to control 60% of school children's symptoms. This drug works by inhibiting the mast cell allergic response in the linings of the bronchi. Swelling and mucus production are inhibited, as is smooth muscle irritation and spasm. Another group of drugs that produce a relaxation of smooth muscle are the xanthines, theophylline and aminophylline. Anti-inflammatory drugs are indicated in more severe conditions. Corticosteroids are potent anti-inflammatory agents.

PERSON CENTRED STUDY 2

Jamie is 5 years old. He is the youngest child in a family of four children and is younger than his nearest sibling by 6 years. He has had repeated admissions for wheezy attacks, each time recovering in 24 hours after nebulised salbutamol therapy. His mother is very protective of him and will not insist on Jamie doing anything he does not wish to do. On visiting this family at home the community nurse reports that the father's business is mink farming and the pelts are stored all over the house. The nurse has started a support programme for Jamie and his parents but considers them to be a long-term project! The care to date has been to introduce the use of a spacer for his medication and some behaviour intervention support.

1. Explain the side effects of salbutamol therapy.
2. What changes are occurring in Jamie's lungs when he has a wheezy attack?

🔑 KEY POINTS

- For oxygen to reach the cells so that oxidation can take place ventilation, diffusion and perfusion are required.
- Physiology of breathing changes with age; patients' particular parameters and disease processes should be understood when supervising medication compliance.
- Medication for respiratory conditions is often inhaled; it may affect other body systems.
- Hypoxia has effects on cardiovascular and renal functions.
- Inflammatory conditions cause much morbidity; over-the-counter medications are available, but asthma needs medically supervised treatment

- Acute infections of the respiratory tract are usually caused by bacteria or viruses.
- Tuberculosis is a chronic infection that has recently re-emerged in crowded and poor living conditions; medication includes vaccination of newborn babies and health care workers.
- Chronic airway disease must be addressed in the younger age group as 'prevention is better than cure'. Bronchitis, asthma and emphysema lead to lung damage over time.
- Oxygen therapy is part of the nurse's role in hospital and in the community; safety precautions are essential.
- Living is killing you – free radicals damage cells. Dietary changes may be the key to a healthy future.

MULTIPLE CHOICE QUESTIONS

Choose the correct answers.

1. Respiration may be affected by
   a. any change in arterial carbon dioxide levels in the cerebrospinal fluid
   b. the acidity of arterial blood
   c. metabolic alkalosis from frequent ingestion of sodium bicarbonate
   d. prolonged vomiting
   e. diuretic therapy

2. The inflammation of airways leads to
   a. emphysema
   b. thick secretions
   c. narrowed airways
   d. 'thrush'
   e. cor pulmonale

3. The antibiotics used to treat tuberculosis are
   a. amoxycillin
   b. rifampicin
   c. chloramphenicol
   d. isoniazid
   e. streptomycin

4. The side effects of salbutamol therapy are
   a. urine retention
   b. glaucoma
   c. fine tremor
   d. raised pulse rate
   e. skin flushing

5. The safety precautions for oxygen delivery include
   a. wearing of gloves
   b. avoidance of naked flames
   c. using the black-shouldered cylinder
   d. always using the low pressure gauge
   e. always administering at a flow of 20 l/min

6. Chronic bronchitis is treated with
   a. physiotherapy
   b. antibiotics
   c. oxygen therapy
   d. regular bronchoscopy
   e. vincristine

7. A cough can be alleviated with codeine linctus because
   a. it acts on the 'cough centre' in the brain
   b. it liquefies mucus
   c. it kills the bacteria in the throat
   d. it soothes the mucosal irritation
   e. it enhances phagocytic activity

8. Babies breathe through their mouths at
   a. 4 weeks
   b. 9 months
   c. 18 months
   d. 2 years

9. Old people have difficulty in gaseous exchange because
   a. they sleep propped up at night
   b. they have lost alveolar wall tissue
   c. they have lost elasticity in the chest wall tissue
   d. they breathe more shallowly
   e. they have poor neural coordination

10. Sodium cromoglycate is useful for
    a. fungal infections
    b. excess mucus production
    c. antigen–antibody reactions
    d. exercise-induced asthma
    e. croup

REFERENCES

Brody TM, Larner J, Minneman KP, Neu HC. *Human pharmacology: molecular to clinical.* St Louis: Mosby, 1994.

Carter B. *Manual of paediatric intensive care nursing.* London: Chapman and Hall, 1996.

Campbell S, Glasper E. *Children's nursing.* St. Louis: Mosby, 1995.

Coakes R, Sellors P. *An outline of ophthalmology.* London: Butterworth Heinemann, 1992.

Cooksey S. Managing chemotherapy for tuberculosis. *Nurs Times* 1995; **91(35):**32-33.

Day M. Up in the air. *Nurs Times* 1995; **91(23):**14-15.

Dodd M. Nebuliser therapy: what nurses and parents need to know. *Nurs Stand* 1996; **10:**39-42.

Downie G, Mackenzie J, Williams A. *Pharmacology and drug management for nurses.* Edinburgh: Churchill Livingstone, 1995.

Halliwell B. Free radicals and vascular disease: how much do we know? *Br Med J* 1993; **307:**885.

Henney CR, Dow RJ, MacConnachie A. *Drugs in nursing practice, 5th ed.* Edinburgh: Churchill Livingstone, 1995.

Hopkins S. *Drugs and pharmacology for nurses.* Edinburgh: Churchill Livingstone, 1992.

Hopkins S. Advances in the treatment of cystic fibrosis. *Nurs Times* 1995; **91(39):**40-41.

Gardner M. *Handbook of neonatal intensive care.* London: Mosby, 1989.

Laurence DR, Bennett PN. *Clinical pharmacology.* Edinburgh: Churchill Livingstone, 1993.

Lissauer T, Clayden G. *Illustrated textbook of paediatrics.* London: Mosby, 1997.

Marieb E. *Human anatomy and physiology, 2nd ed.* Redwood City, CA: Benjamin Cummings, 1992.

McCance KL, Huether SE: *Pathophysiology: the biologic basis for disease in adults and children, 2nd ed.* St. Louis: Mosby, 1998.

McKenry L, Salerno E. *Pharmacology in nursing.* London: Mosby, 1995.

McLeod J, Edwards C, Bouchier I. *Davidson's principles and practice of medicine, 15th ed.* Edinburgh: Churchill Livingstone, 1987.

Miller H. Respiratory syncytial virus and the use of ribavirin. *Maternal and Child Nursing* 1992; **17:**238-241.

Muzulu S. Antioxidants in diabetes and cardiovascular disease. *Pract Diabetes Int* 1996; **13:**70.

Nowak T, Handford A. *Essentials of pathophysiology.* Dubuque: WC Brown, 1994.

Page C. *Integrated Pharmacology.* London: Mosby, 1997

Parfitt VJ, Newrick PG, Bolton CH, *et al.* Effects of moderate dose (400 IU/day) oral vitamin E supplementation on plasma lipoproteins and lipid peroxidation in IDDM. *Pract Diabetes Int* 1996; **13:**72-74.

Payling K. Prevention better than cure *Nurs Times* 1997; **93(29):**80-82.

Pears JS. Educational review: antioxidants. *Proc R Coll Phys Edinburgh* 1995; **25:**544-549.

Peloquin C, Berning S. Tuberculosis and multi-drug resistant tuberculosis in children. *Pediatr Nurs* 1995; **21:**566.

Phelan P. Asthma in children: epidemiology. *Br Med J* 1994; **308:**1584-1585.

Porth CM. *Pathophysiology: concepts of altered health states.* Philadelphia: JB Lippincott, 1994.

Rang HP, Dale MM, Ritter JM. *Pharmacology, 3rd ed.* Edinburgh: Churchill Livingstone, 1995.

Rees J, Price J (1995) Asthma in children: treatment. *British Medical Journal* 310: 1522-1527.

Seeley R, Stephens T, Tate P. *Anatomy and physiology, 3rd ed.* St. Louis: Mosby, 1995.

Shaw T. Tuberculosis: the history of incidence and treatment. *Nurs Times* 1995; **91(38):**27-29.

Sittlington N, Tubman R, Halliday H. Surfactant replacement therapy for severe neonatal respiratory distress syndrome: implications for nursing care. *Midwifery* 1991; **7:**20-24.

Smith H. How bacteria cause disease. *Biol Sci Rev* 1995; **Jan:**2-6.

Soyseth V, Kongerud J, Haarr D. Relation of exposure to airway irritants in infancy to prevalence of bronchial hyper-responsiveness in school children. *Br Med J* 1995; **345:**217-220.

Spector WG. *An introduction to general pathology, 3rd ed.* Edinburgh: Churchill Livingstone, 1989.

Stern M, Alton E. Gene therapy for cystic fibrosis. *Maternal Child Health* 1996; **July/August:**170-173.

Stevens A, Lowe J. *Pathology.* London: Mosby, 1995.

Thompson J. Sign of the times. *Nurs Times* 1993; **89(35):**18-19.

Thomson A. Human recombinant DNAse in cystic fibrosis. *J R Soc Med* 1995; **88(Suppl 25):**24-29.

Walker G. *ABPI data sheet compendium.* London: Datapharm Publications, 1995.

Whatling J. Managing chronic obstructive disease. *Nurs Stand* 1995; **9:**

DRUGS AND CARDIOVASCULAR DISORDERS

INTRODUCTION

The function of the cardiovascular system is to ensure an adequate circulation of blood to the tissues of the body at all times and thus to transport substances to and from the individual cells as required. It delivers oxygen, nutrients, metabolites, hormones, neurochemicals, proteins and blood cells through the body and carries metabolic waste to the kidneys and lungs for excretion (McCance and Huether 1998). The cardiovascular system consists of the heart, blood vessels and the blood. This chapter is divided into three discrete sections, dealing with each of the above in turn.

THE HEART

The heart consists of two pumps in series: one pump propels blood through the lungs for exchange of oxygen and carbon dioxide (the pulmonary circulation) and the other pump propels blood to all other tissues of the body (the systemic circulation). The flow of blood through the heart is unidirectional, this is achieved by the appropriate arrangement of flap valves. Although the cardiac output is intermittent, continuous flow to the body tissues occurs by distension of the aorta and its branches during ventricular contraction (systole) and by elastic recoil of the walls of the large arteries with forward propulsion of the blood during ventricular relaxation (diastole).

More than 40% of patients admitted to medical wards in the United Kingdom have some form of heart disease (Souhami and Moxham, 1990). In the West approximately 50% of deaths are related to cardiovascular disease (Kumar and Clark, 1996). For the purposes of this chapter the following classification of heart disease has been used:
- Deficiency in blood supply to the myocardium.
- Disturbances in conduction and cardiac rhythm.
- Cardiac failure.
- Inflammatory diseases that may result in structural changes within the heart.
- Valvular heart disease.

DEFICIENCY IN THE BLOOD SUPPLY TO THE MYOCARDIUM

An imbalance between the supply of oxygen and essential nutrients to the myocardium and the demand for these substances results in myocardial ischaemia. Ischaemic heart disease is the most common type of cardiac disease and the leading cause of death in the western world, accounting for about 30% of all male deaths and 23% of all female deaths (Stevens and Lowe, 1995).

The main cause of ischaemic heart disease, also called coronary artery disease, is an obstruction in the coronary arteries, which results in a reduction in the blood flow to a region of the myocardium. This obstruction is most commonly caused by atheroma (**Fig. 12.1**) but may also be the result of a thrombus or embolism. A decrease in the flow of oxygenated blood to the myocardium, as in anaemia or hypotension or vasomotor spasm of the coronary vessels, may also result in myocardial ischaemia.

Atheroma is the accumulation of lipid rich materials in the intima of medium-sized arteries and is characterised by the development of atherosclerotic plaques. Such plaques consist of a necrotic core, rich in cholesterol and other lipids, surrounded by smooth muscle cells and fibrous tissue.

Because of its work requirement and consequent greater bulk the myocardium of the left ventricle has a much higher oxygen demand and is therefore more prone to ischaemia than the right ventricle (Stevens and Lowe, 1995).

Four main syndromes are the result of atherosclerosis of the coronary arteries: chronic manifestation causes stable angina; acute manifestations cause unstable angina, myocardial infarction and sudden cardiac death.

ANGINA

Stable angina is caused by a reduced blood flow in atherosclerotic coronary arteries. Angina is episodic chest pain that occurs in response to increased myocardial work, in the presence of impaired perfusion by blood. The pain usually occurs with exercise or stress and is relieved by rest.

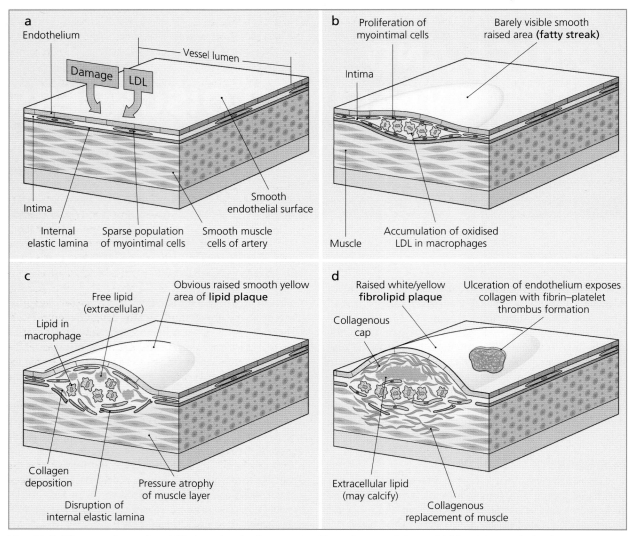

Fig. 12.1 Atheroma formation. LDL: low density lipoprotein. (From Stevens & Lowe 1995, with permission.)

Unstable angina (crescendo angina) is a progressive form of angina in which pain occurs more frequently and becomes more severe over time. The attack may appear during rest and may last longer. This condition may be the result of fissuring of atheromatous plaques, which results in a deep cleft in a lipid rich plaque that either precipitates thrombus formation in the lumen or causes bleeding into the body of the plaque (Stevens and Lowe, 1995).

Pathophysiology

When coronary blood flow is inadequate hypoxia causes an accumulation of pain-producing substances such as lactic acid, kinins and prostaglandins. These products then stimulate the cardiac sensory nerve endings, which transmit the impulses to the central nervous system and produce the typical anginal pain response (McKenry and Salerno, 1995).

Unstable angina is best managed in hospital because of the unpredictable and potentially threatening nature of this condition. Aspirin (page 196) and heparin (page 212) have been shown to reduce the mortality and morbidity of unstable angina (Theroux *et al.*, 1988; FRISC Study Group, 1996). Heparin therapy is indicated in this patient group, as one of the goals of therapy is to prevent myocardial infarction by preventing extension of the thrombus. The role of other anti-platelet agents, such as the glycoprotein IIb/IIIa receptor inhibitors, are actively being examined (Jennings, 1997).

Pharmacological management

Only aspirin and lipid-lowering therapy have been shown to reduce mortality, whereas other treatments such as the nitrates, calcium-channel blockers and beta-blockers have favourable effects on symptoms and exercise tolerance. Many patients are prescribed a combination of two agents.

This enables them to receive the benefits of both therapies but with a reduced likelihood of side effects because the dose of each agent is lower than might be required for monotherapy. Therapy will need to be tailored to individual needs to take account of coexisting conditions such as hypertension or cardiac failure (Jennings, 1997) (**Fig. 12.2**).

Hormonal status influences the development of heart disease in women. Early studies demonstrated that among groups of women of the same age, post-menopausal women were at a higher risk of heart disease than women with functioning ovaries. The use of hormone replacement therapy after the menopause appears to reduce the risk of heart disease (Stampfer and Colditz, 1991). It is unclear precisely why oestrogen may have beneficial effects but the following are thought to be important factors:
• Beneficial lipid changes.
• Direct effect on the blood vessel wall.
• Positive influence on insulin metabolism.
• Redistribution of body fat (an indicator of risk).
• Effects on clotting factors (Abernethy, 1997).

Nitrates

Nitrates are used in the acute treatment of anginal attacks and the long-term prophylactic management of angina. They reduce myocardial oxygen demand by causing peripheral dilatation. Their primary action is to relax vascular (and particularly venous) smooth muscle. The pooling of blood in the veins decreases the amount of blood returning to the heart (preload) and the result is a reduction in cardiac work. Nitrates, therefore, reduce the demand for myocardial oxygen by decreasing left ventricular volume.

Arterial dilatation lowers the blood pressure and also results in a more efficient distribution of blood in the myocardium (McKenry and Salerno, 1995). Dilatation occurs only in normal vessels but this will cause a redistribution of coronary blood flow and increase collateral flow, particularly to ischaemic regions.

Nitrates are metabolised in vascular smooth muscle (Jennings, 1997); they are converted to the nitrate ion, which generates nitric oxide. The latter is thought to be the 'endogenous nitrate', endothelial-derived relaxant factor, which plays an important part in mediating vasodilatation.

Glyceryl trinitrate is used to reduce the pain of angina. For acute attacks a sublingual tablet, 500–600 μg is placed under the tongue and sucked vigorously; alternatively, one metered dose, 400 μg, is sprayed into the mouth. Sublingual glyceryl trinitrate is rapidly absorbed and gives almost instantaneous high serum drug concentrations. Glyceryl trinitrate undergoes extensive first pass metabolism and therefore has very little activity when taken orally.

For prophylaxis of angina glyceryl trinitrate may be taken in the following ways:
• As a nitrolingual spray, 400 μg per metered dose.
• Sublingually, one tablet (300–600 μg) held under the tongue immediately before exercise.
• Buccal route, one tablet of 1, 2, 3 or 5 mg stuck to the gum (**Fig. 12.3**).
• Topical route, one dose of ointment 2%, measured on a special ruler or one skin patch, 5 mg or 10 mg applied to the skin.

The duration of action depends on the nitrate used and the mode of delivery. Nitrates delivered via the buccal and sublingual routes are effective within 1–2 minutes, making them useful in the acute situation. Furthermore, if side effects occur they can be rapidly and easily terminated by removing the tablet, which is not the case with glyceryl trinitrate spray. However, the glyceryl trinitrate spray formulations have advantages in that they are stable for up to 2 years and have a rapid onset of action.

Glyceryl trinitrate has only a short-acting effect of approximately 20–30 minutes. However, the use of skin patches provides 24-hour therapeutic concentrations. Nitroglycerine transdermal patches are pockets of medication containing nitroglycerine, glycerine, water, polyvinyl alcohol and several other ingredients surrounded by a bandage.

The side effects of glyceryl trinitrate are flushing, pounding or pulsating headache, syncope and hypotension, which are all caused by the vasodilator effects of the drug. Patients between the ages of 18 and 59 years are more likely to complain of flushing than older patients. This may be the result of a more sensitive autonomic nervous system (Kuhn, 1994).

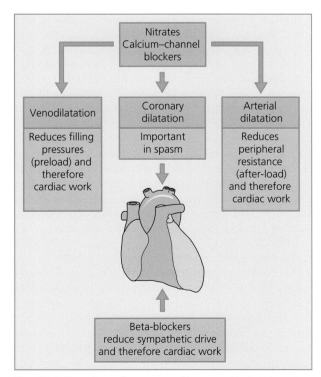

Fig. 12.2 Overview of common drugs used in treatment of angina pectoris

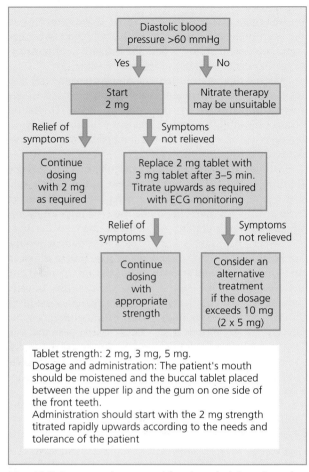

Fig. 12.3 An example protocol for the administration of buccal GTN to patients with unstable angina.

These effects may diminish with continued use of the drug. If they occur while sublingual tablets are sucked during an acute attack the patient should be instructed to terminate the action of the drug by spitting out or swallowing the tablet once the angina is relieved. A patient should be informed that if the angina pain persists after one or two doses of glyceryl trinitrate they must seek medical advice.

Patients must be made aware that glyceryl trinitrate tablets deteriorate with age and may become ineffective. A loss of the bitter taste in the mouth may be an indication of this. The expiry date on the packaging should be noted (Henney *et al.*, 1995).

Isosorbide dinitrate reduces heart work in a similar manner to glyceryl trinitrate. It is sprayed into the mouth, chewed or allowed to dissolve under the tongue in the treatment of angina pectoris or it is taken orally as prophylaxis. Isosorbide dinitrate has a long duration of action, which may be up to 12 hours with slow-release preparations. A disadvantage of this drug is that it is partially metabolised in the liver after absorption thus reducing the amount of systemically available drug. Doses therefore need to be sufficiently large to offset the first pass metabolism.

The usual oral adult dose prescribed for the prevention of angina is 10 mg three or four times a day or 20 mg twice a day of the sustained-release preparation. In an acute attack one to three metered doses of 1.25 mg may be sprayed into the mouth or 5 mg taken sublingually or chewed. Isosorbide may be administered by continuous intravenous infusion to patients suffering from acute unstable angina to reduce the possibility of cardiac failure but the dose must be carefully titrated against the cardiac output of the individual (Henney *et al.*, 1995).

Isosorbide mononitrate is one of the active metabolites of isosorbide dinitrate; it passes through the liver after absorption without being substantially metabolised. It is therefore often preferred to isosorbide dinitrate for oral use, primarily for the prophylaxis of angina pectoris, because its effects are more predictable. It is rapidly absorbed and excreted by the kidneys.

The isosorbide mononitrate dose usually prescribed is 20–40 mg three times daily. However, a single daily dose of from 25 mg up to 60 mg, carefully titrated against individual needs, may be taken using sustained-release preparations, which are available in both tablet (40 mg or 60 mg) and capsule (25 mg or 60 mg) form (Henney *et al.*, 1995). The duration of a 20 mg dose is about 8 hours.

The side effects of isosorbide are the same as those of glyceryl trinitrate. Administration of nitrates with alcohol, antihypertensive agents or other vasodilators may result in enhanced hypotensive effects. Caution should also be exercised in giving high doses of nitrates to the elderly or patients with pronounced renal or hepatic impairment.

When increased dosage is necessary to obtain an effect previously obtained by a smaller dosage, tolerance is said to have developed. Nitrate tolerance refers to the loss of anti-anginal efficacy despite constant plasma levels of nitrate (Downie *et al.*, 1995). Tolerance to nitrates is more pronounced in arteries than veins, which may explain why hypotension after taking nitrates is uncommon. Tolerance is particularly associated with continuous exposure to high circulating concentrations of nitrates. When concentrations are allowed to fall for part of the day tolerance is much less likely. Thus tolerance may be a greater problem with patches providing 24-hour therapeutic concentrations.

Calcium-channel blocking agents or agonists

These constitute an important class of drug that reduces myocardial work directly and in many cases also indirectly by causing vasodilatation. All calcium-channel blockers have different pharmacological effects while sharing the ability to block competitively the slow channel influx of calcium into active cells. The effects of calcium-channel blockers are greatest in cells that depend on intracellular influx of calcium ions for activation (Kuhn, 1994).

In the myocardium of the heart and vascular smooth muscle an essential step in the process of contraction is the entry of calcium ions into cells. In the myocardium the calcium ions cause the contractile muscle proteins, actin and myosin, to interact, thus leading to a shortening of the fibres and an increase in myocardial wall tension. The degree of this contractility (or positive inotropic state) is regulated by the amount of calcium ions that reach the contractile proteins, not only from outside the cells but also from 'activator' calcium ions released from an intracellular calcium pool in the sarcoplasmic reticulum. The calcium-channel blockers decrease the force of myocardial contraction by blocking or diminishing the flow of calcium ions through the slow channels of the cell membrane; in turn the diminished flow fails to trigger the release of large amounts of calcium from the sarcoplasmic reticulum within the cell required for contraction (**Fig. 12.4**).

In vascular smooth muscle the calcium-channel blockers also result in a depressed interaction between actin and myosin, producing a decreased force of smooth muscle contraction. As a consequence, coronary artery dilatation occurs, which lowers coronary resistance and improves blood flow through collateral vessels and oxygen delivery to ischaemic areas of the heart.

In the cardiac conduction system (sinoatrial and atrioventricular nodes) calcium-channel blockers decrease the spontaneous depolarisation of the sino-atrial node and decreases conduction in the atrioventricular node. The result is a decrease in heart rate, that is, a negative inotropic effect.

Calcium-channel blockers also inhibit the contraction of the smooth muscle of peripheral arterioles. This results in widespread reduction in peripheral vascular resistance

and therefore blood pressure (blood pressure = cardiac output × peripheral resistance). This haemodynamic change reduces afterload, which also decreases oxygen demands of the heart. This indirectly provides a beneficial effect in the management of angina. To date numerous calcium antagonists have been developed and many are available in the United Kingdom.

Verapamil has the most pronounced effect upon the atrioventricular node conduction and is the drug of choice for patients with supraventricular tachycardia with or without anginal symptoms. It decreases the oxygen requirement of the myocardium and reduces peripheral resistance, and is therefore useful in the treatment of angina. The oral dose for the prophylaxis of angina is 40–120 mg three times a day.

Verapamil should not be administered to patients who are receiving, or who have in the immediate past received, beta-blocking drugs as the combination of the two can lead to a complete cessation of heart function. As verapamil can produce hypotension, the patient should be supine if the drug is administered intravenously. The main side effects of oral therapy are nausea and vomiting and constipation. However, the elderly are more susceptible to these drugs and may demonstrate side effects such as increased weakness, dizziness, fainting episodes and falls.

Dihydropyridines – nifedipine, nicardipine and amlodipine

These act as potent peripheral vasodilators but have little effect on the sino-atrial or atrioventricular nodes. They decrease the work done by the heart by decreasing its activity and reducing the pressure against which it has to work by peripheral vasodilatation. These properties make them useful in the treatment of angina pectoris. They are useful as adjuncts to beta-blockers for patients with severe symptoms and as an alternative treatment for those who are intolerant of beta-blockers.

Nifedipine relaxes vascular smooth muscle and dilates coronary and peripheral arteries. It has more influence on vessels and less on the myocardium than does verapamil. It may be used prophylactically by administering 10 mg three times a day, which may be increased to 20 mg three times a day if necessary. A capsule may be bitten and placed under the tongue to produce a more rapid onset of effect in the treatment of an acute attack (Henney *et al.*, 1995). Headaches and flushing may be expected in patients on this drug. Lethargy and tiredness may also occur. Occasionally angina may be paradoxically exacerbated in which case the use of the drug should be stopped immediately.

Nicardipine has similar effects to those of nifedipine and may produce less reduction of myocardial contractility. The dose is 20–40 mg three times daily or 30–60 mg sustained-release capsules twice daily.

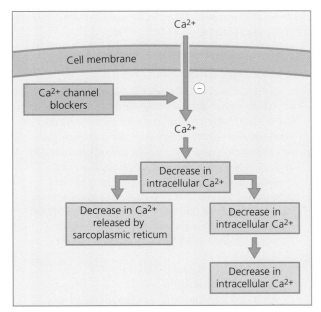

Fig. 12.4 Action of calcium-channel blockers.

Amlodipine also resembles nifedipine and nicardipine in its effects and does not reduce myocardial contractility. It has a longer duration of action and can be given as a single daily dose of 5–10 mg. The side effects are headache, flushing, dizziness and oedema.

β-adrenoceptor blocking drugs

Adrenaline and noradrenaline (catecholamines), which are produced by the adrenal glands and at sympathetic nerve endings, exert their physiological effects via α- and β-adreno-ceptors. These β-adrenoceptors are widely distributed throughout the body and can be divided into two groups:
- β_1 receptors, which predominate in the heart.
- β_2 receptors, which are found mainly in the bronchi and the blood vessels.

Beta-adrenergic blocking agents compete with the catecholamines for available β receptor sites. Several beta-blocking agents, namely atenolol, acebutolol, esmolol, betaxolol, bisoprolol and metoprolol, are said to be cardioselective. This means that they have the ability to antagonise the actions of the catecholamines at β_1 receptors at smaller doses than that at which they block β_2 receptors. However, they are not cardiospecific in that they do have a small effect on airway resistance and are therefore not free of side effects. Pharmacologically, the β_1-adrenergic blocking action in the heart decreases heart rate, conduction velocity, myocardial contractility and cardiac output.

The anti-anginal effects produced by the beta-blockers are primarily caused by their ability to lower the myocardial oxygen requirements, particularly during stress or physical exertion. They reduce the cardiac output and limit the work of the heart during exercise. In the treatment of angina continuous 24-hour beta-blockade is desirable and may readily be achieved by frequent low doses of conventional tablets or a slow-release tablet once daily. There are numerous beta-blocking drugs available with different proportions of β_1 to β_2 antagonist activity. Two beta-blocking drugs that are in common use are atenolol and bisoprodol.

Atenolol is a cardioselective beta-blocker. It is particularly long acting and single daily doses of 100–200 mg in adults are usually adequate. Atenolol is a useful drug in patients who have experienced central nervous system side effects from other beta-blockers, for example nightmares and hallucinations.

Bisoprodol is a beta-blocking drug that is reported to have a degree of cardioselectivity far in excess of other drugs in this category. It has a long duration of action and is required to be taken once daily only. The usual dose lies in the range 5–20 mg for treatment of angina pectoris. Despite its high degree of cardioselectivity it should nonetheless be used with caution in patients with asthma and chronic severe obstructive airways disease.

Potassium-channel activators

Nicorandil is a new anti-anginal agent; it is a potassium-channel promoter with nitrate properties. It reduces pre-load and afterload without affecting conduction or contractility. It is indicated for the prevention and long-term treatment of angina pectoris. Although tolerance is less likely to develop than with conventional nitrates, nico-randil, because of its nitrate effects, cannot be substituted for nitrates in patients intolerant of nitrates. Consequently its place in therapy is currently uncertain (Jennings,1997). The initial dose is 5–10 mg daily, rising to a maximum of 60 mg daily. The side effects are headache, palpitations and dizziness.

MYOCARDIAL INFARCTION

A myocardial infarct is an area of necrosis of heart muscle resulting from a sudden, absolute or relative reduction in the coronary blood supply (Underwood, 1996). The most frequent symptom of acute myocardial infarction is severe chest pain. This often develops suddenly but may build up gradually and last for several hours. Pain is usually accompanied by profuse sweating, nausea and vomiting. The location and size of the infarct depends on the site of the coronary artery occlusion and the anatomical pattern of the blood supply.

Pathophysiology

Myocardial infarction almost always occurs in patients with coronary atheroma and is caused by sudden coronary thrombosis. This usually develops at the site of a fissure or rupture of the intimal surface of an atheromatous plaque. Haemorrhage may occur into a plaque and local coronary spasm may occur. Sometimes thrombosis results from stasis at a critical stenosis or in association with coronary artery spasm (Kumar and Clark, 1996).

PERSON CENTRED STUDY 1

Mr George Thomas, a 45-year-old Systems Analyst, has been admitted to the Accident and Emergency department of a large city hospital complaining of severe central chest pain. An ECG confirms a diagnosis of myocardial infarction. In the brief medical history obtained from Mr Thomas it was determined that he was also suffering from a peptic ulcer for which he had been prescribed cimetidine and an antacid. The doctor who examined Mr Thomas decided to administer streptokinase IV.

1. What will be a major concern for Mr Thomas's safety?
2. What assessments will Mr Thomas require to monitor his condition?

The interruption of the blood supply to the myocardium results in prolonged ischaemia, which causes infarction and leads to irreversible hypoxia and cellular death. Cardiac cells can withstand ischaemic conditions for about 20 minutes before cellular death takes place but electrocardiographic (ECG) changes can be seen after 30–60 seconds (Huether and McCance, 1998). Myocardial oxygen reserves are used up very quickly after complete cessation of blood flow and the affected myocardium becomes cyanotic and cooler. Myocardial cells deprived of the necessary oxygen and nutrients lose contractility thereby reducing the pumping ability of the heart. Oxygen deprivation is also accompanied by electrolyte disturbances, specifically the loss of potassium, calcium and magnesium from cells. Significant arterial occlusion causes the myocardial cells to release adrenalin and noradrenalin, predisposing the individual to serious imbalances of sympathetic and parasympathetic function, irregular heart beats and heart failure.

Pharmacological management (symptom relief and management of a life-threatening event)
Fibrinolytic agents

Arterial thrombosis, such as may occur in the coronary arteries, is partly caused by an aggregation of platelets, which ultimately forms a plug in the blood vessel. Fibrin is laid down to reinforce the platelets and to form a thrombus. Thrombolytic enzymes dissolve clots through activation of the endogenous fibrinolytic system. Fibrinolytic drugs assist the conversion of plasma proteins and tissue plasminogen to plasmin, which degrades fibrin and breaks up the thrombus.

Thrombolytic therapy is the only available treatment that directly influences the outcome of myocardial infarction by reducing the size of the infarct. There are three thrombolytic drugs that are indicated for the acute treatment of myocardial infarction: streptokinase, alteplase and anistreplase. They act by dissolving clots in the coronary arteries thus allowing reperfusion of cardiac muscle, reduction in infarct size and a reduction in mortality (Henney et al.,1995). The contraindications to fibrinolytic therapy are as follows:

• History of cerebrovascular disease.
• Uncontrolled hypertension.
• Known bleeding diathesis.
• Recent major surgery or trauma.
• Active peptic ulceration.
• Acute pancreatitis or bacterial endocarditis.
• Severe liver disease.
• During menstruation.

The sooner fibrinolytic therapy is used from the onset of chest pain (0–6 hours) the better the results, although some benefit is obtained up to 24 hours later. If given within 60 minutes of infarction myocardial salvage is possible; later administration results in improved infarct healing and reduction of infarct extension. The therapy is still more effective when used in combination with aspirin 150 mg daily (particularly streptokinase).

Streptokinase is an enzyme that stimulates the action of the fibrinolytic system. It is not fibrin selective and therefore creates a systemic lytic state. It is administered intravenously in 50–200 ml saline, 5% glucose or haemaccel. Adults who have suffered an acute myocardial infarction may receive a single dose of 1.5 million international units (i.u.) given over 1 hour.

Early reactions to the drug include headache, back pain and allergic anaphylactic reactions with flushing and dyspnoea. Streptokinase is allergenic because it is a metabolic product of β-haemolytic streptococci and therefore antigenic. As a foreign protein, streptokinase has the ability to cause resistance through the development of antibodies. The incidence of allergic reaction can be reduced by administering the drug slowly and giving corticosteroids prophylactically. Therapy can be administered again if needed within 24 hours. After the second dose within the first 24 hours, streptokinase cannot be repeated for 6–12 months, depending upon the preparation used, by which time the antibodies are gone. Also, if a patient has suffered a recent streptococcal infection that has produced high anti-streptokinase titres (e.g. rheumatic fever, acute glomerulonephritis), this may be considered a contraindication to treatment with streptokinase.

Alteplase is a naturally occurring substance: it is a form of human plasminogen activator with a selective fibrinolytic action on blood-clot bound plasminogen. This drug is non-allergenic because it is manufactured using recombinant DNA technology from human tissue cultures. After an acute myocardial infarction adults should receive a total dose of 100 mg, equivalent to 58 million i.u. intravenously over a 3-hour period. Patients weighing less than 67 kg should receive a dose of 1.5 mg/kg. Treatment should be initiated within 6 hours of the infarction.

Systemic side effects that may occur as a result of therapy are gastrointestinal or genitourinary bleeding, intracerebral haemorrhage, retroperitoneal bleeding, surface bleeding and nausea and vomiting. There may also be an accelerated idioventricular rhythm associated with the reperfusion of the coronary artery.

Anistreplase (anisoylated plasminogen-streptokinase activator complex; APSAC) is a derivative and modified version of streptokinase that produces thrombolysis at the site of the clot but remains inactive in the systemic circulation. It is therefore more clot specific than streptokinase. In addition, anistreplase has a longer duration of action than streptokinase, producing more lasting thrombus dissolution. However, it also predisposes the patient to more bleeding complications without overcoming the allergic reactions associated with streptokinase (Albarran and Kapeluch, 1994). It is given as a single dose of 30 units within 6 hours of infarction. As the most common and serious complication after administration of these drugs is bleeding, careful control of any bleeding by pressure at the administration site is essential.

Aspirin

Oral aspirin therapy, 75–300 mg daily, should accompany the fibrinolytic therapy and be continued for a minimum of 4 weeks after infarction, as shown by the International Study of Infarct Survival (ISIS) trial (1992), as it adds considerably to the effectiveness of thrombolytic therapy in increasing survival. Aspirin has an anti-platelet action. It irreversibly blocks the synthesis of a prostaglandin, thromboxane A2, by the platelet in response to injury to the vascular epithelium. In the presence of thromboxane, platelets adhere to form a platelet plug, which under normal circumstances reduces bleeding and promotes blood clotting. Aspirin is so potent that it can inhibit platelet aggregation and prevent clotting at low concentrations. Aspirin can also be used in the primary prevention of myocardial infarction in patients with symptoms of ischaemic heart disease and secondary prevention of re-infarction and sudden death in the period after a myocardial infarction (Henney *et al.*, 1995).

Some patients with peptic ulceration or bleeding tendencies will not be candidates for aspirin therapy, but many with 'indigestion' will tolerate treatment while also taking an H_2 blocker, a compromise in which there is likely to be significant benefit from aspirin treatment (Jennings, 1997).

Analgesia

The most frequent symptom of acute myocardial infarction is severe chest pain. This often develops suddenly but may build up gradually, and generally lasts for several hours. It may be described as heavy or crushing. Radiation to the neck, jaw, back, shoulder or left arm is common. Prompt and effective pain management is vital, not just for the patient's comfort but because the emotional stress caused by the pain may extend the original infarct by increasing myocardial oxygen demand (Cornock, 1996). Pain should therefore be treated promptly with opiates such as **morphine** (10–20 mg intravenously) or **diamorphine** (5–10 mg intravenously) combined with an antiemetic. These drugs combine sedation with an advantageous vasodilatory action that improves haemodynamics. They reduce ventricular preload by increasing venous capacitance and ventricular afterload by mild arterial vasodilatation, hence reducing myocardial oxygen demands. The side effect of respiratory depression is rare with acute myocardial infarction. Opioid induced nausea and vomiting is treated using cyclizine (50 mg intravenously) or metoclopramide (10 mg intravenously).

Persistent pain can be treated with nitrates. If there is no hypotension, sublingual glyceryl trinitrate can be administered (page 191). Alternatively, if the haemodynamic situation is unstable, a continuous infusion of either isosorbide dinitrate (page 192) or glyceryl trinitrate can be considered. Intravenous nitroglycerine may alleviate symptoms of refractory angina (angina that does not respond to normal therapy) and improve blood flow to ischaemic tissue early in a myocardial infarction. Nitrates also have the advantage of causing a reduction in preload and afterload. Calcium antagonist drugs are effective in improving cardiac pain but their use has not been associated with any improvement in infarction mortality.

Oxygen is usually given routinely because during an acute myocardial infarction the arterial partial pressure of oxygen is reduced. Supplemental oxygen will increase arterial oxygen content and deliver more oxygen to the ischaemic myocardium. Oxygen may be given to patients with acute infarction to counteract the hypoxaemic effects of pulmonary oedema. However, many patients are not hypoxaemic and in these patients oxygen delivery to the tissues will not be improved by this treatment.

Anticoagulant therapy

Heparin (page 212) is regularly prescribed for the prevention of thromboembolic complications that result from a myocardial infarction. It is administered subcutaneously in a dose of 5000 units every 8–12 hours. Clotting times are not usually estimated when heparin is given by this route as it does not achieve a full anticoagulant effect but still proves useful in the prevention of thromboembolism.

Pharmacological management (limiting change by increasing circulation to heart and decreasing workload)

Nitrates and **calcium antagonists** may be prescribed for the long-term prophylactic management of angina pectoris. Calcium-channel blockers may reduce cardiac events after a myocardial infarction. However, they are not suitable for patients demonstrating symptoms of cardiac failure. For the action of these drugs refer to the section on angina.

Angiotensin-converting enzyme inhibitors can be used to prevent left ventricular dysfunction after a myocardial infarction. For the action of these drugs refer to pages 215 and 216.

Anti-lipid agents

High serum cholesterol is a known risk factor for the development of cardiovascular diseases such as angina, acute myocardial infarction and hypertension. Therefore, reducing an elevated serum cholesterol level with either diet or drug therapy reduces the risk of death from cardiovascular disease. There is increasingly convincing evidence that raised triglyceride levels are themselves a major causative factor in coronary heart disease and are particularly important in the development of this disease in men under 60 years of age (Assmann *et al.*, 1996). Other evidence suggests that reducing the level of low density lipoproteins (LDL) lowers the risk of coronary heart disease (Joliffe, 1997), whereas a low level of high density lipoproteins (HDLs) increases the risk (Assmann *et al.*, 1996). McCarthy (1997) suggests that myocardial ischaemia might be reduced in 4–6 months by lipid lowering drugs. Many of the medications available interfere with the normal metabolism of cholesterol, lipoproteins or triglycerides and this interference ultimately reduces blood lipids.

Cholesterol-lowering drugs

Bile acid sequestrants such as cholestyramine, colestipol and probucol inhibit the reabsorption of bile acids in the intestine thus causing an increase in the faecal excretion of these acids. By increasing the excretion of bile acids, these compounds increase the hepatic conversion of cholesterol to bile acids, which leads to lowered serum cholesterol levels. A fall in LDL is apparent in 4–7 days and a 15–20% or more decline in cholesterol levels is evident in approximately 1 month (Kuhn, 1994).

Cholestyramine is an anionic ion exchange resin that absorbs and combines with bile salts in exchange for chloride, forming an insoluble, non absorbable complex that is excreted in faeces. It is available in powder form and is a particularly unpleasant preparation for patients to consume. It should be mixed with any liquid or high moisture content food to disguise the taste. For the treatment of hyperlipidaemia the usual dose is of the order 3–6 sachets (12–24 g) daily, taken as a single dose or in up to four divided doses.

Cholestyramine should not be given concurrently with other drugs, particularly acidic drugs, because of its ability to bind with them. Specifically, cholestyramine may interfere with the absorption of oral anticoagulants, digitalis, iron preparations, thyroid products, thiazide diuretics and phenylbutazone. As the drug interferes with fat absorption, it may reduce the absorption of the fat soluble vitamins A, D, E and K. This may result in a vitamin deficiency and parenteral vitamin supplementation may be required. The most frequent side effects are gastrointestinal upsets and constipation. Therefore, the addition of fibre to the diet is recommended. As the drug is not absorbed, systemic toxicity does not occur.

Colestipol is very similar to cholestyramine. It is administered in 15–30 g dosages, divided into two to four equal portions.

Probucol is indicated as an adjunctive therapy to reduce serum cholesterol. The plasma levels of LDL are lowered by 10–15% when accompanied by an appropriate diet. Probucol may also lower the level of circulating HDLs. Probucol also has an antioxidant effect, which may prove to be its main mechanism in preventing atheroma formation.

Unoxidised LDL is prevented from binding with the macrophages of the endothelium and thus atheroma formation does not occur.

The adult dose is 500 mg twice daily. Probucol should be taken with food, when maximum absorption occurs. Some recipients may develop hypersensitivity reactions, including dizziness, palpitations and syncope. Gastrointestinal upsets are the most common side effects of this drug and may include diarrhoea, flatulence, abdominal pain and nausea.

HMG-CoA reductase inhibitors: pravastatin and simvastatin

The 3-hydroxy-3-methylglutaryl coenzyme A (HMG-CoA) reductase inhibitors prevent the synthesis of cholesterol. They decrease the levels of plasma cholesterol and LDLs by 20–40%. The reduction in levels of lipoproteins occurs as a result of decreased synthesis and enhanced removal of LDL by the LDL receptor pathway in the liver. The levels of HDLs also increase during therapy.

Pravastatin is administered in an active form and is generally prescribed for patients with a blood cholesterol in excess of 7–8 mmol/l or triglyceride levels above 3 mmol/l. For adults a single evening dose of 10–40 mg is given, which is effective within 2–4 weeks of commencing therapy. Patients receiving warfarin should have their anticoagulant status checked after starting pravastatin therapy as lipid lowering drugs can increase the risk of bleeding. Mild side effects that may occur are listed below.

Simvastatin is activated by extensive first-pass metabolism in the liver to form active metabolites. The initial adult dose of 10 mg is administered at night, adjusted at intervals of not less than 4 weeks. The range of dosage is 10–40 mg. Side effects that may occur are headache, fatigue and mild gastrointestinal symptoms such as constipation, flatulence, nausea, dyspepsia and abdominal cramps. Liver enzyme levels are increased in 2–3% of patients. Liver transaminase levels should be monitored for elevation for at least the first 15 months of therapy. No evidence of liver dysfunction has been observed and liver function returns to normal after discontinuation of the drug (Kuhn, 1994). When these drugs are discontinued the serum cholesterol levels return to pretreatment levels.

Triglyceride-lowering agents

These include fibric acid drugs – clofibrate, gemfibrozil and nicotinic acid.

Clofibrate has a number of complex and as yet not clearly defined actions on body metabolism. Its overall effect is to reduce blood cholesterol. It inhibits the hepatic synthesis of cholesterol and appears to enhance the intravascular conversion of very low density lipoproteins (VLDL) to LDL. It also increases the biliary secretion of cholesterol, and the presence of gall stones is therefore a contraindication. The prescribed dose is 2 g daily with regular checks on the plasma lipid levels. The side effects are transient nausea and abdominal discomfort.

Gemfibrozil is a derivative of isobutyric acid and it appears to act by inhibiting VLDL synthesis. It decreases serum triglycerides by 40–55% and VLDL by 40%, with a variable reduction in total cholesterol levels. Gemfibrozil may increase HDL by 17–25% with the possible benefit of inhibiting the atherosclerotic process. It is used in the management of familial hyperlipidaemias of types IIa, IIb, III, IV and V in patients in whom dietary measures alone are inadequate. The dosage for adults is 1200–1500 mg daily in two or three divided doses. The drug should be taken with meals if gastrointestinal symptoms occur. Gemfibrozil is generally well tolerated; the most common side effects include disturbance of the gastrointestinal tract followed by fatigue, eczema, rash, vertigo and headache. It may produce sexual impotence in men and should be avoided in patients with liver disease (including alcoholism), gall stones or severe renal disease.

Nicotinic acid inhibits lipolysis in adipose tissue, increases hepatic de-esterification of triglycerides and increases the activity of lipoprotein lipase. It also decreases the hepatic synthesis of LDL and consistently increases the level of HDL. Nicotinic acid is used as adjunctive therapy in the treatment of hypertriglyceridaemia and hypercholesterolaemia. The adult dosage is 300–600 mg daily in three divided doses after meals to avoid gastrointestinal irritation. This may be increased to 6 g daily over 2–4 weeks. The side effects include flushing and dizziness, faintness and pruritis. The side effects may sometimes be reduced by taking aspirin 75 mg half an hour before a dose.

DISTURBANCES IN CARDIAC RHYTHM AND CONDUCTION

A **cardiac arrhythmia** may be defined as any deviation from the normal rhythm of the heartbeat and is caused by a disorder that modifies the electrophysiological properties of the cells of the conduction system or of cardiac muscle cells. Disorders of cardiac rhythm arise as a result of **automaticity** (an abnormal spontaneous initiation of an impulse) or **conductivity** (an abnormality in the conduction of an impulse). In some conditions a combination of both processes may occur (McKenry and Salerno, 1995).

There are two main types of arrhythmia:
- Bradycardia, when the heart rate is slow, less than 60 beats per minute (bpm). The slower the heart rate the more likely the arrhythmia will be symptomatic.
- Tachycardia, when the heart rate is fast, more than 100 bpm. Tachycardias are more symptomatic when the arrhythmia is fast and sustained. Tachycardias are subdivided into supraventricular tachycardias, which

arise from the atrium or atrioventricular junction, and ventricular tachycardias, which arise from the ventricles.

SINUS BRADYCARDIA

This is defined as a sinus rate of less than 60 bpm during the day or less than 50 bpm at night. It is usually asymptomatic unless the rate is very low. It is normal in athletes and in the elderly. The causes may include:
- Hypothermia, hypothyroidism, cholestatic jaundice and raised intracranial pressure.
- Drug therapy with beta-blockers, digitalis and other antiarrhythmic drugs.
- Acute ischaemia and infarction of the sinus node.
- Chronic degenerative changes such as fibrosis of the atrium and sinus node.

Pathophysiology

Bradycardias lower cardiac output by reducing the frequency of ventricular ejection. As cardiac output falls, arterial pressure and peripheral perfusion decrease. This results in faintness, dizziness, chest pain and, eventually, lapses in consciousness and collapse.

Pharmacological management

The treatment of acute symptomatic sinus bradycardia is by the administration of atropine; if the arrhythmia persists a cardiac pacemaker is required.

Atropine sulphate competes for acetylcholine receptors at parasympathetic neuroeffector sites and therefore increases heart rate by blocking vagal stimulation in the heart. The recommended dosage is usually 600 µg administered intravenously.

SINUS TACHYCARDIA

Sinus tachycardia is defined as a sinus rate acceleration to more than 100 bpm. The causes may include fever, exercise, emotion, pregnancy, anaemia, thyrotoxicosis, catecholamine excess and cardiac failure with compensatory sinus tachycardia.

Pathophysiology

Tachycardias lower cardiac output by reducing ventricular filling time and stroke volume thereby resulting in similar signs and symptoms as with bradycardias (see above).

Pharmacological management

The mainstay of treatment involves correction of the condition causing the tachycardia. If necessary beta-blockers may be used to slow the sinus rate. An account of the action of β-adrenoceptor blocking compounds is detailed on page 194.

Antiarrhythmic agents

Antiarrhythmic drugs restrict cardiac electrical activity to normal conduction pathways and decrease abnormally fast heart rates. They may therefore be prescribed for conditions in which there is a pathological tachycardia.

Antiarrhythmic drugs may be classified in a number of ways:
• Their anatomical site of action, for example those that act on supraventricular arrhythmias.
• Their clinical range of activity.
• The Vaughan–Williams classification (**Table 12.1**), which classifies drugs into four distinct classes according to their effects on the electrical behaviour of myocardial cells during activity, namely, the action potential (**Fig. 12.5**).

SUPRAVENTRICULAR ARRHYTHMIAS

These conditions arise in the atria or atrioventricular node and include the following disorders:
• **Supraventricular tachycardias.**
• **Atrial fibrillation.**
• **Atrial flutter.**

Pathophysiology

Supraventricular tachycardias are usually caused by a rapid circular movement within the atrioventricular node, which fires off ventricular contractions via the bundle of His at about 160 bpm. This is known as the re-entrant phenomenon. The symptoms are commonly those of an unpleasant awareness of rapid heart beats or palpitations in the chest. The treatment of this condition involves the use of drugs that slow conduction in the atrioventricular node or bundle of His (see Pharmacological Management section below).

Atrial fibrillation is a condition in which each individual bundle of muscle fibres in the atria contracts individually at a rate of about 450 contractions per minute.

Vaughan–Williams classification	
Class 1	Drugs which contain agents that interfere with the rapid sodium current, with the slowing of conduction or an increase in the refractory period, or both. These agents usually have anaesthetic properties and membrane stabilising activity. They are subdivided according to their influence on duration of the action potential, which may lengthen, (group 1A) or shorten (group 1B), or be unaffected (group 1C).
Class 2	Drugs with anti-sympathetic activity and reduce the potential for arrhythmias to develop in response to the catecholamines.
Class 3	Agents which prolong the duration of the action potential and the effective refractory period in both atrial and ventricular tissue
Class 4	Calcium antagonists such as verapamil inhibit the trans membrane flow of calcium ions. Calcium ions play an essential part in the process of contraction of vascular and myocardial smooth muscle. In the heart this occurs during phase 2 (plateau) of the action potential. The entry of calcium ions into the cells causes fibre shortening and an increase in myocardial wall tension. The degree of this contraction, or positive inotropic state, is regulated by the amount of calcium ions that reach the contractile proteins. Calcium antagonists block the entry of calcium ions through the slow calcium channels and as a result increase the effective refractory period of the AV node and slow the conduction rate between the atria and the ventricles.

Table 12.1 Vaughan–Williams classification

Fig. 12.5 Phases of an action potential and the ion exchanges that take place

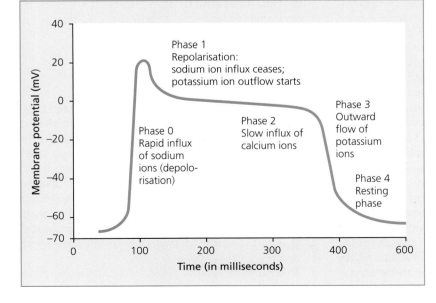

This results in complete disorganisation of atrial contraction and bombardment of the ventricles, via the bundle of His, with rapid irregular stimuli. Consequently the ventricles are unable either to fill properly with blood or to contract satisfactorily. The loss of efficient atrial contraction predisposes to stasis of blood in the atria; this encourages the formation of thrombi, which pose the threat of systemic embolisation. Atrial fibrillation is probably the commonest of the arrhythmias and one that may be paroxysmal or permanent. There are many causes of atrial fibrillation but the most common underlying condition is probably hypertension.

Atrial flutter is closely allied to atrial fibrillation but is much less common. This a rhythm disturbance almost always associated with organic heart disease. The atrial rate varies between 280 and 350 bpm. Under theses circumstances the ventricles are unable to keep up with the atria and only respond to every other or every third atrial contraction. This is known as 2:1 or 3:1 heart block.

Pharmacological management

Cardiac glycosides are often the treatment of choice in slowing ventricular response in atrial flutter or atrial fibrillation. Digitalis acts by means of vagal stimulation on the atrioventricular node to slow conduction, therefore fewer impulses get through to the ventricles. For the detailed action of these drugs please refer to the section on cardiac failure, page 204.

Verapamil – Class 4 antiarrhythmic agent – is a drug usually effective for supraventricular tachycardias. Calcium plays a major role in the mechanical and electrical capabilities of the heart. Electrically, calcium is needed for conduction through the sino-atrial and atrioventricular nodes. The calcium antagonist exerts its major antiarrhythmic effect by slowing conduction and increasing the effective refractory period. Verapamil also interferes with the re-entry of impulses at the atrioventricular node, which is helpful in restoring sinus rhythm in patients with paroxysmal supraventricular tachycardia and Wolff–Parkinson–White syndrome (see below). Verapamil is not effective in the treatment of ventricular arrhythmias. An initial intravenous dose of 5 mg is administered. This may be repeated after intervals of 5–10 minutes until the dysrhythmia is controlled, and may be followed by oral therapy. It cannot be injected into patients recently treated with beta-blockers because of the risk of hypotension and asystole.

Adenosine is a naturally occurring purine nucleotide. It is a potent atrioventricular nodal blocking agent and is used to terminate paroxysmal supraventricular tachycardia. It is given intravenously and its action begins very rapidly and only lasts for a short period, but this is generally sufficient to restore sinus rhythm. The suggested dosage schedule is 3 mg over 2 seconds with cardiac monitoring, then if necessary followed by 6 mg after 1–2 minutes, and then by 12 mg after a further 1–2 minutes, given rapidly.

Adenosine should only be administered in a monitored environment, that is, the Accident and Emergency Department or Coronary Care Unit. The patient may experience flushing, chest pain and dyspnoea coming on immediately after injection and lasting for up to 30 seconds. It is administered cautiously to patients with asthma as bronchospasm may occur.

The major advantage of adenosine is that, unlike verapamil, it can be given to a patient with a broad complex tachycardia of uncertain cause. The ventricular response in supraventricular tachycardia will be slowed but a ventricular tachycardia will continue unchanged. Also, adenosine does not cause significant inotropic effects that may result in reduced cardiac output and low blood pressure. It can be given safely to patients on beta-blockers.

Wolff–Parkinson–White syndrome

The Wolff–Parkinson–White syndrome is a congenital abnormality that occurs in about 0.2% of the population. It is caused by an extra or accessory conducting system between the atria and the ventricles. It is associated with supraventricular arrhythmias caused by re-entry (i.e. down one bundle and up the other) and atrial fibrillation, which are occasionally dangerous. In the treatment of these arrhythmias the accessory bundle may not respond to drugs in the same way as a normal conducting system. Digoxin and verapamil enhance rather than depress conduction through the accessory bundle and are therefore contraindicated. Amiodarone, disopyramide or flecainide are prescribed, depending on the circumstances. When the arrhythmia is caused by a circular movement, as in supraventricular tachycardia, drugs that slow conduction in the atrioventricular node or the bundle of His are used.

VENTRICULAR ARRHYTHMIAS

These include the following conditions:
- Ventricular premature beats.
- Ventricular tachycardia.
- Ventricular fibrillation.

Pathophysiology

Ventricular premature beats may be uncomfortable, especially when frequent. The patient may complain of extra beats, missed beats or heavy beats because it may be the premature beat, the post ectopic pause or the next sinus beat that is noticed. The pulse is irregular because of premature beats. After the premature beat there is usually a complete compensatory pause because the timing of sinus rhythm is not influenced by the premature beat. Treatment of ventricular ectopics may be necessary because of symptoms or because they may provoke or threaten to provoke more serious arrhythmias.

Ventricular tachycardia is defined as three or more ventricular beats per minute. The pulse rate may be between 120 and 220 bpm. Treatment may be urgent, depending on the haemodynamic situation. If the cardiac output and blood pressure are very depressed, emergency cardioversion may be necessary. However, if the cardiac output and blood pressure are well maintained, intravenous therapy with class 1 drugs is generally prescribed.

Ventricular fibrillation is characterised by rapid, irregular and uncoordinated electrical activity within the ventricles, probably caused by re-entry circuits within localised areas of myocardium. This very rapid and irregular ventricular activation has no mechanical effect and cardiac output ceases, leading to unconsciousness within seconds. Ventricular fibrillation rarely reverses spontaneously. The only effective treatment is electrical defibrillation, or, on rare occasions, intravenous bretylium 5–10 mg/kg over 5 minutes.

Pharmacological management

Drugs that may be used in the treatment of supraventricular and ventricular arrhythmias are as follows:

Class 1 Antiarrhythmic agents

Class 1a – Disopyramide decreases the excitability of cardiac muscle and decreases the conduction velocity. It also prolongs the refractory period. It suppresses the frequency of ectopic ventricular beats and the frequency and duration of self-limiting bursts of ventricular tachycardia. It has an anticholinergic effect and a significant negative inotropic effect. It also causes peripheral vasoconstriction.

The adult dosage is 300–800 mg daily in divided oral doses, or 250–375 mg daily of modified-release tablets. The maximum oral dose is 800 mg.

Disopyramide is well absorbed, with peak serum levels occurring 0.5–3 hours after oral administration. It is metabolised in the liver and excreted in the urine. Disopyramide should therefore be administered cautiously to persons with hepatic or renal failure. Serum potassium levels should be within normal limits before disopyramide therapy is started as the drug may be ineffective in hypokalaemia and its toxicity enhanced with hyperkalaemia.

Disopyramide is contraindicated in sinus bradycardia, heart failure or severe left ventricular dysfunction. The negative inotropic effect may cause hypotension and aggravate cardiac failure. The patient may suffer from urinary retention, dry mouth and blurred vision because of the anticholinergic effect of the drug. Glaucoma may also be precipitated.

Class 1b – Lignocaine remains a first-line drug in the treatment of ventricular arrhythmias as it suppresses the conduction of electrical impulses through cardiac muscle and suppresses the excitability of the ventricular muscle with only moderate depression of the action of the heart. For arrhythmic management lignocaine must be given intravenously. An initial dose of 100 mg is rapidly distributed throughout the body and is only effective for approximately 10 minutes. It may be followed by either a second dose of 100 mg and/or an infusion of 2–4 mg/minute to achieve a constant therapeutic effect.

Class 1c – Flecainide is used for serious symptomatic ventricular arrhythmias and paroxysmal atrial fibrillation. It delays intracardiac conduction in the atrioventricular node and bundle of His. Flecainide can be administered by intravenous injection, over 10–30 minutes, in a dose regime of 2 mg/kg body weight to a maximum dosage of 150 mg. This dose should be halved in the elderly. It can also be given orally in doses of 100–200 mg daily and reduced after 3 days to the minimum effective dose.

Class 2 antiarrhythmic agents

Beta-adrenoceptor blocking compounds prevent the stimulation of adrenergic receptors by adrenaline; this reduces the excitability of the heart and thus stops arrhythmias caused by an excitable focus or by a supraventricular focus circular movement, as in tachycardia. However, as a consequence of reducing the adrenergic drive to the heart and depressing heart muscle, beta-blocking agents may exacerbate or precipitate heart failure in recipients whose hearts are under stress from disease. A full detailed account of the action of these drugs is considered on page 194.

Bretylium tosylate has a suppressant effect on the heart muscle and its conducting tissues. It is now rarely used as a first choice but may be considered for ventricular arrhythmias resistant to other treatments. The dosage is 5 mg/kg intramuscularly, 6–8 hourly. It may also be given by slow intravenous injection in doses of 5–10 mg/kg, repeated as required. The side effects include nausea, vomiting and severe hypotension.

Class 3 antiarrhythmic agents

Amiodarone is effective in both ventricular and supraventricular arrhythmias. It acts by prolonging the refractory period of heart muscle. It also inhibits fast sodium channels. Amiodarone may exhibit noncompetitive alpha-blocking effects and mild negative inotropic effects when given intravenously, and coronary artery vasodilatation when given orally. It is thought to be of particular value in the treatment of paroxysmal arrhythmias associated with the Wolff–Parkinson–White syndrome as it has an inhibiting effect on both the anomalous and normal conduction pathways.

It is administered orally; a typical dose regime would be an initial loading regime of 200 mg three times a day for 1 week. This regime may be extended if a response is not achieved. The dose is then gradually reduced until the patient is receiving a maintenance dose of generally 200 mg daily or the minimum required to control the arrhythmia. This unusual dosage scheme is required because amiodarone is very readily bound to the tissues and only when these binding sites have been saturated does it produce an effect upon the heart. Amiodarone can also be administered intravenously, but it must be given over at least 20 minutes and preferably longer via a central venous line otherwise it may cause a considerable fall in blood pressure; the dose is 5 mg/kg body weight. The patient should receive cardiac monitoring while the drug is administered and should not receive more than 1.2 g in 24 hours.

Amiodarone is slowly absorbed at widely varying rates. The onset of action after oral administration is 1–3 weeks. It also has a long half-life and the effects can be seen months after the drug is withdrawn.

Adverse effects are common and to some extent may limit the use of the drug. It may cause a photosensitivity rash and blueish-grey pigmentation of exposed areas. Patients should be advised to shield their skin from sunlight, and to wear hats and long sleeves and to use sunscreen preparations. The drug contains a high concentration of iodine and may cause hypothyroidism and thyrotoxicosis, and thyroid function tests should be performed at 6-monthly intervals on patients receiving long-term therapy. In addition, during prolonged therapy microcrystalline deposits of the drug may develop in the cornea of the eye, which may produce visual impairment. Amiodarone increases the serum level of digoxin and potentiates the action of warfarin.

CARDIAC FAILURE

Cardiac failure complicates virtually all forms of severe cardiac disease. It exists when the heart is unable to maintain sufficient cardiac output to meet the demands of the body. The exact underlying biochemical and structural abnormalities in cardiac failure are imperfectly understood. Current research aims to define the normal and abnormal distribution of molecules that affect myocardial contractility; such molecules include angiotensin-converting enzyme (ACE), angiotensin and its various receptors, and certain forms of nitric oxide synthase (Underwood, 1996). The practical manifestations are acute heart failure, chronic heart failure and cardiogenic shock (circulatory collapse).

ACUTE HEART FAILURE
Acute failure is a sudden event that leads to the abrupt deterioration of left ventricular function and the development of pulmonary oedema. It is most commonly caused by coronary artery disease (usually a myocardial infarction), when there is extensive loss of ventricular muscle, and arrhythmias (frequently atrial fibrillation). The condition may also occur with rupture of the atrioventricular septum, which produces a ventricular septal defect, or because of acute valvular regurgitation.

Pathophysiology
When the heart fails, considerable changes occur within the heart and peripheral vascular system in response to the haemodynamic changes associated with heart failure. These physiological changes, which include ventricular dilatation,

ventricular hypertrophy and neurohormonal activation (activation of the sympathetic nervous system and renin–angiotensin mechanism), are compensatory and attempt to maintain cardiac output and peripheral perfusion.

The clinical manifestations of acute heart failure are the result of pulmonary vascular congestion and inadequate perfusion of the systemic circulation. Individuals experience dyspnoea, cough of frothy sputum and decreased urine output.

Dyspnoea is usually the first symptom of acute left ventricular failure and results from an abrupt rise in pulmonary venous pressure. This leads to a massive transudation of fluid from the capillaries to the interstitial fluid of the lung and alveoli. This increase in fluid content of the lungs is at the expense of air volume. Pulmonary oedema leads to the formation of frothy sputum. A reduced cardiac output leads to a diminished renal perfusion. This will result in a reduction in urine output and activation of the renin–angiotensin mechanism, enhancing fluid retention.

Pharmacological management
The pharmacological management of acute heart failure may involve the administration of the following drugs.

Diuretic therapy
These form the main basis of treatment. A loop diuretic such as frusemide, 40–80 mg, or bumetanide, 1–2 mg, administered intravenously will relieve pulmonary oedema rapidly by means of arteriolar vasodilatation, which reduces afterload, and then diuresis 5–30 minutes after administration. Loop diuretics act on the ascending limb of the loop of Henle, where normally about 20% of the filtered sodium is reabsorbed. They reduce sodium and chloride reabsorption and therefore water reabsorption. They cause a brisk and generally short-lived diuresis as the concentrating power of the kidney is reduced. These agents also produce marked potassium loss and promote hyperuricaemia.

Morphine 10 mg or **diamorphine** 5 mg administered intravenously sedates the patient and also reduces the congestion in the lungs by dilating the veins. If necessary they may be combined with an antiemetic to control vomiting. They must be used with care in patients who are cyanosed, as depression of respiration may occur.

Vasodilators
If diuretics are not sufficient to control heart failure, the addition of vasodilators may be beneficial. Venodilators such as the short- and long-acting nitrates (e.g. glyceryl trinitrate and isosorbide mononitrate, pages 191–192) act by reducing the preload and lowering venous pressure with resulting reduction in pulmonary and independent oedema.

Inotropic agents
In acute heart failure digoxin (page 204) would only be prescribed if the patient was in atrial fibrillation with a rapid ventricular rate.

Oxygen

Oxygen may be prescribed at full concentration if cyanosis is a marked feature, unless the patient has concurrent chronic respiratory disease, in which case the concentration should be controlled.

CHRONIC HEART FAILURE

This is a chronic condition characterised by a low cardiac output with the retention of sodium and water (**Fig. 12.6**). Valvular defects, such as mitral stenosis and some forms of mitral incompetence, may develop over years and the patient may describe only a very gradual worsening of symptoms.

Pathophysiology

The salt and water retention that occurs in chronic cardiac failure is a response to the activation of the renin–angiotensin mechanism to a falling cardiac output (see **Fig. 12.6**). This increased salt and water retention further increases venous pressure, which in the early stages of heart failure improves cardiac output by the Starling mechanism. This produces an increase in venous return, an increase in venous preload and eventually volume overloading of the ventricles. Veins are the reservoir for an increased blood volume and in established heart failure there is widespread congestion of systemic veins, which leads to systemic oedema.

Pharmacological management

The principles of treatment may vary according to the condition of the patient. If the heart is in sinus rhythm, diuretics and vasodilators will be prescribed first to unload the heart. When there is cardiomegaly and a gallop rhythm, digoxin may also be administered to stimulate the heart. However, recently, the treatment of heart failure has been revolutionised by ACE inhibitors, which have been shown to improve signs and symptoms in all grades of heart failure (Colquhoun, 1997).

Diuretic therapy

Diuretic therapy is an effective symptomatic treatment for heart failure. Diuretics will reduce the preload and alleviate the breathlessness. The choice of diuretic is often determined by the degree of heart failure. **Figure 12.7** shows the sites of action of the main types of diuretics.

    Thiazide diuretics, such as bendrofluazide 2.5–10 mg daily, are more effective in mild heart failure. They act on the distal convoluted tubule of the nephron, reducing sodium absorption. They have a gentle action but a greater

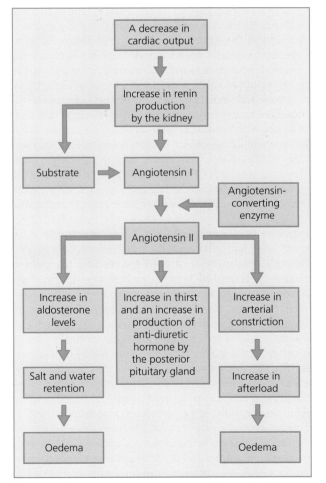

Fig. 12.6 The renin-angiotensin system in cardiac failure

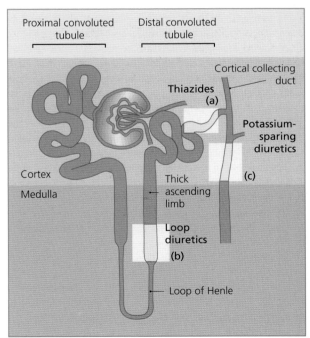

Fig. 12.7 The sites of action of thiazides, loop diuretics and potassium sparing diuretics in the kidney. (From Page 1997, with permission.)

tendency to hypokalaemia than loop agents. Other side effects include rash and thrombocytopenia.

Potassium-sparing diuretics such as spironolactone are specific competitive antagonists to aldosterone, producing a weak diuresis but with a potassium-sparing action. Amiloride and triamterene act at the distal tubule preventing potassium secretion in exchange for sodium. These drugs are weak diuretics but are useful in combination with more powerful loop diuretics. They should be avoided in the presence of renal failure. A detailed action of these drugs is available in Chapter 15.

Mild heart failure is generally managed with an oral thiazide; it may be combined with a potassium-sparing diuretic to avoid the development of hypokalaemia. More severe heart failure requires loop diuretics (see above) often with the addition of a thiazide (e.g. metolazone) to maintain diuresis.

Angiotensin-converting enzyme inhibitors

One of the main haemodynamic disturbances in heart failure is the angiotensin-II-mediated increase in systemic vascular resistance, which produces an increase in the left ventricular afterload and the left ventricular filling pressure (preload). This is caused by a retention of sodium mediated by excess aldosterone (see **Fig. 12.6**). The ACE inhibitors were specifically manufactured to inhibit the renin–angiotensin system by blocking the conversion of angiotensin I to its active form angiotensin II. Therefore a decrease in angiotensin II concentration will lead to a reduction of afterload and preload in the short and long term.

Angiotensin-converting enzyme inhibitors are used in the treatment of heart failure, either as an adjunct to diuretic therapy or in patients in whom there is no response to diuretics. Dilatation of the arterioles reduces the load on the heart and improves its function (Downie *et al.*, 1995). The proven beneficial effects of ACE inhibitors are a reduction in dyspnoea, an increase in exercise ability and an increase in life expectancy in all grades of heart failure.

Enalapril has been demonstrated to decrease mortality in patients with acute and chronic congestive cardiac failure as it decreases the heart size and reduces the need for other drugs for heart failure (Kuhn, 1994). The dose range is from 10 to 40 mg, administered daily as a single dose.

Please refer to the section on hypertension (page 213) for an explanation of the action and names of the remaining drugs within this category.

Vasodilator therapy

Treatment with other vasodilators should be considered when ACE inhibitors cannot be tolerated (Colquhoun, 1997). Vasodilators can be used to reduce preload by dilating venous capacitance vessels or afterload by dilating arterioles. Patients whose symptoms reflect increased preload (venous congestion) should respond better to a venodilator, whereas patients with depressed left ventricular function and symptoms of low output should respond better to an arteriolar dilator. However, as the two conditions often go together, a mixture of drugs may be required.

Alpha-adrenergic blockers, for example prazosin (page 216), and direct smooth muscle relaxants, for example hydralazine (page 217), are potent **arteriolar vasodilators**. The reduction in afterload they produce causes an increase in cardiac output.

Inotropic agents

Drugs that have a positive inotropic effect can be classified as follows:
- Digitalis glycosides.
- Beta-adrenergic agonists.

Digitalis glycosides – digoxin is the most common glycoside in use. It is of particular benefit in congestive heart failure associated with atrial fibrillation.

The effects of digoxin in the failing heart are:
- Increased force of contraction of the ventricular muscle. Digoxin acts as a positive inotrope by competitive inhibition of sodium-potassium ATPase, producing high intracellular levels of sodium. The intracellular sodium is exchanged for extracellular calcium. High intracellular levels of calcium ions allow increased binding of contractile proteins actin and myosin, enhancing the force of cardiac contractility and cardiac output (Kumar and Clark, 1996).
- Slowing of the heart rate, partially through increased activity of the vagus nerve and partly through a direct action on the sino-atrial node.
- Depression of conduction in the atrioventricular node and the bundle of His. This action does not affect the heart in sinus rhythm, but in atrial fibrillation it decreases the number of impulses reaching the ventricles from the fibrillating atria, and thus decreases the rate of contraction.

Digoxin can be administered orally, by injection or as an elixir. After administration the drug is slowly distributed throughout a number of body tissues and the desired plasma concentration is only slowly achieved. Therefore, if rapid control is necessary a high initial or 'loading' dose should be given. The amount given and the route of administration depend upon the age, weight and renal function of the patient. In elderly patients and patients with impaired renal function digoxin may accumulate, resulting in serious toxicity (**Warning Box 12.1**). There is only a small difference between the therapeutic dose and the toxic dose, therefore careful titration of the dose is required in conjunction with the monitoring of serum levels and avoidance of hypokalaemia. In patients with fluctuating renal function the administration of the liver-metabolised digitoxin may be preferable. **Figure 12.8** illustrates how certain drugs may interact with digoxin and other digitalis glycosides to enhance the potential for cardiotoxicity.

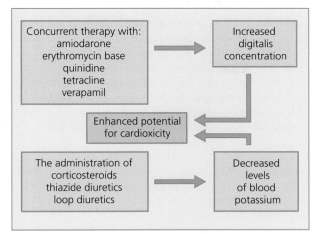

Fig. 12.8 Drugs interacting with digoxin and other digitalis glycosides

12.1 COMMON MANIFESTATIONS OF DIGOXIN OVERDOSE

- Undue slowing of the heart because of an excessive effect on the conducting system.
- Coupled beats, which can be felt at the wrist as a double pulsation followed by a pause. These are caused by ventricular extrasystoles following normal beats and result from increased excitability of the ventricles.
- Nausea and later vomiting caused by stimulation of the vomiting centre in the medulla by digitalis.
- Central nervous system effects that may include headache, fatigue, confusion, blurred vision, alteration of colour perception and halos on dark objects.

12.1 INTERACTIONS IN THE ELDERLY

A variety of drugs used by the elderly decrease absorption of digoxin from the intestines, including magnesium-containing antacids, anti-diarrhoeal suspensions containing kaolin, and antibiotics (especially oral aminoglycosides). Drugs that induce liver enzymes, such as barbiturates, anti-epileptics, antihistamines, phenylbutazone and rifampicin, can increase digoxin metabolism and dosage requirements. Cardiac glycosides interact with any drug or circumstance that alters the level of potassium in bodily fluids. Hyperkalaemia can increase both benefits and side effects of digoxin, whereas hypokalaemia increases positive and negative effects. Drugs that most often alter potassium levels are diuretics, which cause hypokalaemia, and ACE inhibitors and potassium-sparing diuretics, which cause hyperkalaemia.
One of the effects of digoxin on the heart is that it decreases conductance, thereby increasing conduction delays and possibly inducing heart block. Many anti-dysrhythmic drugs also have this action and will add to the blocking action of digoxin.

Adrenergic agonists

Dopamine and dobutamine are adrenergic agonists, but are only effective intravenously.

Dopamine is a naturally occurring substance that is changed to noradrenaline in the body. It is a β_1 stimulant; it also increases the release of noradrenaline in the heart, thus causing the heart to contract more powerfully. In addition, because of its unselective action on the adrenergic system, in lower doses it stimulates receptors in the renal blood vessels, causing them to dilate, thus improving renal perfusion and urinary output.

The adult intravenous dosage is initially 2–5 µg/kg per minute, increasing by 1–4 µg/kg per minute every 15–30 minutes until an adequate effect is achieved. Doses of up to 50 µg/kg per minute have been used but the average dosage is 9 µg/kg per minute. However, high doses of dopamine may produce a reversal in effect – peripheral vasoconstriction, hypertension, cardiac conduction defects and reduced renal blood flow.

This drug is rarely used outside intensive or coronary care units as a major problem with administration is an increase in heart rate that may progress to fatal cardiac tachyarrythmias. Cardiac monitoring is therefore obligatory.

Dobutamine is a selective agonist of the β_1 receptor, increasing intracellular cyclic AMP, which in turn increases calcium availability for the contractile process. It stimulates the heart muscle and leads to an increase in the force of contraction, thus improving cardiac output. It has no effect on the kidneys.

Dobutamine is administered intravenously by infusion. The adult dosage is 2.5–10 µg/kg per minute. Doses of up to 40 µg/kg per minute can be prescribed if the lower dosage fails to produce a reasonable effect. Cardiac monitoring during administration is essential as this drug may produce an increase in heart rate leading to fatal cardiac tachyarrythmias.

CARDIOGENIC SHOCK

Cardiogenic shock is an extreme type of cardiac failure with a high mortality rate: approximately 90%. Its most common cause is a myocardial infarction, but it may also result from a sudden reduction in blood volume, usually as a result of bleeding. Sometimes both causes may be combined, as in septicaemia, when bacterial toxins damage the heart, dilate the blood vessels and cause leakage of fluid from the circulation.

Pathophysiology

Cardiogenic shock is manifested by a severe failure of tissue perfusion, usually characterised by hypotension, low cardiac output, tachycardia and signs of poor tissue perfusion such as oliguria, cold, pale extremities and poor cerebral function. The hypotension caused by pump failure results in a reduction of coronary flow, which results in further impairment of pump action. It is this vicious downward spiral that is responsible for the high mortality rate.

Pharmacological management

If the main fault is pump failure, drugs can be administered to increase the force of contraction of the heart muscle (positive inotropic effect) and thus improve cardiac output and circulation and raise blood pressure. Digitalis is not effective in these circumstances as it may precipitate dangerous cardiac arrhythmias. The most commonly used drugs are dopamine and dobutamine (page 205). The patient will require continuous administration of 60% oxygen, and also analgesia for pain relief.

INFLAMMATORY DISEASES OF THE HEART

In any tissue the inflammatory process may result in destruction of normal functional tissue followed by its replacement with scar tissue, which is fibrous in nature and less specialised.

INFECTIVE ENDOCARDITIS

This is a general term used to describe inflammation of the endocardium – especially the cardiac valves. The disease may occasionally occur as a fulminating or acute infection, but more commonly it runs an insidious course and is known as subacute (bacterial) endocarditis (Kumar and Clark,1996). Many organisms can cause infective endocarditis, the most common ones being *Streptococcus viridans*, *Streptococcus faecalis* and *Staphylococcus aureus*. However, infective endocarditis can also be caused by *Staphylococcus epidermidis*, *Histoplasma*, *Brucella*, *Candida* and *Aspergillis*.

Pathophysiology

The pathogenesis of infective endocarditis is a complex process that requires at least three critical elements. First the endocardium, most commonly the heart valves, must sustain endothelial damage to facilitate microorganism colonisation. This damage exposes the endothelial basement membrane, which contains a type of collagen that attracts platelets and therefore stimulates thrombus formation on the membrane. Second, bloodborne microorganisms must adhere to the damaged endocardial surface. Microorganisms

may enter the bloodstream as a result of minor procedures such as dental extraction or bladder catheterisation or they may spread from uncomplicated respiratory or skin infections. The adherence of microorganisms to the endocardial surface is facilitated by the coexistence of nonbacterial thrombotic endocarditis. Third, the adherent organisms must proliferate and promote the propagation of infective endocardial vegetation (Huether and McCance, 1998).

Pharmacological management

Infective endocarditis is treated with bactericidal antibiotics chosen on the basis of the results of blood culture and an antibiotic sensitivity assessment. The antibiotics are administered intravenously and treatment continues for a minimum of 6 weeks. Serum levels should be measured to ensure that sufficient bactericidal activity is present to inhibit the growth of the organism. Bacteriostatic antibiotics and bacteriostatic levels of bactericidal antibiotics are not sufficient, even with the host's natural defences, to eradicate the organism (Souhami and Moxham, 1990).

MYOCARDITIS

This condition can be idiopathic or infective. A definitive aetiology with isolation of viruses or bacteria is uncommon. Regardless of the aetiology, myocarditis may proceed to cardiomyopathy and myocardial dysfunction.

Pathophysiology

This is an inflammatory response resulting mainly from infection. The main presenting features of myocarditis are a febrile illness accompanied by acute unexplained heart failure, cardiac arrhythmias and chest pain. The chest pain usually results from a myopericarditis. An arrhythmia, such as frequent ectopic beats, is probably the most frequent manifestation of a mild attack of myocarditis and may occur after an attack of influenza.

Pharmacological management

The drug treatment of myocarditis includes eradication of any infection, the management of cardiac failure (page 203) and the treatment of cardiac arrhythmias (page 198).

PERICARDITIS

Pericardial disease is often a localised manifestation of another disorder. Acute pericarditis has numerous aetiologies but coxsackie viral infections and myocardial infarction are the commonest causes in the United Kingdom. Other causes include uraemia, connective tissue disease, trauma, post-pericardiotomy, rheumatic fever, tuberculosis and malignancy.

Pathophysiology

Whatever the aetiology, the pericardial membrane becomes inflamed and roughened and an exudate may develop. The symptoms include sudden onset of severe chest pain that is substernal and sharp and worsens with respiratory movements. Physical examination often reveals a low-grade pyrexia and sinus tachycardia. A friction rub, a short, scratchy, grating sensation, caused by the roughened pericardial membranes rubbing against each other, may be heard at the cardiac apex.

Pharmacological management

The drug treatment of this condition may include anti-inflammatory medication such as oral aspirin, naproxen or indomethacin (chapter 18) to alleviate the pericardial pain. Infective pericarditis demands prompt diagnostic aspiration and identification of the infective agent, with appropriate chemotherapy. Occasionally, if the pericarditis is severe or recurrent, systemic corticosteroids may be required.

CARDIOMYOPATHY

The cardiomyopathies are a broad group of cardiac disorders that are usually non inflammatory but manifest as myocardial dysfunction not associated with hypertension, coronary heart disease or rheumatic heart disease (Vardaxis, 1995). These idiopathic conditions are classified according to their clinical presentation:
• Dilated cardiomyopathy – ventricular dilatation.
• Hypertrophic cardiomyopathy – myocardial hypertrophy.
• Restrictive cardiomyopathy – impaired ventricular filling.

DILATED (CONGESTIVE) CARDIOMYOPATHY

Dilated cardiomyopathies constitute over 50% of the patients diagnosed with cardiomyopathy. The cause is usually not identifiable as an identical clinical, histological and pathological picture can arise after damage to the heart from toxins, from drugs used in cancer chemotherapy or as the result of an attack of acute myocarditis. Chronic alcoholism is associated with dilated cardiomyopathy, and, as alcohol has a suppressant effect on the heart, it is thought to be an aetiological agent in many cases.

Pathophysiology

Dilated cardiomyopathy is characterised by dilatation and grossly impaired systolic function of the left ventricle and/or right ventricle. The basic problem is diminished myocardial contractility, which is reflected in the diminished systolic performance of the heart. Presymptomatic dilated cardiomyopathy may be present for several years. Later the symptoms depend upon the relative degree of right and left heart failure. Atrial fibrillation and thromboembolism are frequent complications. The most common symptoms are dyspnoea and fatigue. Palpitations are common and associated dysrhythmias may cause dizziness.

Pharmacological management

The management of this condition involves the treatment of heart failure (page 203) and arrhythmias (page 198). The treatment consists of salt restriction and the prescription of cardiac glycosides (page 204), vasodilators and diuretics (chapter 15). The vasodilators are administered to combat congestion. Venous dilatation reduces preload by promoting peripheral venous pooling, thereby decreasing central blood volume and alleviating pulmonary congestion. Arterial dilatation reduces afterload, making it easier for the failing left ventricle to eject blood. Anticoagulant therapy (page 212) is given to prevent pulmonary and systemic embolism. Corticosteroids (chapters 3 and 5) and immunosuppressants (chapter 5) can benefit individuals with inflammatory disease. Cardiac arrhythmias are treated conventionally, but as most antiarrhythmic agents are myocardial depressant they have to be used very carefully in the presence of heart failure.

HYPERTROPHIC CARDIOMYOPATHY

There is a familial incidence of hypertrophic cardiomyopathy. It is sometimes inherited as an autosomal dominant condition. The condition may be mild and show only on echocardiographic examination. Some cases have associated triggers for left ventricular hypertrophy such as hypertension or aortic valve disease, but there is usually no obvious cause.

Pathophysiology

Hypertrophic cardiomyopathy is characterised by marked hypertrophy of the left and/or right ventricle, particularly the intraventricular septum, in the absence of cardiac or systemic cause. This results in small ventricular cavities and a hypercontracting left ventricle, with or without subaortic stenosis and obstruction. Patients may present with a diastolic murmur because the posterior cusp of the mitral valve is abnormal. Alternatively sufferers may have chest pain, palpitations and dyspnoea

Pharmacological management

Patients with this condition are generally treated with antiarrhythmic drugs (page 201), although sudden death caused by ventricular arrhythmias is a continual threat. Beta-blockers (page 194) may be prescribed to abolish outflow obstruction and to help in the management of heart failure. Calcium antagonists (page 192) are sometimes prescribed to reduce ventricular hypertrophy, but results are variable. Both types of drug slow the heart rate and aid diastolic function.

RESTRICTIVE CARDIOMYOPATHY

This is a condition in which ventricular filling is restricted. Conditions associated with this form of cardiomyopathy are amyloidosis, sarcoidosis, Loeffler's endocarditis and endomyocardial fibrosis.

Pathophysiology

Restrictive cardiomyopathy is characterised by very high filling pressure to the ventricles. This results from rigidity of the walls because of infiltration of the myocardium with abnormal tissue, such as with amyloidosis, haemochromatosis or glycogen storage disease. The overall clinical and haemodynamic picture mimics and may be confused with that of constrictive pericarditis. The most common clinical manifestation of restrictive cardiomyopathy is congestive cardiac failure, particularly right heart failure. Cardiomegaly, arrhythmias and thrombus formation are common.

Pharmacological management
There is no specific treatment for this condition, but cardiac failure and embolic problems should be treated.

RHEUMATIC FEVER
Rheumatic fever is an inflammatory disease that occurs in children and young adults as a result of an infection with a group A streptococci. It affects the heart, skin, joints and central nervous system.

Pathophysiology
Rheumatic fever is thought to develop because of an autoimmune reaction triggered by the infecting streptococcus. All three layers of the heart may be affected. The characteristic lesion of rheumatoid carditis is the Aschoff nodule, a granulomatous lesion with a central necrotic area that occurs in the myocardium, particularly just below the endocardium in the left ventricle. Small vegetations may grow on the endocardium, particularly on the heart valves. This leads to some degree of valvular regurgitation. There may also be pericardial involvement; an acute pericarditis is characterised by a serofibrinous effusion.

The arthritis associated with rheumatic fever is classically a fleeting polyarthritis affecting large joints such as the knees, elbows and wrists. The joints are swollen, red and tender.

Pharmacological management
The streptococcal infection should be treated with antibiotics such as phenoxymethylpenicillin 500 mg in four daily oral doses for one week. These antibiotics should be administered even if nasal or pharyngeal swabs do not culture the streptococci. A sulphonamide may be used if the patient is allergic to penicillin.

A high dose of aspirin (chapter 18) is prescribed to the level of tolerance determined by the level of tinnitus to reduce the inflammation. If carditis is present systemic corticosteroids may be prescribed (chapters 3 and 5). Prednisolone 60–120 mg in four divided doses each day is administered until the clinical syndrome has improved and the erythrocyte sedimentation rate has returned to normal levels. The steroid therapy is then tailed off over 2–4 weeks.

VALVULAR HEART DISEASE

The normal function of cardiac valves is to prevent retrograde flow of blood between the atria and the ventricles, and between the ventricles and the aorta or pulmonary artery. Pathological problems may result from:
- Valvular stenosis in which the valve becomes thickened or calcified and obstructs the normal flow of blood into a chamber or a vessel.
- Valvular incompetence (also called regurgitation or insufficiency), in which valves lose their normal function as valves and fail to prevent the reflux of blood after contraction of an individual cardiac chamber.
- Vegetations, in which infective or thrombotic nodules that can fragment and embolise form on the valves.

MITRAL STENOSIS
The mitral valve is positioned between the left atrium and ventricle. It prevents backflow into the atrium when the left ventricle is contracting. The primary abnormality in mitral stenosis is a mechanical obstruction to the emptying of the left atrium.

Pathophysiology
When the normal mitral valve orifice of 5 cm^2 is reduced to approximately 1 cm^2, severe mitral stenosis is present. To maintain a sufficient cardiac output left atrial pressure increases and left atrial hypertrophy and dilatation occurs. Consequently, pulmonary venous, pulmonary arterial and right heart pressure also increase. The increase in pulmonary venous pressure is followed by the development of pulmonary oedema. Pulmonary hypertension leads to right ventricular hypertrophy, dilatation and ultimately failure. Atrial fibrillation often complicates mitral stenosis through rheumatic valvulitis.

Pharmacological management
The early symptoms of mild mitral stenosis such as mild dyspnoea can be treated with low doses of diuretics (chapter 15). The onset of atrial fibrillation requires treatment with digoxin (page 204) and anticoagulant therapy (page 212) to prevent atrial thrombus and systemic embolisation.

MITRAL INCOMPETENCE
This is one of the commonest valvular lesions. Any disease that causes dilatation of the left ventricle may cause mild regurgitation but the most common causes are rheumatic heart disease and a prolapsing mitral valve.

Pathophysiology
Mitral incompetence leads to regurgitation of blood into the left atrium, producing left atrial dilatation. If the condition develops over time there is only a small increase in

left atrial pressure as the regurgitant flow is accommodated by the large left atrium. In acute mitral regurgitation the normal compliance of the left atrium does not allow much dilatation and the left atrial pressure rises. This, in turn, leads to an increase in pulmonary pressure and the development of pulmonary oedema.

Pharmacological management

The evidence of progressive cardiac enlargement generally warrants surgical intervention by mitral valve repair or replacement. In patients who are not considered appropriate for surgical intervention or in whom surgery will be considered at a later date, management usually involves treatment with ACE inhibitors (page 215) for the cardiac failure, diuretics to alleviate the pulmonary oedema and possibly anticoagulants (page 212) to prevent the formation of a thrombus and systemic embolisation.

AORTIC STENOSIS

The aortic valve guards the base of the aorta issuing from the left ventricle and prevents backflow into the left ventricle after contraction. There are three main causes of aortic stenosis: congenital aortic valve stenosis, rheumatic fever and the wear and tear of age, which may lead to arteriosclerotic degeneration and calcification of the aortic valve.

Pathophysiology

Stenosis of the aortic valve leads to obstruction of left ventricular emptying, which in turn leads to the development of increased left ventricular pressure and compensatory left ventricular hypertrophy. This results in relative ischaemia of the left ventricular myocardium, and consequent angina, arrythmias and left ventricular failure. The obstruction to left ventricular emptying is more severe on exercise. Normally, exercise causes a many fold increase in cardiac output but when there is severe narrowing of the aortic valve orifice the cardiac output can hardly increase. Thus, the blood pressure falls, coronary ischaemia worsens, the myocardium fails and cardiac arrhythmias develop.

Pharmacological management

Patients with aortic stenosis should be advised not to over exert themselves or to partake in strenuous physical games. Angina is best treated with β-adrenoceptor blocking agents (page 194) because vasodilators such as glyceryl trinitrate or isosorbide dinitrate may aggravate exertional syncope (abrupt episodes of faintness). Antibiotic prophylaxis against infective endocarditis is essential. The treatment of heart failure would be as outlined on page 203.

TRICUSPID STENOSIS

The tricuspid valve is located at the junction of the right atrium and ventricle. It prevents backflow into the atrium when the right ventricle is contracting. Tricuspid stenosis is an uncommon valve lesion, which is seen much more in women than men. It is usually caused by rheumatic heart disease and is frequently associated with mitral and/or aortic valve disease.

Pathophysiology

Tricuspid valve stenosis results in a reduced cardiac output, which is restored towards normal when the right atrial pressure increases. The resulting systemic venous congestion produces hepatomegaly, ascites and dependent oedema.

Pharmacological management

The medical management of this condition involves the administration of diuretic therapy and a salt restriction in the diet to reduce the dependent oedema. Many patients require surgical intervention in the form of a valvotomy or a valve replacement.

BLOOD VESSELS

In order to fulfill their role the blood vessels must:
- Ensure delivery of blood to all tissues.
- Be flexible and adaptable so that blood flow can be varied according to the metabolic requirements of the individual tissues or the body as a whole.
- Convert a pulsatile blood flow in the arteries into a steady flow in the capillaries to facilitate optimum transfer of substances to and from the cells.
- Return blood to the heart.

Disturbances of the circulation within the vascular system may originate in the arterial or venous system. Vascular conditions may be chronic, developing slowly over a considerable period, or they may be sudden or acute. This section includes arterial disorders, venous disorders and hypertension.

ARTERIAL DISORDERS

Blood moves rapidly through the aorta and its arterial branches. These branches narrow and their walls become thinner as they approach the periphery. They also change histologically. The aorta is predominantly elastic in structure, but the peripheral arteries become more muscular until at the arterioles the muscular layer predominates. In the large arteries frictional resistance is relatively small and pressures are only slightly less than the aorta. The small arteries, however, offer moderate resistance to blood flow. This resistance reaches a maximum level in the arterioles. The adjustment in the degree of contraction of the circular muscles of the arterioles permits regulation of blood flow and aids in the control of arterial blood pressure.

ACUTE ARTERIAL OCCLUSION

This is a condition in which there is a sudden partial or complete obstruction of an artery reducing or stopping the blood supply to the affected area. It is serious because there is no time to develop a collateral circulation to the tissues supplied by the artery.

Pathophysiology

Acute occlusion occurs as a result of external compression, or a thrombosis or an embolism originating in the heart. Arterial thrombosis occurs within an artery in which there is narrowing of the lumen as a result of atherosclerotic changes. The stasis in blood flow predisposes to the formation of the clot, partially or completely blocking the vessel.

Arterial embolism is the blocking of an artery by a foreign mass that has been carried by the bloodstream until it reaches an artery too small for it to pass through. Most frequently it is a thrombus that breaks loose from its site of origin, but it may also consist of air, fragments of vegetations from diseased heart valves, atherosclerotic plaques or small masses of tissue or cancerous cells. The effects of an embolism are determined by the localisation of the embolus. Emboli tend to lodge in bifurcations of major arteries, including the aorta, the iliac, femoral and popliteal arteries.

Acute arterial occlusion is usually a complication of heart disease: ischaemic heart disease with or without infarction, atrial fibrillation or rheumatic heart disease. Trauma or arterial spasm as a result of arterial cannulation are other causes.

Occlusion in the extremities causes sudden onset of extreme pain with numbness, tingling, pallor, weakness and coldness. These changes are followed rapidly by cyanosis, mottling and loss of sensory, reflex and motor function. Pulses are absent below the level of the occlusion.

Pharmacological management

The treatment of acute arterial occlusion is aimed at restoring blood flow. The mainstay of treatment is the surgical removal of the thrombus (thrombectomy) or embolism (embolectomy). Thrombolytic therapy in the form of alteplase (tissue plasminogen activator) may be administered to some patients via an intra-arterial catheter introduced into the middle of the thrombus in an attempt to dissolve the clot. Anticoagulant therapy (heparin) is usually given to prevent enlargement of a thrombus and formation or extension of an embolus. Heparin is also administered prophylactically to all patients postoperatively. An account of the action of heparin is detailed on page 212 and thrombolytic therapy on page 195.

CHRONIC ARTERIAL OCCLUSION

This most frequently develops as a result of gradual changes in the walls of vessels, causing narrowing of the lumen. It may also be functional in origin: a hyperactivity of the sympathetic nervous system may cause an excessive vasoconstriction. Gradual occlusion of the vessels allows for collateral circulation to be established, lessening the problem of deprivation in the tissues distal to the occlusion. The arteries of the extremities are a frequent site of chronic occlusion, therefore the following conditions have been considered in this section:

• Peripheral vascular (arterial) disease.
• Raynaud's disease.
• Buerger's disease.

PERIPHERAL VASCULAR DISEASE

This is characterised by ischaemia of the lower limbs that results from a narrowing of the peripheral arteries and a gradual reduction in blood supply. Most patients with peripheral arterial disease benefit from measures such as cessation of smoking and a walking exercise regime. Vasodilators and viscosity-reducing drugs may also be prescribed.

Pathophysiology

Most symptomatic peripheral arterial disease is caused by atheromatous plaque formation, with subsequent stenosis, occlusion or embolisation of the vessel. The iliofemoral and popliteal arteries are most commonly involved. A reduced blood flow leads to hypoxia of the calf muscles when their oxygen demands are high, for example while walking briskly or running. The patient complains of cramp-like pains in the calf muscle on exercise, which disappear after rest. This phenomenon is known as intermittent claudication. A more severe reduction in blood flow can produce similar changes at rest and there are associated skin changes. There is hair loss and the skin is smooth, shiny and slow to heal if traumatised. Complete occlusion, usually by thrombus deposition on the atheroma, produces gangrene and manifests as blueish purple, painful discoloration of the skin, followed by progressive blackening of the tissues. The toes are involved first, but the changes progress proximally until a line becomes demarcated where oxygenation is just adequate.

Pharmacological management

Peripheral vasodilators improve blood flow to distal tissue and reduce vasospasm.

Dipyridamole (Persantin) is the drug most commonly prescribed for this condition. It dilates peripheral blood vessels and decreases platelet aggregation, adhesion and survival. Dipyridamole increases intracellular levels of cyclic AMP by inhibiting cyclic nucleotide phosphodiesterase. This may potentiate the effect of prostacyclin to antagonise platelet stickiness and therefore decrease platelet adhesion to thrombogenic surfaces. The normal adult dosage is 300–600 mg daily in three or four separate doses. With oral therapy, hypotension (manifest by dizziness and fainting) may occur. Dipyridamole can also be administered intravenously; the recommended dosage is 0.56 mg/kg over 4 minutes. A bitter taste in the mouth, facial flushing and hypotension may occur after an intravenous dose.

Nifedipine (page 193) dilates peripheral blood vessels and is often the drug of choice for patients with concurrent ischaemic heart disease and in whom beta-blockers would be contraindicated. It improves peripheral perfusion in patients with vascular insufficiency.

Anti-platelet therapy – junior aspirin 75 mg once daily is prescribed as a viscosity-reducing drug. This action of aspirin is detailed on page 196.

RAYNAUD'S DISEASE

This is a functional disorder caused by intense vasospasm of the arteries and arterioles in the fingers and, less often, in the toes. It is a primary vasospastic disorder of unknown origin. Raynaud's disease is seen most frequently in otherwise healthy young women, and it is often precipitated by exposure to cold or strong emotions.

Pathophysiology

The clinical manifestations of these vasospastic attacks caused by ischaemia are:

- Changes in skin colour that progress from pallor to cyanosis.
- A sensation of cold.
- Changes in the sensory perception such as numbness or tingling (Huether and McCance, 1998).

After the ischaemic episode, there is a period of hyperaemia with intense redness, throbbing and parasthesias. During the attack there may be slight swelling. With repeated episodes of ischaemia the nails may become brittle and the skin over the tips of the affected fingers may become thickened.

Pharmacological management

The treatment of this condition is limited to prevention or alleviation of the vasospasm. Stimuli that trigger attacks are avoided and sufferers are encouraged to stop smoking cigarettes to eliminate the vasoconstricting effects of nicotine. If the attacks of vasospasm become frequent or prolonged, drug therapy may be required. **Nifedipine** (page 193), because of the properties stated above, is generally the vasodilator of choice in patients with this condition. **Calcium antagonists** (page 192) may be prescribed to decrease vasospasm caused by vascular reactivity from vascular influx.

BUERGER'S DISEASE (THROMBOANGIITIS OBLITERANS)

This is considered to be an accelerated form of atheroma affecting young men of 20–40 years of age who smoke or chew tobacco heavily. The cause of Buerger's disease is unknown.

Pathophysiology

It is an inflammatory disease of the peripheral arteries that causes thrombus formation and sometimes vasospasm of

arterial segments. The disorder affects medium-sized arteries, usually the plantar and digital vessels in the foot and lower leg. Arteries in the arm and hand may also be affected. Although primarily an arterial disorder, the inflammatory process often extends to involve adjacent veins and nerves.

Pharmacological management

The most important part of treatment is cessation of smoking. All other measures are aimed at improving circulation to the feet and hands and preventing tissue injury.

Vasodilators, most commonly **nifedipine** (page 193), are prescribed to alleviate vasospasm. Aspirin (page 196) may also be prescribed for its antithrombotic effects. The adverse effects associated with aspirin (gastrointestinal bleeding and possible exacerbation of peptic ulcers) are rare and insignificant at low antithrombotic doses.

KAWASAKI DISEASE

Kawasaki disease (mucocutaneous lymph node syndrome) is a systemic vasculitis usually found in children under 5 years of age. It is usually self-limiting but those aged under 1 year are at a high risk of heart involvement (Wong, 1999). The incidence in the United Kingdom is 3.3 per 100 000, one-third of the incidence found in the United States and one-thirtieth of that found in Japan (Curtis, 1997). The most important complication is coronary arteritis, which may lead to the development of aneurysms and scarring, with accelerated atherosclerosis.

Pathophysiology

The disease is diagnosed on five criteria, which may develop sequentially. These are fever for 5 days or more, bilateral conjunctivitis, polymorphous rash, reddened and cracked lips, tongue and oral pharynx, reddening of hands and feet and cervical lymphadenopathy. Several factors support an infectious cause; a bacterial superantigen toxin similar to those responsible for the staphylococcal and streptococcal toxic shock syndromes appears to be the most likely hypothesis. Kawasaki disease is seen seasonally, often in winter and spring.

Pharmacological management

Intravenous immunoglobulin may be given in the first 10 days, which will relieve the inflammation and symptoms. A single high dose of 2 g/kg is currently advised. To counteract thrombus formation, aspirin may be given regularly. This drug is not usually prescribed for children under 12 years because of the risk of the development of Reye's syndrome. High doses of aspirin are recommended in the acute stage of the disease. The usual dose is 100 mg/kg per day in four divided doses (in Japan the dose is 30 mg/kg per day). After this phase low doses of 3–5 mg/kg per day are given for 2 months. Corticosteroids are not given for this inflammatory condition as they are thought to increase the likelihood of coronary artery aneurysm (Payling, 1997).

VENOUS DISORDERS

The venous system acts as a collecting system, returning blood from the capillary networks to the heart passively down a pressure gradient. The capillaries merge to form venules, which in turn unite to form larger but fewer veins, which amalgamate finally into the vena cavae.

VENOUS THROMBOSIS

Occlusion of veins by thrombi is very common. As many as 65% of people with lower extremity trauma develop deep vein thrombosis (Geerts, 1994). The process of thrombus formation in the veins is the same as that of thrombus formation in the arteries. However, venous thrombi are more common than arterial thrombi because venous flow and pressure are lower.

Pathophysiology

Three factors predisposing to thrombus formation within the veins are:

• Abnormalities or damage within the vein wall caused by trauma or intravenous medications.
• Venous stasis caused by immobility, age and left ventricular failure.
• Hypercoagulability of the blood, such as that seen in pregnancy, oral contraceptive use, coagulation disorders and some cancers.

The inflammatory response triggered by the clotting cascade causes extreme tenderness, swelling and redness in the area of the thrombus formation. The major danger associated with deep vein thrombosis is that a portion of the thrombus will embolise to the lungs causing a pulmonary embolus.

Pharmacological management

The treatment of this condition is by anticoagulant therapy.

Heparin is a naturally occurring antithrombin – a specialised protein that prolongs the bleeding time in the presence of a plasma cofactor. Heparin occurs normally complexed to histamine as a macromolecule in mast cells. It is an injectable, rapidly acting anticoagulant that is used acutely to interfere with the formation of thrombi.

Various clotting factors and hence clot formation are inhibited because:

• Thrombin is bound in an inactive complex so preventing the conversion of fibrinogen to fibrin.
• Activated Factor X is neutralised so preventing the conversion of prothrombin to thrombin.
• Platelet aggregation is inhibited as is the binding of fibrinogen to platelet aggregates.

Heparin must be administered parenterally either in a deep cutaneous site or intravenously, because the drug does not readily cross membranes. For the treatment of venous thrombosis heparin may be administered by continuous or intermittent intravenous infusion. A typical regime would be a bolus injection of 5000 IU followed by a continual infusion of 24 000–48 000 IU over 24 hours, sufficient to maintain a partial thromboplastin time of 2–3 times the normal.

As with all anticoagulant therapy there are two major risks to patients: overcoagulation with resultant bleeding, or undercoagulation with failure to treat the problem of thrombosis effectively. When the symptoms of overcoagulation do occur the effect of heparin may be rapidly reversed by the administration of protamine sulphate. Careful monitoring of bleeding time is required to minimise this problem. Administration of heparin is contraindicated in patients with blood clotting disorders and in those who have a history of peptic ulceration or uncontrolled hypertension.

Warfarin inhibits the synthesis of clotting factors produced by the liver from vitamin K and therefore reduces the ability of the blood to clot. Oral anticoagulation is instituted after several days of heparin administration, with the heparin being discontinued once a prothrombin ratio of 2.5:3.0 is achieved. Unlike heparin, the anticoagulant effects of warfarin are not observed until 8–12 hours after administration. The general principle of warfarin administration is to give a loading dose over 48 hours and subsequently to adjust the dosage to the requirements of the individual as gauged from the results of clotting tests. Oral anticoagulation is generally continued for several months, unless recurrent deep vein thromboses are a problem, in which case lifelong anticoagulation may be considered. A typical adult regime would be a loading dose of 10–20 mg on the first day followed by 10 mg on the second day. The dosage on the third day depends on the results of the clotting test used. These blood tests would be carried out on a regular basis and the results would determine the maintenance dose prescribed.

The occurrence of haemorrhage in a patient on warfarin is an indication for immediate withdrawal of the drug and if necessary the patient may be prescribed vitamin K which accelerates the return to normal clotting function. Warfarin is also contraindicated in patients with severe liver or kidney disease, haemorrhagic conditions or uncontrolled hypertension. It should be used with great caution immediately after surgery or labour. A number of drug interactions that potentiate or attenuate the anticoagulant effect of warfarin have been identified. A summary of the most important of these interactions is shown in **Figure 12.9**.

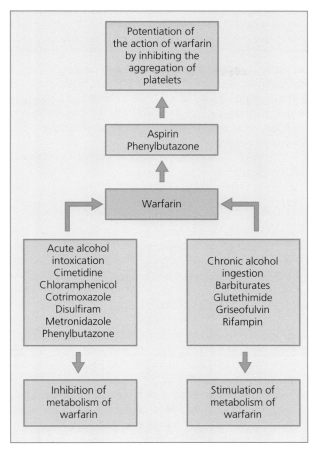

Fig. 12.9 Drugs affecting the anticoagulant effect of warfarin

VARICOSE VEINS

A varicose vein is a vein in which blood has pooled. The veins are dilated and tortuous, varying in size from large palpable bunches to mere discoloured superficial spider bursts on the skin.

Pathophysiology

Varicose veins are caused by:
- Trauma to the vein (typically the saphenous vein in the leg) that results in damage to one or more valves.
- Gradual venous distension caused by a combination of standing for long periods, which reduces the action of the muscle pump, and the action of gravity on the blood within the veins.

The veins are thin-walled, highly distensible vessels. Normally the valves prevent the backflow and pooling of blood. If a valve is damaged and thus permits backflow, the affected section of the vein is subjected to the pressure exerted by the extra volume of blood under the influence of gravity. The vein swells as it becomes engorged and the surrounding tissue becomes oedematous because of the increased hydrostatic pressure pushing plasma through the stretched vein wall.

Valvular incompetence is caused by venous distension that develops over time in individuals who regularly stand for long periods, wear constricting garments, or cross their legs at the knee. Distension progresses until the pressure in the vein is such that it damages the valves, rendering them incompetent. Damaged valves cannot maintain normal venous pressure, which causes an increase in hydrostatic pressure. As the vein distends further it becomes tortuous and oedema develops in the extremity.

Pharmacological management

Sclerosing agents are used to treat varicose veins. The agent most commonly used is sodium tetradecyl sulphate in various concentrations. Sodium tetradecyl sulphate is injected into the lumen of an isolated segment of emptied superficial vein, which causes irritation of the lining of the vessel, damages the endothelial cells and causes the blood to clot and form a thrombus. The injection is followed by immediate continuous compression to keep the resulting thrombus to a minimum and the subsequent formation of scar tissue within the vein produces a fibrous cord and permanent obliteration. Noncompressed veins permit the formation of a large thrombus and produce less fibrosis within the vein.

HYPERTENSION

Hypertension is defined as consistent elevation of systemic arterial blood pressure (Huether and McCance, 1998). Hypertension is caused by increases in cardiac output or total peripheral resistance, or both. Individuals may have combined systolic and diastolic hypertension or isolated systolic hypertension, which is a manifestation of increased cardiac output, rigidity of the aorta or both. In the majority of patients in whom no specific cause can be found for the raised blood pressure, this is diagnosed as primary hypertension (also called essential or idiopathic hypertension). Secondary hypertension may result from several underlying conditions such as renal hypertension, adrenal cortical and medullary tumours, coarctation of the aorta or steroid therapy. Hypertension can be further classified dynamically into benign hypertension, in which there is gradual organ damage, and malignant hypertension, in which there is severe and often acute renal, retinal and cerebral damage.

Pathophysiology

The causes of primary hypertension are complex and largely unknown. It is known, however, that a number of factors interact and produce long-term elevations of blood pressure; these factors include haemodynamic, neural, hormonal and renal mechanisms.

Arterial blood pressure is the product of cardiac output and peripheral resistance. Therefore all forms of hypertension involve haemodynamic mechanisms –

Paul Sandford, aged 37 years, is diagnosed with essential hypertension. His blood pressure has been ranging between 148 and 176 systolic and 95 and 115 diastolic. His average blood pressure is 155/100. There is a strong family history of hypertension and stroke on both sides of the family. Paul is married with two children age 7 and 11 years. He works full time as a loading dock supervisor for a long distance haulage company. His elevated blood pressure was discovered during a routine medical examination. He reports no other symptoms and an extensive physical examination reveals no evidence of renal insufficiency or retinopathy.

Paul is prescribed atenolol, 50 mg daily and a bendrofluazide 2.5 mg daily.

Over the next two years Mr Sandford experiences a gradual increase in his blood pressure and his medication is changed to Captopril 25 mg three times daily.

1. How will the atenolol and the bendrofluazide contribute to the control of Mr Sandford's blood pressure?
2. What will Mr Sandford need to know about taking his medications, avoiding adverse reactions and side-effects he may experience?
3. In addition to drug therapy, what non-pharmacological measures could you teach Mr Sandford to help lower his blood pressure?
4. What does Mr Sandford need to know about taking Captopril in order to achieve maximum therapeutic effect?

either an increase in cardiac output, which would lead to an increasing systolic blood pressure, an increase in peripheral resistance, which would lead to an increase in diastolic blood pressure, or a combination of the two. Many other factors, such as the autonomic nervous system, the electrolyte composition of intracellular and extracellular fluids, the kidneys, cell membrane transport mechanisms and hormones, play a role in regulating the haemodynamic mechanisms that control blood pressure.

The effects associated with primary and secondary hypertension can be explained as the increased wear and tear on the heart and the blood vessels. Chronic hypertension damages the walls of the systemic blood vessels. Prolonged vasoconstriction and high pressures within these vessels stimulate thickening and strengthening to withstand the stress. Arterial smooth muscle undergoes hypertrophy and hyperplasia. Eventually, the lumens of the tunica intima and tunica media narrow permanently.

The increase in the workload of the left ventricle as it pumps against the elevated pressures in the systemic circulation is the stimulus for ventricular muscle hypertrophy, and it increases the need of the heart for oxygen. If the increased work demands exceed the heart's compensatory efforts, heart failure occurs because the heart can no longer pump effectively.

Pharmacological management

Hypertension needs to be treated as serious cardiovascular complications may result. When the cause of the hypertension cannot be removed or lifestyle modifications such as weight reduction, regular physical activity or reduction of sodium intake have been unsuccessful, high blood pressure is treated with antihypertensive agents.

Antihypertensive therapy

The aim of antihypertensive treatment is to reduce the blood pressure to within normal limits. The methods by which antihypertensive agents are effective are based upon the fact that blood pressure depends on:
- Peripheral vascular resistance.
- Cardiac output.
- The volume of blood within the circulation.

Therefore by decreasing one of these it is possible to lower the blood pressure.

The British Hypertensive Society recommends antihypertensive therapy for patients whose diastolic blood pressure averages 100 mmHg or higher when measured on three different occasions or 100–109 mmHg when measured repeatedly over 4–6 months (Sever *et al.*, 1993).

There is a wide choice of well-established drug treatments. The major guidelines describe five groups of first-line antihypertensive drugs: diuretics, beta-blockers, ACE inhibitors, calcium antagonists and alpha-blockers (Chalmers, 1996).

Diuretic therapy

Thiazide diuretics are regarded as the first choice of diuretic in the treatment of hypertension. The hypotensive effect of thiazides relies on their promotion of salt and water loss and arteriolar dilatation, leading to a reduced resistance (**Fig. 12.10**). Only low doses are needed to produce a maximal hypotensive effect and this minimises the incidence of side effects such as hypokalaemia, hyperuricaemia, glucose intolerance, insulin resistance, impotence and elevation of serum calcium and cholesterol. The drugs most commonly used are **bendrofluazide 2.5–5 mg** and **hydrochlorothiazide 25–50 mg** because they are safe, inexpensive and allow once daily dosing. They are usually now used at low dose with either a beta-blocker or an ACE inhibitor.

Beta-adrenoceptor blocking agents

The mechanism by which beta-blockers lower blood pressure is complex. The most probable mechanisms of action include a reduction in cardiac output, a reduction in plasma renin activity, the release of vasodilator prostaglandins and a central nervous system sympatholytic action (Kuhn, 1994) (**Fig. 12.11**). Beta-blockers can be prescribed on their own but are often administered in combination with diuretics.

The advantages of beta-blockers in treating hypertension include once-a-day dosing for many patients and relief from anxiety-related symptoms. However, the disadvantage of using beta-blockers include side effects such as bronchospasm, masked hypoglycaemia in the diabetic, heart failure, impotence, cold extremities, and an increase in triglycerides with a decrease in HDLs. In general, the more selective beta-blockers are now used: atenolol, metoprolol and bisoprolol (page 194).

Angiotensin-converting enzyme inhibitors

The renin–angiotensin–aldosterone system (**Fig. 12.12**) is of primary importance in the control of blood pressure, body fluid volume and myocardial function. Drugs that act as antagonists to this system are valuable therapeutic agents in the control of hypertension and cardiac failure (Feely, 1994).

Angiotensin-converting enzyme (ACE) inhibitors act by inhibiting the enzyme dipeptidyl carboxypeptidase that converts angiotensin I to angiotensin II. Because angiotensin II is a powerful vasoconstrictor, interfering with its production can reduce total peripheral resistance and hence blood pressure. In addition, angiotensin II acts on the adrenal cortex to stimulate the release of

12.2 BETA-BLOCKERS AND THIAZIDES

Beta-blockers and thiazides are the first-line choice in patients aged over 65 years. The rationale for this is their proven efficacy in the prevention of stroke and myocardial infarction, along with minimal side effects (Kinirons and Jackson, 1997).

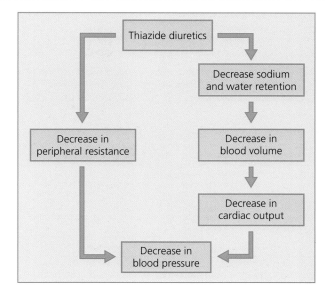

Fig. 12.10 The action of thiazide diuretics to reduce blood pressure

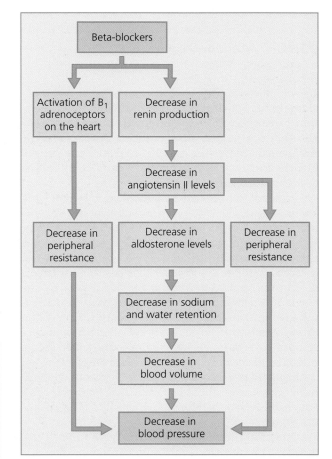

Fig. 12.11 The action of beta-blockers to reduce blood pressure

215

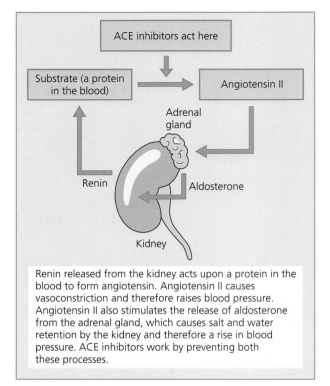

Renin released from the kidney acts upon a protein in the blood to form angiotensin. Angiotensin II causes vasoconstriction and therefore raises blood pressure. Angiotensin II also stimulates the release of aldosterone from the adrenal gland, which causes salt and water retention by the kidney and therefore a rise in blood pressure. ACE inhibitors work by preventing both these processes.

Fig. 12.12 The site of action of ACE inhibitors

aldosterone, which increases sodium and water retention. Therefore ACE inhibitors also inhibit the re-absorption of water, thus reducing blood pressure. Angiotensin-converting enzyme inhibitors also prevent bradykinin (a powerful vasodilator) from being broken down by angiotensin II.

Captopril was the first ACE inhibitor to be developed and is still used to treat patients with hypertension and heart failure. It can be used in reduced dosages in patients with renal failure when a loop diuretic is generally administered concurrently (Kuhn, 1994). Captopril is well absorbed from the gut although it is best administered 1 hour before meals as the presence of food reduces absorption to 50% (Downie *et al.*, 1995). The normal dose range is 6.25–25 mg twice daily. Treatment is started at a low dosage to minimise hypotension; diuretic therapy should be stopped 2–3 days before commencing treatment to minimise the risk of a rapid fall in blood pressure.

Enalapril is a long-acting ACE inhibitor used to treat mild to severe essential hypertension. Enalapril has a long half-life and therefore requires only a daily dose of 2.5–20 mg.

Other ACE inhibitors are available and their usual dosage ranges are listed in the summary box below.

Angiotensin-converting enzyme inhibitors have been found to cause serious side effects and therefore patients should be monitored closely. The most important side effect of these drugs is a persistent dry cough, often troublesome at night; this affects 10–20% of patients. The reason appears to be that once ACE, which is also present in lung tissue, is blocked, the formation of irritant substances – kinins and prostaglandins – follows. This may be associated with voice change and throat discomfort. Rashes, often with pruritis, are common and may be accompanied by fever and eosinophilia. Taste disturbance, usually transient, occurs in about 5% of patients.

Other side effects include proteinuria and neutropenia (which may progress to agranulocytosis).

Angiotensin-converting enzyme inhibitors may also cause an elevation of liver enzymes, transient elevations of blood urea nitrogen and serum creatinine and potassium concentrations. Consequently, ACE inhibitors are given cautiously to patients with impaired renal function and it is essential to measure serum creatinine and potassium levels before and during treatment.

Current ACE inhibitors enhance the hypotensive effects of diuretics and other antihypertensive agents. Potassium-sparing diuretics and potassium supplements should only be given to hypokalaemic patients as they may interact with the ACE inhibitors to produce a significant increase in serum potassium.

There are several newer drugs now available, including a new class of drugs, the angiotensin II receptor agonists – **losartan and valsartan**. They have properties similar to those of the ACE inhibitors. However, unlike ACE inhibitors, they do not inhibit the breakdown of bradykinin and other kinins, and consequently do not appear to cause the persistent dry cough that commonly complicates ACE inhibitor therapy. However, their place in the drug management of hypertension has yet to be determined.

Alpha-adrenoceptor blocking drugs (prazosin, terazosin and doxazosin)

These drugs relax the arterial smooth muscle by blocking the α_1-adrenergic receptors and reducing total peripheral resistance (**Fig. 12.13**). They increase venous capacitance by dilating venous vessels, thereby reducing preload, and

12.1 ACE INHIBITORS AND THEIR DOSAGE	
Cilazapril	1–5 mg daily
Lisinopril	2.5–20 mg daily
Quinapril	5–40 mg daily
Moexipril hydrochloride	15–30 mg daily
Perindopril	2–8 mg daily
Ramipril	2.5–5 mg daily
Trandolapril	1–2 mg daily

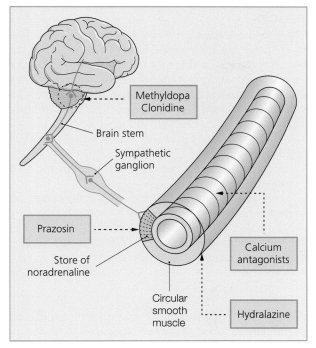

Fig. 12.13 The site of action of some antihypertensive drugs

dilating the arterial bed, which also reduces the afterload. Heart rate, renal blood flow and glomerular filtration are not significantly changed, but because fluid retention occurs these drugs are often given concurrently with a diuretic.

Prazosin – the dosage is 1 mg daily initially, increased as required up to a maximum of 20 mg daily.

Terazosin – the dosage is 1 mg at night initially, slowly increased up to 10 mg as a single daily dose. A small dose is required initially to avoid episodes of syncope during early treatment. Reduced doses are indicated when terazosin is prescribed with thiazide diuretics or other anti-hypertensive agents.

Doxazosin – the dosage is 1 mg initially, slowly increased after 7–14 days to 2 mg daily, up to a daily maximum of 16 mg, usually in association with other antihyertensive drugs.

The advantages of the alpha-adrenergic blockers are that they lack the side effects of sedation and a dry mouth, they decrease peripheral resistance with a fall in cardiac output, and they may benefit plasma lipid levels. However, the first dose may produce hypotension, the patient may experience a general lassitude and a tolerance may develop.

Calcium-channel blockers

These are effective drugs, particularly in more severe hypertension. They block the entry of calcium ions into the muscle cells in the arterial walls, resulting in relaxation of the muscle and dilatation of the arteries. There are three major types: the nifedipine type of drug, the verapamil type of drug and diltiazem. The most widely used ones are nifedipine and the longer-acting amlodipine. Diltiazem is not widely used in the United Kingdom for the treatment of hypertension.

Nifedipine lowers raised blood pressure by its action on peripheral blood vessels, which results in vasodilatation. The normal dosage when using the drug as an antihypertensive agent is 20–40 mg as 'Retard' tablets taken twice a day. Slow-release capsules may be taken once a day in a dose of 30 mg, and up to 90–100 mg if necessary.

Amlodipine possesses the same properties as nifedipine but is longer acting. The normal adult dosage is a single daily dose, which may be doubled depending upon the response of the individual patient.

Verapamil reduces peripheral resistance by causing peripheral vasodilatation, and therefore it reduces blood pressure. The oral antihypertensive dose is in the range of 120–160 mg daily. Verapamil should not be given to patients who are receiving, or who have in the immediate past received, beta-blocking drugs, as the combination of these two can lead to a complete cessation of heart function.

Direct vasodilators – diazoxide, hydralazine and minoxidil

Diazoxide is used in the acute treatment of hypertension associated with renal disease. It is a potent vasodilator drug, its effect being mainly on the arterioles. It is only effective when administered intravenously and, as it is rapidly inactivated, it must be given rapidly, that is, in less than 30 seconds. A dosage of up to 150 mg may be administered in this manner. Patients should be lying flat during administration. The duration of action is 4–6 hours.

Hydralazine has a direct action on arterioles causing them to dilate (**Fig. 12.13**). Administration of the drug often leads to a degree of fluid retention and tachycardia and therefore it is often given along with thiazide diuretics and/or beta-blockers. It may be administered by slow intravenous injection or infusion, 20–40 mg, in hypertensive emergencies, or orally, 25–50 mg, two to three times a day.

Minoxidil directly relaxes arteriolar smooth muscle, causing vasodilatation. It is used for patients with severe hypertension not responsive to other therapy. The normal dosage is 5–50 mg daily. The side effects are weight gain, breast tenderness and tachycardia. Almost all patients experience hypertrichosis (increased body hair) and should be warned accordingly.

Centrally acting antihypertensive drugs

Methyldopa reduces the blood pressure through a direct action on the centres that control blood pressure in the brain (see **Fig. 12.13**). Methyldopa is converted in the body to methylnoradrenaline, which stimulates the alpha-adrenergic receptors in the central nervous system. This results in decreased activity of the central nervous system. Vascular peripheral tone and arteriolar vasoconstriction are decreased, which lowers standing and supine blood pressures. Although methyldopa is effective and easy to use, in that the fall in blood pressure is not precipitous, it is no longer widely given because of the number of side effects (detailed in **Table 12.2**). However, it is safe in asthmatics, cardiac failure and pregnancy.

Clonidine stimulates alpha-adrenergic receptors in the medulla (see **Fig. 12.13**) resulting in decreased sympathetic tone and resistance in the peripheral arterioles, which lowers the standing and supine blood pressure and decreases heart rate and cardiac output. It also produces peripheral vasodilatation. The side effects of clonidine are detailed in **Table 12.2**. The oral dosage is 150–300 µg daily initially, increased up to 1.2 mg daily.

Adrenergic neuron-blocking drugs

Guanethidine, **bethanidine** and **debrisoquine** prevent the release of noradrenaline from postganglionic adrenergic neurons. Guanethidine also depletes the nerve endings of noradrenaline. These drugs do not control supine blood pressure and therefore may cause postural hypotension. They are rarely used now, only in combination with other therapy in resistant hypertension.

BLOOD

The blood is a transport medium which carries a wide variety of substances that are involved in all aspects of cell function. It provides a medium for internal transport, defence against infection by foreign organisms, protection from injury and haemorrhage and maintenance of body temperature. The blood is composed of three types of blood cells:

- Erythrocytes or red blood cells, which transport oxygen and carbon dioxide.
- Leucocytes or white blood cells, which defend the body against infections.
- Thrombocytes or platelets, which are necessary for blood coagulation.

This section includes erythrocyte disorders, coagulation disorders and leucocyte disorders.

ERYTHROCYTE DISORDERS

Alteration of erythrocyte function involves either insufficient or excessive numbers of erythrocytes in the circulation, or the normal number of cells with abnormal components (McCance and Huether, 1998).

The side effects of clonidine and methyldopa	
Clonidine	Methyldopa
1. There is no doubt that the most important fact to remember about this drug is that if it is stopped suddenly serious rebound hypertension may occur within 24 hours. Therefore the drug should never be stopped suddenly unless the patient is under constant medical supervision. 2. Clonidine may worsen symptoms of depression and therefore is relatively contraindicated in depressed patients. 3. Recognised side effects include bradycardia, headache, sleep disturbances, nausea, constipation and impotence in males. Facial pallor has also been noted. 4. Dry mouth, sedation and postural hypotension commonly occur during the early stages of treatment. 5. Rarely a Raynaud's type phenomenon with cyanosis, pallor and paraesthesia of the extremities may develop rapidly at the commencement of treatment.	Although methyldopa is a very effective drug in the treatment of hypertension, the major problem with its use is the large number of potentially serious side-effects which may occur, and it is in the early detection of these side-effects that the nurse can make a major contribution. 1. Neurological side-effects: Depression is by far the most important, but paraesthesia, Parkinsonism, involuntary muscle twitching, nightmares, confusion, light-headedness and dizziness may also occur. 2. Cardiovascular: Postural hypotension, fluid retention, worsening of existing angina and bradycardia. 3. Gastrointestinal: Nausea, vomiting, distension, excess flatus, constipation, dry mouth, black tongue and very rarely pancreatitis. 4. Blood: Haemolytic anaemia, leucopenia, granulocytopenia, thrombocytopenia. 5. Other side-effects include nasal stuffiness, a raised blood urea, gynaecomastia/ galactorrhoea, impotence in males, loss of libido, skin rashes, drug fever and abnormal liver function tests.

Table 12.2 The side effects of clonidine and methyldopa

ANAEMIA

This condition is characterised by a reduction in the total number of circulating erythrocytes or a decrease in the quantity or quality of haemoglobin. True anaemia arises when there is an imbalance between red cell production and red cell destruction. The causes of anaemia are:
- Impaired erythrocyte production.
- Increased erythrocyte destruction.
- Blood loss.
- A combination of the three.

Anaemia is classified after haematological investigation on the basis of cellular structure, specifically the red cell size (anicytosis) and haemoglobin content (poikilocytosis).

IRON DEFICIENCY ANAEMIA

Iron deficiency anaemia develops when there is inadequate iron for haemoglobin synthesis. The causes of iron deficiency include:
- Blood loss.
- Increased demands, such as growth and pregnancy.
- Decreased absorption, for example after gastrectomy.
- Poor dietary intake.

Pathophysiology

The total amount of body iron is 3.0–4.5 g; two-thirds of it occurs in the blood in the form of haemoglobin and myoglobin and in iron-containing enzymes. The remaining one-third represents stored iron, present in the form of soluble ferritin and insoluble haemosiderin. The average Western diet contains 10–15 mg iron per day and about 10% of this is absorbed. In iron deficiency, absorption is increased and may be as high as 30% of the total ingested. Iron enters the mucosal cells of the upper small intestine and is bound to apoferritin for transport to the inner membrane of the mucosal cell, where it is given up to plasma transferrin. The level of transferrin saturation thus regulates absorption. Iron is lost from the body in sweat, urine and desquamated cells, and in breast milk, but most of the iron released from red blood cells is recycled.

When iron loss exceeds iron absorption the iron stores become depleted; the transferrin saturation in the blood drops. When this falls below 10%, abnormal, iron-deficient erythropoiesis occurs. The erythrocytes become microcytic, that is abnormally small and hypochromic, and contain abnormally reduced amounts of haemoglobin.

Pharmacological management

Oral iron preparations

The treatment of iron deficiency anaemia requires identification and correction of the cause whenever possible. The deficiency may be corrected by administering dietary supplements, provided absorption is normal. When iron is administered to a person with hypochromic anaemia,

haematocrit and haemoglobin levels begin to rise in 3 days with a maximum response in 2–4 weeks. Oral iron therapy may be administered as ferrous fumarate, ferrous gluconate or ferrous sulphate (**Table 12.3**).

Parenteral iron preparations

It may be necessary to administer parenteral iron when the patient cannot tolerate or absorb oral iron. The response to parenteral iron is no faster than that to oral iron. Intramuscular iron is generally given as an iron–sorbitol–citric acid complex. Iron dextran can be given intravenously to correct the deficiency in a single infusion but this therapy can be hazardous. The toxic effects of parenteral administration of iron include pain at the injection site, temporary or permanent discoloration of the skin at the injection site, headache, nausea and vomiting, fever and urticaria. Parenteral iron may be deposited in the pancreas or liver and may cause haemochromatosis.

Iron antidote

Desferrioxamine is a chelating agent with a specific affinity for ferric iron. It is used to treat iron overload, which may have resulted from overtreatment with iron preparations, multiple blood transfusions or iron poisoning, a relatively common occurrence in children.

THE MEGALOBLASTIC ANAEMIAS

The megaloblastic anaemias are caused by impaired DNA synthesis and are almost always caused by a deficiency of folate or vitamin B_{12}. As a result erythrocytes die prematurely, which leads to fewer circulating mature erythrocytes, hence the anaemia. These anaemias are characterised by abnormal morphology of all cell lines within the bone marrow and blood. Defective DNA synthesis in megaloblastic anaemias causes cell growth to proceed at unequal rates and DNA replication and cell division to be blocked or delayed. The end result is an over production of haemoglobin during delayed cell division, which creates a larger than normal (macrocytic) erythrocyte. The conditions included in this category are pernicious anaemia and folic acid deficiency.

PERNICIOUS ANAEMIA

This is a chronic condition caused by malabsorption of vitamin B_{12}. It is most common in late adult life and rare in individuals under 30 years or age.

Pathophysiology

Pernicious anaemia is a condition in which the mature red cells are irregular in size and shape and reduced in number as a result of a deficiency of vitamin B_{12}. Folic acid and vitamin B_{12} are essential cofactors for blood cell production. Vitamin B_{12} is necessary for DNA synthesis. The causes of pernicious anaemia are shown in **Figure 12.14**. In addition to the megaloblastic anaemia, a deficiency

Oral iron therapy			
	Ferrous fumarate	**Ferrous gluconate**	**Ferrous sulphate**
Action	Replaces iron stores needed for red blood cell development, energy and O_2 transport, utilisation; drug contains 33% iron	Replaces iron stores needed for red blood cell development; drug contains 11.6% iron	Replaces iron stores needed for red blood cell development; drug contains 20% iron
Dosage & routes	Adult: By mouth, 300–600 mg of ferrous fumarate (100–200 mg of elemental iron) daily Full term infant and child: By mouth, 2.5–5 ml of ferrous fumarate syrup (22.5–45 mg of elemental iron) twice daily Premature infant: 0.6 ml/kg daily of syrup (5.4 mg/kg of elemental iron). Increase to 2.4 ml/kg daily (21.6 mg/kg of elemental iron)	Therapeutic, Adult: By mouth 300–600 mg 3 times a day Therapeutic, Child 6–12 yrs: By mouth 300–900 mg daily Prophylactic, Adult: By mouth, 600 mg daily Prophylactic, Child 6–12 yrs: By mouth, 300 mg daily	Therapeutic, Adult: By mouth 200–600 mg daily in divided doses: Therapeutic, Child 6–12 yrs: By mouth 540 mg in divided doses Therapeutic, Child 1–5 yrs: By mouth 360 mg in divided doses Therapeutic, Child less than 1 year: By mouth, 180 mg in divided doses Prophylactic, Adult: By mouth, 200 mg daily
Side effects	GI: Nausea, constipation, epigastric pain, black and red tarry stools, vomiting, diarrhoea INTEG: Temporary discolouration of tooth enamel	GI: Nausea, constipation, epigastric pain, black and red tarry stools, vomiting, diarrhoea INTEG: Temporarily discoloured tooth enamel, eyes	GI: Nausea, constipation, epigastric pain, black and red tarry stools, vomiting, diarrhoea INTEG: Temporarily discoloured tooth enamel, eyes
Contraindications	Hypersensitivity, ulcerative colitis/regional enteritis, haemosiderosis/haemo–chromatosis, active peptic ulcer disease, haemolytic anaemia, anaemia (long term)		

Table 12.3 Oral iron therapy

of vitamin B_{12} will lead to degenerative changes in the nervous system.

Pharmacological management

The treatment of this condition is the administration of vitamin B_{12} in the form of hydroxocobalamin. Initial treatment is generally 1 mg by intramuscular injection repeated at 2–3 day intervals until a dose of 5 mg has been given. A course of oral iron therapy may also be prescribed to supply the increased number of mature red cells. Thereafter the maintenance dose of hydroxocobalamin is 1 mg every 3 months. Unless the cause of the pernicious anaemia is dietary insufficiency, the lack of vitamin B_{12} will be permanent and the replacement therapy must continue for life.

FOLIC ACID DEFICIENCY

This condition is most commonly the result of malnutrition. It is most prevalent in the elderly The causes of folic acid deficiency are listed in **Box 12.2**.

Pathophysiology

Folates are required for DNA synthesis. Folic acid is the parent compound of the folates, which facilitates the transfer of 1-carbon units necessary in the synthesis of purine and pyrimidine bases. Folates are found in fresh fruit and vegetables, liver and kidney, and are destroyed by thorough cooking. Folate is absorbed in the upper small intestine and stored in a number of tissues, most particularly in the liver.

Pharmacological management

The underlying cause of folate deficiency must be found and treated. The deficiency is treated with folic acid supplements, 5–15 mg/day, which is usually adequate even in malabsorptive states. Folic acid should not be given alone in megaloblastic anaemia until vitamin B_{12} deficiency has been excluded, as folate administration may precipitate neurological changes in vitamin B_{12} deficiency.

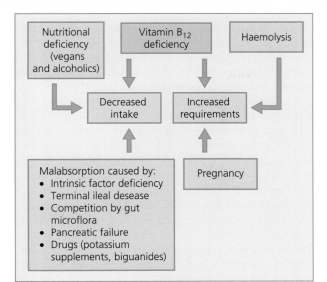

Fig. 12.14 The causes of pernicious anaemia

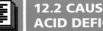

12.2 CAUSES OF FOLIC ACID DEFICIENCY

- Malnutrition, which may result from poor diet, overcooking of food, alcoholism
- Malabsorption, e.g. coeliac disease, tropical sprue, Crohn's disease, gastrectomy
- Increased requirements, e.g. pregnancy and lactation, prematurity, growth spurts
- Pathological conditions, e.g. haemolytic anaemias, myelofibrosis, malignancy, extensive severe inflammatory disease (psoriasis or dermatitis), dialysis
- Drugs, e.g. anti-convulsants

THE HYPOPLASTIC ANAEMIAS

The hypoplastic or aplastic anaemias are a group of disorders in which there is pancytopenia (anaemia, neutropenia and thrombocytopenia) resulting from bone marrow hypoplasia of varying severity.

Pathophysiology

Hypoplastic anaemia is a condition in which haematopoietic bone marrow or erythrocyte stem cells are underdeveloped, defective or absent. The decrease in the number of blood cells may lead to pancytopenia, in which all three types of blood cells are reduced or absent. An immune mechanism is probably responsible for most cases of idiopathic, acquired aplastic anaemia; immune suppression of stem cells by T suppressor cells has been implicated in many of the cases.

Secondary aplastic anaemia is the result of direct damage to the bone marrow caused by drugs, radiation, chemicals or infection.

Pharmacological management

The effective management of this condition is dependent on aggressive supportive care, including the administration of antibiotic therapy, the transfusion of red cells and platelets and the administration of drugs given specifically to treat the condition.

Androgen therapy is a traditional treatment of aplastic anaemia, continued for at least 3–6 months. The drug of choice is oxymathalone as it is less virilising than the testosterone derivatives. The recommended dosage for adults is 2–5 mg/kg body weight daily and for children 2–4 mg/kg body weight daily in divided doses. The dose should be adjusted within this range according to individual response.

Intensive immunosuppression usually consists of high-dose steroids, antilymphocyte globulin and cyclosporin used alone or in combination. Steroids are used to treat children with congenital pure red cell aplasia (Diamond–Blackfan syndrome).

Recombinant haemopoietic growth factors are being used in aplastic anaemia to prevent infective deaths in the early stages of treatment. It is unlikely that the use of haemopoietic growth factors will be effective as primary treatment for severe aplastic anaemia.

HAEMOLYTIC ANAEMIAS

The haemolytic anaemias are those in which a major feature is a reduction in the red cell life span. There are both inherited and acquired forms of these types of anaemias; the clinical and haematological pictures vary depending on the rate and quantity of erythrocyte destruction and the ability of the bone marrow to undergo compensatory hyperplasia.

SICKLE CELL ANAEMIA

Sickle cell disease is an inherited disease that develops in people who have sickle cell haemoglobin instead of the normal adult haemoglobin in their erythrocytes.

Pathophysiology

The most important structural abnormality of the haemoglobin chain is sickle cell haemoglobin (haemoglobin S). The normal adult haemoglobin (haemoglobin A) has two polypeptide chains: the α- and β-chains. Haemoglobin S results from a single base mutation of adenine to thymine, which produces a substitution of valine for glutamine at the sixth codon of the β-globin chain. In the homozygous state (sickle cell anaemia) both genes are abnormal (haemoglobin SS), whereas in the heterozygous state only one chromosome carries the abnormal gene (sickle cell trait haemoglobin AS). As the synthesis of fetal haemoglobin (haemoglobin F) is normal, the disease does not usually manifest itself until the haemoglobin F decreases to adult level at about 6 months of age.

Deoxygenated haemoglobin S molecules are insoluble and polymerise. The flexibility of the cells is decreased and they become rigid and take up the characteristic sickle appearance. Sickling is initially reversible by oxygenation, but each episode causes more membrane damage, leading to irreversible changes. Sickle cells are easily damaged and have a lifespan of only about 7 days compared with the 120 days of normal red cells. The accelerated destruction of spent red blood cells causes haemolytic anaemia, jaundice and the formation of gallstones. Because the bone marrow is working so hard to replace cells, a trivial insult, such as a minor infection, can have a major effect and precipitate a severe aplastic crisis. Sickled cells are rigid and circulate very slowly compared with normal red blood cells and tend to aggregate in and block small vessels. Cells and tissues supplied by these vessels are liable to become infected or infarcted. The course of sickle-cell disease is characterised by episodes of painful crisis caused by vessel occlusion or bone marrow suppression.

Pharmacological management

The symptoms of sickle cell anaemia may vary from a mild asymptomatic disorder to a severe haemolytic anaemia and recurrent severe painful crisis. Therefore the 'steady state anaemia' requires no treatment. Acute attacks require supportive therapy with intravenous fluids, oxygen, antibiotics and analgesia. The antibiotics are administered prophylactically as such patients are very susceptible to infection, particularly with *Streptococcus pneumoniae*, which can cause a fatal meningitis or pneumonia. Osteomyelitis can also occur in necrotic bone, caused by *Salmonella*. Regular blood transfusions are given only if the patient is suffering from severe anaemia or is having frequent crises to suppress the production of haemoglobin S. Analgesia is administered for episodes of pain, which are usually localised to the abdomen or some part of the skeleton, and which may last from a few hours to a few days.

Research is being carried out to find a way to increase production of haemoglobin F to reduce the number of sickle cells and sickle cell crises. Hydroxyurea in combination with recombinant human erythropoietin and butyrate are currently being investigated.

THALASSAEMIA

The thalassaemias are anaemias originally found in people living on the shores of the Mediterranean, but are now known to affect people all over the world. Thalassaemia is an inherited disorder in which there is a reduced synthesis of one or more globin chains.

Pathophysiology

Normally there is a balanced (1:1) production of α- and β-haemoglobin chains. The defective synthesis of globin chains in thalassaemia causes imbalanced globin chain production, leading to precipitation of globin chains within the red cell precursors and resulting in ineffective erythropoiesis. The precipitation of globin chains in mature red blood cells leads to haemolysis.

Pharmacological management

The aims of treatment are to suppress ineffective erythropoiesis, prevent bony deformities and allow normal activity and development. Blood transfusion may be required every 4–6 weeks. Febrile transfusion reactions can be prevented by the use of leucocyte-depleted blood. Transfusion haemosiderosis (iron overload caused by repeated transfusions) may damage the endocrine glands, pancreas, liver and myocardium by the time the patients reach adolescence. **Desferrioxamine**, an iron-chelating agent, can be administered parenterally. It binds iron ions (particularly ferric ions) and aluminium ions to form a water-soluble complex that is removed by the kidneys. It is given overnight as a subcutaneous infusion on 5–7 nights each week. Ascorbic acid, 200 mg daily, is prescribed as it increases the urinary excretion of iron in response to desferrioxamine.

PLATELET (COAGULATION) DISORDERS

Alterations of platelets and coagulation affect haemostasis, either by preventing it from causing internal or external haemorrhage or causing internal or external haemorrhage to occur when it is not needed. Diffuse internal haemorrhage that is visible through the skin causes a discoloration identified as purpura.

THROMBOCYTOPENIA

Thrombocytopenia is a decrease in the number of circulating platelets and may be caused by decreased production or increased destruction. In children and adults the disease is characterised by a sudden onset of purpura, easy bruising and frequent epistaxis.

Pathophysiology

Thrombocytopenia is caused by the immune destruction of platelets. The sensitised platelets are removed by the reticuloendothelial system. There are two distinct clinical syndromes: acute and chronic autoimmune thrombocytopenic purpura.

Acute autoimmune thrombocytopenic purpura is usually seen in children, often after a viral infection. It has been suggested that the thrombocytopenia results from the deposition of immune complexes on the platelets, but the acute development of platelet autoantibodies is probably responsible for the shortened platelet survival time.

Chronic autoimmune thrombocytopenic purpura is characteristically seen in adult women. It is usually idiopathic but may occur in association with other autoimmune disorders such as systemic lupus erythematosus and thyroid disease, and in patients with chronic lymphocytic leukaemia. Platelet autoantibodies are detected in approximately 60–70% of patients.

Pharmacological management
In adults, if the platelet count is very low, the treatment may involve a trial of corticosteroids (chapters 3 and 5). However, the dose required is often very high and produces unacceptable side effects. Splenectomy is a beneficial form of treatment in many patients as it removes a major site of reticuloendothelial platelet destruction. In splenectomy-resistant patients immunosuppression with azathioprine, cyclophosphamide or chlorambucil may be of value.

Azathioprine produces immunosuppression by incorporating itself into the normal production pathway for purine nucleotides, which form the building blocks of DNA and RNA. This creates a faulty end-product that results in a cell that cannot function in the normal immune response. It is usually given in a dose of 1.5–2.5 mg/kg daily in divided doses. Nausea, vomiting and diarrhoea may occur, usually starting early during the course of treatment and may ultimately necessitate the withdrawal of the drug; herpes zoster infection may also occur. However, the combination of azathioprine with a corticosteroid drug usually permits the use of lower doses of both drugs while maintaining their clinical effect.

Cyclophosphamide is a member of the nitrogen mustard group. It is converted by the liver to a number of highly reactive metabolites which interfere with the enzyme systems essential for cell growth. It also has an immunosuppressant action and may be used at a dose of 1–1.5 mg/kg daily for autoimmune conditions such as this. It is a toxic drug and regular blood counts should be carried out.

Chlorambucil is another member of the nitrogen mustard group with an immunosuppressant action. The dosage would be 200–300 μg/kg per day. Side-effects apart from marrow suppression are uncommon but the higher doses required to produce immunosuppression may result in nausea and vomiting.

THROMBOCYTOSIS
Thrombocytosis is defined as a platelet count greater than 400 000/mm³ blood. It may be primary or secondary and is usually asymptomatic until the count exceeds 1 million/mm³ blood. At that point intravascular clot formation (thrombosis), haemorrhage or other abnormalities can occur.

Pathophysiology
Primary thrombocytosis is a myeloproliferative condition in which platelets are produced in greater numbers than normal. The bone marrow of individuals with this disorder is characterised by hyperplasia of the megakaryocytes.

Pharmacological management
The treatment of primary thrombocytosis is problematic and not well defined. The treatment of choice is platelet-pheresis in conjunction with myelosuppressive therapy.

DISSEMINATED INTRAVASCULAR COAGULATION (DIC)
This is a condition in which a combination of haemorrhage and thrombosis is a secondary development in a serious primary illness. It may be seen as a complication in many disorders, including any condition associated with extensive tissue damage, severe infection, severe trauma, burns and extensive metastatic disease.

Pathophysiology
The process involves diffuse traumatisation of tissue cells and/or blood platelets by the primary disorder; this causes the release of thromboplastin, which triggers the clotting process. The activation of coagulation in the microcirculation leads to the formation of microthrombi in numerous organs and to the consumption of clotting factors and platelets in the process of clot formation, in turn leading to a haemorrhagic diathesis. The presence of fibrin degradation products exacerbates the bleeding tendency by inhibiting the polymerisation of fibrin (**Fig. 12.15**).

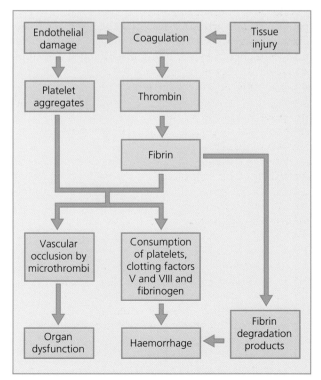

Fig. 12.15 Disseminated intravascular coagulation

Pharmacological management

The treatment of the underlying cause is most important and may be all that is necessary in nonbleeding patients. Transfusion of platelet concentrates, fresh-frozen plasma, cryoprecipitate and red cell concentrates may be indicated in patients who are bleeding. The use of heparin to prevent intravascular coagulation remains controversial and is given rarely.

HAEMOPHILIA A

This is an X-linked recessive disorder, which affects boys and men and is transmitted by female carriers. It is a coagulation disorder that occurs as a result of a deficiency of factor VIII (antihaemophiliac factor).

Pathophysiology

The clinical severity of haemophilia A is very variable and is dependent on the level of factor VIII. Levels of less than 1% are associated with frequent spontaneous bleeding from early life and levels of less than 5% are associated with severe bleeding after injury.

Pharmacological management

Bleeding episodes require prompt treatment by factor VIII replacement, given as cryoprecipitate or freeze-dried factor VIII concentrate. Each bag of cryoprecipitate also contains high levels of fibrin and the development of hyperfibrinogenaemia can therefore limit its continued use after major surgery or trauma.

Bleeding episodes, particularly into joints, are very painful and adequate analgesia must be given. Oral antifibrinolytic agents, such as transexamic acid, which impair fibrin dissolution by inhibiting plasminogen activation and fibrinolysis, may aid haemostasis, and are particularly useful in mild haemophiliacs after dental procedures. For minor procedures and as prophylaxis before minor surgery in very mild haemophiliacs, DDAVP (1-deamino-8-D-arginine vasopressin) may circumvent the need for factor VIII, as it produces a rise in factor VIII proportional to the initial level.

LEUCOCYTE DISORDERS

LEUKAEMIA

This is a malignant disorder of blood and blood-forming organs that causes an accumulation of dysfunctional cells and a loss of cell division regulation. The common pathological feature of all forms of leukaemia is an uncontrolled proliferation of leucocytes, causing an overcrowding of bone marrow and decreased production and function of normal haemopoietic cells. Please refer to Chapter 6 *Drugs and neoplastic disorders* for a detailed account of the pathophysiology and pharmacological management of these disorders.

HODGKIN'S DISEASE

Hodgkin's disease is a clinically and histologically distinct malignant lymphoma, although the cell of origin is uncertain. Lymphomas are tumours of primary lymphoid tissue (thymus and bone marrow) or secondary tissue (lymph nodes, spleen, tonsils and intestinal lymphoid tissue). Please refer to Chapter 6 *Drugs and neoplastic disorders* for a detailed account of the pathophysiology and pharmacological management of this disorder and also other forms of lymphoma including **Non-Hodgkin's lymphoma** and **Burkitt's lymphoma**.

KEY POINTS

- Angina and/or myocardial infarction may be treated by nitrates, calcium-channel blockers, dihydropyridines, β-adrenoceptor blocking agents and potassium channel activators.
- Fibrinolytic agents, aspirin and analgesia are used in the symptom relief and management of myocardial infarction.
- A high serum cholesterol level increases the risk of developing ischaemic heart disease; anti-lipid therapy has a key role in the long-term management of cardiovascular disease.
- Cardiac arrhythmias are of two types: bradycardia (heart rate less than 60 bpm) and tachycardia (heart rate greater than 100 bpm).
- Antiarrhythmic agents restrict cardiac electrical activity to normal conduction pathways and decrease abnormally fast heart rates.
- The Vaughan–Williams classification separates antiarrythmic drugs into four categories according to their effects on the electrical behaviour of myocardial cells during the action potential.
- Acute heart failure occurs when left ventricular function deteriorates and pulmonary oedema develops; chronic heart failure develops over time – cardiac output is low and sodium and water are retained.
- Acute heart failure is treated by diuretics to reduce the pulmonary oedema; diamorphine for sedation and the relief of lung congestion; nitrates to lower venous pressure and reduce cardiac preload and digoxin and oxygen when appropriate.
- Treatment of chronic heart failure varies; angiotensin-converting enzyme inhibitors improve signs and symptoms in all grades of heart failure.
- Inflammatory diseases of the heart are treated with antibiotics to eradicate bacterial infection, anti-inflammatory medication and, if required, drugs used in the management of cardiac failure or cardiac arrhythmias.
- The cardiomyopathies are a broad group of idiopathic cardiac disorders that are classified according to their clinical presentation.
- Chronic arterial occlusion may be treated with vasodilators such as dipyridamole, a peripheral dilator, and viscosity-reducing drugs such as aspirin. Nifedipine is the drug of choice for Raynaud's or Buerger's disease.

- Venous thrombosis is treated by anticoagulant therapy, principally heparin and warfarin.
- Hypertension is defined as a consistent elevation of systemic arterial blood pressure. Primary hypertension is when no specific cause can be found for the raised blood pressure whereas secondary hypertension results from an underlying condition such as renal hypertension, adrenal cortical and medullary tumours, coarctation of the aorta or steroid therapy.
- Antihypertension agents include diuretic therapy, β-adrenoceptor blockers, ACE inhibitiors, α-adrenoceptor blocking agents, direct vasodilators, methyldopa, clonidine and angiotensin II receptor agonists.
- Anaemia occurs when erythrocytes or haemoglobin levels are depleted through iron loss (iron deficiency anaemia), lack of vitamin B_{12} or folate (pernicious anaemia) or bone marrow hyperplasia (hypoplastic anaemia).
- Iron deficiency anaemia is treated by correction of the cause whenever possible and administration of oral iron.
- Pernicious anaemia is treated by the administration of vitamin B_{12} in the form of hydroxocobalamin.
- The effective management of hypoplastic anaemias includes antibiotic therapy and the transfusion of red cells and platelets, and drugs such as steroids, immunoglobulins and androgen therapy.
- The main platelet disorders are thrombocytopenia (a decrease in the number of circulating platelets), thrombocytosis (an increase in the number of circulating platelets) and disseminated intravascular coagulation, a condition in which a combination of haemorrhage and thrombosis complicates another disorder.
- Thrombocytopenia may treated by corticosteroids if the platelet count is very low, a splenectomy or immunosuppression with azathioprine, cyclophosphamide or chlorambucil. Patients with thrombocytosis in whom thrombotic events have occurred may be treated with aspirin.
- The clinical severity haemophilia is variable and depends on the level of factor VIII; bleeding may be spontaneous or the result of injury. Treatment is with factor VIII replacement. Oral anti-fibrinolytic episodes impair fibrin dissolution and may aid haemostasis.

MULTIPLE CHOICE QUESTIONS

Choose the correct answers.

1. The main function of anticoagulant therapy is to:
   a. stimulate fibrinolysis
   b. dissolve existing clots
   c. retard the clotting process
   d. dissolve clotting factors
   e. to inhibit platelet aggregation

2. Simvastatin has the following action in the treatment of hyperlipidaemia:
   a. it inhibits lipolysis in adipose tissue
   b. it decreases hepatic synthesis of high density lipoproteins
   c. it inhibits the hepatic synthesis of cholesterol
   d. it decreases biliary excretion of triglycerides
   e. it increases biliary excretion of cholesterol

3. Nitrates are effective in the treatment of angina because they:
   a. relax vascular smooth muscle
   b. relax skeletal muscle tissue
   c. constrict cerebral blood vessels
   d. increase myocardial oxygen demand
   e. constrict peripheral blood vessels

4. The administration of ACE inhibitors leads to:
   a. decreased blood pressure
   b. decreased aldosterone levels
   c. increased levels of bradykinin
   d. increased cardiac performance
   e. all of the above

5. Which of the following adverse effects is associated with glycerol trinitrate:
   a. hypertension
   b. throbbing headache
   c. bradycardia
   d. sexual dysfunction
   e. anaemia

6. Which of the following is **not** a potential side-effect of beta-adrenoceptor blocking drugs:
   a. bronchospasm
   b. vasoconstriction
   c. tachycardia
   d. nausea and vomiting
   e. dizziness

7. All of the following statements about calcium channel blockers are true except that:
   a. they decrease peripheral vascular resistance
   b. they increase coronary blood flow
   c. they decrease cardiac afterload
   d. they decrease serum calcium ion concentration
   e. they may cause hypotension

8. The major side-effect from oral iron therapy is:
   a. hypokalaemia
   b. hypertension
   c. gastro-intestinal irritation
   d. headaches
   e. urticaria

9. Which of the following is a potential cause of folic acid deficiency:
   a. alcoholism
   b. tropical sprue
   c. psoriasis
   d. renal dialysis
   e. all of the above

10. Which of the following is not an acceptable treatment for haemophilia:
    a. aspirin
    b. freeze dried factor VIII
    c. tranexamic acid
    d. 1-deamino-8-D-arginine vasopressin
    e. cryoprecipitate factor VIII

REFERENCES

Abernethy K. The menopause and hormone replacement therapy. *Nurs Stand* 1997, **11:** 1249-1256.

Albarran J, Kapeluch H. The role of the nurse in thrombolytic therapy. *Br J Nurs* 1994, **3:**104-109.

Assman G, Schulte H, Von Eckardson A, Huang Y (1996) High density lipoprotein cholesterol is a predictor of coronary heart disease risk. The PROCAM experience and pathological implications for reverse cholesterol transport. *Atherosclerosis* July 1996; **124:**511-520.

CAF. *Contact a Family*. London: Contact a Family, 1997.

Chalmers J. Treatment guidelines in hypertension: current limitations and future solutions. *J Hypertension* 1996; **14:**53-58.

Colquhoun M. Better treatment and diagnosis in chronic heart failure. *Practitioner* 1997; **241:**647-652.

Cornock M. Psychological approaches to cardiac pain. *Nurs Stand* 1996; **11:** 1234-1238.

Curtis N. Kawasaki disease. *Br Med J* 1997; **315:**322-323.

Downie G, MacKenzie J, Williams A. *Pharmacology and pharmacological management for nurses*. Edinburgh: Churchill Livingstone, 1995.

Feely J. *New drugs*. London: British Medical Journal, 1994.

FRISC Study Group. Low molecular weight heparin during instability in coronary artery disease. *Lancet* 1996; **347:**561-568.

Geerts WH. A prospective study of venous thromboembolism after major trauma. *N Engl J Med* 1994; **331:**1601.

Henney CR, Dow RJ, MacConnachie AM. *Drugs in nursing practice*. Edinburgh: Churchill Livingstone, 1995.

Huether SE, McCance KL. *Understanding pathophysiology*. London: Mosby, 1998.

ISIS-3. A randomised comparison of streptokinase vs. tissue plasminogen activator vs. anistreplase and of aspirin plus heparin vs. heparin alone among 41,299 cases of suspected acute myocardial infarction. *Lancet* 1992, **339:** 1-16.

Jennings K. Current management of angina. *Practitioner* 1997, **241:**668-672.

Joliffe P. Blood lipids and CHD: making a difference. *Practitioner* 1997; **241:**677-684.

Kinirons M, Jackson S. Hypertension in the elderly. *Practitioner* 1997, **241:**686-690.

Kuhn MA. *Pharmacotherapeutics: a nursing process approach, 3rd ed*. Philadelphia: FA Davis, 1994.

Kumar P, Clark M. *Clinical medicine, 3rd ed*. London: WB Saunders, 1996.

McCarthy M. Heart ischaemia rapidly reduced by lipid lowering. *Lancet* 1997; **349:**332.

McKenry L, Salerno E. *Pharmacology in nursing*. London: Mosby, 1995.

Page C. *Integrated Pharmacology*. London: Mosby, 1997.

Payling KJ. Kawasaki disease. *Prof Nurse* 1997; **13:**108-109.

Sever P, Beevers G, Bulpitt C. Management guidelines in essential hypertension: report of the second working party of the British Hypertensive Society. *Br Med J* 1993; **306:**983-987.

Souhami RL, Moxham J, eds. *Textbook of medicine*. Edinburgh: Churchill Livingstone, 1990.

Stampfer MJ, Colditz GA. Oestrogen replacement therapy and coronary heart disease: a quantitative assessment of the epidemiological evidence. *Prev Med* 1991; **20:**47-63.

Stevens A, Lowe J. *Pathology*. London: Mosby, 1995.

Theroux P, Quimet H, McCann J. Aspirin, heparin or both to treat unstable angina. *New Engl J Med* 1988; **3:**1105-1111.

Underwood JCE. *General and systematic pathology*. Edinburgh: Churchill Livingstone, 1996.

Vardaxis NJ. *Pathology for the health sciences*. London: Churchill Livingstone, 1995.

Wong D. *Nursing Care of Infants and Children, 6th Ed*. London: Mosby, 1999.

13 Barbara Worster
DRUGS AND MUSCULOSKELETAL DISORDERS

INTRODUCTION

The way an individual functions in daily life, moves about or manipulates objects physically depends upon the integrity of the musculoskeletal system. The musculoskeletal system is actually two separate systems that work together intricately: the muscles, including tendons and ligaments, and the bones, including joints. Each of the systems contributes to mobility. The skeleton supports the body and provides leverage to the skeletal muscles so that movement of various parts of the body is possible. Movement is accomplished by contraction of the skeletal muscles and bending or rotation at the joints (McCance and Huether, 1998).

This chapter covers diseases of the joint, bone disorders and diseases affecting skeletal muscle. Musculoskeletal injuries include fractures, dislocations, sprains and strains. Alterations in bones, joints and muscles may be caused by metabolic disorders, infections, inflammatory or non-inflammatory diseases or tumours

DISEASES OF THE JOINT

A joint may be referred to as an articulation; the ends of the bones involved in the joint are the articular surfaces. Joints permit mobility, but not all junctions between bones are designed to allow movement. At one extreme, the cranial sutures in adults are rigidly fixed, whereas at the other, the shoulder joint has an almost unlimited range of movement.

Joints have a rich innervation, usually derived from nerves supplying the adjacent muscular tissue. This arrangement allows a local reflex arc to be established between movement in an individual joint and the actions of the surrounding muscles. There are many sensory nerve endings in the fibrous capsule of joints and in the bone underlying the articular surfaces. In contrast, the synovial membrane has no specialised sensory receptors apart from those associated with adjacent blood vessels and is therefore relatively insensitive to pain. However, any substantial pathological process involving a joint is likely to cause inflammatory cell infiltration and oedema of the adjacent joint capsule, if not the articular surfaces themselves. This results in pain and the subsequent limitation of movement (Underwood, 1996).

The diseases of the joints are forms of arthritis. Most of these disorders can be placed into two main categories: inflammatory joint disease and non-inflammatory joint disease, of which degenerative joint disease (osteoarthritis) is the most prevalent.

OSTEOARTHRITIS

Osteoarthritis is the commonest type of arthritis, occurring in about 20% of the population as a whole and in 50% of those aged over 60 years. It is a disease of cartilage, which becomes eroded and progressively thinned as the disease proceeds (**Fig. 13.1**) (Kumar and Clark, 1996).

Pathophysiology

Early in the disease process the articular cartilage loses its glistening appearance, becoming a yellowish or brownish grey. As the disease progresses surface areas of the articular cartilage flake off and deep layers develop longitudinal fissures. Over time the cartilage becomes thin and may wear away completely, leaving the underlying bone (subchondral bone) unprotected. Erosion of the articular cartilage allows cartilage-coated osteophytes to grow outwards from the underlying bone and alter the bone contours and bone anatomy. As the osteophytes enlarge small pieces of the bony projections may break off and irritate the synovial membrane, resulting in inflammation (synovitis) and joint effusion (McCance and Huether, 1998). The synovial membrane is heavily infiltrated with mononuclear cells (Underwood, 1996).

The pattern of development of this disease is additive. It moves slowly from joint to joint and in most cases also progresses very slowly within individual joints. Its greatest impact is on weight-bearing joints such as the hips and the knees.

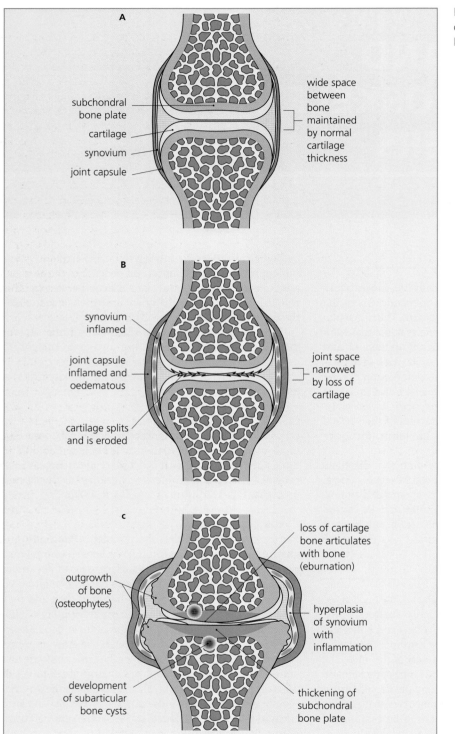

Fig 13.1 Pathological changes in osteoarthritis. (From Stevens & Lowe 1995, with permission.)

Labels for panel A:
- subchondral bone plate
- cartilage
- synovium
- joint capsule
- wide space between bone maintained by normal cartilage thickness

Labels for panel B:
- synovium inflamed
- joint capsule inflamed and oedematous
- cartilage splits and is eroded
- joint space narrowed by loss of cartilage

Labels for panel C:
- outgrowth of bone (osteophytes)
- development of subarticular bone cysts
- loss of cartilage bone articulates with bone (eburnation)
- hyperplasia of synovium with inflammation
- thickening of subchondral bone plate

There are three main types of treatment for osteoarthritis, which help to relieve pain and improve joint function: drugs, physical therapies such as topical heat and exercise and surgery to replace the affected joint.

Pharmacological management

Unfortunately there is no specific therapy to control the disease process. There is, however, research into methods of healing the cartilage defects in osteoarthritis: see *Cartilage Growth Factor in Osteoarthritis* overleaf.

Analgesics will almost certainly be prescribed to alleviate the pain, which is a result of stimulation of the nerve endings in the joint capsule and synovium. The pain is often aggravated by use and relieved by rest. A detailed account of the action of drugs prescribed to alleviate pain can be found in Chapter 18.

Non-steroidal anti-inflammatory drugs (NSAIDs) may also be prescribed to reduce the swelling produced by the inflammation and to reduce pain. Non-steroidal anti-inflammatory drugs have an analgesic, anti-inflammatory and antipyretic effect. A detailed account of the action and side effects of NSAIDs is given in Chapter 18 *Pharmacological management of pain*.

Cartilage growth factor in osteoarthritis

A number of investigators are currently involved in studies of 'chondro-protective agents', which prevent, retard or reverse anatomical changes in the disease process. The chondro-protective mechanisms include inhibition of cartilage degradative metalloproteases, or stimulation of chondrocyte proliferation and matrix synthesis. Researchers Ernst Hunziker of the University of Bern, Switzerland, and Lawrence Rosenberg of the Montefiore Medical Center, New York, USA, 1996 recently reported on the use of a cartilage growth factor substance called transforming growth factor-β (TGF-β) in the triggering of repair in experimentally induced cartilage defects in white rabbits. Using several different forms of TGF-β, they found a way to induce cartilage repair that resembled normal hyaline cartilage, with good results persisting 1 year after surgery.

Similar studies investigating cellular replacement derived from cartilage, periosteum or bone marrow mesenchymal stem cells are also being carried out. At present these treatments have not been studied in humans and are not approved or available for the treatment of osteoarthritis. However, these studies based on significant advances in the understanding of cartilage biochemistry and pathophysiology suggest that the development of specific approaches to the treatment of osteoarthritis will be possible in the future.

RHEUMATOID ARTHRITIS

Rheumatoid arthritis is a chronic systemic disease that produces:
• A symmetrical inflammatory polyarteritis.
• Extra-articular involvement. Inflammatory lesions can develop in many tissues, including the heart and pericardium, blood vessels, lungs, skin, subcutaneous tissues and the eye.
• Progressive joint damage causing severe disability.

The aetiology of rheumatoid arthritis is unknown, but toxic substances produced by the inflammatory reaction in the synovium are thought to lead to the destruction of cartilage, the characteristic feature of progressing rheumatoid arthritis (**Fig. 13.2**).

Pathophysiology

Rheumatoid arthritis is considered to be an autoimmune disease for a number of reasons: immune complexes are found in the synovial fluid and circulation, locally synthesised immunoglobulins and lymphokines are found in the synovial fluid, cell-mediated immunity is defective and rheumatoid arthritis is associated with other organ-specific autoimmune diseases. A likely hypothesis for the chronicity of the inflammatory process is that a persistent foreign antigen, possibly a bacteria or a virus, is taken up by the macrophages but not destroyed or removed, and leads to a systemic inflammatory reaction (Kumar and Clark, 1996).

The evidence suggests that microvascular injury and mild synovial cell proliferation are the first lesions and that small vessels are obliterated. Synovial inflammation occurs when immune complexes in the blood and synovial tissue trigger the inflammatory response, chiefly by activating the plasma protein complement. Complement activation stimulates the release of kinins and prostaglandins, which in turn increases the permeability of blood vessels in the synovial membranes and attracts leucocytes and lymphocytes to the synovial membrane (Huether and McCance, 1998).

Inflammatory and immune processes result in swelling of the synovial membrane and hypoplastic thickening as the cells proliferate and enlarge abnormally. As synovial inflammation progresses to involve its blood vessels, small venules become occluded by the hypertrophied endothelial cells, fibrin, platelets and inflammatory cells, which decreases vascular flow to the synovial tissue. A compromised circulation, coupled with increased metabolic needs because of hypertrophy and hyperplasia, causes hypoxia and metabolic acidosis. Acidosis stimulates the release of hydrolytic enzymes from synovial cells into the surrounding tissue, initiating the erosion of articular cartilage and inflammation in the supporting ligaments and tendons (Huether and McCance, 1998).

Pharmacological management

It is important to remember that drug treatment is just one component in the total management of the disease (see **Summary Box 1**). The general principle of drug therapy is to use the least number of agents in the lowest effective dosage. Drug regimes must be tailored to the needs of individual patients as indications for a specific drug may vary throughout the course of the disease.

There is no cure for rheumatoid arthritis, therefore the aims of treatment are to reduce inflammation, maintain function and prevent deformities while maintaining quality of life. Successful management requires early diagnosis and aggressive treatment before functional impairment and irreversible joint damage has occurred. The drugs used can be classified into groups (see **Summary Box 2**).

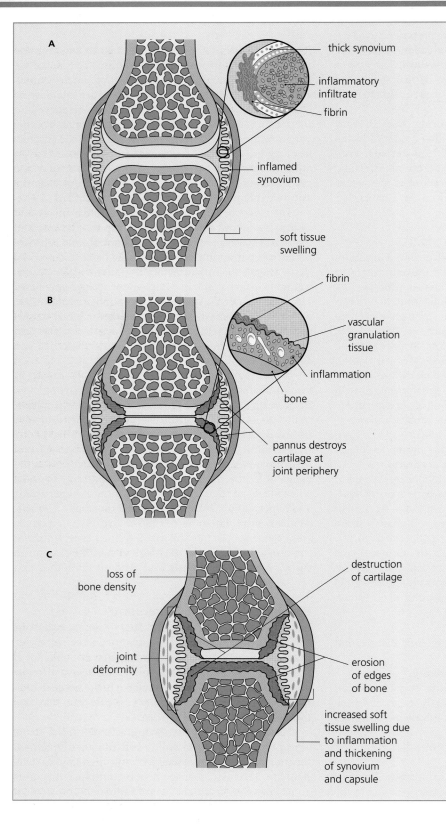

Fig 13.2 Rheumatoid arthritis. (From Stevens & Lowe 1995, with permission.)

A

thick synovium

inflammatory infiltrate

fibrin

inflamed synovium

soft tissue swelling

B

fibrin

vascular granulation tissue

inflammation

bone

pannus destroys cartilage at joint periphery

C

loss of bone density

destruction of cartilage

joint deformity

erosion of edges of bone

increased soft tissue swelling due to inflammation and thickening of synovium and capsule

13.1 PRINCIPLES OF MANAGEMENT OF RHEUMATOID ARTHRITIS

Drug therapy.
Splinting.
Exercises to maintain joint mobility.
Physiotherapy.
Explanation and reassurance.
Home appliances to reduce dependence on others.
Physical treatments such as heat, ice and wax baths.

13.2 DRUGS USED IN THE TREATMENT OF RHEUMATOID ARTHRITIS

Simple analgesics e.g. paracetamol.
Non-steroidal anti-inflammatory drugs e.g. aspirin, indomethacin and ibuprofen.
Pure anti-inflammatory drugs – corticosteroids.
Disease-modifying anti-rheumatic drugs (DMARDs) – gold and penicillamine.
Anti-inflammatory immunosuppressives – azathioprine.
Intra-articular radioactive colloids.

Non-steroidal anti-inflammatory drugs

Group	Examples
Salicylates	Aspirin Benorylate Diflunisal
Propionic acid derivative	Diclofenac Fenbrufen Fenoprofen Ibuprofen Ketoprofen Naproxen
Anthranillic acid	Mefenamic acid
Pyrazolones	Azapropazone Phenylbutazone
Cyclic acetic acids	Etodolac Indomethacin Sulindac
Oxicams	Piroxicam Tenoxicam

Table 13.1 Non-steroidal anti-inflammatory drugs

Simple analgesics

At an early stage in mild rheumatoid arthritis all that may be required to alleviate the pain is a simple analgesic such as paracetamol, dihydrocodeine or buprenorphine. However, these drugs have no anti-inflammatory action so their use is limited.

Non-steroidal anti-inflammatory drugs

There are two main actions of the NSAIDs: an analgesic effect and an anti-inflammatory effect. The analgesic action occurs quickly and recedes within a few hours whereas the anti-inflammatory effect builds up over a period of days and requires regular dosage. This makes NSAIDs particularly useful for the treatment of continuous or regular pain associated with the inflammation of rheumatoid arthritis. There is a large number of NSAIDs to select from. The main groups of NSAIDs are shown in **Table 13.1** and the formulation and side effects of the commonly used NSAIDs in **Table 13.2**. Although the differences in the anti-inflammatory activity is minimal between the various NSAIDs, the differences between individual patient responses may be considerable. The main differences between NSAIDs are in the potency and the incidence and type of side effects. In general, the more potent the drug the greater the incidence of side effects.

It is believed that NSAIDs produce their anti-inflammatory effect by the inhibition of prostaglandin synthesis (**Fig. 13.3**). Prostaglandins are synthesised by virtually every tissue and there are over 20 different naturally occurring prostaglandins, which are widely distributed throughout the body. They are very potent chemicals with a broad range of activities, which include:

• Inhibition of gastric secretion.
• Bronchial relaxation.
• Vasodilator and hypotensive activity.
• Mediation of some aspects of inflammation.
• Contraction of the iris.

The release of prostaglandins may be stimulated by hormones, the nervous system or mechanical damage.

Prostaglandins are formed in the body by the enzymatic oxygenation of arachidonic and linoleic acid by cyclo-oxygenase. Two distinct forms of this enzyme, COX-1 and COX-2, are now recognised. COX-1 is involved in the production of prostaglandins in the gastrointestinal tract, kidneys and platelets. Prostaglandins in the gastrointestinal tract have an important protective role in the maintenance of microvascular integrity, the regulation of cell division and production of mucus. In contrast, COX-2 is involved in the process of inflammation (see **Fig. 13.3**) (Hayllar and Bjarnason, 1995).

In rheumatoid arthritis it appears that control over the balanced production of prostaglandins is lost to some extent, and this results in excessive production of prostaglandins involved in inflammation. The NSAIDs

	The formulation and side effects of the commonly used NSAIDs	
Drug	Formulation	Action / Side effects
Ibuprofen	Tablets, capsules, syrup, granules	A weak anti-inflammatory activity but fewer side effects than others.
Naproxen	Tablets, suspension, suppositories	Often the first choice as it combines good efficacy with a low incidence of side effects.
Diclofenac sodium	Tablets, controlled-release tablets, injection, suppositories	The action and side effects are similar to naproxen.
Indomethacin	Capsules, controlled-release capsules, suspension	Action equal to or superior to that of naproxen, but the incidence of side effects is higher, including headaches, dizziness and gastrointestinal disturbances.
Benorylate	Tablets, suspension	This is a paracetamol-aspirin ester and can be useful for patients experiencing dyspepsia with other NSAIDs. The side effects include tinnitus, dizziness and mental confusion. Care must be taken not to increase the side effects with purchased drugs containing aspirin.
Sulindac	Tablets	Similar in effect to naproxen but does not inhibit renal prostaglandins and therefore may be a safer option for patients with renal impairment.
Fenbrufen	Tablets, effervescent tablets, capsules	Less gastrointestinal bleeding but a high risk of skin rashes.
Ketoprofen	Capsules, controlled-release capsules, suppositories, injection, gel	The controlled-release preparation is claimed to cause less gastrointestinal irritation.

Table 13.2 The formulation and side effects of the commonly used NSAIDs

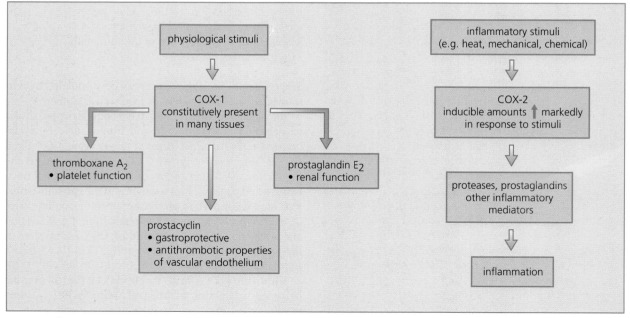

Fig 13.3 The two cyclo-oxygenase isoforms COX-1 and COX-2. (From Page 1997, with permission.)

block the action of the enzyme cyclo-oxygenase, which effectively reduces the synthesis of prostaglandins. The undesirable effects of NSAIDs on the kidneys and gastro-intestinal tract (damage to the gastrointestinal mucosa, peptic erosions and ulceration, gastrointestinal bleeding) are thought to be caused by the inhibition of COX-1, whereas the beneficial anti-inflammatory effects are thought to be attributable to the inhibition of COX-2 (Hayllar and Bjarnason, 1995).

Although it is preferable to avoid them in patients with current or previous gastrointestinal bleeding or ulceration, patients with rheumatoid arthritis are usually dependent on NSAIDs for effective relief of pain and stiffness. The administration of histamine H_2-receptor-blocking drugs or misoprostol may permit the long-term administration of NSAIDs without gastrointestinal problems (**Table 13.3**).

Both diclofenac sodium and naproxen are available in a form combined with misoprostol. **Arthrotec** tablets consist of diclofenac sodium 50 mg and misoprostol 200 µg. **Naprotec** tablets consist of naproxen 500 mg and misoprostol 200 µg. The misoprostol is for prophylaxis against NSAID-induced gastro-duodenal ulceration. The side effects of misoprostol include diarrhoea, nausea, vomiting, flatulence, dyspepsia and abdominal pain, menorrhagia, dizziness and rashes. It is contraindicated in pregnancy or while breast feeding.

Care should be taken when administering NSAIDs to asthmatic patients because one of the side effects of NSAIDs as a result of reduced prostaglandin synthesis is bronchospasm. Some of the important points to take into account when administering NSAIDs to the elderly are outlined in **Box 13.1**.

Meloxicam is a new NSAID that exerts its action by inhibition of cyclo-oxygenases, the enzymes that convert arachidonic acid to prostaglandins (see **Fig. 13.1**). However, it demonstrates a high degree of selectivity for COX-2 inhibition and therefore combines the beneficial effects of NSAIDs with a lowered incidence of the common side effects associated with inhibition of COX-1 (Engelhardt, 1996). The meloxicam dosage for patients with rheumatoid arthritis is a single daily dose of 15 mg (tablets or suppositories), which may be reduced to 7.5 mg daily depending on the therapeutic response.

Aspirin was the traditional first choice anti-inflammatory analgesic for rheumatoid arthritis, but most physicians now prefer to start treatment with another NSAID that may be better tolerated and more convenient for the patient.

In regular high dosage aspirin has about the same anti-inflammatory effect as other NSAIDs. The required dose for active inflammatory joint disease is at least 3.6 g daily. There is little anti-inflammatory effect with less than 3 g daily. Gastrointestinal side effects such as nausea, dyspepsia, gastric ulceration and bleeding may occur with any dose of aspirin but anti-inflammatory doses are associated with a much higher risk of these side effects. Anti-inflammatory

Drugs administered to prevent the gastrointestinal side effects of NSAIDs	
Drug	Action
Misoprostol	This drug is a synthetic prostaglandin analogue. It inhibits gastric acid secretion, protects the gastroduodenal mucosa, and increases bicarbonate and mucus production.
H_2-receptor antagonists (cimetidine, ranitidine famotidine nizatidine)	These drugs reduce gastric acid output as a result of H_2-receptor blockade and therefore prevent the development of or heal gastric or duodenal ulceration.

Table 13.3 Drugs administered to prevent the gastrointestinal side effects of NSAIDs

13.1 THE ADMINISTRATION OF NSAIDS TO THE ELDERLY WITH ARTHRITIS

Because of the increased susceptibility of the elderly to the side effects of NSAIDs the following recommendations are made:

For osteoarthritis measures such as weight reduction, heat, exercise and use of aids should be tried first.

For osteoarthritis and rheumatoid arthritis avoid giving an NSAID unless paracetamol administered alone, or with a low-dose opioid analgesic, has failed to relieve the pain adequately.

When a paracetamol preparation has failed to relieve the pain adequately a very low dose of an NSAID (generally ibuprofen) can be added.

If an NSAID is considered necessary the patient must be monitored carefully for 4 weeks for gastrointestinal bleeding. This also applies when changing the patient from one NSAID to another.

Two NSAIDs should not be administered simultaneously.

doses of aspirin may also lead to the development of mild chronic salicylate intoxication (salicylism), characterised by dizziness, tinnitus and deafness.

Corticosteroids

Corticosteroids are undoubtedly the most powerful agents in suppressing the inflammation of arthritis but, because of the side effects associated with their long-term use and because of disease rebound upon withdrawal, they are reserved for:

- Patients unresponsive to other treatments.
- The elderly with very active disease.
- When rapid relief is required in younger patients before slower acting drugs begin to work.

Also there is little evidence that corticosteroids affect the ultimate course of rheumatoid disease, including joint destruction.

Corticosteroids can be administered orally or by intravenous or intra-articular injection. For oral administration, soluble or enteric-coated prednisolone is usually the drug of choice; the smallest dose (e.g. 5–10 mg/day) that produces a beneficial effect is given. Large bolus doses (e.g. methylprednisolone up to 1 g on 3 consecutive days) can be given intravenously. This form of steroid therapy is used to suppress highly active inflammatory disease and is only given to patients commencing disease-modifying anti-rheumatic drugs; it has no place in the routine management of the disease. It appears to shorten the time taken to achieve a response from the disease-modifying drugs.

Intra-articular injections of corticosteroids are given to relieve pain, prevent recurrent effusion, increase mobility and reduce deformity in one or a few joints. Hydrocortisone acetate or triamcinolone hexacetonide are commonly prescribed, the dose depending upon the size of the joint. Stringent aseptic precautions are required to minimise the risk of septic arthritis. Although most peripheral joints can be so treated, this therapy should only be considered when one or two joints are actively inflamed and others are under good control from general treatment.

Deflazacort is a newly introduced corticosteroid with a high glucocorticoid activity; it is derived from prednisolone. It is recommended for use in diabetic patients who require steroid treatment for rheumatoid arthritis because it has a less adverse effect on glucose metabolism in that it does not produce a significant deterioration in blood glucose tolerance by increasing hepatic production and decreasing peripheral utilisation of glucose. Initially, in an acute situation the dose may be up to 120 mg daily, with a maintenance dose of 3–18 mg daily.

Deflazocort may also be recommended for postmenopausal women because it is claimed to reduce the incidence of osteoporosis caused by a decrease in bone reabsorption. It has been reported that deflazacort is less suppressive on the intestinal absorption of calcium and it minimises the secondary hyperparathyroidism and hypercalciuria characteristic of patients receiving glucocorticoid therapy (Osvaldo *et al.*, 1992).

A double-blind study of deflazacort and prednisolone was carried out in patients with chronic inflammatory disorders (Gray *et al.*, 1991). Deflazacort was found to be an effective anti-inflammatory corticosteroid with a therapeutic potency 83% that of prednisolone. However, it was less effective than prednisolone in stimulating daily calcium loss and inhibiting endogenous cortisol secretion.

Please refer to Chapter 3 for a detailed account of the action and side effects of steroids.

Disease-modifying anti-rheumatic drugs

Disease-modifying anti-rheumatic drugs (DMARDs) include penicillamine, gold salts, chloroquine, hydrochloroquine and sulphasalazine, and are drugs that may suppress the disease process in rheumatoid arthritis. The indications for this type of more specific anti-rheumatic treatment are:
- Progressive disease.
- Troublesome extra-articular problems.
- Failure of NSAIDs to control symptoms.
- Excessive corticosteroid requirements.

The current trend is to use these drugs very early in the treatment of rheumatoid arthritis with the aim of controlling the disease process before structural damage appears in the joints. The characteristics of long-term suppressive therapy are:
- A slow action – these drugs only start to work after 4–6 weeks and take 6 months to produce their full effect. For this reason treatment with NSAIDs should be continued for 2–3 months.
- An improvement in joint symptoms is accompanied by a fall in the erythrocyte sedimentation rate and the titre of rheumatoid factor.
- Very effective suppression or complete remission of the disease can be achieved, delaying or preventing joint destruction.

The exact anti-inflammatory mechanism of **gold therapy (sodium aurothiomalate)** is unknown, but these drugs appear to suppress the synovitis of the acute stage of rheumatoid disease. Proposed mechanisms of action include inhibition of prostaglandin synthesis, inhibition of various enzyme systems, suppression of the phagocytic action of macrophages and leucocytes and alteration of the immune response (McKenry and Salerno, 1995). Gold salts bind to the products of the immune response such as immunoglobulins and complement and in doing so may modify the autoimmune process that underlies rheumatoid arthritis.

Sodium aurothiomalate is administered weekly by deep intramuscular injection. The initial dose is 10 mg and this can be slowly increased to 50 mg weekly and continued until a remission occurs or until a total dose of 1 g has been given. After remission, 20–50 mg may be given every 2–4 weeks for many months. Blood and urine tests are essential after each injection because two of the serious side effects of the drug include renal toxicity and blood dyscrasias such as agranulocytosis, thrombocytopenia and aplastic anaemia. Other possible serious side effects include skin eruptions and pulmonary fibrosis. The early side effects that may precede the more life-threatening side effects are a dry cough or progressive breathlessness, a metallic taste in the mouth, a painful mouth or tongue, mouth ulcers, bleeding gums and nose bleeds.

Penicillamine is a chelating agent for heavy metals such as mercury, lead, copper and iron. The metals are made more soluble so that they can be readily excreted by the kidneys. The mechanism of action of penicillamine as an anti-rheumatic agent is unknown. It has been proposed that penicillamine may improve lymphocyte function. It also reduces the level of rheumatoid factor (antibody) and immune complexes located in the serum and synovial fluid, but overall it does not significantly reduce the absolute levels of serum immunoglobulins. The relationship of these effects to rheumatoid arthritis is unknown (McKenry and Salerno, 1995).

The initial adult dosage is 125–250 mg per day and this is gradually increased until a reponse is obtained. Usually the required dose is in the range of 500–750 mg per day, although the response may take several weeks to develop. After maintaining patients on these high doses for several months it is often possible to reduce the maintenance dose without loss of effect. Penicillamine should never be given to patients who are already receiving gold treatment or anti-malarial treatment. The side effects of this drug include headache, sore throat, fever, skin rash, nausea, pruritis, muscle and joint pain and altered taste sensitivity. Routine checks of white cell and platelet counts and urine tests for albumin should be performed at weekly intervals because the more serious side effects of penicillamine include leucopenia, agranulocytosis, thrombocytopenia, proteinuria and nephrotic syndrome.

As the mode of action of these drugs is unknown it is impossible to predict which patient will respond to a particular compound. It may be necessary to try several. The most effective drug in this category is penicillamine. Hydroxychloroquine, sulphasalazine and auranofin are less effective but safer. Intramuscular gold is as effective as penicillamine but because of the inconvenience of injections and the frequency of side effects, which produce a low ultimate success rate, it is less frequently used (**Table 13.4**).

Sulphasalazine is an anti-inflammatory agent that can be used as a disease-modifying agent in the treatment of rheumatoid arthritis. It is a combination of two drugs: an anti-inflammatory salicylic acid derivative and an anti-infective sulphonamide derivative, sulphapyridine. More information about this drug can be found in **Table 13.4**.

Immunosuppressive drugs

When used in rheumatoid arthritis, immunosuppressants are useful alternatives in patients who have failed to respond to the more specific anti-rheumatic drugs such as gold or penicillamine. The theory of their use for this purpose is to reduce the body's autoimmune response to its own tissue. If the rheumatoid antibodies can be suppressed there is reason to hope that the disease process can be controlled; cytotoxic drugs such as azathioprine, methotrexate, cyclosporin and cyclophosphamide, which are active against lymphocytes (antibody-forming cells), have proved useful.

Drugs used in long-term suppressive therapy for rheumatoid arthritis			
Drug	**Formulation**	**Dose**	**General information**
Auranofin (oral gold)	Tablets, 3 mg	3 mg twice daily. The dose can be increased to 9 mg daily if there is no response at 6 months on 6 mg	Less effective but safer than injectable gold. It exhibits similar side effects to the injectable form. The most common side effect is diarrhoea.
Chloroquine	Tablets, syrup, injection	150 mg daily	The action is similar to gold and penicillamine but is better tolerated. The use is limited by ocular toxicity. Corneal opacities, reversible on discontinuation of therapy, have been reported in 20–40% of patients. Retinopathy, linked to the size of the daily dose, may occur. All patients should have a full ophthalmic examination before commencement of treatment and subsequently at regular intervals. Other side effects include gastrointestinal disturbances, depigmentation, skin reactions and loss of hair.
Hydroxychloroquine	Tablets	400 mg daily initially; a maintenance dose of 200–400 mg	
Sulphasalazine	Enteric coated tablets	Initially 500 mg daily; maximum 2–3 g daily	The effectiveness is similar to gold and penicillamine. The side effects are also similar but include mild depression and male infertility. Full blood counts and liver function tests are required throughout therapy. Allergy is common and sulphasalazine should not be given to patients allergic to sulphonamides or aspirin. Discolours urine and may stain soft contact lenses yellow.

Table 13.4 Drugs used in long-term suppressive therapy for rheumatoid arthritis

Azathioprine is often the drug of choice. Azathioprine incorporates itself into the normal production pathway for purine nucleotides, which form the building blocks of DNA and RNA. These substances are vital to the synthesis of such cells as lymphocytes. Thus when azathioprine incorporates itself into the normal pathway for the production of DNA and RNA, it creates a faulty end product that results in a cell that cannot function in the normal immune response.

It is usually given in a dosage of 1.5–2.5 mg/kg daily in divided doses. The patient requires regular blood counts to detect possible neutropenia and/or thrombocytopenia, which are usually resolved by reducing the dosage. Nausea, vomiting and diarrhoea may occur, usually starting early during the course of treatment, and may ultimately necessitate the withdrawal of the drug; herpes zoster infection may also occur.

Methotrexate is also effective in the treatment of rheumatoid arthritis. It acts by inhibiting the enzyme dihydrofolate reductase, which converts folic acid into its biologically active form, folinic acid, which is needed for cell growth and reproduction. It is usually given in an initial dose of 2.5 mg once a week, increased slowly to a maximum dosage of 15–20 mg once a week subject to the results of regular blood tests and liver function tests.

Cyclosporin is now licensed for severe active rheumatoid arthritis when conventional therapy is ineffective or inappropriate. There is evidence that cyclosporin may retard the rate of the erosive process. Cyclosporin is a fungal metabolite and potent immunosuppressant that is virtually non-myelotoxic but is markedly nephrotoxic. It acts on human T lymphocytes, which undergo a complex change during the development of the normal immune response.

A typical dosage is 2.5–5 mg/kg daily in two divided doses. Cyclosporin is contraindicated in rheumatoid arthritis patients who have abnormal renal function, uncontrolled hypertension or infection or malignancy. The serum creatinine levels must be measured at least twice before the commencement of treatment and monitored every 2 weeks for the first 3 months of treatment and then every 4 weeks, or more frequently if the patient is receiving concomitant NSAIDs. Hepatic function must also be monitored if the patient is receiving concomitant NSAIDs.

Cyclophosphamide is a member of the nitrogen mustard group. It is converted by the liver to a number of highly reactive metabolites that interfere with the enzyme systems essential for cell growth. It may be used at a dose of 1–1.5 mg/kg daily for rheumatoid arthritis with severe systemic manifestations. It is a toxic drug and regular blood counts should be carried out.

JUVENILE CHRONIC ARTHRITIS

Juvenile chronic arthritis (JCA) is a generic term that covers several overlapping conditions, including Still's disease (systemic JCA), pauciarticular JCA and polyarticular-onset JCA. The aim of the treatment of JCA is to achieve a state in which the child can live at home with minimal residual joint deformity. Daily exercises are important and night splints are used during the acute phase of the disease. Drugs form only part of the treatment

Pathophysiology

The basic pathophysiology of JCA is the same as that of adult rheumatoid arthritis. However, JCA has three distinct modes of onset: arthritis in fewer than five joints (oligoarthritis), arthritis in more than five joints (polyarthritis) and systemic disease. Juvenile chronic arthritis affects primarily the large joints, and subluxation and ankylosis of the cervical spine are common.

Pharmacological management

Aspirin usually controls the fever and pain, reduces the inflammation and is therefore often the drug of choice. However, because of the association with Reye's syndrome, the prescription must be licensed by the paediatric consultant responsible for the child. It is given at approximately 90 mg/kg body weight per day in divided doses. This

---

PERSON CENTRED STUDY 1

Mrs Jane Arthur, aged 52 years, is an insulin-dependent diabetic who has suffered from rheumatoid arthritis for 6 years. For the first 5 years after diagnosis she was treated successfully with an NSAID, naproxen, which she combined with mistoprostol. Throughout this period she remained active and was able to continue working as a shop assistant in the local supermarket. Over the past 6 months, however, the rheumatiod arthritis has become progressively worse and the naproxen is failing to control the symptoms. Jane is finding it increasingly difficult to continue with her job. After a consultation with the rheumatologist, Jane was prescribed auranofin (gold salts).

1. Explain why until recently naproxen was an effective form of treatment for Jane's rheumatoid arthritis.
2. Why did Jane have to continue to take the naproxen for 3 months after commencing the gold therapy?
3. What side effects may Jane experience as a result of taking the auranofin?
4. Why do you think corticosteriods may be contraindicated in the treatment of Jane's rheumatoid arthritis?

produces a blood salicylate level of about 25 mg/100 ml. Blood levels should be monitored regularly and the child observed for signs of toxicity, overbreathing, drowsiness or vomiting.

Non-steroidal anti-inflammatory drugs such as naproxen may be preferred to reduce the pain and inflammation because of the side effects associated with the administration of aspirin in children. The dosage is 10 mg/kg daily in two divided doses. The actions of NSAIDs are discussed on page 233.

Gold and **penicillamine** may be prescribed if the disease progresses (pages 236–237). For a child the initial dose of penicillamine is 50 mg daily given before food for 1 month. This dosage is then increased at 4-week intervals to a maintenance dose of 15–20 mg/kg daily. Oral gold therapy (auranofin) is not recommended for children but sodium aurothiomalate can be administered by deep intramuscular injection. Children may be given 1 mg/kg of sodium aurothiomalate weekly to a maximum of 50 mg weekly, the intervals being gradually increased to 4 weeks according to the response; an initial test dose is given corresponding to between one-tenth and one-fifth of the calculated dose.

Corticosteroids are rarely used in the treatment of this disease as they do not influence the ultimate prognosis or prevent complications, and can cause alarming iatrogenic effects that cannot be justified in a disease with a good prognosis. They may, however, be indicated in severe systemic disease, chronic iridocyclitis that does not respond to local steroids and progressive disease that is resistant to other drugs. Alternate day dosage is preferred; this allows for some skeletal growth and does not suppress growth spurts, sexual maturation or reaction to stress.

Deflazacort is effective in controlling disease activity in children with JCA who are receiving long-term steroid therapy. In contrast to prednisolone, it allows lumbar spine mineral growth to occur appropriately in relation to somatic growth, against the background of variable growth impairment that inevitably occurs in JCA (Loftus *et al.*, 1993).

Children receiving steroid therapy will require annual physical and developmental checks. Refer to Chapter 3 for a full account of the action and side effects of steroids.

INFECTIVE ARTHRITIS

Arthritis may arise from direct infection of joints by microorganisms, or as a reaction to a preceding infection. Infection must be considered in all cases of acute arthritis, particularly when only one joint is affected. A delay in treatment may lead to permanent joint damage or septicaemia (Souhami and Moxham, 1990). If its presence is suspected, synovial fluid will need to be obtained for culture. The two forms of infective arthritis considered in this section are septic arthritis and Lyme arthritis.

SEPTIC ARTHRITIS

Septic arthritis is the result of bloodborne spread from a focus of infection elsewhere. It is a form of infective arthritis that results from infection of the joints with pyogenic organisms, of which *Staphylococcus aureus* is the most common. It can also be caused by other types of staphylococci, streptococci, *Neisseria* or Gram-negative bacilli.

Pathophysiology

Organisms reach the joint in septic arthritis via the bloodstream, sometimes from an identifiable site of infection such as otitis media or a boil. Less commonly, infection spreads from osteomyelitis adjacent to the joint, or the organism is introduced directly as a result of trauma, surgery or intra-articular injection. Septic arthritis particularly occurs at the extremes of life and in immunologically compromised individuals.

Pharmacological management

Antibiotic therapy should be started immediately the diagnosis is made, as cartilage destruction can occur within a few days of the onset of joint infection. The choice of antibiotic will depend upon the organism concerned. However, 'blind' therapy should commence immediately with a slow intravenous infusion of flucloxacillin, 500 mg every 6 hours, together with clindamycin, 300 mg intravenously every 6 hours, or Fucidic acid, 500 mg by mouth every 8 hours. Flucloxacillin is a bactericidal antibiotic that interferes with bacterial cell wall synthesis. Clindamycin has a bacteriostatic action, in that it inhibits further growth and multiplication of bacterial microorganisms. Fucidic acid is an antibiotic that has been found to be particularly effective against staphylococcal infections. It is good at penetrating most tissues, including bone.

Changes in therapy can be made once the sensitivities of the offending organisms are known. Drug concentrations within the joint are generally adequate when antibiotics are given systemically, and intra-articular therapy is not required. The joint should also be splinted. The more specific types of bacterial arthritis are listed below:

- Gonococcal arthritis. The most common pattern of joint involvement is a migratory polyarthritis associated with tenosynovitis, with the synovitis localising in one or two joints. Penicillin remains the treatment of choice and generally benzylpenicillin is given intravenously until there is a clinical response. Occasionally the infection is caused by strains of gonococci resistant to penicillin and cephaloridine. For such patients spectinomycin, a bacteriostatic antibiotic, or the cephalosporins, a group of antibiotics with a bactericidal action, should be given.
- Meningococcal arthritis usually occurs as part of a generalised meningococcal septicaemia. It is a migratory polyarthritis and organisms cannot generally be isolated from the joint. Treatment is with penicillin.
- Tuberculous arthritis. Only about 1% of all patients with tuberculosis have skeletal involvement; of these, approximately 50% have spinal disease, 30% infection of hips or knees and 20% infection of other joints, particularly the sacroiliac joints. Treatment is with anti-tuberculous therapy.

LYME ARTHRITIS

This is a form of infective arthritis caused by a spiral bacterium, *Borrelia bungdorferi*, which is transmitted by the bite of infected body lice or ticks.

Pathophysiology

The disease characteristically begins around the bitten site as a typical red skin lesion, termed erythema chronicum migrans, with about one-half the cases also showing multiple, annular expanding secondary lesions. The arthritis develops typically weeks or months after the initial infection, commonly in the knee or other large joints and temporomandibular joints.

Pharmacological management

Tetracyclines are the recommended drugs for the treatment of Lyme disease and early treatment prevents joint involvement and the systemic complications. The tetracycline group of antibiotics have a broad spectrum of activity and are bacteriostatic. The mechanism of action is by interfering with the synthesis of proteins necessary for growth and division of bacterial cells. The dosage will depend on the specific drug within the tetracycline group.

ANKYLOSING SPONDYLITIS

Ankylosing spondylitis is a relatively uncommon chronic inflammatory joint disease characterised by stiffening and fusion (ankylosis) of the spine and sacroiliac joints. It is a systemic, immune inflammatory disease. The cause of ankylosing spondylitis is unknown, but the disease is strongly associated with the presence of histocompatability antigen HLA-B27 on the chromosomes of affected individuals, suggesting a genetic predisposition.

Pathophysiology

Ankylosing spondylitis begins with inflammation of the fibrocartilage in cartilaginous joints, primarily the vertebrae. The fibrous tissue of the joint capsule, the cartilage that surrounds the intervertebral discs, the entheses (the ligamentous attachment to bone), and periosteum are infiltrated by inflammatory cells. As inflammatory cells, macrophages and lymphocytes infiltrate and erode bone and fibrocartilage in joint structures, repair begins with the proliferation of fibroblasts, which synthesise and secrete collagen. The collagen becomes organised into fibrous scar tissue that eventually undergoes calcification and ossification. Over time, all the cartilaginous structures of the joint are replaced by ossified scar tissue, causing the joint to fuse and lose flexibility (McCance and Huether, 1998).

The earliest changes are often in the sacroiliac joints, and the resulting sacroileitis often produces the first symptoms of pelvic and back pain, with pain in the buttocks often radiating down both legs. The lesions strongly associated with ankylosing spondylitis are:

- Chronic inflammatory changes in the entheses, progressing to bone alkylosis.
- Peripheral polyarthritis; the joints of the lower limbs are particularly affected.
- Anterior uveitis affecting the iris and ciliary body of the eye.
- Aortic incompetence.
- Inflammatory bowel disease.

In all but the mild cases there is progressive limitation of spinal movement over the course of a few years. In severe cases the spine becomes completely fused.

Pharmacological management

A long-term programme of active mobilisation in combination with anti-inflammatory drug therapy is the mainstay of treatment. An exercise programme is essential to maintain movement, relieve symptoms and prevent deformity, particularly kyphosis.

Non-steroidal anti-inflammatory drugs are a very effective treatment for this condition, with slow-release indomethacin, 75 mg given at night, often being the best choice. It is particularly useful in relieving pain at night and morning stiffness. Other NSAIDs that may be prescribed for this condition are piroxicam and fenbrufen. The action of NSAIDs are discussed in Chapter 18.

Sulphasalazine (see **Table 13.4**) is useful as a long-term suppressive drug in the more severe cases.

Azathioprine (page 238) may be useful in the treatment of peripheral arthritis but not for spondylitis.

GOUT

Gout is a metabolic disorder in which there is an increase in the amount of uric acid in the body; the resulting deposition of urate crystals in joints and other tissues produces a painful inflammatory response. The increased production of uric acid may result from increased cell turnover, for example in tumours, or a decrease in the renal excretion of uric acid, or both. **Summary Box 3** lists certain drugs that may precipitate an attack of gout.

13.3 DRUGS CAUSING HYPERURICAEMIA AND GOUT

Thiazide and loop diuretics can precipitate an attack of gout by inhibiting the tubular secretion of uric acid. Aspirin in low doses inhibits the tubular secretion of uric acid.

Cytotoxic drugs causing a high rate of cell death may increase purine production with a consequent increase in the production of uric acid, which may result in an acute attack of gout.

Pathophysiology

The pathophysiology of gout is closely linked to purine metabolism and kidney function. Uric acid is a breakdown product of purine (nucleic acid) metabolism. Most uric acid is excreted by the kidneys. In the blood, most uric acid is in the form of monosodium urate. In patients with gout the monosodium concentration may be very high, forming a supersaturated solution, thus risking urate crystal deposition in the tissue, which causes:
• Tophi (subcutaneous nodular deposits of urate crystals).
• Synovitis and arthritis.
• Renal disease and calculi.

The exact process by which crystals of monosodium urate are deposited in the joints and induce gouty arthritis are unknown. However, several mechanisms may be involved:
• Monosodium urate precipitates at the periphery of the body, where lower body temperatures may reduce its solubility.
• Decreased albumin levels cause a decrease in urate solubility.
• Changes in ion concentration and decreases of pH may enhance urate deposition.
• Trauma may promote urate crystal precipitation (McCance and Huether, 1998).

Gout most commonly affects the metatarsophalangeal joint of the first toe. The onset of gout is sudden and manifests as an acute inflammatory monoarthritis and the affected joint or joints are warm, tender and extremely painful. There may be an associated pyrexia, and the white cell count and erythrocyte sedimentation rate are generally raised.

Pharmacological management

Treatment of acute gout is with NSAIDs. Indomethacin is generally the drug of choice at a dose of 50 mg three or four times daily, which should produce substantial relief within 24–48 hours. The dose should then be reduced to 25 mg three or four times daily. The attack should resolve completely within a few weeks. Other anti-inflammatory drugs can be used in the management of acute attacks such as azapropazone (standard dose 600 mg twice daily), diclofenac, naproxen and ketoprofen. The action and side effects of NSAIDs are discussed earlier in this Chapter and in Chapter 18.

Colchinine is specific and effective in gout. It has a prophylactic, suppressive effect that helps to reduce the incidence of acute gouty attacks. It interferes with the uptake of uric acid crystals by the white cells in gouty joints. The result is a rapid reduction in the inflammation and the symptom of pain is relieved. Colchinine is administered orally and is rapidly absorbed from the gastrointestinal tract. However, the use of oral colchinine is very limited by the frequent occurrence of side effects such as nausea,

abdominal pain and diarrhoea, which may necessitate the withdrawal of treatment. The oral dose is 1 mg initially followed by 500 µg every 2–3 hours until relief of pain is obtained, or vomiting or diarrhoea occurs or until a total dose of 10 mg has been reached. The course should not be repeated within 3 days. It is important to remember that aspirin and salicylates should not be prescribed as they induce hyperuricaemia.

Long-term management

A single attack of gout does not justify preventative treatment. Simple measures to reduce uric acid levels in such patients include:
• Weight loss in obese patients.
• Reduction in alcohol intake.
• Avoidance of food and drinks containing high levels of purine, e.g. game and lager.
• A good fluid intake
• Review of the need for salicylates and thiazide diuretics, which cause hyperuricaemia.

The indications for long-term therapy include recurrent attacks, tophi or chronic gouty arthritis and renal disease; it is also given in the long-term for prophylaxis when treating malignant disease. The long-term management and prophylaxis of gout can be achieved in two ways: blocking the production of uric acid by the administration of a xanthine oxidase inhibitor such as allopurinol, and increasing the rate of excretion of uric acid by the administration of a uricoscuric drug such as probencid or sulphinpyrazone (**Fig. 13.4**).

Allopurinol acts by inhibiting one of the enzymes that takes part in the production of uric acid from its constituent chemicals and therefore reduces the total amount of uric acid produced. Treatment with allopurinol should not be commenced until 4 weeks after the last acute attack as it may precipitate another attack. Also when allopurinol treatment is commenced the blood urate level is likely to fall. It has been found that any change in blood urate level may lead to an acute attack of gout. To prevent this a prophylactic anti-inflammatory or colchinine should be prescribed concomitantly for the first 3 months.

Allopurinol is given orally, the usual dose being 300 mg daily, which should be sufficient to bring the serum urate down to normal levels. For patients with renal disease the dose is 100 mg daily. It is well tolerated and side effects are uncommon but it may cause a skin rash, in which case it should be withdrawn and only re-introduced with caution.

Probencid acts directly on the kidney tubules and promotes the excretion of uric acid and urate from these tubules. This drug should be commenced at low dosage, usually 250 mg twice daily, in order not to overload the excreted urine with acid. This can be aided by increasing the fluid intake to a minimum of 2 l daily and neutralising

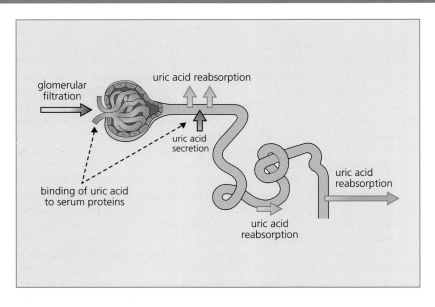

Fig 13.4 Uric acid secretion and reabsorption in the kidney. (From Page 1997, with permission.)

the acidic urine with potassium citrate or sodium bicarbonate mixtures. The dosage is increased after the first week to 500 mg twice daily. Up to 2 g per day may be given in 2–4 divided doses when necessary, with a subsequent reduction if the serum uric acid can be maintained at a normal range. Side effects are infrequent but occasionally include anorexia, nausea, vomiting, headache and frequency of micturition. More rarely, allergic reactions to this drug may occur; these include anaphylactic shock, dermatitis, pruritis, fever and sore gums.

Probencid may also precipitate an acute attack of gout at the onset of treatment, therefore it is common practice to administer concurrent therapy with an anti-inflammatory drug at the beginning of treatment. **It should be noted** that aspirin blocks the effect of probencid and therefore it should not be taken in addition to the prescribed medication.

Sulphinpyrazone increases the urinary excretion of uric acid. The initial dosage is 100–200 mg daily, taken with meals or milk, as sulphinpyrazone may occasionally produce gastrointestinal upset and gastric bleeding. The dosage is gradually increased over 1 week until the daily dose of 600 mg is reached. After the blood urate concentration has been controlled the maintenance dose may be reduced to as low as 200 mg/day.

BONE DISORDERS

Bones give form to the body, support tissues and permit movement by providing points of attachment for muscles. Many bones meet in moveable joints that determine the type and extent of movement possible. Bones protect many of the body's vital organs: the bones of the skull protect the brain; the thoracic cage, the heart and lungs and the bones of the pelvis, the reproductive and urinary organs.

PERSON CENTRED STUDY 2

Mr James Rudge, aged 59 years, has been diagnosed with acute gout. Mr Rudge is employed as a lorry driver for a road haulage company. He takes very little exercise, enjoys his food and likes to spend his spare time in the pub drinking lager with his friends. Consequently for a man of his height (5 feet 8 inches), at 17 stones, he is very overweight. Mr Rudge was diagnosed as having mild hypertension 6 months earlier, for which his GP prescribed bendrofluazide, 2.5 mg daily.

Mr Rudge is prescribed a 4-day course of indomethacin, 50 mg, four times daily for the gout.

Over the next 4 months Mr Rudge experiences recurrent attacks of gout, for which he is prescribed allopurinol, 300 mg daily.

1. What information should Mr Rudge be given about the possible side effects of indomethacin?
2. What advice should be given to Mr Rudge to reduce his uric acid levels and hopefully prevent further attacks?
3. The GP changes the prescription for hypertension to enalapril, 5 mg daily. Why is this change necessary?
4. Why is Mr Rudge also prescribed a further course of indomethacin?

The marrow cavities within certain bones serve as sites of blood cell formation. In adults, blood cells originate exclusively in marrow cavities of the skull, vertebrae, ribs, sternum, shoulders and pelvis. Bones also have a crucial role in mineral homeostasis, storing calcium, phosphate, carbonate and magnesium, the minerals that are essential for the proper working of many delicate cellular mechanisms. The exchange of calcium between bone and plasma is 10–15 mmol daily and over 1 year 20% of bone calcium is exchanged. Therefore minor imbalances in control of the remodelling processes can lead to substantial changes in bone mass or mineralisation over the years.

Bone forms 25% of the weight of a normal adult. Although the major growth is in childhood, in the adult bone is not a static framework; there is a continuous process of bone remodelling, with bone formation by osteoblasts and bone reabsorption by osteoclasts.

OSTEOMYELITIS

Osteomyelitis is the result of a bacterial infection of bone. The commonest causative organisms are *S. aureus*, *Mycobacterium tuberculosis*, *Escherichia coli*, pneumococcus or group A streptococcus.

Pathophysiology

The pathological features of bone infection are similar to those in any other body tissue. The invading pathogen initially provokes an intense inflammatory response that is characterised by vascular engorgement, oedema, leucocyte activity and abscess formation in the metaphysis of the bone, the section of the shaft immediately adjacent to the epiphyseal plate. The rich capillary network and large venous channels in this area may favour the deposition of circulating microorganisms and their subsequent growth.

Because of the accumulation of debris caused by infection, the periosteum may separate and form a shell of new bone around the infected portion of the shaft. Lifting of the periosteum disrupts blood vessels that enter bone through the periosteum, which deprives the underlying bone of its blood supply; this leads to necrosis and death of the area of bone infected, producing sequestrum, an area of devitalised bone. Lifting the periosteum also stimulates an intense osteoblastic response. Osteoblasts lay down a layer of new bone that can partially or completely surround the infected bone, called an involucrum.

Pharmacological management

The treatment of osteomyelitis is with immobilisation and antibiotic therapy or, in the case of tuberculous osteomyelitis, antitubercular drugs. (The actions of antitubercular drugs are discussed in Chapter 5 *Drugs and immunological disorders*). Wherever possible a precise bacteriological diagnosis must be made and treatment continued for several weeks. Most patients experience localised bone pain and therefore require appropriate analgesic therapy for pain relief.

NEOPLASTIC BONE DISEASES

Many different types of bone tumour involve the skeleton. Bone tumours may originate from bone cells, cartilage, fibrous tissue, marrow or vascular tissue. The malignant tumours of bone are shown in **Table 13.5**. The most common tumours are metastases from the bronchus, breast and prostate. The symptoms experienced are usually related to the anatomical position of the tumour, with local bone pain over the area. Systemic symptoms, including malaise, pyrexia and aches and pains occur, and are sometimes related to the hypercalcaemia.

The general pathological features of bone tumours include bone destruction, erosion or expansion of the cortex and the periosteal response to the changes in the underlying bone. Benign bone tumours, because they usually have a symmetric controlled growth pattern, tend to compress and displace neighbouring normal bone tissue, which weakens the bone structure until it is incapable of withstanding the stress of ordinary use, leading to a pathological fracture. Malignant tumours invade adjacent normal bone tissue by producing substances that promote reabsorption by increasing osteoclast activity or by interfering with the blood supply to the bone.

The treatment is usually symptomatic, with analgesics and anti-inflammatory drugs. Local radiotherapy over bony metastases may, however, be the best way of relieving pain. Depending on the tumour, cytotoxic chemotherapy is occasionally helpful. Some tumours are hormone dependent and a remission can be obtained by hormone therapy.

OSTEOSARCOMA

This is a highly malignant primary bone neoplasm. It is the most prevalent bone tumour in the first two decades of life. The tumour occurs primarily in the long bones of the extremities.

Pathophysiology

Osteosarcoma is a malignant bone-forming tumour. Osteosarcomas usually arise in the epiphyseal region of

Malignant neoplasms of bone	
Metastases (osteolytic)	Bronchus Breast Prostate Thyroid Kidney
Multiple myeloma	
Primary bone tumours	Osteosarcomas Fibrosarcomas Chondromas Ewing's tumour

Table 13.5 Malignant neoplasms of bone

243

long bones and consist of malignant osteoblasts, which make osteoid. Typically the tumour may also contain chondroid (cartilage) and fibrinoid tissue, which may form the bulk of the tumour. The osteoid is deposited in thick masses between the trabeculae of callus, which infiltrate the normal compact bone, destroy it, and replace it with dense callus and masses of osteoid. Bone tissue produced by osteosarcomas never matures into compact bone. Local invasion occurs when the tumour breaks through the bone and the periosteal surroundings and invades soft tissues, including the nerves and blood vessels around the joint.

Pharmacological management

The use of cytotoxic drugs has contributed to improving the survival rate for this cancer. Chemotherapy is given as the initial treatment before surgery, using a combination of cytotoxic drugs.

The optimum drug combination and best overall treatment times are determined by controlled trials. Modern adjuvant programmes typically use cisplatin, doxorubicin and high-dose methotrexate. Ifosfamide is also active. Chemotherapy is given at intervals of 3–4 weeks, and at least three cycles are given before surgery. The resultant shrinking of the tumour may make it possible for the surgeon to resect the tumour and replace the removed bone with a metal prosthesis, so retaining the limb. Chemotherapy is continued postoperatively.

Cisplatin is a cytotoxic agent that contains platinum bound in an organic complex. The action is linked with drug-induced changes in DNA structure that inhibit cell development. The doses are highly variable and dependent on local treatment protocols and also on whether the patient is receiving concomitant therapy.

All patients treated with this drug suffer from anorexia, nausea and vomiting. Bone marrow suppression may occur, leading to anaemia, haemorrhage caused by thrombocytopenia and infection as a result of suppression of white cell function. Cisplatin is particularly nephrotoxic and a progressive fall in renal function may occur. Other side effects include tinnitus, hearing loss, peripheral neuropathy and abnormal liver and cardiac function. Anaphylactic reaction may occur within minutes of drug administration.

Doxorubicin is an anthracycline antibiotic that is used in oncological practice for its cytotoxic effects. It inhibits the division of cells, particularly those of rapidly multiplying malignant tumours. The drug is administered intravenously but the doses are highly variable and depend on local treatment protocols and the use of concomitant therapy. The drug is extremely caustic and must be given in a fast-running infusion to prevent severe local effects.

An important side effect peculiar to this type of antibiotic is its cardiotoxicity. Initially tachycardia develops but this can progress to gross cardiomyopathy, resulting in cardiac failure and death. Bone marrow suppression produces anaemia, leucopenia and thrombocytopenia with a resultant increased risk of severe infection and haemorrhage. Gastrointestinal side effects such as oral ulceration, nausea, vomiting and diarrhoea may occur. The drug usually produces a red discoloration of the urine.

All cells require the vitamin folic acid for growth. Folic acid is converted by a number of enzymatic steps in the cell to its biologically active form, folinic acid. **Methotrexate** blocks this conversion and therefore reduces cell growth and multiplication by depriving the cell of folinic acid. The role of intra-arterial administration of high-dose methotrexate in the treatment of osteosarcoma is still being assessed. Although high response rates are claimed it is not clear whether these are better than with the same doses and schedules given intravenously.

The principal toxic effects of methotrexate are suppression of the bone marrow and gastrointestinal disturbance, with one of the earliest manifestations being oral soreness progressing to ulceration.

Ifosfamide is a derivative of cyclophosphamide and is therefore a member of the nitrogen mustard group. It is converted by the liver to a number of highly reactive metabolites. These metabolites interfere with the enzyme systems essential for cell growth and therefore diminish tumour growth.

CHONDROSARCOMA

This is the second most common bone tumour, but it occurs later in life than osteosarcoma. The tumour is usually slow growing. It occurs most often in the diaphysis or metaphysis of the long bones, especially the femur, and in the bones of the pelvis.

Pathophysiology

A chondrosarcoma is a large, ill defined malignant tumour that infiltrates trabeculae in spongy bone. This tumour occurs in any bone preformed in cartilage and it remains cartilaginous throughout its evolution, producing collagen and cartilage matrix.

The tumour contains large lobules of hyaline cartilage that are separated by bands of fibrous tissue and anaplastic cells. The tumour expands and enlarges the contour of the bone, causes extensive erosion of the cortex and expands into the soft tissues.

Pharmacological management

The mainstay of treatment is surgery, with complete removal of the tumour and associated soft tissues. Cytotoxic chemotherapy only has a small part to play in the treatment of this tumour. From the little evidence available, the tumour appears to be resistant to cytotoxic drugs. However, in a high-grade tumour in a young person, cytotoxic drugs such as cisplatin, doxorubicin and ifosfamide may be used in a similar way to that of osteosarcoma.

EWING'S SARCOMA

This is a round cell tumour of bone, the aetiology of which is unknown. This neoplasm is believed to arise from cells of the reticuloendothelial system in the bone marrow.

Pathophysiology

The tumour usually arises in the midshaft positions in the long bones, occasionally the pelvis and other flat bones. Histologically, it consists of small round cells. The tumour typically permeates the medullary and cortical bone. Metastases to the lung frequently occur.

Pharmacological management

This tumour is highly radiosensitive, therefore surgery or radiotherapy are used for local control and chemotherapy is always administered adjuvantly, both before and after local therapy, to destroy clinical or subclinical metastatic disease. The most useful agents are doxorubicin, cyclophosphamide, vincristine, actinomycin D and ifosfamide. Responses are also seen with etoposide, methotrexate and nitrosureas. A variety of different combinations of these drugs is in use, with none showing a clear superiority (Souhami and Tobias, 1998). It is probable that all first-line agents should be used and that the dose of drugs should be kept as high as possible. In recent years the tendency has been to use chemotherapy very intensively over a period of 9–12 months.

Doxorubicin – refer to the section on osteosarcoma.

Cyclophosphamide is a member of the nitrogen mustard group. It is converted by the liver to a number of highly reactive metabolites that interfere with the enzyme system essential for cell growth and thus diminish tumour growth. Cyclophosphamide may be given orally or intravenously. The dosage depends on many factors, including the state of the patient and coincident administration of other cytotoxic drugs.

It is essential that all patients receiving cyclophosphamide should maintain an adequate fluid intake as this has been shown to reduce the incidence of haemorrhagic cystitis, which results from an irritant effect on the bladder surface caused by metabolites. Common side effects of the drug include bone marrow suppression, with the white cells being more commonly affected than the platelets, gastrointestinal toxicity and alopecia. Cyclophosphamide enhances the effect of oral anti-diabetic therapy and therefore should be used with caution in diabetics.

Ifosfamide – refer to the section on osteosarcoma.

Vincristine is a cytotoxic drug, the action of which is not completely understood. It has, however, been shown to interfere with the synthesis of DNA and RNA and to affect chromosome multiplication, all of which are necessary for cell division. The difference between therapeutic and toxic doses of vincristine is very small. It is therefore important to establish carefully the dosage requirements for individual patients.

The most important side effect of vincristine is neurotoxicity, which most frequently manifests as a peripheral neuropathy, sensory, motor or mixed. The initial symptoms may be slight and include numbness and tingling of the fingers and toes. Subsequently, tendon reflexes may disappear. The most common side effects include diplopia and malaise but gastrointestinal side effects may occur and include anorexia, nausea, vomiting and constipation or diarrhoea.

Actinomycin D is a derivative of a group of antibiotics. It acts by combining with DNA thus blocking the process of cell duplication. The drug is always given by intravenous injection and is a strong irritant if it escapes from the vein. The usual adult dosage is 0.5 mg daily and courses are up to 5 days in duration. These courses may be repeated at intervals of several weeks.

The side effects, which may be delayed for days or even weeks after finishing a course of actinomycin D, include bone marrow depression, ulcerative stomatitis, dysphagia, alopecia, erythema, fever, hypocalcaemia, myalgia, malaise and gastrointestinal symptoms.

A detailed account of the action and side effects of many of the cytotoxic agents mentioned in this section can be found in Chapter 6 *Drugs and neoplastic disorders*.

MULTIPLE MYELOMA

This is a malignancy derived from plasma cells, that is, cells that develop from B lymphocytes and produce immunoglobulins (antibodies). Although the origin of this tumour is from haemopoietic tissue of the bone marrow, it is most often included by convention with primary malignancies of bone. The tumour occurs in many sites around the body and the bones commonly involved are the lower vertebral column, ribs, skull, pelvis, femur and clavicle.

There is a detailed account of the pathophysiology and pharmacological management of this disorder in Chapter 6 *Drugs and neoplastic disorders*.

OSTEOPOROSIS

This is a condition in which there is a reduction in the total bone mass, which causes weakening. However, the bone that remains is normal histologically and biochemically. Osteoporosis results from the progressive imbalance between bone reabsorption and bone formation that is a feature of the normal ageing process (**Fig. 13.5**). Therefore some degree of osteoporosis is inevitable in the elderly, but the disease assumes particular significance when complications such as fractures result. Osteoporosis is also a complication of steroid therapy and Cushing's syndrome, and is associated with alcoholism, diabetes, liver disease and smoking. Localised osteoporosis is inevitable after immobilisation of any part of the skeleton (**Fig. 13.6**).

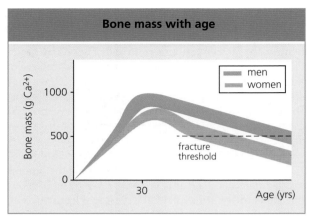

Bone mass with age

Bone mass (g Ca²⁺)

— men
— women

1000

500

fracture
threshold

0

30

Age (yrs)

Fig 13.5 Bone mass with age. (From Page 1997, with permission.)

Pathophysiology

Whatever the cause, osteoporosis develops when the remodelling cycle – the process of bone reabsorption and bone formation – is disrupted, leading to an imbalance in the coupling process. The condition is thought to arise from an initial episode of increased bone reabsorption, which is followed by an inadequate reactive bone deposition. A new equilibrium is reached in which there is

reabsorption and deposition of bone, but in this new state there is less bone overall. Osteoporotic bones are lighter in weight, less dense radiographically and show thinning of the cortex. The bony trabeculae are thinner and there may be a decreased number of osteoblasts, or an increased number of osteoclasts actively reabsorbing bone. The blood levels of calcium, phosphate and alkaline phosphatase are normal, whereas the urine levels of calcium are increased.

Pharmacological management

The treatment of established osteoporosis is, unfortunately, often unsatisfactory because bone mass has already been lost. Prophylaxis for high-risk individuals is, therefore, preferable. The goals of osteoporosis treatment are to slow down the rate of calcium and bone loss and to stop the disease before it progresses too far.

Oestrogen therapy

There is, however, good evidence that osteoporosis is reduced in women treated with oestrogens (hormone replacement therapy – HRT), which inhibit bone reabsorption from the time of the menopause. Important new findings suggest that oestrogen may prevent excessive bone loss before and after the menopause by limiting osteoclast life span through promotion of apoptosis.

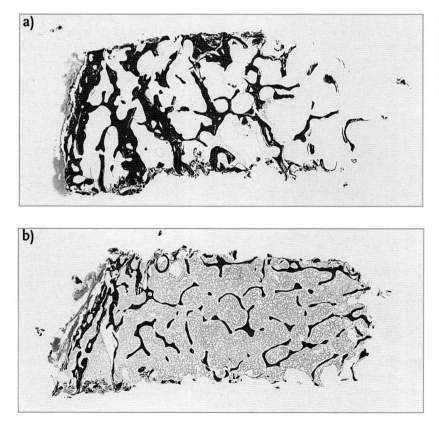

Fig 13.6 Osteoporosis. (From Stevens & Lowe 1995, with permission.)
(a) Micrograph of normal bone;
(b) Micrograph of bone from a patient with osteoporosis (the calcified bone is stained black).

Synthetic oestrogen can be administered orally or transdermally and is metabolised by the liver and peripheral tissues more slowly than naturally occurring oestrogen. The synthetic oestrogens are also generally fat soluble and are stored in adipose tissue, from which they are released. They therefore have a prolonged action and potency compared with natural oestrogens. Transdermal therapy provides relatively low systemic levels of oestradiol and is much less likely than oral therapy to increase cardiovascular risk.

For women who still have their uterus, a progesterone is usually included with the oestrogen therapy, as the combination therapy reduces the risk of endometrial carcinoma associated with oestrogen treatment. A monthly course consists of an oestrogen given for 3 weeks followed by a progestogen for 5 days; the course is restarted after 2 days rest. A convenient alternative is oestrogen in which an oestrogen is given throughout the cycle and a progestogen for the last 12 days. As mentioned above, oestrogens can also be given as a patch applied to the skin. The patch available in the United Kingdom contains oestradiol, which diffuses through the skin and is effective for 3–4 days, after which the patch is replaced. Cyclical progestogen treatment causing monthly bleeding is still required.

For women who have had a hysterectomy, unopposed oestrogen therapy is recommended, as progesterone may unfavourably alter the high-density to low-density lipoprotein ratio. Typical preparations include ethinyloestradiol 5–15 μg/day, or conjugated oestrogens 625 μg/day, administered orally.

Tibolone is a synthetic compound described as a gonadomimetic steroid as it has oestrogenic and progestogenic properties. It controls postmenopausal symptoms and limits osteoporosis without stimulating the endometrium, and thus it eliminates the risk of endometrial carcinoma.

The disadvantages of oestrogen treatment include irregular vaginal bleeding, a slightly increased risk of venous thrombosis and a possible increase in carcinoma of the body of the uterus.

Calcium supplements

Regular exercise and increased dietary intake of calcium (at least 25–50 mMol per day) also have beneficial effects. If this calcium intake is not achieved the diet may be supplemented with calcium chloride, calcium gluconate or calcium lactate tablets, 20 mmol daily. However, calcium alone will not retard the rapid bone loss.

Bisphosphonates

Alendronic acid and disodium etidronate may have an important role in the treatment of osteoporosis as they inhibit bone reabsorption by binding to calcium crystals forming a coating which prevents the access of osteoclasts to the bone (see page 249).

Calcitonin

Calcitonin is a viable therapeutic option for patients in whom oestrogens are contraindicated or for patients intolerant to oestrogen side effects or regimes. A form of calcitonin derived from pig thyroid tissue or salcatonin derived from salmon may be prescribed. Calcitonin is a hormone secreted by the parathyroid glands that regulates bone turnover (**Fig. 13.7**). It does so by lowering plasma calcium and phosphate levels, and by antagonising the actions of parathyroid hormone on bone. It may be beneficial to patients with osteoporosis because it inhibits the activity of the osteoclast bone cells, which continuously digest bone to release free calcium and phosphate. However, these drugs remain under investigation and the field is changing rapidly.

RICKETS AND OSTEOMALACIA

Osteomalacia is characterised by inadequate mineralisation of the organic matrix of the skeleton. Rickets is the name given to osteomalacia that affects the growing skeleton of children, resulting in characteristic deformities. In the adult, osteomalacia may produce bone and muscle pain and tenderness, often as a result of subclinical fractures.

Pathophysiology

The causes of osteomalacia include:
- Dietary deficiency of vitamin D.
- Deficiency of vitamin D metabolites as a result of skin pigmentation or inadequate exposure to sunlight.

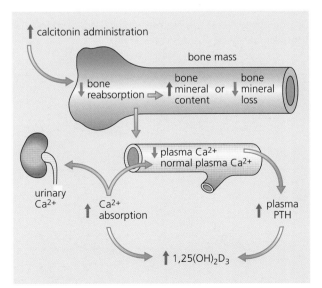

Fig 13.7 The effect of calcitonin on bone and calcium homeostasis. PTH: parathryoid hormone; 1,25(OH)$_2$D$_3$, 1,25-dihydroxyvitamin D$_3$. (From Page 1997, with permission.)

- Intestinal malabsorption as a result of coeliac disease, Crohn's disease or extensive surgical resection of the small intestine.
- Renal or hepatic disease, because the liver and kidneys play an important role in the metabolism of vitamin D. **Figure 13.8** illustrates the metabolism of vitamin D.

Pharmacological management

The simplest treatments are exposure to sunlight and oral vitamin D_2 supplements such as calciferol, which is a mixture of ergocalciferol and cholecalciferol. The initial dose can be between 500 and 5000 units (5000 units equals 125 µg) daily, depending upon the severity of the deficiency state and the age of the patient. The dose should be carefully monitored by regular estimation of blood calcium levels. Hypervitaminosis D manifests with nausea and vomiting and other features of hypercalcaemia. Intramuscular injection can overcome problems associated with malabsorption. The usual treatment for vitamin D deficiency in renal disease is 1α-hydroxy-cholecalciferol (alfacalidol) 1 µg daily; $1,25(OH)_2D_3$ (calcitriol) is also available for anephric patients.

PAGET'S DISEASE

Essentially, this is a condition of bone remodelling, although the metabolic changes are considerable. Recent evidence involving apparent viral inclusion bodies suggests a possible 'slow viral' aetiology, for which canine distemper virus is a prime candidate. This condition causes uncontrolled bone turnover, with local excessive osteoclastic reabsorption followed by disordered osteoblastic activity; this leads to abundant new bone formation that is structurally abnormal and weak. The commonest sites that are affected by the disease are the femur, pelvis, tibia, skull and lumbosacral spine (Underwood, 1996).

Pathophysiology

Most cases are entirely asymptomatic, but clinical features of the disease may include:
- Bone pain, generally in the spine or pelvis.
- Apparent joint pain, when the area of bone involvement is close to a joint.
- Bone deformities, particularly bowed tibia and skull changes.
- Patients with extensive Paget's disease commonly have general malaise and lethargy.
- Complications such as deafness as a result of cranial nerve compression, a modest increase in cardiac output as a result of vascular shunting of blood through diseased bone, fracture through abnormal bone structure and, rarely, osteogenic sarcoma.

Pharmacological management

When asymptomatic, Paget's disease requires no treatment. The development of pain is the usual indication for treatment, which may include:
- Simple analgesics or NSAIDs, which may be sufficient to control the pain.
- Calcitonin.
- Bisphosphonates.

Calcitonin

Calcitonin given by repeated injection was the first treatment to have any real beneficial effect, either on deep-seated bone pain or on the course of the disease. The hormone acts by binding to surface receptors on osteoclasts and inhibiting their bone reabsorbing function. There is an abrupt reduction in bone reabsorption, whereas bone formation continues; thus the administration of this treatment to a severely affected patient with extensive disease leads to a transient fall in serum calcium concentration.

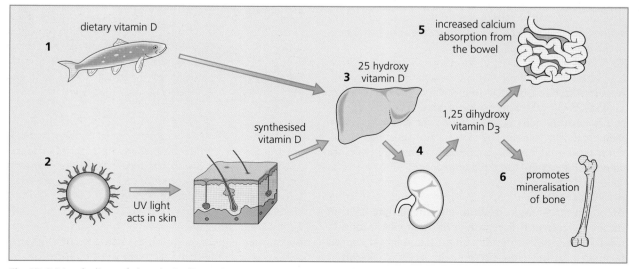

Fig 13.8 Metabolism of vitamin D. (From Stevens & Lowe 1995, with permission.)

The required dose is 50–100 IU given three times per week by subcutaneous injection. The hydroxyproline and plasma alkaline phosphatase fall as a consequence of the treatment, but rarely dramatically, and an improvement in bone structure and recalcification occurs. The side effects of calcitonin are frequent and include flushing, palpitations, headache and malaise shortly after each injection. Unfortunately, after approximately 1 year of treatment, antibody formation to the salmon or porcine calcitonin is a further difficulty.

Biphosphonates (formerly diphosphonates)

These are absorbed onto the calcium-containing crystals in bone and slow their rate of formation and dissolution. Therefore, by reducing bone turnover biphosphonates relieve pain and reduce hypercalcaemia.

Disodium etidronate administered orally at 5 mg/kg as a single daily dose over 6 months reduces osteoclastic activity and frequently induces a remission of up to 2 years. The serum alkaline phosphatase level falls, reflecting the effect of the drug. This drug should be given on an empty stomach as absorption is erratic. High doses may lead to osteomalacia and pathological fractures.

Disodium pamidronate, as with other biphosphonates, is poorly and erratically absorbed by mouth and causes gastrointestinal side effects when given orally. Patients with severe Paget's disease may benefit from short intravenous courses under supervision, which produce a dramatic response and may be followed by a prolonged remission. The dosage for Paget's disease is usually a single dose of approximately 30 mg weekly. Pamidronate is an irritant and therefore should be administered by slow intravenous infusion via a cannula in a relatively large vein. In the early stages, pamidronate treatment is commonly followed by an increase in bone pain and by mild, transient fever; however, this is quickly followed by symptomatic improvement and a reduction in bone pain.

DISEASES OF SKELETAL MUSCLE

The skeletal muscles are made up of millions of individual fibres that, by the process of contraction and relaxation, do the work necessary to complete movements as varied as a ballerina's pirouette or an artist's deft stroke. Muscle constitutes approximately 40% of an adult body weight and 50% of a child's body weight. Muscle consists of 75% water, 20% protein and 5% inorganic compounds. Thirty-two per cent of all protein stores for energy and metabolism is contained within muscle (McCance and Huether, 1998).

The disorders that primarily impair skeletal muscle are collectively known as myopathies. Primary myopathies are caused by intrinsic defects within the muscle fibre and secondary myopathies arise as a sequel to endocrine, metabolic or vascular disorders. Myositis is the term used to describe an inflammatory muscle myopathy and myotonia

a defect of the muscle membrane. The disorders included in this section are muscle membrane abnormalities and inflammatory muscle diseases.

MUSCLE MEMBRANE ABNORMALITIES

Two defects of the muscle membrane have been linked to clinical syndromes: the hyperexcitable membrane seen in the myotonic disorders and the intermittently unresponsive membrane seen in the periodic paralyses.

MYOTONIAS

Myotonia is a delayed relaxation after voluntary muscle contraction. It is seen in several disorders: myotonia congenital (Thomsen's disease), myotonic muscular dystrophy and some forms of periodic paralysis (see below).

Pathophysiology

Myotonia is caused by prolonged depolarisation of the muscle membrane. It is considered to be the result of an abnormality of the muscle fibre, particularly of chloride conduction in the fibre membrane. Grip, ocular movements, eye closure, chewing, swallowing and movements of trunk and distal limb muscles may be affected and the abnormality is often made worse by cold and inactivity.

Pharmacological management

Treatment of myotonia is by the use of drugs that reduce muscle fibre excitability such as procainamide and some other antiarrhythmic agents, for example phenytoin and quinidine preparations. Prednisolone and acetazolamide, a carbonic anhydrase inhibitor, have also been used but with less consistent results. Tricyclic antidepressants have produced benefit in some patients and more recently a small number of patients have improved using calcium-channel blockers such as nifedipine or verapamil.

PERIODIC PARALYSES

These are rare membrane disorders characterised by intermittent flaccid muscle weakness and alteration in serum potassium levels. Periodic paralysis is triggered by exercise and any process or medication that increases serum potassium. The paralysis, which leaves the individual flaccid and weak, does not affect the respiratory muscles.

HYPOKALAEMIC PERIODIC PARALYSIS

This is usually inherited as an autosomal dominant trait. It is a condition in which an inadequate amount of potassium is found in the circulatory bloodstream; causes include starvation, treatment of diabetic acidosis, adrenal tumour or diuretic therapy.

Pathophysiology

Hypokalaemic periodic paralysis is characterised by generalised weakness (including speech and bulbar muscles) that often starts after a heavy carbohydrate meal or after a period of rest after exertion. The attacks may last for several hours and during an attack the serum potassium may be as low as 3.0 mmol/l.

Pharmacological management

The weakness responds to the administration of oral or intravenous potassium chloride. A similar weakness may occur in hypokalaemia caused by diuretic therapy and may also occur during thyrotoxicosis.

HYPERKALAEMIC PERIODIC PARALYSIS

Again, this is usually inherited as an autosomal dominant trait and is characterised by sudden attacks of muscle weakness that are sometimes precipitated by exercise.

Pathophysiology

During an attack the muscle membrane is unresponsive to neural stimuli; the resting membrane potential is increased from −90 to −45 mV and the serum potassium is raised.

Pharmacological management

The attacks of muscle weakness are terminated by the administration of intravenous calcium gluconate or calcium chloride to restore normal neuromuscular activity. Because calcium influences the threshold potential, changes in extracellular fluid calcium concentration can override the effects of hyperkalaemia.

INFLAMMATORY MUSCLE DISEASE – MYOSITIS

Myositis is encountered in a variety of different settings and there are many causative agents of muscle inflammation (**Table 13.6**). Infection may be seen as a secondary involvement of muscle in the course of a systemic infection or, less commonly, the muscle may be involved in the infective process primarily. Alternatively, many muscles around the body are inflamed in the course of noninfectious, autoimmune inflammatory conditions, generally specified by the term polymyositis (Vardaxis, 1995).

In the United Kingdom **bacterial myositis**, specifically clostridial myositis, develops in dirty wounds with anaerobic conditions. *Clostridium perfringens* produces a toxin and enzymes that cause necrosis of muscle, with inflammation and haemorrhage. Urgent treatment with penicillin and surgical debridement is necessary.

Parasitic myositis may also cause considerable damage and inflammation in muscle, especially *Trichinella spiralis* infestation, trichiniasis. This is associated with the consumption of undercooked or raw infected meats, especially pork.

Pathophysiology

Trichinella spiralis invades the muscle and the damage in the muscle is enzymatic, as the organism is a tissue liquifier; it secretes lytic enzymes that kill and lyse the muscle cells.

Pharmacological management

Treatment is with thiabendazole, an anthelmintic drug that is used in the United Kingdom and in tropical countries for the treatment of trichinosis. It eradicates adult worms from the gut lumen but does not affect larvae. The dosage given depends upon the weight of the patient and is calculated using the formula 25 mg/kg. Two doses are given each day for 2–4 successive days. Alternatively, a single dose of 50 mg/kg may be given, but this produces a higher incidence of side effects. These are common and include anorexia, nausea, vomiting, dizziness, diarrhoea, epigastric pain, pruritis, weariness, giddiness, headache and drowsiness. A hypersensitivity to the drug may result in fever, facial flushing, chills and, more rarely, anaphylactic shock.

Steroids (see above and Chapter 3) should also be administered to those who have marked systemic upset and muscle tenderness.

POLYMYOSITIS

This term refers to a group of conditions the cardinal feature of which is a myopathy. Some forms of polymyositis are associated with malignancy.

The categories of inflammatory muscle disease	
Infective causes	
Bacterial	Clostridial myositis (gas gangrene) Staphylococcal myositis
Viral	Post-viral myalgia Influenza myositis Coxsackie A & B Echo
Parasitic	Cysticercosis Trichinosis Toxoplasmosis Trypanosomiasis
Unknown causes	Polymyositis Dermatomyositis Polymyositis with connective tissue disease Sarcoidosis Other granulomatous myositis Eosinophilic polymyositis

Table 13.6 The categories of inflammatory muscle disease

Pathophysiology

The typical presentation of polymyositis is a history of several weeks' progressive, painful, proximal upper and lower limb weakness. Dysphagia and other bulbar involvement is common, together with respiratory muscle weakness. In addition to muscle pain, arthralgia is common and the patient may also complain of general malaise and fever. A muscle biopsy shows inflammatory infiltrate with lymphocytes and plasma cells, and a variable degree of necrosis and phagocytosis of muscle fibres.

Pharmacological Management

Treatment is with corticosteroids (Chapter 3), usually prednisolone at a dose of 60–80 mg daily. Azathioprine or cyclophosphamide may also be prescribed. Most patients begin to improve within 2–3 weeks and for most of them polymyositis without associated disease runs a course of a few months to 2 years.

KEY POINTS

- In osteoarthritis the cartilage becomes eroded and progressively thinned as the disease progresses.
- Rheumatoid arthritis is a chronic systemic disease that produces a symmetrical inflammatory polyarteritis, inflammatory lesions in tissues such as the heart, blood vessels, lungs, skin and the eye, and progressive joint damage that leads to severe disability.
- Infective arthritis may be the result of a direct infection of the joints by microorganisms or may be a reaction to a preceding infection.
- Ankylosing spondylitis is an inflammatory disorder of spinal joints.
- Gout is a metabolic disorder; excess uric acid is deposited as urate crystals in joints and other tissues, producing an inflammatory response.
- Osteoporosis describes a reduction in the total bone mass, resulting in weakness.
- Biphosphonates and calcitonin may be prescribed in the treatment of osteoporosis and Paget's disease.
- Myotonia is caused by prolonged depolarisation of the muscle membrane; treatment is with drugs that reduce muscle fibre excitability.
- Bacterial myositis requires urgent treatment with antibiotics; parasitic myositosis is treated with thiabendazole, an antihelminthic drug.

MULTIPLE CHOICE QUESTIONS

1. Prostaglandins are very potent chemicals with a broad range of activities. Which of the following statements about prostaglandins is incorrect?
   a. they inhibit gastric secretion
   b. they cause peripheral vasodilatation
   c. they are responsible for the mediation of some aspects of inflammation
   d. they cause bronchoconstriction
   e. they cause contraction of the iris

2. Which of the following statements concerning gold salts is correct?
   a. they may provide immediate relief of arthritic pain
   b. they act by inhibiting prostaglandin synthesis
   c. they frequently cause dermatitis of the skin or mucous membranes
   d. they are drugs of first choice in treating arthritis
   e. they must all be given intramuscularly

3. Which of the following statements about colchinine is correct?
   a. it is used in the treatment of chronic gout
   b. it can cause serious gastrointestinal problems
   c. it has general use as an anti-inflammatory drug
   d. it blocks further synthesis of uric acid
   e. it acts to promote the secretion of uric acid

4. Allopurinol
   a. increases uric acid levels in the blood
   b. increases the excretion of uric acid
   c. is used prophylactically to reduce the number of acute gouty attacks
   d. is a toxic compound with a high frequency of adverse effects
   e. reduces the total amount of uric acid produced

5. Which of the following adverse effects is **not** associated with the administration of oral disodium pamidronate?
   a. nausea and vomiting
   b. transient fever
   c. bone pain
   d. hypercalcaemia
   e. abdominal pain

6. Which of the following is not a clinical manifestation of polymyositis?
   a. dysphasia
   b. respiratory muscle weakness
   c. arthralgia
   d. general malaise
   e. fever

7. All of the following may cause osteomalacia except
   a. renal disease
   b. overexposure to sunlight
   c. Crohn's disease
   d. dietary deficiency of vitamin D
   e. surgical resection of the small intestine

8. Which of the following statements concerning the treatment of osteoporosis is incorrect?
   a. Oestrogen and progesterone is only recommended for women who still have a uterus.
   b. The side-effects of oestrogen therapy may include an increased risk of venous thrombosis and carcinoma of the uterus.
   c. An increased intake of dietary calcium will retard the rapid bone loss of osteoporosis.
   d. Biphosphonates accumulate in the area of bone remodelling, bind to calcium crystals forming a coating and prevent the access of osteoclasts to the bone.
   e. Calcitonin inhibits bone reabsorption by reducing the activity of the osteoclasts.

9. In which of the following conditions would aspirin be contraindicated?
   a. juvenile chronic arthritis
   b. fever
   c. myalgia
   d. ischaemic heart disease
   e. peptic ulceration

10. Which of the following are correctly paired?
    a. indomethacin: causes frontal headaches
    b. fenbrufen: high risk of skin rashes
    c. meloxicam: causes a high level of gastrointestinal irritation
    d. sulindac: a safer option for patients with renal impairment.
    e. benorylate: must not be taken with other drugs containing aspirin

REFERENCES

Engelhardt G. Pharmacology of meloxicam, a new non-steroidal anti-inflammatory drug with improved safety profile through preferential inhibition of COX-2. *Br J Rheumatol* 1996; **35(suppl 1):**4-12.

Gray RS, Doherty SM, Galloway J, Coulton L, DeBroe M, Kansis JA. A double blind study of deflazacort and prednisolone in patients with chronic inflammatory disorders. *Arthritis Rheum* 1991; **34:**287-295.

Hayllar J, Bjarnason I. NSAIDs, cox-2 inhibitors and the gut. *Lancet* 1995; **346:**521-522.

Hunziker EB, Rosenberg LC. Repair of partial-thickness defects in articular cartilage: cell recruitment from the synovial membrane. *Journal of Bone and Joint Surgery (American Volume)* 1996; **78-A65:** p721-733

Kumar P, Clark M. Clinical medicine, 3rd ed. London: WB Saunders, 1996.

Loftus JK, Reeve J, Hesp R, David J, Ansell BM, Woo PMM. Deflazacort in juvenile chronic arthritis. *J Rheumatol* 1993; **20(suppl):**3740-3742.

McCance SE, Huether KL. *Understanding pathophysiology.* London: Mosby, 1996.

McKenry LM, Salerno E. Pharmacology in nursing. London: Mosby, 1995.

Osvaldo DM, Barreira JR, Zanchetta JA, Maldonado-Cocco CE, Bogado ON, Sebastian DF, Augusto MR, Redondo G, Lazaro A. Effect of low doses of deflazocort and prednisolone on bone mineral content in premenopausal rheumatoid arthritis. *J Rheumatol* 1992; **19:**1520-1526.

Page C. *Integrated Pharmacology.* London: Mosby, 1997

Souhami RL, Moxham J, ed. *Textbook of medicine.* Edinburgh: Churchill Livingstone, 1990.

Souhami R, Tobias J. *Cancer and its management,* 3rd Ed, Oxford: Blackwell Science, 1998.

Stevens A, Lowe J. *Pathology.* London: Mosby, 1995.

Underwood JCE, ed. *General and systematic pathology.* Edinburgh: Churchill Livingstone, 1996.

Vardaxis NJ. *Pathology for health sciences.* Edinburgh: Churchill Livingstone, 1995.

14 Janet MacGregor
DRUGS AND GASTROINTESTINAL DISORDERS

INTRODUCTION

The gastrointestinal tract is a muscular tube that extends from mouth to anus and is controlled by the autonomic nervous system (the intrinsic nerves of the enteric nervous system) throughout its length. Also hormones and neural activity in the cerebrum affect its activity at many sections of its length. Its function is to break down ingested nutrients, change them into a suitable state for absorption into the blood transport system and eliminate the waste (McCance and Huether, 1998). Associated organs that assist in this process are the liver, gall bladder and pancreas (**Fig. 14.1**).

Disorders of the gastrointestinal tract and associated organs are many and varied depending on the site, aetiology and whether they are secondary to malfunction in other body systems. For example, brain tumours may promote vomiting by local inflammatory effect on the vomiting centre so a medication that reduces this oedema, such as dexamethasone 16 mg daily, may be the drug of choice.

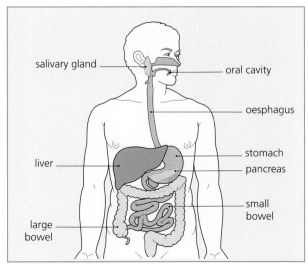

Fig 14.1 Structure of the alimentary tract. (From Page 1997, with permission.)

Psychological distress may result in gastric ulceration, which can be controlled with adrenergic blocking agents such as propranolol 80 mg twice daily.

Gastrointestinal tract disease is common throughout the world. In the tropics, parasites, roundworms and hookworms are frequently the cause of extensive morbidity among those already weakened by poor diet. Anthelmintics are a diverse group of drugs specific to the infestation. Threadworms are seen in children in the United Kingdom and these can be treated with piperazine 50–75 mg/kg daily in two treatments of 1 week's duration, separated by 1 week of rest (Trounce, 1988). In the United Kingdom gastrointestinal tract complaints constitute 11% of general practitioners' work and treatment costs equal those of the maternity services (Jones *et al.*, 1985).

Drugs can affect the motility, digestion, secretion and absorption processes of the stomach and intestine. In addition, nutrients are increasingly being used to prevent gut pathology, address deficiencies and treat many physical and psychological abnormalities. Iron-rich foods are now recommended for weaning diets in early childhood to prevent the development of anaemia seen increasingly in the United Kingdom (Griffiths *et al.*, 1995). Dietary fibre in the adult population may prevent colon cancer, diverticulitis, haemorrhoids and gall stones (Brody *et al.*, 1994). Vitamin and mineral supplements have been shown to reduce anti-social behaviour and increase intellectual ability (Brown, 1996). Reference to nutrition is made in all chapters in this book in which the use of dietary supplements is part of treatments.

There are three major types of gastrointestinal medications. The first are designed to help restore or maintain the protective lining by reducing gastric acidity or inflammatory processes. These drugs may be administered orally as liquids, suspensions, gels and powders to act directly on the stomach lining to neutralise acid or by intravenous or intramuscular injection to act systemically.

The second type affect the motility of the muscular tube. Prokinetic drugs increase the gastrointestinal contractions and propulsion by increasing cholinergic stimuli at the smooth muscle M_2 receptors, mimicking the action of the parasympathetic nervous system. Opioids, conversely, reduce transit time through the bowel by increasing the slower segmenting contractions in the small and large bowel thus increasing resistance to flow through the lumen. Some medications act centrally at sites in the brain and spinal cord, others act locally on the submucosal plexus to inhibit secretion and promote net absorption (Brody *et al.*, 1994).

The third type acts on the colon to improve bowel emptying in a variety of ways. They are classified in five major categories: bulk-forming agents, faecal softeners, hyperosmolar or saline solutions, lubricants and stimulant or irritant laxatives. Other medications involve those that improve mouth or anus comfort, reduce gas production, replace digestive enzymes and promote or reduce nausea and vomiting.

The gastrointestinal system is innervated by the autonomic nervous system, so medications for this nervous network will have numerous effects. Sympathetic nervous system activity may produce a variety of symptoms in the gut in anxiety and shock. It may reduce blood flow to the glands so saliva becomes reduced and sticky, inhibit peristalsis and secretion in the bowel, stimulate glycogenolysis in the liver and reduce insulin secretion. Anxiolytics and/or coping strategies can act centrally (see Chapter 7 *Drugs and psychological disorders*, more specific α-receptor or β-receptor blocking agents can reverse the constriction effects on the blood vessels in the stomach and intestine (Garbett, 1995).

GLOSSARY OF TERMS

UPPER GASTROINTESTINAL TRACT ABNORMALITIES

Symptoms of upper gastrointestinal tract abnormalities include:

- Anorexia, i.e. lack of desire to eat.
- Nausea, defined as a subjective experience that is an unpleasant but not painful sensation associated with the back of the throat and the gut and giving rise to the feeling that vomiting is imminent (Hawthorn, 1995).
- Halitosis: faeculent smelling breath may indicate intestinal obstruction; ammoniate odour, liver failure; 'new-mown hay' or 'pear drops' may indicate diabetes mellitus; or particular food and drink e.g. garlic or alcohol may produce a characteristic smell of the breath (Hinchliff *et al.*, 1996).
- Dysphagia, i.e. difficulty in swallowing, may be alleviated by antimuscarinic drugs such as merbentyl.
- Retching is defined as a rhythmic movement of stomach contents from stomach to lower oesophagus. This usually occurs in bursts immediately before vomiting. It is sometimes called 'dry heaves'; retching is essentially breathing against a closed glottis. The external intercostal muscles, the diaphragm and abdominal muscles contract together to cause rhythmic decrease in intrathoracic pressure with

concomitant increases in abdominal pressure (Hawthorn, 1995). A diffuse sympathetic discharge causes tachycardia, tachypnoea and sweating. The parasympathetic system mediates copious salivation, increased gastric motility and relaxed oesophageal sphincters.

- Vomiting (emesis) is defined as the forceful emptying of stomach and intestinal content (chyme) through the mouth. A powerful contraction of the rectus abdominus muscle and the external muscles overlying the stomach and a relaxation of the upper oesophageal sphincter and peri-oesophageal diaphragm occurs. The stomach becomes quite flaccid and still, whereas pressures in the abdomen and thorax rise.
- Reflux is when chyme moves from stomach to oesophagus.
- Belching describes the forceful expulsion of gas from stomach through mouth.
- Dyspepsia (heartburn) is when acid from stomach irritates the lower oesophagus. It should not be confused with the referred pain from heart, i.e. angina and infarction.
- Achalasia is when the oesophagus dilates and becomes hypertrophied. This results from degeneration of the ganglionic nerve supply of the oesophagus. It may also result from damage to the swallowing centre in the medulla, poliomyelitis, polymyosis and scleroderma.
- Haematemesis describes bloody vomitus. Blood is either fresh and bright red or digested and dark and grainy with 'coffee grounds' appearance.
- Dumping syndrome describes the rapid emptying of hypertonic chyme from the surgically reduced stomach into the small intestine 10–20 minutes after eating. This rapid distension stimulates the sympathetic nerve endings. In addition, the sudden high osmotic gradient within the small intestine causes shift of fluid from the vascular compartment to the intestine lumen. Plasma volume decreases causing vasomotor responses of raised pulse, lowered blood pressure, weakness, pallor, sweating and dizziness. Rapid distension of the intestine produces a feeling of epigastric fullness, cramping, nausea, vomiting and diarrhoea. Late dumping syndrome occurs 1–2 hours after eating a high carbohydrate meal. Hypoglycaemia symptoms result because large amounts of insulin are secreted in response to the rapid absorption of glucose and consequent hyperglycaemia after a meal. Dumping syndrome is managed by dietary manipulation.
- Itching skin from jaundice caused by raised bile levels in the bloodstream if liver or gall bladder dysfunction inhibits the excretion of bile into the small intestine.
- Weight loss reflects the inability of nutrients to enter the cells (Garbett, 1995).

LOWER GASTROINTESTINAL TRACT ABNORMALITIES

Symptoms of lower gastrointestinal tract abnormalities include:

- Altered bowel habit, i.e. constipation or diarrhoea. Constipation is defined as difficult or infrequent defecation. It must be individually defined as number of bowel movements per week, hard stools and difficult evacuation. Diarrhoea is defined as the increase in volume, frequency or fluidity of stool (McCance and Huether, 1998). The World Health Organization definition is 6–8 movements in 24 hours.

- Abdominal distension from activity within the gut or peripheral to it in the abdominal cavity.
- Flatulence is gas produced in the lumen of the gut. Anaerobic bacteria *Bacteroides fragilis* and *Clostridium perfringens*, and aerobic bacteria *Enterobacter aerogenes* and *Escherichia coli* break down some food products and synthesise vitamin K, thiamine, folic acid and riboflavin. This fermentation also produces gases called flatus; this consists of nitrogen, carbon dioxide, hydrogen, methane and hydrogen sulphide. The normal daily production is 500–700 ml (Garbett, 1995).
- Tenesmus is straining at stool.
- Malaena describes black sticky tarry stools. They are foul smelling because of the digestion of blood in the gastrointestinal tract. This should not to be confused with the effects of patients taking iron supplements by mouth.
- Bleeding from the rectum (haematochezia), is characterised by fresh bright blood passed, mucus in the stool, normal-looking stools that have occult blood detectable by a laboratory test, weight loss and anaemia.

SYMPTOMS LINKED WITH DISORDERS OF THE GASTROINTESTINAL TRACT

DRY MOUTH
Normally the three pairs of salivary glands produce secretions under the control of the parasympathetic fibres of the glossopharyngeal and facial nerves. They keep the mouth wet and the saliva contains salivary amylase and IgA antibodies. If these secretions dry up, infections quickly establish themselves. A compound thymol glycerin mouthwash can act as a mild antiseptic or chlorhexidine gluconate in a 0.2% solution may be used. Sodium bicarbonate 0.25 teaspoonful in 50 ml water is useful to remove dry mucus in patients who cannot use a toothbrush.

VOMITING
The external intercostal muscles, the diaphragm and abdominal muscles contract together to cause a rhythmic decrease in intrathoracic pressure with concomitant increases in intra-abdominal pressure (Hawthorn, 1995). A diffuse sympathetic discharge causes tachycardia, tachypnoea and sweats. The parasympathetic system mediates copious salivation, increased gastric motility and relaxed oesophageal sphincters. Vomiting may then cause forceful emptying of the stomach and duodenal contents (chyme) through the mouth. A powerful contraction of the rectus abdominus muscle and the external muscles overlying the stomach and a relaxation of the upper oesophageal sphincter and

peri-oesophseal diagram occurs. The stomach becomes quite flaccid and motionless; pressures in the abdomen and thorax rise. Gastric acid decreases and salivation increases, the patient appears pale, can experience cold sweats, may have a tachycardia and feel cold and clammy. This is the result of raised sympathetic nervous system activity. The effects are a reduction of urine production, glucose utilisation and end-tidal carbon dioxide production, and an increase in lactic dehydrogenase levels, blood pH and plasma antidiuretic hormone (vasopressin) by 20–50 fold.

In some circumstances, for example paediatric surgery, good preparation can reduce postoperative nausea (Grunberg and Hesluth, 1993). The reduction of anxiety, transporting patients in a semi-recumbent position, controlled sitting up after anaesthetic and small frequent fluid intake 2 hours after the operation can also reduce the experience of this debilitating sensation. Perhaps the greatest advance in the treatment of nausea and vomiting has been in the care of patients. Similarly, the care of those cancer patients who are terminally ill and those who undergo chemotherapy has improved. The vomit reflex (**Figs. 14.2** and **14.3**) is complex and the medications for its control numerous.

Pharmacological management of vomiting
Serotonin production is 80–90% from the chromaffin cells of the gastrointestinal mucosa, especially in the duodenum and stomach. Serotonin, or 5-hydroxytryptamine (5-HT), is formed from the amino acid tryptophan obtained from the diet. It is a neurotransmitter that works in many ways on tissues in the body; by March 1994 seven groups of receptors for this chemical had been identified and research continues (Hawthorn 1995). It is the 5-HT 3 receptor that is involved in vomiting. Chemotherapy, radiotherapy, surgical procedures and vomiting itself stimulate the release of 5-HT from the gut mucosa, which then activates afferent nerve terminals to initiate vomiting. It may also activate central brain receptors in the nucleus of the solitary tract via the vagus nerve pathway and the area posterna via the blood circulation. Thus, drugs which block 5-HT production, such as **ondansetron**, are highly effective. This 5-HT 3 receptor antagonist may act locally on the vagal afferent terminals or centrally in the brain to prevent processing of information received. Ondansetron can be given orally as a 'loading' dose of 8 mg 1–2 hours before treatment or intravenously immediately before treatment, and thereafter 8 mg 12 hourly for 5 days. Children need 5 mg/m² body surface area (Cook and Gallagher, 1996).

Dopamine D_2 is involved in the control of gastric motility. Dopamine receptor antagonists increase peristalsis and thus reduce reflux and facilitate gastric emptying. Dopamine receptors are found in the chemoreceptor trigger zone (CTZ), the nucleus tractus solitarius (NTS) and all over the central nervous system, including the extrapyramidal system, which controls voluntary motor activity and muscle tone (**Fig. 14.4**). They are also found in

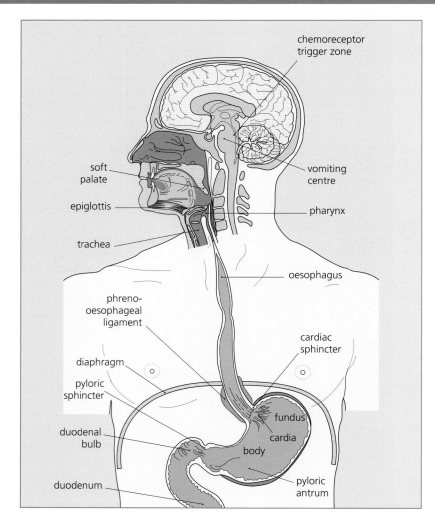

Fig 14.2 The major visceral and central structures involved in the vomiting reflex. (From Page 1997, with permission.)

the pelvic nerve networks and thus may explain the nausea and vomiting experienced by women undergoing gynaecological surgery (Berkley *et al.*, 1990). Side effects of these drugs are hypotension, sedation, agitation and extrapyramidal reactions in young children. Other extrapyramidal reactions from the side effects of dopamine antagonists are outlined below:

- Feeling of swelling tongue.
- Back teeth grind.
- Jaw 'locks'.
- Restlessness.
- Akathisia (involuntary limb shaking).
- Oculocrisis (spasm of eyeball muscles).
- Torticollis (spasm of neck and face muscles, causing head to twist).

The butyrophenones, **haloperidol** 20–100 mg daily in divided doses (25–50 μg/kg for children) and **droperidol** 5 mg intravenously or intramuscularly for adults and 0.02–0.075 mg/kg for children, are dopamine receptor antagonists acting on the CTZ centrally. These drugs block

nerve messages at synapses. Droperidol is less effective in premenopausal women because of an oestrogen effect (Linblad *et al.*, 1990).

Domperidone acts peripherally in the gut therefore has fewer side effects than those medications that act centrally. It is not licensed in the United Kingdom for intravenous use because of its cardiac effects, but oral and rectal preparations are available. This drug is used widely in postoperative nausea and vomiting (PONV) and patient-controlled analgesia (PCA) in gynaecological surgery (Grunberg and Hesluth, 1993).

Metoclopramide acts centrally, blocking dopamine receptors in the CTZ and peripherally to increase gastric and small intestine transit time. However, it is a dangerous drug to use immediately after gut surgery as it stimulates mobility. At high doses it is a serotonin$_3$ receptor antagonist and is best used in continuous infusion to maintain serum levels of 850–1000 ng/ml (Assaf *et al.*, 1974). **Cisapride** also increases gut motility and promotes the release of acetylcholine in the gut wall. This drug is best used for gastric stasis and oesophageal reflux.

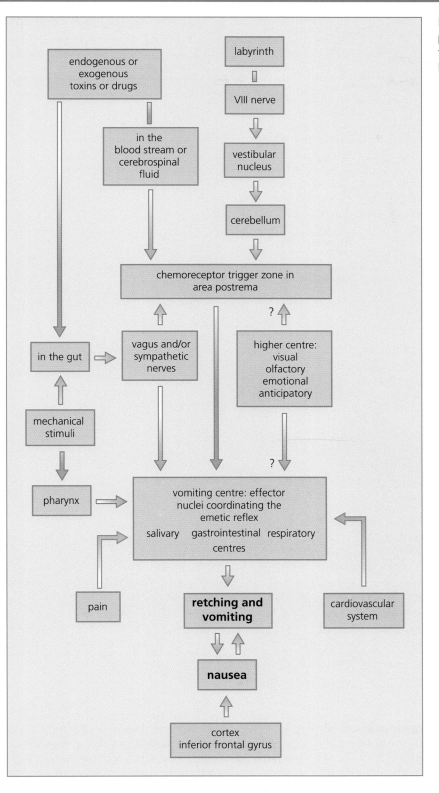

Fig 14.3 The major emetic stimuli, pathways and structures mediating the emetic reflex and nausea. (From Page 1997, with permission.)

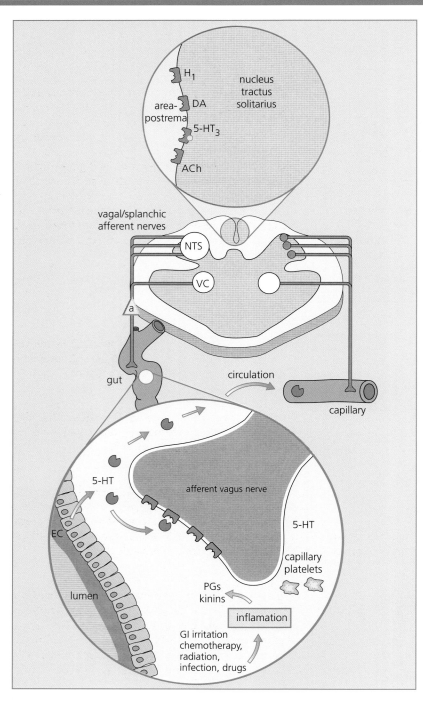

Fig 14.4 Chemical transmitters mediating emetic stimuli. ACh: acetylcholine; 5-HT: serotonin; ECs: enterochromaffin cells; GI: gastrointestinal; PGs: prostaglandins; VC: vomiting centre; NTS, nucleus tractus solitarius. (From Page 1997, with permission.)

Phenothiazines, for example **Chlorpromazine** can be used in terminal conditions. For adults the dose is 25–50 mg by deep intra-muscular injections 3–4 hourly, 10–25 mg 4–6 hourly by mouth or 100 mg 6–8 hourly rectally. For children the doses are lower and are titrated against body weight and age group. Five-hundred micrograms per kilogram every 4–6 hours can be given orally or by deep intra-muscular injection with the maximum dose for 1–5 years of 40 mg and maximum dose for 6–12 years of 75 mg. Phenothiazines block dopamine receptors at the CTZ and are helpful to counteract the effects of chemotherapy, radiotherapy, surgical treatments, vertigo, Ménière's disease and migrane. However, the side-effects must be considered in treating individual patients of hypotension, sedation and extrapyramidial effects. Carers of children should be particularly aware of dystonia as a side effect of phenothiazines.

Prochlorperazine also has the same effects. Anticholinergic medications depress the vomit centre and have an antispasmodic action on the gut. **Hyoscine** 0.4 mg and **atropine** 0.6 mg are commonly used in travel sickness prescriptions. Hyoscine is the most useful for travel sickness and the nausea of terminal cancer, when it can be applied behind the ear by transdermal patch 500 µg every 72 hours. Side effects for both these drugs are dry mouth, visual disturbance and drowsiness. Hyoscine should be used with care in patients with glaucoma and those imbibing quantities of alcohol, as alcohol increases its effect. Atropine is often used preoperatively as it increases gut emptying time thus reducing the chance of inhalation of vomit at intubation. This drug works widely in the body so has many side effects. In children it is known to raise pulse rates, dry the skin and produce flushing; this effect is often misread as a pyrexia.

14.1 ATROPINE – TREAT WITH CAUTION

Some over-the-counter remedies for travellers to purchase freely include combinations of atropine and diphenoxylate. The atropine has an anticholinergic action and is dangerous for sufferers of glaucoma as it dilates the pupils. The diphenoxylate hydrochloride is a narcotic that will cause respiratory depression in overdose.

Antihistamines act on the CTZ and vestibular apparatus. They block histamine receptors that stimulate acid production from the parietal cells and have antimuscarinic properties. They are useful for motion sickness. **Cyclizine** is used, 50 mg three times daily (25 mg in the child), for obstructed intestinal situations. **Promethazine**, 25–50 mg daily (5 mg 6–8 hourly for the child), and **dimenhydrinate** are used to counteract nausea after radiotherapy.

Steroids are routinely prescribed for patients undergoing chemotherapy for cancer. They stabilise cell membranes and decrease permeability of the blood–brain barrier. They inhibit cerebral oedema and raised intracranial pressure caused by the cytotoxic drugs and radiotherapy. They lower the immune response and cause Cushing-like symptoms if used long term. Intravenous or oral **dexamethasone**, 5–20 mg (child 200–500 µg/kg) is given daily in the morning to reduce adrenal suppression and the patient's own cortisone supply (see reference to this function in Chapter 10 *Drugs and endocrine disorders*).

Benzodiazepines are sedative and anxiolytic in their action. **Lorazepam** 1–4 mg daily depresses the subcortical levels of the central nervous system, including the limbic and reticular formation, and thus the psychological stimulus for nausea and vomiting in chemotherapy treatment. Other complementary treatments that target this sensory input include distraction, aromatherapy and visualisation.

Cannabinoids, active agent delta-9-tetrahydrocannabinol, work by their anxiolytic activity and they may have some anti-opioid activity. **Nabilone**, 1–2 mg orally twice a day, is used as a chemotherapy antiemetic as it inhibits the vomit control mechanism in the medulla oblongata.

Natural products such as **feverfew** and **ginger extract**, 6-gingerol, may be useful as adjuncts to antiemetic medication. Feverfew releases serotonin from platelets and ginger is active in the system used for assaying the serotonin$_3$ receptors. A 1 g capsule of ginger given with the premedication can help the nausea experienced in children after grommet insertion and squint surgery.

COMMON DISORDERS OF THE GASTROINTESTINAL TRACT

CONSTIPATION

This is difficult or infrequent defecation. It can be individually defined in terms of the number of bowel movements per week, hard stools and difficult evacuation.

Pathophysiology

Constipation can be caused by a neurogenic disorder, muscle weakness, low-residue diet, emotional upset, an iatrogenic effect or a sedentary lifestyle.

Pharmacological management

Laxatives change faecal consistency, speed the passage of faeces through the colon and aid elimination of stool from the rectum. Types of laxative include bulk-forming preparations, faecal softeners, hyperosmolar or saline solutions, lubricants and stimulants or irritants (**Fig. 14.5**).

Bulk-forming treatments

These are useful in simple constipation of post-partum, elderly and debilitated patients. Also they are helpful in those suffering from diverticulitis. However, these preparations may cause abdominal cramps, diarrhoea or obstruction if the patient is dehydrated. High-bran foods (30 g per day) (Nazarko, 1996), methyl cellulose (3–6 tablets) and ispaghula husk swell on contact with water. As the contents of the colon swell so peristalsis is stimulated in the smooth muscles of the gut. These preparations are also useful in decreasing diarrhoea in some conditions. All these medications should be administered with adequate fluid and be given daily. They should take effect in between 12 hours and 3 days, depending on the preparation and patient.

Faecal softeners

Faecal softeners lower surface tension of the stool thus allowing faecal mass to be penetrated by intestinal fluids.

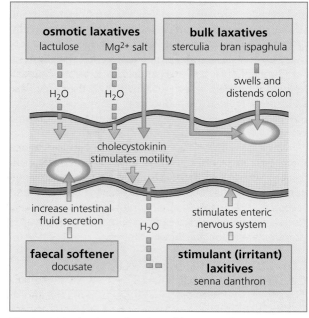

Fig 14.5 Mechanism of action of laxatives. (From Page 1997, with permission.)

They then inhibit fluid and electrolyte reabsorption by the colon, so may cause diarrhoea. They are useful in overcoming constipation caused by delay in rectal emptying, for example postoperatively, post-partum and after rectal surgery, because they reduce straining at stool. These medications should not be used with phenolphthalein as they allow it to be absorbed more quickly and cause liver toxicity. **Docusate sodium** 50–200 mg can be given orally in divided doses or by enema. In terminally ill patients it is commonly given in combination with the stimulant co-danthrusate. Similarly, **poloxamer**, another surface-wetting agent, is given in combination with **danthron** in the **form** of **co-danthramer** (White, 1995).

Hyperosmotic liquids

These produce their effect in the colon by distending the bowel with fluid accumulation, which promotes peristalsis in the same way as the bulk-forming treatments above. **Glycerine** suppositories 4 g are commonly used for a variety of patients. They may produce a cramping feeling as the glycerol has a mildly irritant action. **Lactulose**, 15 ml twice daily, is a sugar that is broken down by bacteria in the large bowel to produce various acids that stimulate peristalsis. The sugar is not absorbed so is safe for the treatment of those with diabetes. In the large doses needed by patients on opioid therapy this medication can make the patients feel bloated so a combination of laxatives is often prescribed (White, 1995). **Magnesium sulphate** 5–10 g in water is poorly absorbed from the gut, acts speedily in 2–4 hours but may cause painful colic. It should be given before

food so that it can pass more quickly through the stomach to reach the large intestine. **Phosphate** enemas should not be used in ulcerative conditions of the large intestine.

Lubricants

Lubricants such as **liquid paraffin**, 15 ml orally three times daily, soften stools and lubricate the contents of the gastrointestinal tract. However, prolonged use may interfere with the absorption of fat soluble vitamins A, D and K. It may be given in the form of an emulsion with magnesium hydroxide, which avoids the unpleasant side effects of anal seepage and lipoid pneumonia (White, 1995). Mineral oil may be given as a retention enema, 120 ml, to soften stools before an irritant evacuant is administered.

Natural stimulant or irritant laxatives

These all contain anthraquinones. After liberation in the intestine they are absorbed into the bloodstream and act on the large intestine muscle, causing an increase in peristalsis. All preparations take 8–12 hours to work and should be taken at bedtime. **Senna** 2–4 tablets or 1–2 teaspoonfuls of granules is commonly used. Artificial agents such as bisacodyl stimulate motor activity as they come into contact with the colon wall – thus they must come into contact with the rectal wall. **Bisacodyl** can be given rectally by suppository (10 mg) or orally 5–10 mg (enteric coated). The tablets should not be taken with antacids as these dissolve the coating and lead to gastric irritation.

DIARRHOEA

Diarrhoea is defined as the increase in volume, frequency or fluidity of stool (McCance and Huether, 1998). The World Health Organization defines diarrhoea as 6–8 bowel movements in 24 hours.

Pathophysiology

Diarrhoea can be acute, secondary to enteric infection, or chronic, secondary to inflammatory bowel disease. The major hazard is loss of fluid and electrolytes. Excessive fluid in the lumen of the gut generates rapid, high-volume flow that overwhelms the capacity of the colon to absorb. Faecal incontinence is experienced by 1–2% of adults.

Pharmacological management

Natural opioids such as morphine and codeine and synthetic opioids such as **loperamide hydrochloride** (2 mg three times per day) act on intestinal nerve endings to decrease secretion and promote mucosal transport out of the lumen. They also act on the central nervous system to alter extrinsic neural influences on the intestine, thus promoting absorption of fluid and electrolytes. Loperamide hydrochloride does not, however, cross the blood–brain barrier and therefore has no central sedating effect. **Codeine phosphate** (10–60 mg 4 hourly) decreases peristalsis and increases bowel tone. Kaolin (10–30 ml 4 hourly) increases the solidity of the stool and raises its resistance to flow. It forms a gel and thus the stool is more formed, but it has no tissue effect.

FLATULENCE

This is the presence of an excessive amount of air or gas in the stomach and intestinal tract. It can cause distension of the organs and in some cases mild to moderate pain.

Pathophysiology

Anaerobic bacteria *B. fragile* and *C. perfringens*, anaerobic *E. aerogenes* and *E. coli* break down some food products and synthesise vitamin K, thiamine, folic acid and riboflavin. This fermentation also produces gas, known as flatus, that consists of nitrogen, carbon dioxide, hydrogen, methane and hydrogen sulphide. Normally, 500–700 ml is produced daily.

Pharmacological management

Treatment of flatulence is usually to adjust the patient's diet, perhaps with restrictions on fibre and aromatic root vegetables. If air swallowing is a cause, the patient is encouraged to stop this habit.

OBESITY

The commonest malnutrition in the West is obesity. This is defined as a body mass index of above 30. This is a common problem in childhood and adolescence; 9.6% of girls and 6.5% of boys are overweight. In adults in 1993, 56% of men and 46% of women were overweight (Hall, 1996).

Pathophysiology

Organic causes such as Cushing's syndrome (see Chapter 10 *Drugs and endocrine disorders*), hypothalamic lesions, hypothyroidism, hyperinsulinism, oopherectomy and genetic transmission must be excluded as underpinning the weight increase before appetite manipulation is commenced. It is probably a multifactorial phenomenon, thus social, psychological and physical measures need to be investigated in its treatment.

Pharmacological management

Current treatments for obesity may include diet manipulation, exercise, behaviour modification, surgery and an emerging use of medications. Historically **dexamphetamine sulphate** (maximum dose 60 mg daily) and **fenfluramine hydrochloride** (60 mg daily for up to 3 months) were the first drugs used to control weight. They increased metabolic rate by increasing the release of noradrenaline and dopamine in the cerebral cortex and reticular activating system. These stimulants often resulted in distressing tachycardia and sleeplessness. Recently, a drug to suppress appetite has been available both in the USA and the United Kingdom. Dexfenfluramine hydrochloride stimulates the production of serotonin in the brain to mimic the feeling of satiety. More recently, a combination of fenfluramine with phentermine has become available; it has the additional chemical that makes the user feel energetic and thus able to burn off calories and lose weight at a faster rate (Millar, 1997).

A second group of drugs act locally in the gut; **acarbose**, 100 mg three times daily, is an amylase inhibitor that interferes with the digestion of sucrose and complex carbohydrates in the small intestine. Tetrahydrolipostatin, a lipase inhibitor, blocks the digestion of lipids. New drugs are being developed to mimic cholecystokinin, which is a naturally produced gut hormone secreted by the columnar cells of the duodenal and jejunal mucosal crypts in response to products of protein digestion and fats entering the duodenum. This chemical reaches the pancreas via the systemic circulation to stimulate the acinar cells to produce digestive enzymes; it is also a neurotransmitter and travels to the area of the hypothalamus called the satiety centre. In addition, it augments secretin, which is secreted from the wall of the duodenum and jejunum in response to chyme entering that area of the gastrointestinal tract. Secretin circulates via the systemic system to the pancreas and stimulates the release of a watery fluid rich in bicarbonate ions that decrease gastric acidity and motility, slowing gastric emptying (Garbett, 1995).

CYSTIC FIBROSIS

This is a genetically transmitted disorder that results in the production of abnormally viscous solutions. Symptoms are produced particularly within the gastrointestinal and respiratory systems.

Pathophysiology

In cystic fibrosis abnormal genetic expression of the cystic fibrosis transmembrane regulator results in a disordered activity of the sodium and chloride ion channels across apical membranes. The dehydrated secretions that are produced then obstruct the secretion of digestive enzymes and hormones by the pancreatic cells. Chronic respiratory infections increase individual calorie requirements to 120–150% of recommended daily allowance. Insufficient bicarbonate in gut secretions results in low enzyme function in the gut, which prevents adequate absorption of fat and protein.

Pharmacological management

Cystic fibrosis patients must be given high-lipase pancreatic enzymes with all their food; pancreatin capsules or powder, vitamins and minerals, especially sodium chloride in hot weather, must be given daily as supplements. **Creon**, 25 000 i.u., is given as enteric-coated capsules with food. The capsule coating dissolves in an environment of pH higher than 5.5, therefore the capsule remains intact in the acid environment of the stomach and releases its active ingredients in the duodenum. This pancrease medication is prescribed individually and the dosage is regulated in relation to stool fat content patient weight. The active ingredients are protease, lipase and amylase. Too high a dose results in a state similar to meconium ileus and damage similar to burns affect the buccal mucosa and skin round the anus. The medication will corrode gastrostomy tubes so, as many children with cystic fibrosis are fed overnight to supplement their poor nutrient absorption, the insertion sites must be inspected regularly (Guy's, Lewisham and St Thomas' Hospital, 1997).

RUMINATION

The regurgitation of small amounts of undigested food with little force after feeding, a condition commonly seen in infants.

Pathophysiology

The regurgitation occurs largely because of cardiac sphincter immaturity and it will usually resolve at 3–4 months of age and when weaning onto solid foods occurs. Sometimes it seems to become habitual.

Pharmacological management

A combination of antacid with alginates, which forms a solid gel when taken into the stomach with 100 ml milk can reduce regurgitation. If reflux occurs, the alkaline antacid protects the mucosa of the lower oesophagus (Trounce,

1988). Simple remedies such as feeding the baby smaller amounts more frequently and sitting the baby up after feeds may be sufficient to control the regurgitation. Other interventions include the use of feed thickeners. Cornflour is no longer recommended as it adds extra calories and may lead to overweight. However, **Carobel** flakes from carob bean gum are frequently used to add to warmed feeds as a thickener. As it has no nutritional value, the preparation does not produce obesity (McQuaid *et al.*, 1996). If, despite the medication, the baby continues to ruminate and fails to thrive, further investigation may be needed.

14.1 COELIAC (GLUTEN-SENSITIVE DISEASE)

All children need adequate calories for optimal growth. Fad diets or cultural requirements may limit choice and nutritional content, which results in poor physical development. Some children may, however, suffer an absorption deficit between 6 months and 2 years of age. In coeliac (gluten sensitive) disease, the ileal villi become flattened and reduced absorption of fats, carbohydrates and vitamins occurs. This disease is usually controlled by a diet which avoids gluten, rather than by pharmacological remedies.

INFLAMMATORY BOWEL DISEASE

Inflammatory conditions of the gastrointestinal tract are the result of infection, ingestion of irritants, trauma and altered autonomic nervous system control. Diverticula are herniations of mucosa through the muscle wall of the sigmoid colon that require an increase in dietary bulk. They can become inflamed (**diverticulitis**) and rupture, requiring surgery.

Ulcerative colitis is an inflammatory process of the lining of the sigmoid colon and rectum.

Pathophysiology

Inflammatory bowel disease may be initiated by infection, genetic make-up or immunological factors. Inflammation occurs at the base of the crypt of Lieberkühn, which leads to the mucosa appearing hyperaemic and ulcerated. The patient complains of fever and abdominal pain, and is generally unwell.

Pharmacological management

Sulphasalazine, 2 g daily, is metabolised by the gastrointestinal bacteria to release 5-aminosalicylate and sulphapyridine, which has local anti-inflammatory action. Patients with inflammatory bowel disease who wear contact lenses and are taking this medication should be aware that

PERSON CENTRED STUDY 2

Mary-Ann is a young lady aged 25 years who has suffered from ulcerative colitis for 10 years. She has recently moved from living with her parents to a flat that she shares with three other women who work in the same organisation. She now complains that her stools have increased to six per day, some having mucus and blood evident. She takes sulphasalazine, 2 g daily, and tries to remain on her diet low in dairy produce, wheat and spices. She has taken codeine 4 hourly for 2 days but this has not relieved her symptoms. She is now embarrassed by her condition as toilet facilities in the flat are shared between four people.

1. What other locally applied medication could be prescribed to alleviate her distress?
2. What is the difference between ulcerative colitis and Crohn's disease?

a side effect of sulphasalazine is to stain contact lenses. **Hydrocortisone** enemas daily decrease inflammation locally by suppressing migration of polymorphonuclear leucocytes and fibroblasts, and by reversing the increased capillary permeability and lysosomal stabilisation (McCance and Huether, 1998).

CROHN'S DISEASE

This condition is a chronic inflammatory bowel disease of unknown origin that affects the large and the small intestine. Diseased segments may be separated by normal bowel segments. Twenty per cent of affected individuals have a positive family history.

Pathophysiology

Crohn's disease is characterised by increased suppressor T cell activity and alterations of immunoglobulin A production. Inflammation starts in the submucosa and spreads to the mucosa and serosa. A typical lesion is a granuloma, which has projections of inflamed tissue surrounded by fibrous scarring.

Pharmacological management

The treatment for Crohn's disease is similar to that for ulcerative colitis and it is sometimes difficult for medical practitioners to differentiate between the two conditions. When there is severe disruption of function in the intestine, vitamin and mineral absorption is reduced. Other body systems are then affected, for example vitamin B_{12} deficiency has an effect on the developing blood cells (see Chapter 12 *Drugs and cardiovascular disorders*).

COMMON DISORDERS CAUSED BY INFECTION

The gastrointestinal tract is in contact with the external environment at both ends. As a result, infective agents may enter the body via either route. The gastrointestinal tract normally repels infection by protective lymphatic tissue and changes of pH throughout its length.

COLD SORES

This is an infection caused by a herpes simplex virus that has an affinity for the skin and nervous system. It usually manifests as small, transient, irritating, painful fluid-filled blisters on the skin and mucous membranes. Cold sores on the lips inhibit ingestion of nutrients.

Pathophysiology

Herpes simplex virus comes in two forms: type 1 and type 2. Type 2 is responsible for genital infection and type 1 is spread by direct contact onto the surface of the lips where there are no sebaceous glands to lubricate this surface and thus protect it. By the age of 25 years 90% of adults have been infected with herpes simplex (Williams, 1994).

Pharmacological management

Herpes simplex infection can be treated with **idoxuridine** 0.1% solution, held in the mouth for 2–3 minutes four times a day for 4 days. **Acyclovir**, which interferes with viral DNA replication, can be applied locally as a 5% cream or systemically, 5 mg/kg given intravenously every 8 hours (child 250 mg/m^2 8 hourly). **Aspirin** helps to reduce pain and swelling, and local anaesthetic ointment such as **lignocaine** gel 2% helps to reduce soreness. Herpes recurs when the individual becomes immunosuppressed, for example when suffering from the common cold or experiencing stressful conditions.

APHTHOUS ULCERATION

Aphthous ulceration in the mouth causes widespread misery and discomfort. Patients can become quite debilitated if they become secondarily infected.

Pathophysiology

The small painful, recurrent oral ulcers are thought to originate from a viral infection.

Pharmacological management

Hydrocortisone lozenges or **tetracycline** mouthwashes may be prescribed for aphthous ulcers. A compound **thymol glycerine** mouthwash can act as a mild antiseptic or chlorhexodine gluconate in solution 0.2% may be used. Sodium bicarbonate 0.25 teaspoonful in 50 ml water is useful to remove dry mucus in patients who are unable to use a toothbrush.

CANDIDA

A common yeast-like fungal infection that can give the symptoms of a sore mouth in all age groups.

Pathophysiology

Candida can be a secondary fungal infestation, which commonly occurs because antibiotics have destroyed natural oral flora, for example after the overenthusiastic use of tetracycline. *Candida* can also occur as a primary infection in those who have low levels of immunity, such as young babies and patients undergoing chemotherapy.

Pharmacological management

Nystatin is used to treat the common secondary effects of fungal infestation because it binds to sterols in the cell membranes of fungi, allowing intracellular components to leak out, thus destroying the microorganism. Nystatin is given in doses of 100 000 i.u. four times daily after food and is continued for 5 days. It may be given by tablet, the softer pastille or as liquid suspension. For maximum results, it must be held as long as possible in the buccal cavity before being swallowed. **Hydrogen peroxide** 6% mouthwash solution can be used to clear ulcer debris crusting. A more recent homeopathic treatment, which also tastes better, is tea tree oil, 2–3 drops in half a cup of warm water to rinse the mouth four times daily.

PEPTIC ULCERS

These have a multifactorial causation that includes increased gastric acid output, the use of non-steroidal anti-inflammatory drugs, *Helicobacter pylori* infection, smoking, gender, genetic predisposition and age. At some time in their lives 5–10% of the world's population are affected and nearly all non-iatrogenic stomach ulcers are caused by *Helicobacter pylori* bacilli (Blaser, 1996).

Pathophysiology

The healthy stomach does not usually harbour infections; however, *Helicobacter pylori* has been shown to be responsible for many cases of gastric ulceration.

There are reports that gastric ulceration is found more frequently in patients with blood group O (Mestrel, 1994). This may be attributed to sugars located in the stomach lining of these individuals, which are precisely those required by the bacillus for attachment to the mucosa. *Helicobacter pylori* lives symbiotically with humans in an oxygen level of 5% (normal for the lining of the antrum of the stomach) and manufactures an enzyme, urease, which cleaves urea to ammonia and carbon dioxide. It is this ammonia that neutralises the stomach hydrochloric acid locally, thus allowing the bacillus to survive. Having attached itself and developed a suitable micro-environment, the bacillus is then thought to produce noxious chemicals that elicit an inflammatory response in the gastric tissue. In this way ideal conditions are produced for replication and colonisation.

It is the local increase of pH in the antrum from ammonia production that stimulates gastrin to be produced from the gastrointestinal cells. This hormone then circulates in the blood to the parietal cells where it liberates histamine to stimulate acid production (**Fig. 14.6**).

Pharmacological management

Since 1910, treatments have focused on the maxim 'no acid – no ulcer'. **Antacids** neutralise hydrochloric acid produced from the parietal cells by raising the pH. However, this stimulates gastrin production by a process of negative feedback and thus more acid is ultimately produced and the stomach motility is increased (Neal, 1992).

Sodium bicarbonate powder, 1–5 g in water (or equivalent dose in 300 mg tablets), reacts with hydrochloric acid to produce carbon dioxide gas, sodium chloride and water. This was used to reduce gastric hyperacidity, but resulted in the patient experiencing flatus and belching. In excess, this treatment may result in systemic alkalosis as it raises plasma bicarbonate, which buffers hydrogen ion concentration. Also it must not be taken with milk as it results in a milk–alkali syndrome.

Magnesium and aluminium salts also neutralise gastric acidity. **Magnesium trisilicate** 1–5 g with water three times daily is commonly used but may cause diarrhoea. Aluminium-containing compounds such as magaldrate 800–1600 mg per dose may be less laxative in their side effects. Both magnesium and aluminium salts interact with many other medications, for example they reduce the therapeutic effect of tetracycline. Absorption of aluminium from antacids may have been involved in the pathogenesis of Alzheimer's disease (McGee *et al.*, 1992) and children have been found to lay down deposits of aluminium in their developing bones.

Some drugs coat the ulcers that have already formed and protect them from acid secretions, thus allowing healing to proceed. **Sucralfate** molecules polymerise in an acidic environment to a sticky gel that coats the base of the ulcer crater. It also inhibits pepsin and gastric juice secretion and absorbs bile salts. Thus this drug is useful for gastric and duodenal ulcer treatment. The dose is 1 g every 4 hours, before meals and at bedtime. It decreases the effect of antacids, however, and interferes with the absorption of tetracycline and cimetidine. Its use is recommended for patients who have suffered cerebral vascular accidents and to prevent stress ulcers in acutely ill patients (Rao and Theodossi, 1992).

Bismuth chelate, 120 mg four times daily, has a toxic effect on the *H. pylori* bacterium and stimulates production of the protective gastric mucosal prostaglandin and secretion of bicarbonate. To be effective it must be taken on an empty stomach; its effect is reduced by antacids, proteins and milk consumed at the same time. Blackening of stool and tongue are normal side effects and must not be confused with the melaena of bleeding ulceration (Kelly, 1994).

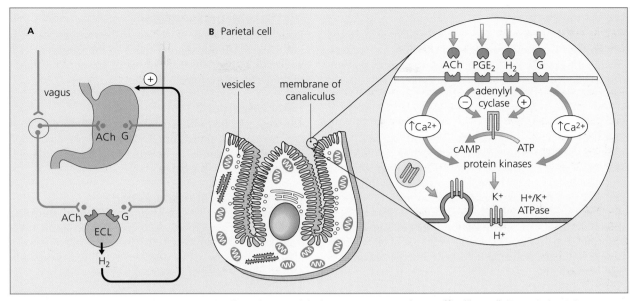

Fig 14.6 Acid secretion from the parietal cell. ACh: acetylcholine; ECL: enterochromaffin-like cell; G: gastrin; PG: prostaglandin. (From Page 1997, with permission.)

Carbenoxolone, a synthetic derivative of liquorice, is believed to increase the quantity and viscosity of mucus production in the stomach. It has an aldosterone-like action, resulting in sodium retention and hypokalaemia, so may exacerbate oedema and hypertension. Potassium supplements and thiazide diuretics may be needed to minimise side effects (Kelly, 1994).

Misoprostol, 400 μg twice daily, is a prostaglandin analogue that enhances cytoprotection. It does this by inhibiting acid production, increasing bicarbonate and mucus secretion and stimulating rapid cell renewal and microcirculation. It is a good maintenance therapy for patients needing regular non-steroidal drug therapy for other diseases (Rao and Theodossi, 1992). It should not be given with magnesium-containing antacids as it compounds a laxative side effect. It should be used with care in women of child-bearing age as it may produce intramenstrual bleeding. It also may compound the pathology of those with cardiovascular disease (Kelly, 1994; Rao and Theodossi, 1992).

Over the past decade drugs that inhibit gastric acid production by blocking acetylcholine receptors have been available. They antagonise cholinergic muscarinic receptor sites (M_1) on histamine-containing paracrine cells in the oxyntic mucosa to inhibit acetylcholine-induced release of histamine; they also block M_3 receptors on parietal cells to inhibit direct acetylcholine-induced acid secretion. However, they have only been able to give symptom relief while being taken and are often not a cure for ulcers. **Cimetidine**, orally 400 mg twice daily or 800 mg at night for 4–6 weeks (or by intravenous or intramuscular injection 200–400 mg), and **ranitidine**, 150 mg twice daily or 300 mg at night for 4–6 weeks (or by the intravenous or intramuscular route 50 mg 6–8 hourly), are drugs that do not block cholinergic receptors or gastrin receptors.

Proton pump inhibitors such as **omeprazole** (20–40 mg once daily for 4–8 weeks) block parietal cell hydrogen–potassium ATPase, which is required for transport of hydrogen ions into the lumen of the stomach. The antibiotic **metronidazole**, 400 mg 8 hourly by mouth, is useful against anaerobic bacteria such as *H. pylori*, and **amoxycillin**, 250 mg 8 hourly, is effective as a broad-spectrum antibiotic; amoxycillin interferes with the cell wall replication of susceptible bacteria, rendering them osmotically unstable and thus liable to swell and burst.

A combined drug regime of omeprazole, bismuth chelate, metronidazole, amoxycillin and sucralfate or the prostaglandin analogue misoprostol will heal 90% of all ulcers (Rao and Theodossi, 1992). However, this therapy is not without risk. Malaise, nausea, diarrhoea, sore mouth, fungal infections and pseudomembranous colitis have been reported. Healthcare workers are reminded to look at the treatments for ulcers holistically and to warn patients on diets that cause over-secretion and hypermobility in the gastrointestinal tract (Kelly, 1994). In addition, smoking reduces the protective bicarbonate secretions from the pancreas thus increasing acidity in the duodenum; the overuse of aspirin, stressful lifestyle and poor coping strategies do likewise. Appropriate counselling can complement the effect of medication. It should be possible in future to vaccinate against peptic ulceration using a vaccine that has now been found safe in phase 2 European–US trials (Voekler, 1996).

GASTROENTERITIS

This is inflammation of the stomach and intestines and accompanies numerous gastrointestinal disorders. Symptoms include nausea, vomiting, abdominal discomfort and diarrhoea. It continues to be a significant cause of morbidity in the United Kingdom.

Pathophysiology

The ileum is a high-alkaline environment, but some bacteria and parasites can survive. *Escherichia coli*, *Shigella* and *Salmonella* commonly produce devastating vomiting and diarrhoea, which can be life threatening in the young and old. Childhood gastroenteritis continues to be a significant cause of morbidity in the United Kingdom. These infections result in inflammation and sloughing of the absorptive brush-border cells, with subsequent impairment of water and electrolyte homeostasis and altered absorption of nutrients.

Pharmacological management

The symptoms of gastroenteritis need to be treated conservatively at first, with rehydration solutions given orally or intravenously. Sodium chloride 3.5 g, sodium bicarbonate 2.5 g, potassium chloride 1.5 g and glucose 20 g made up to 1 l can be titrated against fluid stool loss. For infants with gastroenteritis, present thinking suggests that breast feeding, which supplies the child with surface immunoglobulin A, macrophages and lymphocytes, should be continued. Older children should continue their diet to supply calorific needs. Antibiotics need only be given if sensitivities are defined (Carter, 1995).

OVERUSE OF ORAL ANTIBIOTICS

From 1982 to 1992 there has been a marked rise in the incidence of *Clostridium difficile*, an anaerobic bacillus, in patients over the age of 65 years; it causes antibiotic-associated diarrhoea and may lead to pseudomembranous colitis.

Pathophysiology

The infection occurs when there has been disruption of the gut flora in the colon from the use of broad-spectrum antibiotics. It produces toxins that enter the cells of the gut mucosa and cause inflammation and damage.

Pharmacological management

Treatment is to stop the antibiotic currently being taken by the patient and to give **metronidazole**, 250 mg, and **vancomycin**, 500 mg, every 6 hours if the condition is severe (Gammon, 1995) (see chapter 3 *Classes of drugs*).

Diarrhoea caused by antibiotic therapy can be treated with *Lactobacillus*, a bacteria found in natural yoghurt. This replaces natural gut flora destroyed by oral antiobiotic therapy.

INTESTINAL INFESTATION

Roundworms and hookworms are common causes of extensive morbidity among those in the tropics already weakened by poor diet. Threadworms are seen in children in the United Kingdom.

Pathophysiology

The parasites cause inflammation in the gut mucosa, bleeding and pain. An already immunocompromised individual may become secondarily infected with bacteria that will release toxins into the blood.

Pharmacological management

Parasites can be treated with appropriate anthelmintics. Anthelmintics are a diverse group of drugs specific to the infestation. Threadworms are treated with piperazine 50–75 mg/kg daily in two treatments of 1 week's duration, separated by 1 week of rest.

ANOREXIA NERVOSA

Many young children may have a period of food fads and poor appetite especially after illness. However, serious food refusal is more likely to be seen in older children and young adults. Anorexia nervosa occurs in 1–2 per 1000 adolescent girls, but the incidence has risen in the past 50 years. The peak age for diagnosis is 14 years (Garralda, 1993).

Pathophysiology

The problem appears to be multifactorial in origin; personality, social group, culture, puberty and sexual abuse have been suggested. Family disharmony often underpins the trigger for expression. Anorexia nervosa may be more about weight phobia than appetite (Taylor and Muller, 1995). It is characterised by frequent incidence of voluntary food restriction or starvation, vomiting, purging and increased activity.

Pharmacological management

The treatment must be as an in-patient with forced intravenous and/or enteral feeding if extreme weight loss (80% of weight for age), dehydration, signs of circulatory failure, persistent vomiting and marked depression (seen in 50% of patients) are present. Depression may be treated with **imipramine** (75–200 mg at night for 3 months), which can increase the action of noradrenaline and serotonin in the nerve cells. Other antidepressants such as **amitriptyline** can be used. These drugs take 5 days to achieve a steady blood state and 3 weeks to have a clinical effect. Side effects are sleepiness, thirst and gastrointestinal irritation, therefore they are often prescribed to be taken with milk at night. Forceful control of the diet is taken by carers, and family therapy is initiated to help the patient come to recognise their needs and build self-esteem (Shaw and Lawson, 1994).

BULIMIA NERVOSA

Bulimia nervosa, seen in 1% of young girls and women, is when there are episodes of binge eating followed by self-induced vomiting and purging, and periods of food intake limitation without severe weight loss. It can be treated similarly to anorexia (Brody *et al.*, 1994) (see Chapter 7 *Drugs and psychological disorders*).

HEPATIC DISORDERS

Liver cells carry out a wide variety of metabolic functions. Carbohydrate, protein, fat, alcohol and drugs are metabolised. Hormones, bilirubin and bile salts are produced; vitamins A, D and B_{12}, K and folate and the mineral iron are stored. Any pathology has a wide ranging effect in all body systems and deficits of function require complex replacement therapy. Jaundice results from an increase in bilirubin concentration in body fluids when the liver is not able to transport bilirubin into the bile. It may be the result of liver damage, infection, immaturity or congenital defect. It can be detectable when serum levels exceed 50 mmol/l.

PHENYLKETONURIA

Phenylketonuria is the abnormal presence of phenylketone and other metabolites of phenylalanine. Phenylketonuria has been screened for nationally in the United Kingdom since 1969, 6–10 days after birth (Guthrie test) when the baby is fully established on milk feeds.

Pathophysiology

Phenylketonuria is an autosomal recessive inherited metabolic disorder in which there is a deficiency of the liver enzyme phenylalanine hydroxylase. A positive test shows phenylalanine above the normal range of 30–70 μmol/l; if left, this leads to irreversible nerve damage.

Pharmacological management

The treatment for phenylketonuria is a strict phenylalanine restricted diet using protein substitutes that provide all the other amino acids essential for growth and development. Treatment is recommended for life and specialist advice should be sought in sickness and pregnancy.

HEPATITIS

This is basically an inflammatory condition of the liver and comes in many forms. Severe hepatitis may lead to cirrhosis and chronic liver dysfunction. Vaccination programmes against some forms exist worldwide.

Pathophysiology

The organisms that cause hepatitis A and E are enteric viruses; they spread via the faecal–oral route and are passed to new hosts through faecal contamination of food and water and where there may be poor handwashing techniques by children in nurseries (Campbell and Glasper, 1995). Hepatitis A infects the gut cells and then spreads to the liver via the blood. It causes periportal necrosis and infiltration of mononuclear cells, and is excreted via the bile into the gut and urine, beginning 2 weeks before jaundice is clinically detected (Greenwood *et al.*, 1992).

Pharmacological management

Hepatitis is usually treated by restricting physical activity and social contacts and giving a low fat, high carbohydrate diet. Close contacts can be given passive protection by **human normal immunoglobulin (HNIG)** (250 mg for children up to the age of 9 years and 500 mg for those who are older), which will give protection for 2–6 months. The newer killed vaccine can give protection for up to 10 years after three doses (Robert-Sargeant, 1993).

HEPATITIS B

This is a form of viral hepatitis caused by the hepatitis B virus.

Pathophysiology

The causative organism of hepatitis B is a DNA-containing virus, a double-shelled particle with the outer surface component, the hepatitis B surface antigen (HBsAg), used as the marker that identifies the carrier state or chronic state. Two other antigens of hepatitis B have also been identified: the core antigen (HBcAg) and the e antigen (HBeAg), the latter being an envelope antigen used as the marker of infective ability (Nicoll and Rudd, 1993). This virus is transmitted by blood, sexual activity and during intranatal or postnatal contact between mother and child.

Pharmacological management

Hepatitis B vaccination is now offered to all children born in the USA: at birth, 1 month, 2 months and 12 months, with boosters every 5 years (Nicoll and Rudd, 1993). In the United Kingdom hepatitis B vaccination is recommended for all healthcare workers. The active vaccination which will stimulate the body to make antibodies, is an inactivated preparation derived from the surface antigen of the virus. Two types are available; each contains 20 μg/ml of HBsAg adsorbed on aluminium hydroxide adjuvant. The first is purified from human plasma and the second is created by genetic engineering using a recombinant DNA technique.

For new-born infants and children aged under 12 years, who are not contacts, 0.5 ml of strength 20 μg per ml is repeated three times, for adults the dose is 1 ml three times. A responder, an individual who manufactures their own antibodies in response to the vaccination stimulus, shows post-vaccination antibody levels to HBsAg of more than 10 IU/ml.

Passive immunity, the specific antibody to hepatitis B, is given within 48 hours in emergency situations where there has been contact with hepatitis B and there is not time for the individual to manufacture their own antibodies. Individuals such as newborn babies born to infected mothers would be considered for this type of vaccination.

HEPATITIS DELTA VIRUS

Hepatitis delta virus is part of another virus that cannot replicate without the hepatitis B virus; it infects 50% of those who are chronic carriers of the hepatitis B virus and increases the severity of their clinical symptoms.

Pathophysiology
See section on pathophysiology for hepatitis B.

Pharmacological management
Interferon α may give temporary improvement but only vaccination against the hepatitis B virus will ensure new cases of hepatitis delta virus do not emerge.

HEPATITIS C

Hepatitis C is a type of hepatitis transmitted largely by blood. The disease progresses to chronic hepatitis in up to 50% of the patients acutely infected.

Pathophysiology
Hepatitis C [non A, non B (NANB)] is 90% responsible for transfusion-associated hepatitis and 50% for enteric hepatitis in young adults in the Third World. It is usually mild and does not result in the carrier state. However, it can be fatal to the fetus in the third trimester.

Pharmacological management
The drug used to eradicate this virus is α **interferon**, which occurs naturally in the body but can be prepared commercially. This type of hepatitis virus cannot be prevented by vaccination as it is easily able to change itself; a large number of genetic types have been identified throughout the world (Kings College Hospital, 1996).

Medical treatment and nursing care of all the hepatitis types are aimed towards the relief of discomfort and maintenance of adequate nutrition and hydration. Antiemetics may be used if nausea prevents adequate nourishment. If blood coagulation is significantly impaired, **vitamin K** or blood components may be administered. Treatment with interferon α may give transient histological improvement in liver function (Hazinski, 1992). Ascites may be treated with diuretics such as **spironolactone**, which competes with aldosterone at receptors in the renal tubules and results in the excretion of sodium chloride and water but the retention of potassium and phosphates. Adult dosage is 100–400 mg daily. Steroids reduce inflammation and oedema in the liver, but care must be given with the administration of all medication as the dysfunctioning liver cannot carry out one of its prime functions, namely to detoxify and excrete drugs and poisons.

BILIARY DISORDERS

Some drugs change biliary metabolism. For example, **rifampicin** reduces the conjugation of serum bilirubin and **sulphonamides** and **salicylates** displace unconjugated bilirubin from binding sites on serum albumin, which can cause kernicterus in babies suffering from haemolytic disease. Conjugated bilirubin may also be inhibited from entering the biliary canaliculus and show increased retention in the blood. **Norobiocin, sulphadiazine, oral contraceptives, methyltestosterone,** and **anabolic steroids** act in this way.

The gall bladder receives its autonomic nerve supply mainly from the vagus nerve. The neurotransmitter acetylcholine causes contraction of the gall bladder muscle and increased tone. However, gall bladder contraction and choledochal sphincter opening are mainly caused by the opening effect of cholecystokinin, secreted by the duodenal mucosa in response to food. **Glyceryl trinitrate, secretin, analgesic morphine, pethidine** and **pentazocine** also produce gall bladder contraction.

Acute cholecystitis is a painful condition that is associated with stasis of the biliary system and infection of the contents of the gall bladder. The pain is best treated with **morphine** 10–20 mg (see Chapter 18 *Pharmacological management of pain*) given with **atropine**, 0.6 mg, to counteract the increased contraction of the choledochal sphincter. The antibiotic of choice is **co-trimoxazole**. Other immediate treatment is supportive, for example for jaundice. Elective surgery is planned as soon as the acute phase has settled to remove the gallstones and/or the gall bladder by laparoscopy, laparotomy or lithotripsy of stones via endoscopy (Hinchliff *et al.*, 1996).

GALLSTONES

Gallstones are most common in patients who are obese, middle-aged and female and in those who have gall bladder, pancreas and ileal disease. Gallstones can be dissolved chemically if surgery is risky.

Pathophysiology
There are two types of gallstone: cholesterol and pigmented. The first is formed in bile that is saturated with cholesterol. Crystallisation occurs in the gall bladder that has reduced motility. Gallstones are also formed when liver cells oversecrete cholesterol or have a deficit of controlling enzymes. They are also prevalent when there is diminished secretion of bile acids or decreased reabsorption of bile salts from the ileum.

Pigmented stones are made of cholesterol, calcium bilirubinate and pigmented polymers. They are usually found in biliary infection and when there is unconjugated bilirubin, which precipitates to form stones.

Pharmacological management

Ursodeoxycholic acid desaturates bile from cholesterol in cholesterol gallstones. The recommended dose is 8–12 mg/kg daily at bedtime for 2 years. Diarrhoea and pruritus are unpleasant side effects. Women taking oestrogen preparations for contraception or hormone replacement therapy should be warned that they reduce the effect of this medication.

14.2 EPIDEMIC OF E. COLI IN 1996

Deaths from *Escherichia coli* (*E. coli*) and related gram negative coliform bacteria in the UK in 1996 originated from cooked meats which had been displayed in a shop cabinet. These bacteria normally predominate among the aerobic commensal flora present in the gut in humans and animals, thus handling of cooked meat produce should be carefully undertaken by vendors. Strains of *E. coli* grow at a wide range of temperatures, 15–45°C with some strains surviving at 60°C for fifteen minutes. Re-heating cooked meats in a cool oven may not kill these bacteria and they may multiply rapidly in suitable environments. They cause diarrhoea by adhering to the villi cells of the gut mucosa, inhibiting the absorption of sodium and thus water into the body. Antimicrobial drugs are useful in treatment, drug treatment includes neomycin and other antimicrobal preparations (see chapter 5 on antibiotic therapy). Young children, the elderly and the sick will quickly become dehydrated as water is lost from the body; renal failure was the cause of death in some victims of the 1996 epidemic in UK.

PANCREATIC DISORDERS

PANCREATITIS

This is an inflammatory condition of the pancreas and is typically divided into acute and chronic forms.

Pathophysiology

Acute pancreatitis is an inflammatory process and is characterised by severe abdominal pain radiating to the back, fever, anorexia, nausea and vomiting. There may be jaundice if the common bile duct is obstructed.

Chronic pancreatitis is similar to acute pancreatitis, but is characterised by progressive destruction of the gland. When the cause is alcohol abuse, there may be calcification and scarring of the pancreatic ducts. There is abdominal pain, nausea and vomiting, and steatorrhoea and creatorrhoea caused by the diminished output of pancreatic enzymes.

Pharmacological management

Pancreatitis requires immediate medical treatment for shock, pain and respiratory and renal failure. Gastrointestinal tract feeding is via nasogastric tube or total parenteral nutrition with blood glucose monitoring and **insulin** support. In the medium term removal of gallstones may be required after the acute phase is stabilised; psychosocial support will be needed if the client abuses alcohol. In the long term, pancreatic **enzymes** and **insulin** may be required if the organ is totally destroyed. However, recovery often results in some retention of pancreatic function.

For other conditions of the pancreas see Chapter 10 *Drugs and endocrine disorders.*

🔑 KEY POINTS

- The gastrointestinal tract digests food chemically and mechanically; medication affects both these functions.
- Abnormalities of the gastrointestinal tract may be caused by failures in other body systems.
- Three types of gastrointestinal medications are those that protect the gut lining, change gut motility and improve bowel emptying.
- Many congenital and developmental abnormalities can be improved with medication.
- Inflammation and infection in the intestinal tract can be treated by protecting the gut lining and altering the secretions of gut glands.
- Nausea and vomiting are unpleasant but can usually be addressed with a combination of local and centrally targeted treatments.

- Constipation affects people of all ages; medication combinations that induce water into the bowel, lubricate the stool and increase muscle activity in evacuation are usually successful.
- Eating disorders of obesity and anorexia have a multifactoral origin; medication is only one aspect of treatment.
- Liver damage results in a multitude of symptoms; deficits of function require complex replacement therapy.
- Gall bladder pathology can be improved with a lifelong change in dietary habit; a few conditions need particular medication for adequate function.
- Healthy eating maintains a healthy gut.

MULTIPLE CHOICE QUESTIONS

Choose the correct answers.

1. The gastrointestinal tract may be affected by drugs that
   a. help restore or maintain the protective lining by reducing gastric acidity
   b. may decrease the gastrointestinal contractions and propulsion by increasing cholinergic stimuli at the smooth muscle M_2 receptors
   c. act locally on the submucosal plexus to inhibit secretion and promote net absorption of fluids and electrolytes
   d. are bulk forming agents that reduce gas production
   e. cause rhythmic movement of stomach contents from stomach to lower oesophagus

2. Symptoms that indicate abnormality of the gastrointestinal tract include
   a. vomiting dark grainy digested blood with a 'coffee grounds' appearance
   b. difficulty in swallowing, which may be alleviated by antimuscarinic drugs such as merbentyl
   c. rapid emptying of hypertonic chyme from the stomach into the small intestine 10–20 minutes after eating
   d. gas expelled from stomach through mouth
   e. lack of desire to eat

3. Cystic fibrosis may be treated with
   a. high lipase pancreatic enzymes given with all food
   b. individual calorie requirements to 120–150% of recommended daily allowance
   c. pancrease medication prescribed individually in relation to stool fat content
   d. sodium chloride in cold weather given daily as supplements
   e. drugs designed to release active ingredients in the duodenum and remain intact in the acid environment of the stomach

4. Diseases of the gastrointestinal tract in children may include
   a. failure to thrive because of excessive regurgitation
   b. coeliac gluten sensitivity, which usually develops between the ages of 6 months and 2 years
   c. diabetes mellitus, which may be outgrown by puberty
   d. anatomical abnormalities such as cleft palate, hair lip, tracheo-oesophageal fistula, pyloric stenosis
   e. *Clostridium*, *Enterobacter* and *Escherichia coli* infections which lead to intussusception

5. Inflammatory and infectious diseases of the gastrointestinal tract include
   a. herniations of mucosa through the muscle wall of the sigmoid colon
   b. Crohn's disease, which is an inflammatory process of the lining in the sigmoid colon and rectum
   c. aphthous ulceration, that is, small painful, recurrent oral ulcers, causing widespread morbidity
   d. non-iatrogenic stomach ulcers caused by *Helicobacter pylori*
   e. ulcerative colitis, which is a granuloma with projections of inflamed tissue surrounded by fibrous scarring

6. Treatment for gastric ulceration may include
   a. antacids, which stimulate gastrin production by a process of negative feedback
   b. sucralfate molecules, which polymerise in an acidic environment to a sticky gel that coats the base of the ulcer crater
   c. a vaccine, found safe in Phase 2 European–US trials, which is a recombinant urease with mucosal adjuvant
   d. an enzyme, urease, which cleaves urea to ammonia and carbon dioxide
   e. aluminium-containing compounds such as magaldrate 800–1600 mg per dose

7. Drugs used in the treatment of nausea include
   a. metoclopramide, hyoscine and cisapride in postoperative nausea
   b. herbs such as cannabinoids, feverfew and ginger extract
   c. benzodiazepines, phenothiazines and steroids for chemotherapy
   d. anticholinergic medications and antihistamines for travel sickness
   e. cyclizine, 50 mg three times daily (25 mg in the child), for obstructed intestinal situations

8. Organs associated with the gastrointestinal tract have diseases that affect this system; these include
   a. pancreatitis
   b. hepatitis B
   c. biliary atresia
   d. phenylketonuria
   e. gallstones

9. Hepatitis affects the body in many ways, which include
   a. nausea
   b. ascites
   c. excretion of drugs
   d. bleeding
   e. constipation

10. Foods can cause and cure disease, including
    a. liquorice is believed to increase the quantity and viscosity of mucus production in the stomach
    b. ketotic diet to mimic the effect of fasting and the production of ketotic bodies for myoclonic epilepsy in children
    c. high-gluten foods can cause ileal villi to become flattened and absorption of fats, carbohydrates and vitamins to be reduced in coeliac disease
    d. natural yoghurt, which replaces natural gut flora destroyed by oral antibiotic therapy
    e. green vegetables, which protect against indigestion

REFERENCES

Assaf RAE, Clarke RSJ, Dundee JW, Samuel IO. Studies of drugs given before anaesthesia XXIV: Metoclopramide with morphine and pethidine. *Br J Anaesth* 1974; **46:**514-519.

Berkley KJ, Hotta H, Robbins J, Sat Y. Functional properties of afferent fibres supplying reproductive and other pelvic organs in the pelvic nerves of female rat. *J Neurophysiol* 1990; **63:**256-272.

Blaser M. The bacteria behind ulcers. *Sci Am* February 1996; 92-97.

Brody T, Larner J, Minneman K, Harold C. *Human pharmacology, 2nd ed.* London: Mosby, 1994.

Brown I. Malnutrition, poverty and intellectual development. *Sci Am* February 1996; 26-30.

Carter E. Management of acute childhood gastro-enteritis in the community. *Maternal Child Health* 1995; **November:**365-368.

Campbell S, Glasper EA (Eds). *Whaley & Wong's Children's Nursing.* London: Mosby, 1995.

Cook J, Gallagher A. Evaluation of an anti-emetic protocol. *Paediatr Nurs* 1996; **8:**21-23.

Gammon J. Difficult bug to beat. *Nurs Times* 1995; **91(37):**57-60.

Garbett R. Digestive tract cancers. Professional Development. *Nursing Times* 1995 Unit 23, part 2, pp. 5-8, Vol 91 No. 50.

Garbett R. Digestive tract cancers. Professional Development. *Nursing Times* 1995 Unit 23, part 3, pp. 9-14, Vol 91, No. 51.

Garralda AM. Managing children with psychiatric problems. London: British Medical Journal, 1993.

Greenwood D, Slack R, Peutherer J. *Medical microbiology, 14th ed.* Edinburgh: Churchill Livingstone, 1992.

Griffiths B, Poynor M, O'Connell K. Health education and iron intake of weaning children. *Health Visitor* 1995; **68:**418-419.

Grunberg SM, Hesluth PJ. Control of chemotherapy induced emesis. *New Engl J Med* 1993; **329:**1790-1796.

Guy's, Lewisham and St Thomas' Hospital. *Guy's paediatric formulary.* London: Guy's, Lewisham and St Thomas' Hospital, 1997.

Hall C. Call for radical rethink on treatment of obesity. *Daily Telegraph* 1996; **13 March:**9.

Hawthorn J. *Understanding and management of nausea and vomiting.* Oxford: Blackwell Science, 1995.

Hazinski MF. *Nursing care of the critically ill child, 2nd ed.* London: Mosby, 1992.

Hinchliff S, Montague S, Watson R. *Physiology for nursing practice, 2nd ed.* London: Bailliére Tindall, 1996.

Jones P, Brunt P, Mowat N. *Gastroenterology.* London: Heinemann, 1985.

Kelly J. Drug therapy and peptic ulceration. *Br J Nurs* 1994; **3:**1129-34.

Kings College Hospital. *Children's liver disease.* London: Kings College Hospital, 1996.

Linblad T, Beattie WE, Forrest JB, Buckley DN. Loss of anti-emetic effect of droperidol in menstruating women. *Can J Anaesth* 1990; **37:**5139.

McCance K, Huether S. *Pathophysiology, 2nd ed.* London: Mosby, 1998.

McGee J, Issacson PG, Wright NA. *Oxford textbook of pathology, vol 2b.* Oxford: Oxford University Press, 1992.

McQuaid L, Huband S, Parker E. *Children's nursing.* Edinburgh: Churchill Livingstone, 1996.

Mestrel R. Sugary clues to stomach ulcers. *New Sci* 1994; **141:**15.

Millar S. 'The week': wonder cures may prove a bitter pill to swallow. *Guardian* 1997; **4 January:**5

Nazarko L. Preventing constipation in older people. *Prof Nurse* 1996; **11:**816-820.

Neal MJ. *Medical pharmacology at a glance, 2nd ed.* Oxford: Blackwell Science, 1992.

Nicoll A, Rudd P. *Manual on infections and immunisations in children.* Oxford: Oxford Medical Publishers, 1993.

Page C. *Integrated Pharmacology.* London: Mosby, 1997.

Price SA, Wilson L. *Pathophysiology Clinical Concepts of Disease Processes* 5th Edition, St Louis, Mosby, 1997

Rao KJM, Theodossi A. New treatments for peptic ulcers: are they necessarily better? *Maternal Child Health* 1992; **March:**90-92.

Robert-Sargeant S. RCN update: hepatitis A and B: the nurse's role. *Nurs Stand* 1993; **7(26):**3-8.

Shaw V, Lawson M, eds. *Clinical paediatric dietetics.* Oxford: Blackwell Science, 1994.

Taylor J, Muller D. *Nursing adolescents.* Oxford: Blackwell Science, 1995.

Trounce JR. *Clinical pharmacology for nurses.* Edinburgh: Churchill Livingstone, 1988.

Voekler R. Promising *H. pylori* vaccine. *J Am Med Assoc* 1996; **276:**1461.

White T. Dealing with constipation. *Nurs Times* 1995; **91(14):**57-60.

Williams C. Causes and management of nausea and vomiting. *Nurs Times* 1994; **90(44):**38-41.

15 Sylvia Prosser
DRUGS AND
UROLOGICAL DISORDERS

INTRODUCTION: STRUCTURE AND FUNCTION OF THE KIDNEY

In this chapter, renal physiology is presented in some detail in order to assist the reader's understanding of the effects of renal dysfunction and the rationale for the nursing and pharmacological management of the patient.

The urinary system consists of two major components: the kidneys, which have a range of physiological functions, and the urinary drainage and storage system (**Fig. 15.1**).

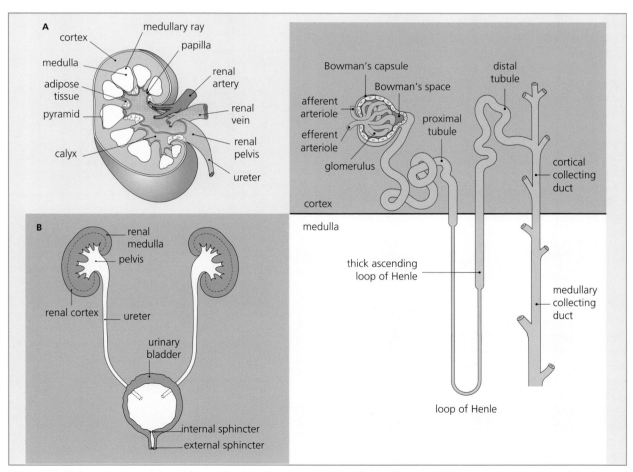

Fig 15.1 (A) The structure of the kidney. (B) Macroscopic structures of the urinary system. (From Page 1997, with permission.)

The effect of drugs within the body is partially determined by the manner in which the kidneys deal with the substances in question. In association with the liver, the kidneys are responsible for the excretion of many chemicals from the body. The concentration mechanism that accompanies the formation of urine results in substantial amounts of drugs or their metabolites being presented to the microstructures that perform the excretory or homeostatic functions of the kidney. In some circumstances, this means that it is possible to use the mechanism to obtain a therapeutic effect. **Penicillin**, for example, is secreted into the proximal tubule and is not reabsorbed into the body; the result is that penicillin-sensitive infections within the nephrons are responsive to penicillin treatment. However, the kidney is so efficient at removing penicillin from the bloodstream, that the dose must be repeated regularly in order to maintain a therapeutic level of the antibiotic in the urinary filtrate. The ability of the kidneys to filter and concentrate chemicals carries the hazard that the tubular structures may be subjected to harmful concentrations of toxins and poisons that cause renal dysfunction (see the discussion of nephropathies later in this chapter). In a similar manner, ingestion of some carcinogens such as products from cigarettes and certain dyes have been implicated in the pathogenesis of neoplasia of the urinary tract, such as carcinoma of the bladder and prostate.

The kidneys are highly active organs. Each contains approximately one million nephrons, not all of which are active at any given time (**Fig. 15.2**). This gives the kidney huge functional reserves. The cells within the nephrons have a high energy expenditure as they function as biochemical pumps. This makes the renal cells vulnerable to the effects of oxygen shortage. The cells of the juxtaglomerular apparatus function as chemical sensors and secrete hormones that maintain optimum conditions for renal activity.

The kidney functions as an organ of excretion and of homeostasis and as an endocrine gland. The mechanisms by which chemicals are filtered from the blood in the glomeruli, and selectively returned to the body according to biochemical need are shown in **Figure 15.2**.

GLOMERULAR FILTRATION

It can be seen from **Figure 15.3** that the arterioles bringing blood into the glomerular capillaries arise from the renal artery. The two renal arteries branch from the descending aorta, and are comparatively short and wide vessels. The importance of this is that blood is delivered to the glomeruli under high pressure. The hydrostatic pressure within the glomeruli is further increased by the efferent arteriole having a narrower lumen than the afferent arteriole. The result is that enhanced filtration occurs, with blood constituents that are of sufficiently small molecular size and of the appropriate electrical polarity to pass through the fenestrations in the glomerular capillaries passing down the

pressure gradient into the Bowman's capsule, and from there into the proximal tubule.

As the filtrate passes along the proximal tubule, the chemical pumps within the cells of the tubular wall return substances to the blood vessels wrapped around the nephron, so causing reabsorption according to bodily need. Most water and electrolytes are returned to the bloodstream via the cells of the proximal tubule. The absorptive cells of the nephron are arranged similarly to those in the small intestine, being positioned on the microvilli, thus producing a 'brush border'.

In the distal tubule, fine tuning of the electrolyte acid–base and water balance takes place. The function has changed from one primarily of excretion to one of maintaining homeostasis. It is at the distal tubular cells that sodium, potassium and hydrogen ions are passed into the urinary filtrate or back into the bloodstream according to the prevailing chemical balance within the body. If the body needs to excrete an accumulation of potassium or hydrogen ions, sodium excretion is inhibited. If sodium overload requires correction, hydrogen and potassium excretion is delayed, so imbalance of a given electrolyte tends to produce a reflex imbalance in the others (see **Fig. 15.3**).

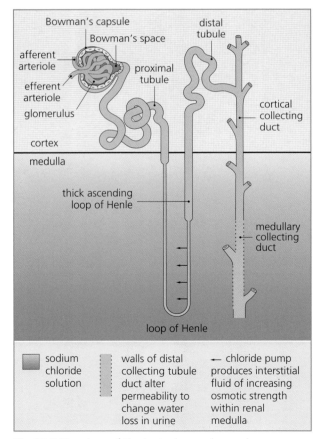

Fig 15.2 Structure of the juxtaglomerular nephron.

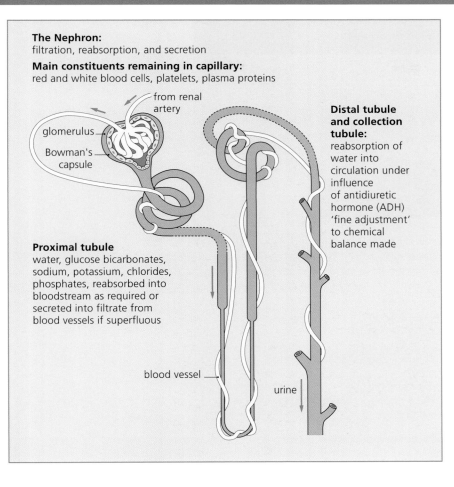

The Nephron:
filtration, reabsorption, and secretion

Main constituents remaining in capillary:
red and white blood cells, platelets, plasma proteins

from renal artery

glomerulus

Bowman's capsule

Distal tubule and collection tubule:
reabsorption of water into circulation under influence of antidiuretic hormone (ADH) 'fine adjustment' to chemical balance made

Proximal tubule
water, glucose bicarbonates, sodium, potassium, chlorides, phosphates, reabsorbed into bloodstream as required or secreted into filtrate from blood vessels if superfluous

blood vessel

urine

Fig 15.3 The nephron: filtration, reabsorption and secretion.

WATER BALANCE

A significant proportion of the water filtered into the Bowman's capsule re-enters the bloodstream as it is reabsorbed in the proximal tubule. The kidney is capable of maintaining a normal water load despite a fluid intake that may be excessive or scarcely adequate. Normal water loss from the renal system is around 1500 ml in 24 hours, but may fall to 500 ml in situations when hydration is poor, or may increase to 4–5 l if fluid intake is high or if a diuretic drives the nephrons to increase water excretion.

15.1

Some drugs change the colour of urine
Dark yellow: fluorescein, riboflavin.
Orange/brown: ibuprofen, phenytoin, sulphamethoxazole, sulphasalazine.
Red: daunorubicin, desferrioxamine, ibuprofen, rifampicin.
Blue-green: amitriptyline, methylene blue, triamterine.

The ability of the kidney to excrete or retain water depends upon the cells of the distal and collecting tubules, which may be made more or less permeable to the passage of water molecules. The distal and collecting tubules have in their walls pores that can be opened or closed according to the amount of antidiuretic hormone present. The interstitial fluid within the kidney has a progressively strong osmotic pressure within the renal medulla. This extracellular fluid behaves like blotting paper: when the pores of the distal and collecting tubule are open, water is attracted into the renal interstitium by osmosis. Water subsequently re-enters the capillaries, again because of osmosis, but this time produced by the effects of the plasma proteins. The renal extracellular fluid has an osmotic gradient because of the effect produced within the loop of Henle. On the ascending limb, particularly near the 'hairpin bend' at the tip of the loop, cells pump chloride ions and some urea molecules into the interstitial space, thus making the extracellular fluid more concentrated. As the distal and collecting tubules pierce through the deep layers of the kidney tissue, they are subjected to osmotic pressure. If the pores are open, water is pulled from the urinary filtrate into the renal interstitium, and then into the bloodstream (**Fig. 15.4**).

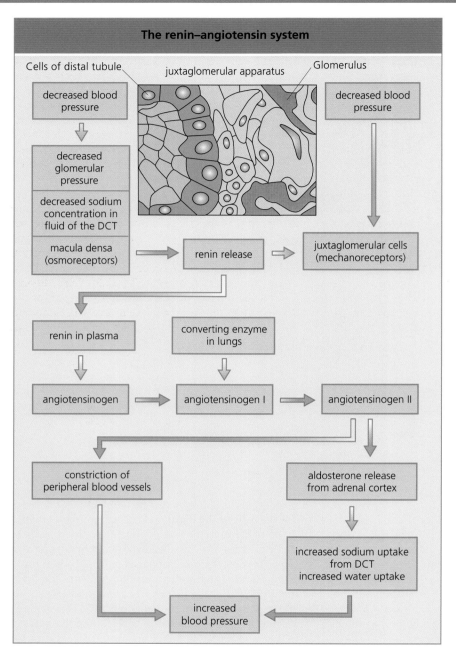

Fig 15.4 The renin–angiotensin system. DCT, distal convoluted tubule.

The renin–angiotensin system

Cells of distal tubule

juxtaglomerular apparatus

Glomerulus

decreased blood pressure

decreased blood pressure

decreased glomerular pressure

decreased sodium concentration in fluid of the DCT

macula densa (osmoreceptors)

renin release

juxtaglomerular cells (mechanoreceptors)

renin in plasma

converting enzyme in lungs

angiotensinogen

angiotensinogen I

angiotensinogen II

constriction of peripheral blood vessels

aldosterone release from adrenal cortex

increased sodium uptake from DCT increased water uptake

increased blood pressure

DISORDERS OF WATER HOMEOSTASIS

The kidneys participate with other structures such as the posterior pituitary, the cardiovascular system and the liver – where plasma proteins are synthesized – to achieve control of body water volume. Water retention produces symptoms such as oedema and circulatory overload and may occur in certain renal disorders such as acute tubular necrosis and chronic renal failure, which are discussed later in this chapter. It is important to be aware that the kidney collaborates with other organs to control the body water load. Although the pathophysiology of oedema may originate from dysfunction in organs other than the kidneys, the pharmacological management is explained here because it is important to understand how various types of diuretics affect different structures within the nephron.

OEDEMA
This is the abnormal accumulation of fluid in interstitial spaces of tissue.

Pathophysiology

When the body retains water inappropriately, the circulatory volume becomes excessive because the proportion of water being transported has increased. One result is that the blood pressure may rise. In addition, the increased water load may cause the normal osmotic mechanisms, which draw water from the extracellular compartment into the circulatory system, to become impaired. Water, which as a by-product of metabolism is constantly excreted from the cells, cannot then pass from the extracellular space into the circulation via the capillaries of the cardiovascular and lymphatic systems. The tissues become engorged with extracellular fluid, which produces the characteristic appearance of tissue oedema. The increased extracellular fluid volume means that the distance over which oxygen, nutrients and metabolites must travel between the cell and the capillaries is increased. As a result, the function of individual cells is at risk of becoming impaired. The consequences of this depend upon the types of tissue affected: in the respiratory system, the functioning of the alveoli may be impaired. In the skin, subcutaneous cells may become ischaemic and the patient be susceptible to tissue breakdown and ulcer formation.

Pharmacological management

It can be seen that, for adequate functioning of body systems and individual cells, excesses in body water content should be corrected. Diuretics may be ordered to treat water overload in a range of conditions. They are also used in treatment of hypertension. The retained water may occur as a result of failure of a system other than kidneys. However, an important principle of diuretic therapy is that, for a diuretic to be effective, the kidney's mechanisms for achieving water excretion must be capable of functioning, even if a certain degree of impairment is present.

Diuresis may be achieved simply by improving the supply of blood to the kidney, as when inotropic drugs are given to increase the force of myocardial contractility (see the section on diuretics in Chapter 3). Diuretics acting directly on renal mechanisms may exert their effect within the glomeruli, the proximal tubule, the loop of Henle or the distal and collecting tubules (**Fig. 15.5**). The additional effects of the diuretic vary according to the part of the nephron influenced. Generally, the nearer to the glomerulus a diuretic exerts its effect, the larger will be the loss of fluid and electrolytes.

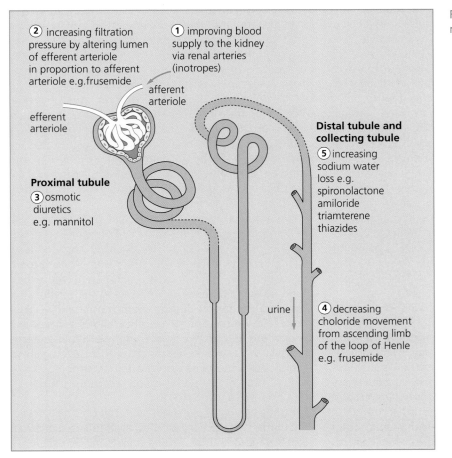

Fig 15.5 Diuretics and the kidney: major sites of action.

② increasing filtration pressure by altering lumen of efferent arteriole in proportion to afferent arteriole e.g. frusemide

① improving blood supply to the kidney via renal arteries (inotropes)

afferent arteriole

efferent arteriole

Proximal tubule
③ osmotic diuretics e.g. mannitol

Distal tubule and collecting tubule
⑤ increasing sodium water loss e.g. spironolactone amiloride triamterene thiazides

urine

④ decreasing choloride movement from ascending limb of the loop of Henle e.g. frusemide

Thiazide diuretics

These diuretics work mainly at the distal tubule and are presented as **hydrochlorothiazide** tablets. The normal dosage for treatment of oedema in adults is 25–100 mg daily, either in one dose or two divided doses (Walker, 1996). Thiazide diuretics are not effective in moderate or severe renal insufficiency. Use of these agents may cause hypokalaemia, hyponatraemia, impaired carbohydrate tolerance, reduced serum magnesium levels and increases in the serum lipoprotein and cholesterol levels. Hyperuricaemia may occur, with gout developing in susceptible individuals.

Metolazone works in a similar way to the thiazides, influencing the distal tubule, but, in addition, sodium reabsorption in the proximal tubule is decreased. The thiazides require adequate renal function in order to be effective; metolazone has an effect even in the presence of marked renal impairment and is sometimes given concurrently with loop diuretics (see below). Hypokalaemia may complicate long-term use of this drug. The dose for mild hypertension is 5 mg daily; for oedema 5–10 mg daily is usually given, although sometimes the dosage is increased to 20 mg daily.

Loop diuretics

These work at a range of sites along the nephron, but their major site of action is the ascending limb of the loop of Henle. A commonly used loop diuretic is **frusemide**. Loop diuretics accelerate secretion by the cells in this location and thus inhibit mobilisation of chloride ions into the renal interstitium. This group of diuretics also induces vasodilatation, both within the kidney by influencing the action of prostaglandin (blood flow is diverted from the renal medulla to the cortex) and systemically by interacting with the renal production of angiotensinogen. The result is a systemic vasodilatation, which is useful in the treatment of patients with cardiac failure as the cardiac preload is reduced (see Chapter 12 *Drugs and cardiovascular disorders*). Loop diuretics are effective even when renal function is impaired: frusemide may be given intravenously to support failing kidneys. The dosage of frusemide varies according to the condition being treated, but a common dosage is 20–40 mg taken as a tablet in the morning. Children may be prescribed frusemide: it is available as a paediatric preparation, usually given in a dosage of 1–3 mg/kg body weight.

Side effects of frusemide include tinnitus or deafness, because the drug is toxic to the eighth cranial nerve if a large dose is rapidly infused; hypokalaemia, for which potassium supplements may be given, and latent diabetes caused by alteration of glucose tolerance. As with any diuretic, dehydration is a hazard, as is exacerbation of urinary retention in patients with prostatic hypertrophy. Patients taking frusemide should be aware that concurrent use of some non-steroidal anti-inflammatory drugs (NSAIDs) can reduce the therapeutic effect of the diuretic.

Elderly patients have slower rates of excretion of frusemide and potassium, so are more susceptible to the toxic effects and are less able to compensate for cardiovascular effects of dehydration.

Potassium-sparing diuretics

Diuretics such as **spironolactone**, **amiloride** and **triamterene** act upon the distal portion of the distal tubule. Potassium-sparing agents are classed as weak diuretics. Because potassium excretion is avoided, the patient's electrolyte levels need to be monitored in order to avoid cardiac arrhythmias as a result of hyperkalaemia. Spironolactone works by competing with the aldosterone receptor sites. It can be administered to children, but is contraindicated in pregnancy because of the risk of feminisation of male fetuses (Walker, 1996). In addition, spironolactone should not be given to people with renal impairment. The normal adult dose ranges between 50 and 200 mg daily.

Amiloride is often used as an adjunct to a stronger diuretic to achieve shifting of the water load while conserving potassium. It is also used for congestive heart failure, the oedema of hepatic cirrhosis and hypertension. When given alone, the dosage should not exceed 20 mg a day. Amiloride alters glucose tolerance and therefore should be discontinued before a diabetic undergoes a glucose tolerance test. It must be given with care in patients with carbon dioxide retention because the respiratory acidosis influences potassium transport into the cells and dangerous hyperkalaemia may develop, exacerbated by the potassium-sparing effect of the diuretic.

Triamterene is also given for oedema or hypertension. When prescribed as the sole diuretic, a dose of 50 mg after food is usually ordered. The dose is reduced to once daily as the patient's condition stabilises. Triamterene raises the serum uric acid levels, so can exacerbate existing gout, and must be given with care to patients with hepatic or renal insufficiency. As with other thiazide diuretics, triamterene can cause hyperglycaemia.

As a general principle, diuretic therapy produces a risk of fluid and electrolyte imbalance and therefore it is useful to monitor the urea, electrolytes and body weight of those taking diuretics. Patients who suffer from stress incontinence or reduced mobility may be tempted to reduce their fluid intake if they fail to understand the relationship between their diuretic therapy and their urine output. They must be made aware of the dangers of allowing themselves to become dehydrated, which will contribute to renal impairment, as will the use of certain NSAIDs in a patient whose renal function is already compromised.

GLOMERULONEPHRITIS

Inflammation of the glomeruli can result from disorders of the immune system or vasculitis; such inflammation can also be caused by drugs, toxins or systemic disease.

Pathophysiology

Acute glomerulonephritis can occur as a sequel to bacterial infection by streptococci or staphylococci, or viral infection by varicella or hepatitis B. Rapidly progressive glomerulonephritis may occur as a result of antibody formation that causes inflammation of the glomerular basement membranes. In rapidly progressive glomerulonephritis, renal failure may develop within weeks or months and the patient commonly develops haematuria, proteinuria, hypertension and oedema.

An example of an autoimmune cause of glomerulonephritis is Goodpasture's syndrome. The inflammatory changes cause a proliferation of inflammatory cells and fibrin deposits within the Bowman's capsule; these deposits are termed crescents because of their characteristic shapes seen on microscopic examination of a renal biopsy specimen. Renal biopsy is associated with a significant risk of haemorrhage because of the number of blood vessels in the kidney, therefore the patient must be observed regularly for signs of shock. Important observations include those of pulse, blood pressure and the urine for fresh blood.

Chronic glomerulonephritis may occur as a result of the deposition of antigen–antibody complexes in the glomerular capillaries, or may result from a specific immune response targeted at the glomerular basement membrane. These events are caused by inappropriate local activation of inflammatory mediators such as complement, which attracts neutrophils and monocytes to the glomeruli;

the complement inflammatory mediators subsequently attack the neutrophils and monocytes, releasing lysozyme and thus producing cellular damage. The tissue damage attracts platelets, which release histamine and serotonin. This has the effect of increasing the permeability of the glomerular membranes and altering the electrical polarity of the capillary membrane, so allowing protein and erythrocytes into the urinary filtrate.

Pharmacological management

Pre-existing bacterial infection is treated with the appropriate antibiotic for the causative microorganism. Patients with rapidly progressive glomerulonephritis may be treated with an anti-inflammatory agent such as prednisolone. Immunosuppressants such as cyclophosphamide or azathioprene may be given to reduce the inflammatory damage produced by an inappropriately activated immune system. Anticoagulants are sometimes given to reduce the local fibrin deposition that tends to obstruct the Bowman's capsule. When the nephritis has occurred as a result of antibody formation, plasmapheresis may additionally be undertaken to remove the antibodies from the plasma (**Table 15.1**).

NEPHROTIC SYNDROME

The nephrotic syndrome occurs when protein loss in the urine causes a fall in the serum albumin sufficient to lower the oncotic pressure in blood vessels so that oedema occurs.

Table 15.1 Examples of nephropathies and their treatment

Nephropathies and their treatment	
Cause	Treatment
Glomerulopathies.	Cause identified and treated.
Acute glomerulonephritis causing inflammatory changes in the glomerular architecture and thus impaired filtration.	Steroids and other immunosuppressives may be given.
Diabetic nephropathy producing thickening of glomerular basement membrane and impaired filtration.	Long-term control of diabetes mellitus.
Acute tubular necrosis e.g. from hypoxia or shock.	When possible, cause must be corrected.
Poisons and drug toxicity.	Supportive or replacement therapy.
Renovascular disease Tubulo-interstitial renal disease, e.g. tuberculosis, tumours, poisons and drug toxicity	When possible, cause must be corrected. Supportive or replacement therapy.of underlying pathology.

Pathophysiology

There are numerous causes of nephrotic syndrome, the most prominent being minimal change nephropathy, which mainly occurs in children. The condition receives its name because very few changes are seen on light microscopy of the renal biopsy specimen. Membranous nephropathy is a commoner cause in adults. Membranous nephropathy can be idiopathic (no identifiable cause and confined to the kidney), or related to a systemic disorder such as carcinoma of the bronchus. The 'membranous' description refers to the specific appearance on renal biopsy. There are many other disorders that cause this syndrome and produce different histological changes, for example, diabetes mellitus, a range of disorders of the glomeruli, amyloidosis, systemic lupus erythematosus, vasculitis and pre-eclampsia. It is also important to note that drugs may be a cause of proteinuria and nephrotic syndrome. This condition can occur in children or adults, and causes a shift in the normal distribution of body water so that the extracellular space becomes overloaded, producing tissue oedema, and hypovolaemia exists in the circulatory system.

Normally, protein molecules do not escape from the glomerular capillaries into the urine. This is because protein molecules of sufficiently small molecular weight to pass through the fenestrations of the glomerular capillary wall are prevented from doing so by electrical repulsion: the plasma proteins and the capillary wall carry the same electrical polarity. When a person develops nephrotic syndrome, pathological changes within the glomerulus are triggered by a disease process. These physiological disturbances alter the relative polarity between the plasma proteins and the capillary endothelium and allow protein molecules to escape into the urinary filtrate. Gross protein loss into the urine occurs and the urine often appears frothy and becomes positive to protein on routine urinalysis. The loss of protein, particularly albumin, from the plasma causes reduction of the oncotic pressure in the circulatory system. As a consequence, the normal mechanism for drawing tissue fluid into the circulatory system from the extracellular space is impaired, and tissue oedema becomes apparent, particularly in the periorbital region on waking after a night's sleep. The reason why oedema of renal origin produces facial oedema and oedema of cardiac origin does not is because oedema secondary to cardiac failure causes breathlessness, which makes the patient seek an upright position to assist breathing. Gravity then ensures that, in oedema of cardiac origin, the oedema is seen in the dependent areas of the body such as the sacrum or feet, rather than in the face.

The loss of plasma proteins into the urinary filtrate causes loss of the normal protein balance within the body. Loss of larger molecular weight proteins such as immunoglobulins produces impaired resistance to infection. The liver synthesises more albumin in an attempt to redress the abnormally low oncotic pressure in the plasma caused by lack of colloid. This hyperactivity is unfortunately not restricted to correcting the plasma protein imbalance; the liver also increases the synthesis of lipoproteins, which tends to produce hyperlipidaemia; and, in addition, blood clotting factors are inappropriately produced, which results in coagulation defects.

The oedema of nephrotic syndrome is further exacerbated by sodium retention, which is the kidney's response to the diminished circulating blood volume. Activation of the renin–angiotensin–aldosterone system (see **Fig. 15.4**) causes the adrenal gland to increase secretion of aldosterone, but this simply serves to make the oedema worse as water is further retained in the extracellular space, rather than in the circulatory system.

Patients with nephrotic syndrome are advised to consume a controlled intake of protein, as what would appear to be a logical diet, including a high intake of protein, is now considered to increase the glomerular permeability to protein (Mouser and Hak, 1996) Sodium intake will also be restricted in an attempt to control the oedema.

Pharmacological management

Loop diuretics plus a potassium-sparing agent such as **spironolactone** may be given to reduce the oedema. In addition to hypovolaemia, there is a risk of patients with nephrotic syndrome suffering infection, clotting anomalies and pathologies subsequent to hyperlipidaemia. The treatment of this syndrome therefore consists of identifying and treating the cause and the widespread effects of the renal pathology. Cholesterol-lowering drugs may be given if the serum low-density lipoprotein levels fail to respond to dietary restriction. Clotting abnormalities may need treatment with anticoagulants (see Chapter 12 *Drugs and cardiovascular disorders*). In order to identify the exact cause of the disorder within the glomeruli, a renal biopsy may be taken. According to the findings from the biopsy, corticosteroids with or without cytotoxic drugs may be given to suppress an inappropriate immune response.

RENAL DISORDERS

As can be seen from the introduction to this chapter, the kidney is a complex organ that has specific prerequisites for normal functioning. The glomeruli require an arterial blood flow that produces sufficient hydrostatic pressure to allow superfiltration to take place. The cells in the walls of the proximal and distal tubules need considerable oxygen and nutrient substrates to produce the ATP to power secretion or selective reabsorption in order to maintain biochemical homeostasis. The glomerular fenestrations and the lumen of the nephrons must be free of obstruction to enable drainage of the filtrate. Nephropathy – malfunctioning of the kidney – will occur if the prerequisites are not met. The treatment of renal dysfunction requires a knowledge of the cause of the problem from clinical history, biochemical investigations, renal imaging and possibly renal biopsy as often the initial disorder must be corrected before the kidneys' powers of recovery can take effect. Pharmacological treatment of renal conditions may therefore involve other body systems or may occur as an adjunct to surgery or renal replacement therapy. In addition, hormone treatment may be needed to counter disorders of the renal endocrine systems. Table 15.1 shows some nephropathies and their treatment.

To promote understanding, the causes of renal dysfunction are often categorised into 'pre-renal'; 'renal' and 'post-renal' events.

PRE-RENAL EVENTS

This category includes disorders of structures that influence renal function before filtration occurs in the glomeruli. Therefore causes of pre-renal events include disordered functioning in body systems outside the urinary tract (**Table 15.2**).

RENAL EVENTS

This category encompasses problems that primarily involve the filtration and absorption mechanisms within the nephrons. Such causes include obstruction within the lumen or the filtration surfaces of the glomeruli; failure of the cells of the renal tubules, or blockage of the lumen of the nephrons.

Drugs and renal toxicity

The kidneys are susceptible to poisoning by a range of substances as outlined at the beginning of this chapter. Drugs given to treat systemic disorders may damage the renal cells.

Amphotericin B disrupts the cell membranes within the renal tubule, causing electrolyte and pH imbalance, failure to concentrate urine, proteinuria and tubular necrosis. Radiographic contrast media can produce nephrotoxic effects by impairing renal perfusion and thus causing damage to the glomerular capillaries and the renal tubule. **Table 15.3** lists nephrotoxic drugs and substances.

Aminoglycosides such as **gentamycin** are nephrotoxic because they become concentrated in the renal cortex. They become attached to the brush-border cells of the proximal tubules and are taken into the tubular cells in lysosomes, which subsequently degenerate to release proteolytic enzymes that destroy the cellular organelles; eventually, necrosis of the cells of the proximal tubule results.

The use of angiotensin-converting enzyme inhibitors (ACE inhibitors) as treatment for hypertension can cause renal damage by reducing the perfusion of the kidney as a result of intrarenal vasoconstriction. This occurs as a misguided corrective renal response to the systemic reduction of the arterial blood pressure. The dilatation of the efferent arterioles reduces the pressure within the glomerular capillaries and therefore impedes the normal glomerular filtration mechanism. Similarly, by altering the action of intrarenal prostaglandins, NSAIDs used for the control of chronic pain may alter the balance of blood vessel control within the kidney and produce ischaemia of renal cells.

Table 15.2 Examples of causes of pre-renal failure and their treatment

Causes of pre-renal failure and their treatment	
Cause	**Treatment**
Decreased renal perfusion: Poor cardiac output	Treatment of cardiac dysfunction (see Chapter 12).
Hypovolaemia	Replace with appropriate fluid (see Chapter 19).
Cardiogenic, oligaemic or bacteraemic shock	Treatment of cause.
Renal cell hypoxia (e.g. shock; hypoxic states)	Treatment of cause; oxygen therapy
Hypotension	Vasoconstrictors; treatment of anaphylaxis or septic states.
Blood vessel obstruction, e.g. renal artery stenosis; diabetic small vessel disease; thrombotic episodes; atherosclerosis	Relief of obstruction; prevention or treatment of underlying pathology.

Examples of nephrotoxic drugs and substances	
Analgesics	NSAIDS Phenacetin
Antibiotics	Amphotericin b Ampicillin Cephalosporins Erythromycin Gentamycin Methacillin Penicillin Rifampin Sulphonamides
Cytotoxic chemotherapy	Cisplatin Cyclophosphamide Daunorubicin Methotrexate
Metals	Gold Mercury Platinum
Psychotropic substances	Cocaine Lithium

Table 15.3 Examples of nephrotoxic drugs and substances

The presence of salicylates from chronic analgesic use causes the cells of the kidney to convert substances such as phenacetin into toxic chemicals. For this reason, it is inadvisable for patients to take a range of 'over-the-counter' analgesics as self-medication for long-standing painful conditions.

The cytotoxic agent **cisplatin** is concentrated in the cells of the proximal tubules and is transformed into a highly reactive chemical that denatures the bases in the DNA molecules of the tubular cells. As a result, these cells break down and the lumen of the nephrons becomes blocked with cellular debris. Cisplatin toxicity is reduced if the patient's water excretion rate is increased so that the contact time between the cisplatin and the tubular cells is minimised. Cisplatin is converted into toxic metabolites less readily if chlorides are available. For this reason, cisplatin is diluted in sodium chloride before administration. **Carboplatin** is now used as it is less nephrotoxic.

POST-RENAL EVENTS

Post-renal causes of kidney dysfunction encompass disorders of the drainage tracts between the renal pelvis and the external urethral orifice (or beyond this if a blocked urinary catheter is responsible for the obstruction). Post-renal events therefore tend to produce stasis in the urinary drainage system, with a consequent dilatation of the drainage structures, and may be accompanied by urinary tract infection. In some cases, the urinary drainage tract becomes blocked by precipitates of substances being excreted in the urine. This causes 'stones' to form in the urinary tract (see the section below describing urinary calculi). Medication may be needed for infection of the urinary tract or obstruction as a result of solid precipitates within the urine.

Treatment of post-renal causes of kidney dysfunction may therefore involve mechanical or surgical decompression of an obstruction, mechanical or chemical lysis of crystals or stones or mechanical, surgical or pharmacological treatment of disorders of micturition (see below).

ACUTE RENAL FAILURE

Acute renal failure has many possible causes. Important principles of treatment therefore include prevention or, if acute renal failure has developed, removal if possible of the causes of the dysfunction.

Pathophysiology

There are two classic phases of acute tubular necrosis – a cause of acute renal failure – the oliguric phase and the diuretic phase. However, not all patients follow the classic pattern, and some may enter the diuretic phase without an identifiable preliminary oliguric episode. During the oliguric phase, it is thought that the failure to produce urine is caused by a combination of mechanisms. First, the renal tubules may become obstructed by tubular cells that have sloughed from the walls of the nephron as a result of cellular necrosis. The result is back pressure that impedes glomerular filtration. The second theory is that the pathological process occurs mainly because the permeability of the tubular cells alters and inappropriate reabsorption of metabolites takes place. The third theory suggests that the glomerular blood flow rate falls and, as a result, the glomerular filtration rate (GFR) becomes insufficient for normal renal functioning.

Pharmacological management in the oliguric phase of acute renal failure

In the oliguric phase, it is important to look out for and prevent water overload, so the urine output should be monitored hourly. Diuretic therapy with **frusemide** may be given to maintain water loss, and measurement of serum urea, creatinine and electrolyte levels is used to estimate the extent of excretory and homeostatic impairment. The serum potassium level is of particular concern as hyperkalaemia is a cause of cardiac arrest if the serum potassium level exceeds 6 mmol/l. If this occurs, the serum potassium must be reduced immediately. This can be achieved by producing a shift of potassium ions from the intravascular to the intracellular compartment. **Insulin** causes transport of potassium as well as glucose into the cells, and so intravenous insulin, within an infusion of glucose to prevent hypoglycaemia, may be given; the serum potassium and glucose levels must be closely monitored. As a temporary measure, the production of alkalosis by the administration of **sodium bicarbonate** also produces a shift of potassium into the cells; however, this is a short-term measure only as sodium overload exacerbates the water retention of oliguric renal failure and, in addition, rapid alteration of the blood pH can cause disequilibration with the pH of the central nervous system tissue fluid (see Chapter 19 *Pharmacological management of medical emergencies*). Hyperkalaemia may also be treated by the use of **calcium resonium**, an ion exchange resin, which binds potassium in the gut and therefore causes a gradual reduction in the hyperkalaemia.

Principles of non-pharmacological management

There are many possible causes of acute renal failure. Important principles of management include recognising when patients are at risk so as to prevent renal failure occurring. If acute renal failure has developed, a principle of treatment is to remove as far as possible the causes of the dysfunction.

Moderate to severe disturbances of blood chemistry or clinical deterioration will require correction by haemofiltration, haemodialysis or occasionally, peritoneal dialysis. Dietary intake of protein, water and electrolytes, all retained when renal function is impaired, may be restricted, although sufficient energy in the form of fats and carbohydrates must be given to compensate for catabolic breakdown of the body proteins.

Occasionally, and especially in non-oliguric acute renal failure, conservative measures may suffice. Water retention may be assessed by daily weighing, and catabolism minimised by encouraging rest, thus controlling the metabolic needs. The uraemic state produces a general toxicity that causes malaise, nausea and neurotoxicity that may result in twitching, drowsiness, convulsions and coma. The patient must therefore be observed carefully for the development of these signs. Hyperventilation may indicate an acidotic state.

Diuretic phase: pathophysiology and general management

As the renal tissue recovers from the insult that caused the acute failure, the urine output may increase dramatically. This is beneficial as water overload will be prevented, although the diuresis produces the risk of dehydration, poor renal perfusion and subsequent deterioration in renal function. It is therefore of paramount importance to keep the patient sufficiently hydrated. This requires a dramatic shift from the principles of management of water overload. A good principal of management for both oliguric and diuretic phases is that the patient will receive a water intake equivalent to the intake of the previous day plus 500 ml. This will provide an appropriate regime irrespective of whether the patient is in an oliguric or diuretic phase. The extra 500 ml covers insensible loss from sweating, exhalation and bowel evacuation and also represents the obligatory loss of 500 ml water that is needed for renal filtration to take place at all. Such a regime will enable a response to be made as the patient's recovery produces a transition from oliguria to diuresis. The diuresis occurs because the distal and collecting tubules have not yet fully recovered and are not responsive to antidiuretic hormone. For this reason, water homeostasis remains impaired for some time, although the rehabilitating tubular cells gradually become able to handle excretion, as will become evident in the improving biochemical results. It is important to watch for inappropriate electrolyte losses, particularly potassium.

The treatment of a person in acute renal failure relies in part on medication, but careful observation and prevention of further biochemical imbalance is vital and this requires an overall understanding of the disordered processes so that the patient's kidneys can be protected from further harm.

Clinical recovery from acute tubular necrosis tends to be rapid. Otherwise, most cases of acute renal failure resolve slowly but completely, taking between 1 and 2 years for the GFR to return to 70–80% normality. In a minority of patients recovery is incomplete and results in a degree of residual renal impairment. A few patients develop chronic renal failure (Mattson Porth, 1994).

PERSON CENTRED STUDY 1

Pratiba is a woman of 56 years of age who had been troubled with arthritic pain in her knee. She had treated this herself with a combination of aspirin and ibuprofen, which she had purchased at the local supermarket. The pain in her knee improved, but she began to feel tired and unwell, with mild swelling of her ankles One morning on waking, she was horrified to find that her eyelids had become swollen. She had a headache and felt slightly nauseated. Her GP had her admitted to the local hospital.

1. Pratiba's friend brings her some grapes and chocolates. Why is she not allowed to eat very many of them?
2. How would you manage Pratiba's fluid intake?
3. Why will the physiotherapist encourage her to practise deep breathing and coughing?
4. Pratiba announces that 'these diuretics are too strong: I have to keep rushing to the toilet carrying this bedpan. It's not doing my knee any good. Perhaps I'm taking too much to drink' What information should she receive?

CHRONIC RENAL FAILURE

Very few people proceed to chronic renal failure from acute renal failure. People in chronic renal failure may be asymptomatic or their symptoms may be those of feeling generally unwell and they may have a reduced or enhanced urine output depending upon the nature of the renal disorder. In untreated chronic renal failure, the body is subjected to the long-term effects of malfunction of the excretory, homeostatic and endocrine activities of the kidney, so in addition to the immediate problems associated with dysfunction of the renal mechanisms, effects upon distant systems and tissues become evident.

Pathophysiology

Chronic renal failure is characterised by a permanent and often progressive rise in the blood urea and creatinine levels. In order for the symptoms of renal failure to become evident, the capacity of the kidney must be reduced to about 25% of the normal (McCance and Huether, 1994). However, if the decrement is slow, symptoms may not become evident until the renal function is around 20–25% of the normal, or sometimes even lower. The serum creatinine, in fact, is often within normal limits until around 60% of the renal function is lost. If there is muscle wasting and therefore low creatinine production, it may be normal or near normal in severe renal failure. The overall loss of functioning nephrons results in the remainder of those that continue to work compensating by hypertrophying. Chronic renal failure may be caused by any of the problems that result in acute renal failure. In addition, a range of disease states such as glomerulopathies; hypertension; diabetes mellitus; polycystic renal disease; systemic lupus erythematosus; vasculitis and renal artery stenosis may cause chronic renal failure. **Fig. 15.6** shows the relationship between hypertension and renal disease.

Pharmacological management
Maintenance of water, electrolyte and acid–base control

The pharmacological treatment of chronic renal failure is directed towards supporting the failing kidneys and correcting associated disorders. Chronic renal failure is characterised by impaired ability to handle sodium and water. Patients whose ability to excrete water is impaired may be prescribed diuretics. The normal GFR in a healthy young man is 120 ml/min/1.73 m^2. The values are slightly less for a woman. When the GFR is reduced to 25 ml/min, loop diuretics such as **frusemide** must be used as thiazides are not effective. Additionally, patients whose chronic renal failure causes oedema because of their inability to control the sodium load need a dietary sodium restriction of around 2 g per 24 hours (known in nursing practice by the phrase 'no added salt').

Chronic renal failure results in disordered acid–base balance, usually a metabolic acidosis. In order to correct this, a buffer such as **sodium bicarbonate** may be prescribed. A suitable buffer is provided by sodium bicarbonate tablets, which provide 4 mEq bicarbonate per 325 mg tablet. To achieve suitable pH control, this would entail taking between 5–10 bicarbonate tablets per day. Interaction between the gastric hydrochloric acid and the sodium bicarbonate tends to produce gastric distension and flatulence because of the production of carbon dioxide.

People with chronic renal failure may develop hyperkalaemia if they are taking potassium-sparing diuretics, a diet with excessive potassium or if they have metabolic acidosis, which causes movement of potassium from the intracellular to the extracellular compartment. The section on acute renal failure above describes treatment of hyperkalaemia. Calcium–potassium ion exchange resin may be administered rectally, but in this form it has a tendency to produce constipation.

RENAL BONE DISEASE

This is a consequence of calcium and phosphate imbalance. In advancing renal failure hydroxylation of vitamin D is impaired, so **1α-hydroxyvitamin D** is often prescribed to offset this. This drug may also be used to try to 'switch off' the abnormally high levels of parathyroid hormone that occur because of the calcium imbalance.

Pathophysiology

Calcium imbalances occur in chronic renal failure because there is a decreased ability to excrete phosphates and so the serum phosphate levels tend to become elevated. The hyperphosphataemia suppresses renal production of 1,25-dihydroxycholecalciferol, which normally activates vitamin D and increases the absorption of calcium from the diet. As a consequence, the serum calcium levels fall, which stimulates the production of parathyroid hormone. Hypocalcaemia is not tolerated by the body because a decrease in plasma calcium impairs myocardial functioning. For this reason, deficits in the plasma calcium are rectified by mobilising ionised calcium from storage in the skeletal system as a result of the increased parathormone production. The removal of calcium from bone produces renal osteodystrophy, with loss of bone strength, an increased tendency to rickets, and painful movement caused by the deposition of some of the mobilised calcium into joint spaces. Control of hyperphosphataemia in mild chronic renal failure can be achieved by reducing the dietary intake of phosphates through the control of protein intake, as foods with high protein content tend also to have high phosphorus levels. Parathyroidectomy may eventually be necessary.

Pharmacological management

If the renal failure deteriorates so that dietary control is insufficient to contain the tendency towards hyperphosphataemia, the phosphate levels must be reduced by

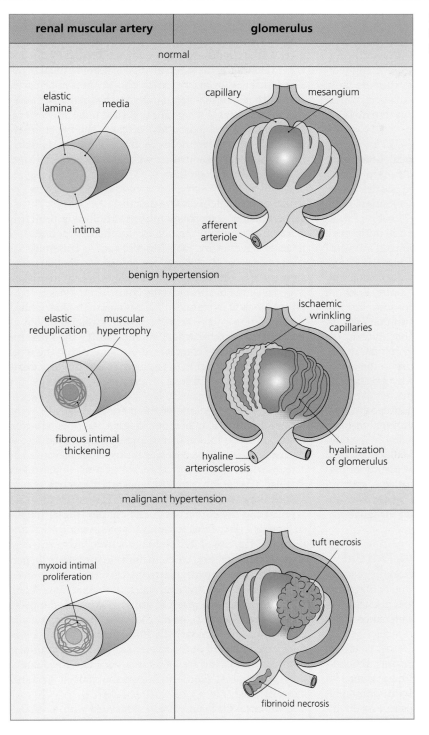

Fig 15.6 Hypertensive renal disease. (From Stevens & Lowe 1995, with permission.)

another method. **Calcium carbonate** or **calcium acetate** is prescribed to bind phosphate in the gut and to provide additional dietary calcium intake. **Aluminium hydroxide** may also be used in low doses, with monitoring of blood levels of aluminium to avoid aluminium toxicity.

CHRONIC RENAL FAILURE AND ERYTHROCYTE PRODUCTION

The cells of the kidney have a substantial demand for oxygen. The kidney functions as an endocrine organ, producing erythropoietin to stimulate the bone marrow to produce more red cells when hypoxia is present.

Pathophysiology

The loss of interstitial cell mass in chronic renal failure results in reduced secretion of erythropoietin, and the toxins produced in uraemia cause an increased fragility of existing red cells. For these two reasons, patients with chronic renal failure have a tendency to be anaemic, which causes the symptomatic pallor and fatigue of uraemia.

Pharmacological management

Genetically engineered erythropoietin – **epoetin beta** – may be administered by intravenous or subcutaneous injection. The preparation is available as a freeze-dried powder that is reconstituted with water for injection or as colourless solution that is supplied in prefilled syringes. The dose varies according to whether the aim of treatment is initial correction of the anaemia or maintenance therapy. The initial dosage varies according to body weight, but usually is 3000–4000 international units per week subcutaneously in 2–3 doses. For people with chronic renal failure, erythropoietin treatment must continue for life, or until a renal transplant becomes available. Erythropoietin therapy carries a small risk of a hypersensitivity reaction, and may be dangerous in a patient with uncontrolled hypertension because the therapy can cause a sudden rise in the blood pressure. Some uraemic patients develop hyperkalaemia in association with erythropoietin treatment.

Because of the complexity of its production, epoetin beta is an expensive preparation. However, replacement therapy is the most effective approach to the correction of the otherwise profound anaemia of chronic renal failure and can produce a marked improvement in the wellbeing of the patient. In addition to its use for uraemic patients, epoetin beta is sometimes prescribed for neonatal anaemia or in the treatment of anaemia in association with malignancy.

HYPERTENSION IN CHRONIC RENAL FAILURE

Hypertension and chronic renal failure are closely related. Hypertension may be the primary disease and damage the kidneys, and conversely, severe chronic renal disease may cause hypertension or contribute to its maintenance.

Pathophysiology

Because of its need for high filtration pressures, the kidney is extremely sensitive to decreases in the pressure of blood in the renal artery. Should blood pressure within the renal microcirculation diminish, or the sodium load fall, the interstitial cells initiate a series of corrective responses to improve the quality of renal perfusion (see **Fig. 15.6**).

Glomerular disorders that result in renal insufficiency may provoke inappropriate mobilisation of the renin–angiotensin–aldosterone mechanism. The natural response of the kidney to inadequate glomerular perfusion is to react as if the problem were caused by systemic hypotension. The arterial blood pressure is increased as a result of a generalised vasoconstriction in response to the activation of angiotensin. Additionally, increased levels of aldosterone increase the circulating blood volume through sodium and water retention. This mechanism is helpful in renal insufficiency caused by hypovolaemic shock, but is not a useful corrective response when the diminished renal perfusion occurs as a result of other causes such as renal artery stenosis or small vessel glomerular disease. The hypertensive patient in renal failure needs control of the inappropriately high systemic blood pressure without further impairment of the intrarenal blood flow.

Pharmacological management

Hypertension associated with renal failure is primarily treated with sodium restriction and thiazide diuretics. If thiazide is ineffective, loop diuretics such as **frusemide** are used in doses of 40–200 mg/day. It is important that potassium-sparing diuretics are not used because of the risk of hyperkalaemia in chronic renal failure. Beta-blockers may be used to treat hypertension in patients with renal failure.

Angiotensin-converting enzyme inhibitors such as **enalapril** are useful when, in addition to the systemic hypertension, there is increased pressure within the renal microvasculature. This is because ACE inhibitors dilate the glomerular efferent arterioles, thus correcting glomerular hypertension. It is likely that ACE inhibitors in addition reduce oedema of the mesangial cells in some forms of glomerular sclerotic disease. Angiotensin-converting enzyme inhibitors are excreted via the kidney, so the patient needs to be observed for hypotension caused by accumulation of the agent as a result of renal impairment. The use of ACE inhibitors in renal artery stenosis is hazardous because the intrarenal blood flow is already compromised by the partial obstruction in the arterial supply, so there is a risk of exacerbating any pre-existing renal dysfunction. The use of ACE inhibitors in renal impairment also carries the risk of contributing further to hyperkalaemia. This is particularly the case in diabetics even when only modest renal impairment is present. When ACE inhibitors are given to patients with moderate to severe renal disease, frequent checks of renal function and electrolytes are necessary. Calcium-channel blockers produce vasodilatation of the afferent and efferent arterioles of the glomeruli and are therefore useful as a preventative measure against glomerular damage caused by renal hypertension.

Patients with hypertension associated with renal failure may also be treated with centrally acting hypotensives such as **methyldopa**, and α-adrenergic blocking agents such as **prazosin** and **doxazosin**.

The treatment of hypertension in patients with renal failure requires the reduction of systemic pressure without causing further injury to the already damaged kidneys. If, in addition to systemic hypertension, raised pressure within the renal microvasculature is present, further damage to glomerular function is a possibility, so antihypertensives that dilate afferent and efferent arterioles are useful. Blood urea and creatinine levels must be monitored to ensure that further deterioration of the renal function as a result of antihypertensive medication is avoided.

End-stage renal failure

When deterioration of renal function is such that coma and death would occur unless the excretory function of the kidney was undertaken artificially, the patient is defined as being in end-stage renal failure. Renal replacement therapy by dialysis in such cases is for life, or until a renal transplant becomes available. Very rarely, recovery of function through reversal of the underlying condition may occur, enabling dialysis to be discontinued. Treatment by dialysis is beyond the scope of this text and the reader is referred to specialist works for further information.

Renal transplantation

Unless the grafted organ originates from a genetically close relative, recipients will require continuing prophylactic immunosuppressant therapy to prevent graft rejection. If an episode of rejection occurs, then anti-rejection therapy must be instituted. Drugs used in prophylactic treatment include oral **prednisolone**, **azathioprene** and **cyclosporin**. New products include **tacrolimus** and **mycophenolate**. Oral prednisolone diminishes the response to inflammatory mediators interleukins 1 and 2, prostaglandins and interferon, and suppresses the activity of cytotoxic T lymphocytes. Azathioprene blocks proliferation of T and B lymphocytes by inhibiting DNA and RNA synthesis; cyclosporin decreases the activation of cytotoxic T lymphocytes and inhibits the effect of interleukins and prostaglandins. Acute rejection episodes are commonly treated with high-dose intravenous **methylprednisolone**. For further discussion of the action of immunosuppressive agents, see Chapter 5 *Drugs and immune disorders*. It is important to remember that patients receiving immunosuppressive therapy are susceptible to infections, which may become overwhelming. In addition, the loss of immune surveillance increases the risk of the development of neoplastic disease.

URINARY TRACT DISORDERS

Infections of the lower urinary tract result in stimulation of the sensory nerves in the bladder mucosa, producing an urge to micturate as soon as urine enters the bladder (urinary frequency). Inflammation of the mucosa may also lead to haematuria, which further worsens the irritability of bladder. Women are particularly susceptible to the development of urinary tract infections because of the shortness of the female urethra and the relative ease with which perineal contaminants may enter the bladder via an ascending

infection. The presence of urinary catheters may predispose to infection and requires particular vigilance (Wilde, 1997).

Urinary tract infections are commonly caused by Gram-negative organisms and may originate at any point within the urinary tract. Some protection is offered against infection because of the bactericidal effect of the low urinary pH and the presence of urea in the urine. Surviving microorganisms tend to be washed towards the urethra, and reflux of urine is prevented by the one-way valve effect at the junction between the ureters and the bladder. Infections of the lower urinary tract may produce the troublesome symptoms of frequency of micturition and dysuria. The patient may complain of pain in the suprapubic area or loin.

ACUTE PYELONEPHRITIS

This is usually the result of an infection that ascends from the lower urinary tract to the kidney. The onset is rapid, characterised by fever, chills, pain in the flank, nausea and urinary frequency. Relapse or re-infection is common.

Pathophysiology

Infection in the renal pelvis or interstitial cells of the kidney may be the result of ureteric reflux, or of spread of the pathogenic organism via the bloodstream from another focus of infection. The renal medulla becomes infiltrated by white blood cells, which contribute to the inflammation and oedema of the cells of the interstitium and renal tubules. The cells of the renal papillae may become necrotic; those of the glomeruli are usually spared. Pus may be observed in the urine. As the infection is contained, healing occurs, but the architecture of the renal tubules may be distorted by scarring.

It is important therefore that patients known to have systemic or urinary tract infections are observed for the signs of renal infections: fever, chills and loin or groin pain. Such signs should be reported and acted upon so as to reduce the risk of permanent renal impairment from scarring as a result of the earlier inflammatory process.

Pharmacological management

Because of the ease with which the kidneys concentrate antibiotics in the urine, lower urinary tract infections may be effectively treated by antibiotic therapy using single doses of **trimethoprim**, 600 mg, or **ciprofloxacin**, 500 mg. More persistent infections, particularly those affecting the upper urinary tract (the ureters and renal pelvis) are treated with 7–10 day courses of trimethoprim, 100 mg at night or 200 mg twice daily according to severity. Pyelonephritis (infection of the renal pelvis) is a more serious condition as there is a risk of damage to the renal tissue and subsequent impairment of kidney function. Fever is present, the patient suffers from loin pain and the urine appears cloudy. Parenteral antibiotics are administered for severe forms of pyelonephritis; aminoglycosides such as **gentamycin**, **trimethoprim**, **Augmentin** and **cephalosporin** or quinolones such as **nalidixic acid** may be prescribed according to the results of urinary culture. In patients with recurrent infections of the urinary tract, prophylactic antibiotics may be used and advice related to personal hygiene may be needed.

URINARY CALCULI

Solid precipitates sometimes develop within the urinary system. These may occur as a result of a urinary tract infection that alters the urinary pH and increases the tendency for urinary precipitates to form. Urinary calculi may result from a metabolic condition producing excessive oxalates, citrates or calcium salts in the urine. The 'stones' may originate from cystine, calcium oxalate (calcareous stones) or from the degradation products of purines, in which case urate stones are produced.

Pathophysiology

Urate calculi are particularly likely to be produced when the pH of the urine is low (less than pH 5.5). Some people are 'stone formers' and need to avoid foods rich in the chemicals that constitute the stones: calcium (milk, cheese, antacids) or oxalates (strawberries, rhubarb, tea, chocolate, peanuts). The secretion of calcium and oxalate into the urine is reduced by thiazide diuretics. The formation of urate calculi as a result of hyperuricaemia is inhibited by **allopurinol**, which is also used as therapy for gout (Laurence and Bennett, 1992). Those people who are predisposed to form urinary calculi are generally advised to maintain a high fluid intake to prevent over concentration of stone-forming inorganic chemicals in the urine.

Pharmacological management

The impaction of calculi in the ureters will result in spasm of the smooth muscle of the ureters (ureteric colic). For this, analgesia is prescribed for the severe pain, and the muscle spasm is treated with an autonomic nervous system ganglion-blocking agent such as **hyoscine butylbromide**, presented in ampoules containing 20 mg/ml or tablets containing 10 mg of the preparation. This acts as a smooth muscle relaxant, reducing the pain and enlarging the lumen of the ureter, which may enable the calculus to be passed in the urine. Should calculus formation occur and the stones not be voided in the urine, treatment is usually to break brittle stones by the use of ultrasound, or to remove them surgically. The aim of treatment in either case is to prevent renal damage caused by obstruction of urinary drainage (obstructive uropathy). Certain types or urinary calculi may be dissolved pharmacologically. **Sodium bicarbonate** may be used to dissolve uric acid stones. In rare instances, D-**penicillinamine** may be given to diminish the formation of calculi in patients with cysteinuria.

PERSON CENTRED STUDY 2

John Brown, a 29-year-old construction worker, was admitted to the Accident and Emergency Department by ambulance, having collapsed at work with severe pain in his left loin, radiating to the groin. The pain made him feel faint and sick. He was restless, sweating and his blood pressure was 90/60 mmHg. He said he had never before experienced such pain, and had up to the present been healthy. He had an abdominal X-ray, which showed no abnormality, but an emergency intravenous urogram showed an obstruction consistent with a calculus in the left ureter. John was given analgesia and admitted to the ward.

1. List, with brief explanations, the renal risk factors that John's history illustrates.
2. John is not keen on 'needles'. What reasons would you give to justify to him the blood tests he needs to have?
3. Explain the observations that would be necessary to monitor John's condition.
4. John's calculus was removed by ultrasound treatment. What is the likelihood of this condition returning?

MICTURITION DISORDERS

The bladder must meet a series of design challenges. It must provide a receptacle for the urine, which drains constantly from the kidneys via the ureters. It must be capable of holding volumes of urine ranging from a few millilitres immediately after voiding to around 300 ml and, when micturition must be delayed, up to 1000 ml. When there is a problem of urinary retention this volume may be doubled or trebled, and still the bladder must remain intact and allow urine to drain from the ureters, but not ascend towards the kidneys. It must be able to withstand the pressure from the surrounding pelvic organs, not leak when intra-abdominal pressure rises during coughing or lifting heavy objects and be capable of voiding at will. The lining of the bladder must be resistant to the damage from the potentially harmful chemicals dissolved in the urine, and the tissue of the bladder must be capable of recovering from minor damage, for instance caused by the presence of a urinary infection.

It can be seen from **Figure 15.1B** that the ureters pierce through the wall of the bladder at an oblique angle. This angle enables the muscular wall of the bladder to create the effect of a one-way valve, enabling urine to pass into the bladder, but not to flow in the opposite direction. The structure of the detrusor muscle and the transitional epithelium of the bladder wall enables distension to occur so that the capacity of the bladder matches that of the volume of urine currently contained within it. As the bladder expands and its volume increases, the intravesical pressure remains unchanged, and the urine remains within the bladder cavity rather than being forced in a retrograde direction towards the kidneys as capacity is approached.

THE MECHANISM OF MICTURITION

As the bladder fills, the muscle of its wall is relaxed and the capacity increases. As the volume of urine within the bladder approaches around 300 ml in an adult, a change occurs in the activity of the detrusor muscle. The parasympathetic nervous system causes peristaltic waves to begin to travel across the surface. This stimulates the sensory nerve endings in the mucosa and the neurons of the micturition centre in the pons. An urge to micturate is registered by the cerebral cortex. If it is not convenient to void the bladder at that time, inhibitory impulses are relayed from the brain via the spinal cord. The peristaltic waves subside and the sensory stimulation is suppressed, so the need to micturate is temporarily forgotten. The detrusor muscle resumes its progressive relaxation, enabling the capacity to enlarge further. Eventually, a threshold volume is reached at which the peristaltic waves and sensory stimulation resume and the need to micturate is now sensed urgently, as the peristalsis causes a rapid increase of pressure within the bladder cavity. This exerts pressure upon the internal urethral sphincter. When it is convenient to micturate, inhibition of the parasympathetic nerves ceases, α_1-adrenoceptors are activated and contraction of the bladder occurs simultaneously with a relaxation of the internal and external urethral sphincters. The bladder empties (**Fig. 15.7**).

DETRUSOR INSTABILITY

This is a condition in which the normal ability to inhibit detrusor peristalsis when it is not convenient to micturate is lost.

Pathophysiology

As the bladder fills, uncoordinated and unsuppressed contraction of the detrusor muscle occurs, which causes urinary urgency and at times, stress incontinence. The pressure within the bladder may rise slightly and the sufferer feels the urge to micturate at an earlier stage of bladder filling than usual. The incidence of detrusor instability tends to increase with age. It is not always apparent why this disturbance of bladder control occurs; in some cases there is no apparent neural disorder or irritation of the bladder mucosa to explain the problem.

Pharmacological management

Pharmacological blockade of the α_1-parasympathetic receptors with antimuscarinic drugs such as **oxybutynin** (orally, 5 mg twice or three times daily) or **propantheline** (in dosages of up to 120 mg in divided doses) may be helpful in controlling this condition. These are anticholinergic drugs, and so may cause drying of the mouth, blurring of vision, constipation, nausea, facial flushing, abdominal distension and hesitancy of micturition. The anticholinergic effects are more pronounced in frail elderly people, and hepatic or renal function may be compromised (Walker, 1997). For these reasons, decisions to treat disorders of micturition with drugs involves a consideration of the relative costs and benefits of medication.

URINARY INCONTINENCE

There are many conditions that result in urinary incontinence and careful assessment of the patient is necessary to establish the likely cause.

Pathophysiology

The predisposing problem may be one of cortical awareness, in which the conscious brain is unable to respond to signals that the bladder is nearing capacity. There may be a problem with the ascending spinal sensory pathway and the descending autonomic pathway, which permit voiding at will. This could be the result of a disorder in the spinal cord or the nerve tracts emerging from the spinal column, which enable the relaxation of the sphincter muscles in

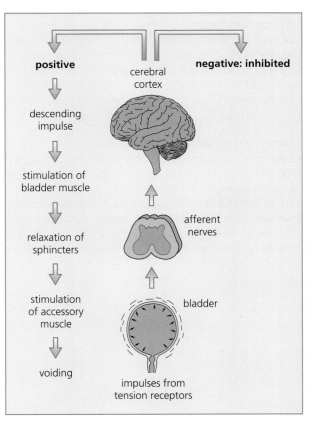

Fig. 15.7 Mechanism of micturition.

synchrony with contraction of the detrusor muscle. The treatment or urinary incontinence depends upon the cause, and for a full discussion of this subject the reader is advised to refer to a specialist text.

Pharmacological management

Pharmacological treatment of urinary incontinence with tricyclic antidepressants such as **amitriptyline**, **nortriptyline** or **imipramine** may be effective. In addition to relieving depression, the tricyclic antidepressants block the parasympathetic nervous system and therefore reduce the readiness of the detrusor muscle to respond to the impulses that initiate micturition. The anticholinergic side effects are similar to those experienced by patients receiving parasympathetic blockade to control detrusor instability.

NOCTURNAL ENURESIS

Urinary incontinence during deep sleep affects some otherwise healthy children. Bedwetting in children who have long passed the preschool milestone, by which time they would usually be able to suppress bladder voiding during sleep and wake to visit the toilet to empty a full bladder, is a source of disruption of the child's normal social patterns. Problems may be posed if the child accepts invitations to sleep away from home and other children become aware of the difficulty.

Pathophysiology

During slow wave sleep, the cerebral cortex fails to register impulses from the micturition centre so the child remains asleep rather than waking to micturate. The reflex to empty the bladder is not suppressed by the higher centres and the distended bladder eventually empties by reflex action (Carlson, 1991).

Pharmacological management

Short-term use of **antidiuretic hormone** nasal spray may retard bladder filling and diminish the problem of bedwetting for specific occasions and tricyclic antidepressants such as **imipramine** in a maximum dosage of 2.5 mg/kg body weight may eliminate it. However, the child usually relapses on ceasing the medication. In addition, the outcomes of overdosage of tricyclic antidepressants make this a hazardous therapy (see Chapter 7 *Drugs and psychological disorders*), and non-pharmacological treatment of nocturnal enuresis is preferable.

URINARY RETENTION

A range of conditions exists that result in urinary retention, but few of these are responsive to pharmacological management.

Pathophysiology

Urinary retention may occur as a result of loss of muscle tone in the bladder. Damage to the neurons of the brain or spinal cord (upper motor neurons) may result in urinary retention because the normal stimulation of the detrusor muscle is lost. This results in the muscle becoming flaccid and the wall subsequently continues to stretch until the bladder is full to capacity.

Pharmacological management

In the older man, the commonest cause of urinary retention is enlargement of the prostate gland, which produces a mechanical obstruction of the outflow tract from the bladder. As a temporary measure, this situation may occasionally be assisted with the use of medication. The use of α_1-adrenoceptor agonists such as **prazosin** or **doxazosin** in low doses will increase the responsiveness of the internal urethral sphincter to parasympathetic impulses to void urine. This will help to overcome the increased resistance in the urethra to the force exerted by the contracting detrusor muscle, and may enable the patient to void his bladder without needing recourse to an indwelling urinary catheter.

Patients with loss of bladder tone caused by upper motor neuron lesions may be helped to void if they are prescribed parasympathomimetic medication to promote sphincter relaxation and detrusor contraction. **Distigmine bromide**, 5 mg daily, potentiates the parasympathetic nervous system because it is an anticholinesterase and thus prevents the breakdown of acetylcholine at parasympathetic nerve endings.

Use of distigmine may cause bradycardia, atrioventricular block, hypotension, bronchospasm, increased salivation and increased respiratory mucosal secretion, so the treatment is not without hazards.

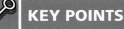

KEY POINTS

- The kidneys play a key role in homeostasis and excretion of toxins, metabolites and drugs.
- The intrarenal blood flow is precisely regulated so as to maintain an appropriate GFR; collapse of this mechanism impairs renal function.
- Diuretics alter water and electrolyte homeostasis; the nearer to the glomerulus a diuretic exerts its effect, the larger will be the loss of fluid and electrolytes.
- Nephrotic syndrome is primarily a disorder of glomerular protein conservation.
- Insufficient arterial blood flow or oxygen levels may cause renal dysfunction.
- Nephrotoxic drugs should not be given to patients with compromised renal function; when this is unavoidable, the patient's renal function must be monitored.
- Obstruction of the urinary tract may cause renal dysfunction.
- It is imperative that the patient with acute tubular necrosis does not become dehydrated.
- The patient in chronic renal failure is likely to require medication to correct disruption of the endocrine functions of the kidney.
- Pharmacological correction of disorders of micturition is associated with hazardous side effects; relative costs may outweigh the benefits.

MULTIPLE CHOICE QUESTIONS

1. Which of the following disorders may be caused by diuretic therapy?
   a. impaired glucose tolerance and hypokalaemia
   b. raised serum lipoprotein and cholesterol levels
   c. dehydration and peripheral vasodilatation
   d. metabolic alkalosis and tinnitus
   e. all of the above

2. A patient with nephrotic syndrome may require
   a. cholesterol-lowering agents
   b. vitamin D
   c. low-protein diet
   d. sodium supplementation
   e. antidiuretic hormone

3. Match the following causes and types of renal dysfunction
   a. hypovolaemia
   b. pyelonephritis
   c. gentamycin toxicity
   d. ureteric calculus
   e. hypoxaemia

   X a post-renal cause
   Y a renal cause
   Z a pre-renal cause

4. A patient has acute renal failure as a result of a period of hypotension. Which of the following medications may be ordered?
   a. ACE inhibitors and loop diuretics
   b. erythropoietin and calcium carbonate
   c. insulin and glucose
   d. antibiotics and renin
   e. clotting factors and potassium supplements

5. Which of the following statements are true in relation to the treatment of hypertension in patients with renal dysfunction?
   a. patients receiving ACE inhibitors should be observed for the development of hypotension
   b. hypertension may affect the systemic circulation and the intrarenal circulation
   c. antihypertensives work by constricting the efferent glomerular arterioles
   d. β-adrenergic blockers are suitable for antihypertensive medication
   e. hypertension may be treated by using drugs that enhance the renin–angiotensin–aldosterone response

6. Infections of the lower urinary tract may be treated effectively by a single dose of a suitable antibiotic because
   a. the urinary flow flushes away the microorganisms
   b. the metabolites dissolved in the urine act as bacterial inhibitors
   c. antibiotics tend to be retained by the body in conditions that affect the urinary tract
   d. the antibiotics used are secreted into the proximal tubule and are therefore concentrated in the urinary filtrate
   e. a large dose of the antibiotic is given

7. Which substances should be avoided by a person with a predisposition to form calcareous precipitates in the urinary tract?
   a. potassium citrate
   b. strawberries
   c. sodium cellulose phosphate
   d. antacids
   e. rhubarb

8. Ureteric reflux is normally prevented by
   a. peristaltic waves in the abdomen
   b. the angle of insertion of the ureters through the musculature of the bladder wall
   c. the flow of urine from the renal pelvis
   d. the distensibility of the urinary bladder
   e the urethral sphincters

9. A patient with hesitancy of micturition caused by neurological impairment as a result of multiple sclerosis may be assisted to void by the administration of
   a. a parasympathetic blocker
   b. an antidepressant
   c. a diuretic
   d. an anticholinesterase
   e. an antispasmodic

10. Jason, aged 7 years, suffers from nocturnal enuresis. He dearly wants to go camping for a weekend with a friend's family. It would be the first time he has been away from home on his own. What suggestions could be made to help him to enjoy his weekend?
    a. his mother could attach a battery to his normal mains-powered early warning buzzer system
    b. his mother could enquire about an antidiuretic hormone nasal spray for him
    c. he could take a course of tricyclic antidepressants
    d. he could try a course of muscle relaxants
    e. he could be prescribed parasympathetic blockers to reduce the urge to micturate

REFERENCES

Carlson NR. *Physiology of behaviour*. Boston: Allyn and Bacon, 1991.

Laurence DR, Bennett PN. *Clinical pharmacology*. Edinburgh: Churchill Livingstone, 1992.

Mattson Porth C. *Pathophysiology: concepts of altered health states*. Philadelphia: JB Lippincott, 1994.

McCance KL, Huether SE, eds. *Pathophysiology: the biologic basis for disease in adults and children*. St Louis: Mosby, 1994.

Mouser JF, Hak LJ. Acute and chronic renal diseases. In: Herfindal ET, Gourlay DR, eds. *Textbook of therapeutics: drug and disease management*. Baltimore: Williams and Wilkins, 1996.

Stevens A, Lowe J. *Pathology*. London: Mosby, 1995.

Walker G. *ABPI compendium of data sheets*. London: Datapharm Publcations Ltd, 1996.

Walker G. *ABPI compendium of data sheets*. London: Datapharm Publcations Ltd, 1997.

Wilde MH. Long term indwelling catheter care: conceptualising the research base. *J Adv Nurs* 1997: **June 25/6:**1252-1261.

16 Janet MacGregor
DRUGS AND REPRODUCTIVE DISORDERS

INTRODUCTION

Reproduction needs genetic material to be available from the male and the female of the species in order that new individuals may be produced. Human reproduction requires highly complex patterns of hypothalamic–pituitary–gonadal function. The gonad has two distinct and functional parts: one develops the germ cell lines, sperm and ova; the other is composed of endocrine cells that secrete sex steroid hormones testosterone, oestradiol and progesterone, and other hormones inhibin, activin, follistatin, anti-müllerian hormone, oocyte meiosis inhibitors, and derivatives of pro-opiomelanocortin, a precursor of adrenocorticotrophic hormone (ACTH) in the pituitary gland. Treatments for reproductive disorders aim to maintain normal development and function of the gonads and related anatomy.

Gonad hormones act locally in paracrine and autocrine fashion to stimulate development and function of the secondary sexual organs essential for support and delivery of sperm and ova to a site for fertilisation. They regulate secretion of the pituitary hormones that control gonad function via negative feedback loops. They modify somatic shape; they regulate certain physiological functions within each gender and support the conceptus in the pregnant female. Sex steroid hormone biosynthesis of androgen follows a common pathway in both sexes in the adrenal cortex.

Sexual identity is governed genetically at conception. The majority of individuals have XX or XY configuration of the sex pairing, which determines the anatomical changes towards female or male genitalia. These changes occur *in utero* at approximately 8 weeks' gestation when, if it is present, the Y chromosome influences the development of the gonads to testes. Otherwise the gonad continues to develop towards an ovary. The structures of the male and female reproductive tracts are outlined in **Figures 16.1** and **16.2**.

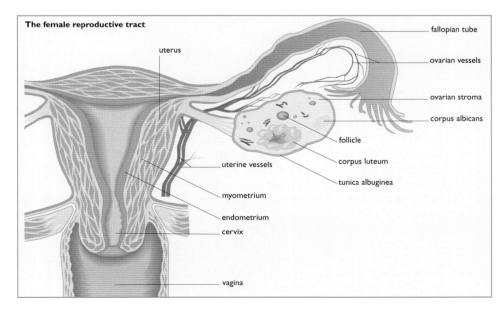

Fig 16.1 Structure of the female reproductive tract. (From Page 1997, with permission.)

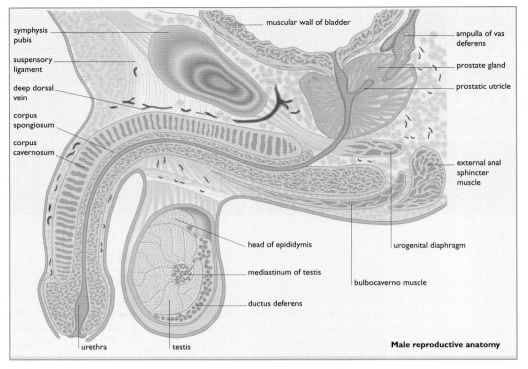

Fig 16.2 Structure of the male reproductive tract. (From Page 1997, with permission.)

symphysis pubis

suspensory ligament

deep dorsal vein

corpus spongiosum

corpus cavernosum

muscular wall of bladder

ampulla of vas deferens

prostate gland

prostatic utricle

external anal sphincter muscle

head of epididymis

mediastinum of testis

ductus deferens

urogenital diaphragm

bulbocaverno muscle

urethra

testis

Male reproductive anatomy

SEX STEROIDS

Oestrogens are used extensively as medications for females requiring chemical contraception and they are now being extensively used as replacement hormone support around the time of the menopause when the naturally occurring hormone, oestrodiol, is being secreted in gradually decreasing amounts by the ageing ovary.

Oestradiol has many effects in the body:
- inhibits bone loss
- stimulates reabsorption of sodium from the renal tubules, which leads to weight gain
- increases hepatic synthesis of binding proteins for thyroid and steroid hormones
- increases synthesis of the renin substrate angiotensinogen,
- increases synthesis of clotting factors 10 and 12, platelet aggregation, decreased anti-thrombin 3 concentration, increased plasminogen concentrations and changes in the fibrinolytic system
- increase of serum triglycerides and high density lipoproteins, decrease in low density lipoproteins
- impairment of glucose tolerance in some women.

Thus, increasing levels of this hormone in the blood can lead to hypertension, venous thrombosis and hyperlipidaemia.

Unwanted side effects of the oestrogens
- Water and sodium retention, weight gain.
- Increased risk of thromboembolism as a result of raised clotting factors 10 and 2, platelet aggregation, decreased anti-thrombin 3 concentration, increased plasminogen concentrations and changes in the fibrinolytic system.
- Rise in concentration of serum triglycerides and high-density lipoproteins, decrease in low-density lipoproteins.
- Impairment of glucose tolerance in some women.

PROGESTERONES
- Progesterone acts on tissues sensitised by oestrogen. It is used in conjunction with oestrogen as a combined oral contraceptive and in hormone replacement therapy (HRT) for women with disturbing symptoms of the menopause who retain their uterus. Central nervous system actions stimulated by progesterone include increased appetite, decreased wakefulness and heightened sensitivity of the respiratory centre to carbon dioxide levels (Berne and Levy, 1996). It is naturally produced by the corpus luteum after ovulation, the luteal phase of the female menstrual cycle (approximately one week), to maintain the lining of the uterus for pregnancy. Specific changes in the uterus include:
- secretion by endometrial cells in preparation for pregnancy
- increase in the endometrium water content
- decreased myometrial contractions.

At other times in the cycle, very low levels of this hormone are produced by the developing follicle and adrenal cortex (Thibodeau and Patton, 1999).

Testosterone derivatives have progesterone-like activity and can be taken orally. The action of **norethisterone, norgestrel, megestrol, levonorgestrel** and **ethynodiol** is primarily to make the cervical mucus inhospitable to sperm, to hinder implantation through effects on the endometrium, and to increase the motility and secretions of the fallopian tubes. Side effects are irregular bleeding, weight gain because of fluid retention, nausea, flushing, dizziness, depression and skin changes; however, this group is useful in that they do not interfere with lactation.

ANDROGENS

Testosterone is a natural androgen synthesised by the interstitial cells of the testis in men and the ovary in women and the adrenal cortex in both sexes. Androgens cause masculinisation and are useful for castrated males and those men who are hypogonadal due to pituitary or testicular disease. They may occasionally be used for women with disseminated cancer of the breast as they oppose growth of the tumour that relies on oestrogen. **Testosterone enanthate** and **propionate** are given preferably by intramuscular depot injection. **Undecenoate** and **mesterolone** are given orally. Androgens are bound to plasma protein and the sex-steroid-binding globulin, and are inactivated in the liver. Synthetic androgens are less rapidly broken down and certain amounts are excreted in the urine unchanged. Treatment with synthetic androgens may inhibit gonadotrophin release and thus fertility, encourage salt and water retention and lead to growth disturbances and acne in children.

Anabolic steroids are modified androgens. **Nandrolone, ethyloestrenol, oxymetholone** and **stanozolol** increase protein synthesis and enhance muscle development. If taken in excess – as done by some athletes to increase strength and performance – they can lead to coronary heart disease, testicular atrophy, sterility, and gynaecomastia in men and hirsutism and acne in women (Rang *et al.*, 1995). Nandrolone, 50 mg every 3 weeks by deep intra-muscular injection, is used in the treatment of some aplastic anaemias and to reduce the itching symptoms in chronic biliary obstruction. Stanozolol, 2.5–10 mg is given to control attacks of hereditary angioedema. This drug has been abused in the past by athletes who wanted to build muscle quickly in order to win events that depend on muscle power.

GONADOTROPHIN-RELEASING HORMONE

Gonadotrophin releasing hormone, produced by the hypothalamus, stimulates the synthesis and secretion of follicle stimulating hormone (FSH) and luteinizing hormone (LH) from the anterior pituitary. Synthetic gonadotrophin-releasing hormone (GnRH) is termed **gonadorelin**. Other GnRH agonists are **leuprorelin, goserelin, buserelin** and **nafarelin**. They are given subcutaneously in a pulsatile fashion to induce ovulation. Interestingly, if given in a continuous release, for example by depot, they inhibit ovulation, desensitising the pituitary gland and inhibiting gonadotrophin generation. In prolonged use they produce hypo-oestrogenism and hot flushes, decreased libido and osteoporosis. Gonadorelin analogues are indicated in endometriosis, where Gestrinone 2.5 mg is given twice weekly for six months. Goserelin 3.6 mg is given every 28 days, by subcutaneous injection into the abdominal wall, for women with advanced breast cancer and males with advanced prostate cancer where it works to increase the FSH and LH surge. This, in turn, increases production of oestrogen or testosterone which will eventually switch off the FSH and LH release.

CONGENITAL DISORDERS

An increase in the number of sex chromosomes does not relate to the severity of defects except in cases of mental retardation, which increases proportionally to each X chromosome present. Fragile X syndrome, caused by mutation in 1:1000, manifests itself in a wide range of learning disabilities and other functional abnormalities. Turner's syndrome is caused by the absence of one X chromosome in girls in 1:2500 and is exhibited in short stature, sexual infantilism and amenorrhoea. Girls with Turner's syndrome require female hormone replacement therapy, **androgen** and **growth hormone** at the age of 10–11 years; **oestrogen** and **progesterone** are required to produce a normal cyclic hormone pattern at the age of 14–15 years.

Klinefelter's syndrome is seen in boys who have one or more additional X chromosomes. They have azoospermia, small testes and poor development of secondary sexual characteristics. **Testosterone** is given to increase masculine appearance and cosmetic surgery is offered for gynaecomastia.

DEVELOPMENTAL DISORDERS

Hypospadias with the urethral opening along the ventral surface of the penis, cryptorchidism, failure of one or both testes to descend into the scrotum and hydrocele, when there is fluid persisting in the processus vaginalis, are all treated by surgery soon after birth.

Female pseudohermaphroditism, male pseudohermaphroditism, true hermaphroditism and mixed ambiguous genitalia are usually the result of virilisation of a female by adrenal androgens *in utero*. The most common, congenital adrenal hyperplasia (CAH), can be an autosomal recessive inherited deficiency of adrenocortical hormones, the effect of a tumour or caused by the mother ingesting steroids during the pregnancy. Treatment is to suppress the high stimulation of the ACTH in the pituitary by the administration of **cortisone**. It is given in divided doses to mimic the diurnal pattern of normal secretion. It should be remembered that in situations of acute stress, for example infection, increased dosage is necessary. Those children suffering from salt-losing CAH require **aldosterone** replacement and supplementary dietary **sodium**. Untreated, CAH results in early sexual maturation but the female does not develop breasts or menarche and is infertile. In the male spermatogenesis does not occur. Because of the early epiphyseal closure in CAH, both sexes are short in stature (Campbell and Glasper, 1995).

Reproduction can only occur once the gonads are mature. This process of maturation occurs in childhood over a period of 2–3 years, known as puberty. Girls enter this phase of development between 8 and 14 years and boys between 10 and 16 years (Coleman and Hendry, 1995). Five per cent of delayed puberty is secondary to some disruption of the hypothalamic–pituitary–gonadal axis or systemic disease. These children can be treated with the appropriate hormone.

Precocious puberty describes the onset of sexual characteristics such as breast development and growth of pubic hair in girls aged less than 8 years and boys aged less than 9 years. This occurs when there is early stimulation of the ovaries or testes by the hypothalamus and pituitary gland. Pseudopuberty occurs when there is excessive sex steroid secretion resulting from a cyst or adrenal gland tumour. Oral medication such as **cyproterone** prevents oestrogen and testosterone stimulating the tissues in both conditions. Children with severe bone advancement may be prescribed **zoladex**, which is a long-acting gonadotrophin analogue that prevents stimulation of the hypothalamus and thus the pituitary secretion of gonadotrophins, three or four times weekly by intramuscular depot injection. The dosage depends upon age, weight, and severity of the condition. Side effects of this treatment may be headaches, acne and menstrual spotting.

Other pathological changes and treatments are now described separately for female and male systems.

DISORDERS OF THE FEMALE REPRODUCTIVE SYSTEM

PREMENSTRUAL SYNDROME

This is described as the cyclical recurrence of physical, psychological and behavioural change in the luteal phase of the menstrual cycle.

Pathophysiology

Fluid retention occurs as a result of steroid hormone fluctuation; lack of vitamin B_6 has also been implicated (Hinchliff and Montague, 1996). There is an endocrine imbalance of progesterone deficiency, oestrogen and progesterone discrepancies, raised aldosterone levels in the luteal phase and raised prolactin. Excessive ACTH from pro-opiomelanocortin causes an endorphin deficiency. There also appears to be an evolutionary phenomenon of sexual hostility to the male after ovulation, confining coitus to the fertile period. Perhaps it is a 'survival of the species' mechanism. Premenstrual tension has also been related to those with a neurotic personality.

Pharmacological management

The treatment of premenstrual tension is with multivitamins, minerals, antidepressants, anti-prostaglandins and alprazolam, an anxiolytic. Pyridoxine (vitamin B_6), 20 mg twice daily, corrects the reduced brain serotonin in sufferers of depression. Pyridoxine may be prescribed to increase the brain levels of dopamine which, in turn, has the effect of lowering levels of prolactin. Unsteadiness, numbness and awkwardness with the hands are signs of pyridoxine toxicity. Recent work on premenstrual tension suggests that progesterone receptors may be involved; when these

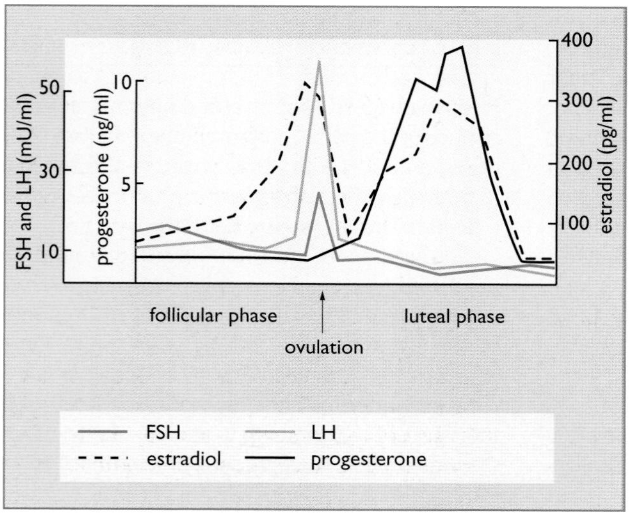

Fig 16.3 Changes in the concentrations of circulating hormones during the menstrual cycle. FSH: follicle stimulating hormone; LH: luteinising hormone. (From Page 1997, with permission.)

are reduced in numbers progesterone cannot enter the cell nucleus. Dydrogesterone, 10 mg twice daily, is given to address progesterone deficiency. Also if adrenaline is present it appears to inhibit the cellular absorption of progesterone. This latter chemical interaction would explain the worsening of symptoms in times of stress. Bromocriptine mesylate, 2.5 mg twice daily, reduces breast pain and elevated serum prolactin (above 60–360 mU/l). This is a dopamine agonist of post-synaptic receptors that inhibits prolactin release. A gynaecological assessment is required annually when this drug is being prescribed. Danazol is a derivative of progesterone and has a partial agonist action for androgen activity. It is a relatively selective inhibitor of follicle-stimulating hormone (FSH) and luteinizing hormone (LH), acting in the mid-menstrual cycle surge. It thus reduces ovarian function, which leads to atrophic changes in the endometrium. Oestrogen, high-dose hormone replacement therapy (HRT), suppresses the cycle and in some patients causes ablation of the ovaries. It is interesting that elimination of the menses will effect a cure. Gamma-linoleic acid (evening primrose oil) has also been successful in the treatment of premenstrual tension in some women. Diuretics may also help with the water retention discomfort and eating small amounts of carbohydrate every 3 hours may counteract the progesterone effect on blood sugar levels.

PRIMARY AMENORRHOEA

This is failure to reach menarche by the age of 16 years. It is not unusual for an adolescent girl to miss a menstrual period when establishing normal menstrual and ovulatory cycles. Delayed menarche is commonly attributed to excessive exercise and reduction in body fat. Surgery can restore normal function if there is a rare case of imperforate hymen or transverse vaginal septum.

Pathophysiology

Primary amenorrhea may be caused by congenital defects in the production of gonadotrophin and thus there is insufficient stimulation for gonad development. For example, Prader–Willi syndrome is a multisystem disorder that includes secondary hypogonadism. Primary hypogonadism, for example Turner's syndrome, may result in a wide range of non-functional female anatomy being present (Nelson and Daniels, 1993). Congenital nervous system defects such as hydrocephalus may affect hypothalamus and pituitary function and thus gonad development. Congenital anatomical malformations of the reproductive tract, when there is no uterus, cannot respond to trophic stimulus. Finally, acquired central nervous system lesions, for example from trauma, may obliterate hypothalamic control.

Pharmacological management

There is currently little to offer girls and women who have an absent or grossly abnormal hypothalamic–pituitary–gonad pathway. Those with Turner's syndrome can now be offered the chance to carry a baby by in-vitro fertilisation and pregnancy-supporting hormonal therapy. This is outside the remit of this text and the reader is advised to refer to specialist works.

PRIMARY DYSMENORRHOEA

Dysmenorrhoea means painful menses and is the leading cause of lost working hours in women; 15% of UK women reduce their workload during menstruation (World Health Organization, 1983). It is directly caused by physical changes such as abnormal contractility of the myometrium, age changes, parity, cigarette smoking, menstrual flow and irregular periods.

Pathophysiology

The aetiology of the symptoms is related to the actions of prostaglandin E_2 and $F_{2\alpha}$, which are formed from the phospholipids of dead cell membranes in the menstruating uterus. Prostaglandin E_2 causes degradation of platelets and is a vasodilator, whereas prostaglandin $F_{2\alpha}$ mediates or potentiates pain sensations and stimulates smooth muscle contraction. Oestrogens can also stimulate synthesis and/or release of prostaglandin $F_{2\alpha}$ and antidiuretic hormone (vasopressin) that cause uterine hyperactivity.

PERSON CENTRED STUDY 1

Ms Jones is a 20-year-old secretary. Every month, just before her period, she suffers pain in her lower abdomen. Lately, the pain has radiated to her back and she has experienced headaches and fainting spells at work. Her mother tells her to take 2 codeine tablets with her cola drink at lunch time or in the train on the way home. She tells her that there is nothing wrong but 'woman's trouble' and that it will pass.

This particular day, Ms Jones passes out at her desk and her boss tells her to go to the firm's surgery. Here, the nurse takes her pulse and blood pressure then weighs her. She checks Ms Jones' history and advises her to eat fewer snack foods and perhaps to walk to and from the station to her home. The doctor reassures her that her contraceptive, micronor, is the best for her, but prescribes mefenamic acid 500 mg three times daily to help the dysmenorrhoea.

1. Explain how dysmenorrhoea occurs and why the contraceptive micronor will be helpful.
2.. Discuss why mefenamic acid will be a better medication than codeine phosphate.

Pharmacological management

Progestin-dominant combination oral contraceptives are often used to alleviate primary dysmenorrhoea (Herfindal and Gourlay, 1996). Combination oral contraceptives are successful in 90% of women, probably because they reduce the amount of endometrium formed and consequently the amount of prostaglandins formed. However, socioeconomic factors such as education, attitude to menstruation, ethnicity and social support are also important (Hewison and Van den Akker, 1996). **Analgesics** (see Chapter 18 *Pharmacological management of pain*) that oppose this prostaglandin effect are aspirin, paracetamol, mefenamic acid, diclofenac sodium and indomethacin. Patients should be told that NSAIDs need not be taken until the onset of symptoms as the half-life of prostaglandins is only minutes (Herfindal and Gourlay, 1996). Beta-receptor stimulator, **ritodrine hydrochloride**, reduces frequency and intensity of uterine contractions by stimulating β_2 receptors in the uterine smooth muscle. The dose should be related to the severity of the symptoms. **Terbutaline sulphate** and **salbutamol** act similarly. A diet low in fat, regular exercise, local heat application, massage and relaxation complement the medications for increased effect.

PRIMARY MENORRHAGIA

Excessive menstrual flow can lead to iron-deficiency anaemia because of a fall in iron stores. Polymenorrhoea describes short regular heavy flows and metrorrhagia irregular, non-cyclical heavy flow.

Pathophysiology

Primary menorrhagia may be caused by endometriosis, cervical polyps, adenomyosis, ovary tumour, pelvic inflammation, an intrauterine device, fibroids, genetic clotting disorders – Von Willebrand's disease, thyroid dysfunction or mental stress (Govan *et al.*, 1993; Nowak and Handford, 1994).

Pharmacological management

Iron stores must be replenished with a course of oral **ferrous sulphate**. A dosage of between 200 and 600 mg may be given daily in divided doses. This medication causes constipation and should be given orally 1 hour before meals with water. **Tranexamic acid** reduces capillary fragility of the basal endometrial arteries and allows thrombosis to occur. It competitively inhibits the activation of plasminogen to plasmin. The dose of 1–1.5 g two, three or four times a day should not be given if the patient has a history of thromboembolic disease.

SECONDARY AMENORRHOEA

This is the absence of menses for three cycles or 6 months in previously menstruating women. Secondary amenorrhoea may be caused by mental stress, metabolic imbalance, for example in disease states of hypothyroidism or hyperthyroidism and severe diabetes mellitus, endocrine changes, defective ovarian follicular growth, follicular cystic disease, weight loss or surgery. If the uterus is removed (**hysterectomy**) bleeding cannot take place as the endometrium is missing. Secondary amenorrhoea also occurs during lactation, and in women nearing the menopause.

Pathophysiology

In 60% of cases of secondary amenorrhoea the cause is mental stress, which results in inhibition of the hypothalamic releasing hormone production; this leads to the absence of FSH and LH and thus loss of the effect of these hormones on ovarian production of oestrogen and progesterone and ultimately the uterine lining (Govan *et al.*, 1993). Other more common causative conditions are described later in the chapter.

Sheehan's syndrome occurs because of ischaemic necrosis of the pituitary after post-partum haemorrhage. **Cushing's syndrome** is caused by excess stimulation of the adrenal cortex and consequently excess steroid production, including oestrogen, and thus amenorrhoea. **Addison's disease** results in destruction of the adrenal glands (autoimmune) and the loss of all adrenal steroid production. Defective ovarian follicular growth may be caused by disappearance of the primordial follicles, no follicular development or autoimmune oophoritis. Another rare condition that may result in secondary amenorrhoea is defective ovarian follicular growth. Follicular cystic disease and elevated and lowered ovarian steroid hormone levels also cause secondary amenorrhoea.

FOLLICULAR CYSTIC DISEASE

The most common ovarian cysts form from Graafian follicles that do not degenerate normally. They continue to secrete oestrogen and progesterone thus anovulatory and irregular cycles accompany their development. Less common is polycystic ovarian disease in which excess androgens are secreted near the time of menarche.

Pathophysiology

It is not clear whether it is the anterior pituitary or the hypothalamus that is malfunctioning in polycystic disease, but, whichever it is, excess androgens are converted by the liver to oestrogens. This raised oestrogen level stimulates the hypothalamus, which in turn stimulates the pituitary to secrete LH, which then induces more androgen and oestrogen to be produced by the ovary. This consistent high level of circulating oestrogen in the blood ensures that no follicles mature or are released (a negative feedback loop), and amenorrhoea persists. The excess androgens are converted by the adipose tissue to more oestrogen, thus the obese patient is more likely to fuel the abnormal situation.

Pharmacological management

Treatment includes progesterone therapy to oppose oestrogen effect and also medication to stimulate ovulation. Clomiphene is the treatment of choice for ovulation stimulation, 50 mg daily for five days, doubling this dose for a further five days if ovulation does not occur. For women who do not wish a pregnancy, a low oestrogen dose oral contraceptive will suppress androgen production and control unwanted symptoms.

Clomiphene citrate increases LH and FSH by stimulating the release of GnRH to speed the maturation of the ovarian follicle, ovulation and development of the corpus luteum; 50 mg/day is given for 5 days from the fifth day of the cycle. This drug is structurally related to stilboestrol, a weak oestrogen. It blocks the hypothalamic oestrogen receptors so that the negative feedback of natural oestrogens is prevented. The pituitary responds by increased secretion of gonadotrophins, which may induce ovulation. The principal adverse effect is multiple pregnancy. Other drugs used in this pathology are **Tamoxifen** which is a non-steroid oestrogen antagonist that acts at target organs and is also used for anovulatory infertility to stimulate gonadotrophin release. (It may also be given for the prevention and treatment of oestrogen-dependent breast cancer.) An hypothalamic hormone **gonadorelin** (synthetic GnRH) releases LH and FSH. It is given to mimic the natural intermittent pulsatile delivery. **Urofollitrophin** is prepared from the urine of postmenopausal women. It contains the pituitary hormone FSH which directly stimulates the development of the ova. **Bromocriptine**, an ergot derivative, is a dopamine receptor agonist that reduces prolactin release. Prolactin antagonises LH releasing hormone in the hypothalamus thus inhibiting pituitary LH and FSH release and ultimately the ovary. The reduction of prolactin allows ovulation to take place (Rutishauser, 1994)

ANOVULATION

This is when the ovaries fail to produce or release mature eggs; there are a number of causes:
- Ovarian immaturity or postmaturity.
- Altered ovarian function as in pregnancy and lactation.
- Primary ovarian dysfunction as in ovarian dysgenesis.
- Disturbance of the interaction of the hypothalamus, pituitary gland and ovary caused by stress or disease.

Pathophysiology

Anovulation may result from decreased gonadotrophin or low levels of central nervous system neurotransmitters.

Pharmacological management

Clomiphene citrate, 50 mg daily for 5 days from the fifth day of the cycle for three cycles, increases LH and FSH, which increase maturation of the ovarian follicles,

ovulation and development of the corpus luteum. Increased prolactin, which also inhibits ovulation, can be treated with **bromocriptine mesylate**, 1–1.25 mg at night, increased to a maximum 30 mg daily in divided doses. It inhibits prolactin release by activating post-synaptic dopamine receptors.

HYPERPROLACTINAEMIA

Endocrine changes such as hyperprolactinaemia, in which prolactin levels rise to 10 times the normal figure (150–400 mU/l), in pregnancy or changes caused by pituitary tumour or primary hypothyroidism may result in secondary amenorrhoea.

Pathophysiology

In hyperprolactinaemia, raised thyroid-releasing hormone stimulates production of prolactin, which suppresses oestrogen. This then leads to a reduction of secretion of GnRH, an absence of the normal LH surge and subsequent amenorrhoea. **Elevated and lowered ovarian steroid hormones** can disrupt feedback systems of the hypothalamic–pituitary–ovarian axis, preventing ovulation.

Pharmacological management

Drug therapy inhibits prolactin with medications that resemble dopamine. **Phenothiazines** block dopamine receptors. **Reserpine** and **methyldopa** deplete dopamine, **bromocriptine** – a semisynthetic ergot alkaloid – opposes prolactin as it resembles dopamine action on the hypothalamic prolactin release inhibiting factor. **Metergoline**, a serotonin antagonist, has the same effect: 2.5 mg is given three times per day. The side effects are nausea, giddiness and syncope.

DYSFUNCTIONAL UTERINE BLEEDING

This is when bleeding occurs but no demonstrable organic cause is present. Most women with dysfunctional bleeding are having anovulatory cycles.

Pathophysiology

This condition occurs secondary to ovarian dysfunction and is the result of either progesterone deficiency or relative oestrogen excess from the granulosa–theca cell complex. This stimulates proliferation and hyperplasia of endometrial glands without stromal support.

Pharmacological management

Therapy for dysfunctional uterine bleeding may consist of **progestin–oestrogen** therapy, cyclic low-dose contraceptives or **medroxyprogesterone acetate**. This inhibits secretion of pituitary gonadotrophins that prevent follicular maturation and ovulation and is given by deep intramuscular injection, 50 mg weekly, or orally, 2.5–10 mg daily for 5–10 days.

MENOPAUSE

The age of onset remains at about 48 years in the United Kingdom (Hinchliff and Montague, 1996) even though the life span of women is increasing to over 80 years. Menopausal symptoms such as hot flushes, vaginal dryness and mood swings may be distressing. It is becoming apparent that many body systems, including the skeleton, cardiovascular system and brain, may be affected by lack of oestrogen.

Pathophysiology

This event results from extinction of oestrogen inhibition on the hypothalamus and pituitary. At menopause, FSH and LH rise and remain high over a period of 10 years before they slowly decline. When oestrogen levels fall too low to stimulate endometrial proliferation, menstrual flow ceases.

Pharmacological management

Medicinal treatments for the menopause should be inexpensive and personally acceptable to promote confidence and compliance over many years. Hormone replacement therapy is an attempt to mimic the sex steroid status in the years between menarche and menopause. It should be non-invasive, with a regime that is easily remembered. It should be at a dose that reduces the symptoms of vasomotor instability and vaginal dryness but that does not cause nausea. Pharmacological action should protect the urethra and skeleton. Finally, it should not facilitate breast or uterine oncogenesis, carbohydrate tolerance or deranged coagulation, but it should promote a lipid profile to protect coronary and cerebral vasculature (Bonnar, 1990).

Oestrogen used for replacement therapy at menopause, or after surgical menopause before the age of 45 years, relieves the symptoms of vasomotor instability (hot flushes) and menopausal vaginitis. There is increasing evidence that it will reduce osteoporosis and the incidence of cerebral vascular accident (CVA) and myocardial infarction (MI). There is some worry, however, of endometrial cancer if oestrogen is not countered by cyclical progesterone and an increased risk of breast cancer if high dose of oestrogen treatment is used. Oestradiol, which mimics the naturally produced hormone, is the best medication for HRT vasomotor instability and dienoestrol cream for vaginal atrophy. Oestradiol transdermal patches are popular as they more closely mimic the endogenous hormone activity because they do not suffer 'first pass' liver metabolism, but there are many routes by which this hormone can be taken according to client preference. Oestradiol 50 µg can be combined with norethisterone 250 µg (per 24 hours) releasing patches to mimic the female cycle and protect the uterus lining. Typically one hormone is taken by two patches 'applied below the waist' weekly for two weeks followed by the second hormone for the same time. Dienoestrol cream should be used sparingly to achieve the

required effect. More than twice-weekly use may cause vaginal tissue hypertrophy.

Ethinyloestradiol enhances liver synthesis of proteins such as sex-steroid-binding globulin, thyroxine-binding globulin, cortisol-binding globulin and raised renin substrate, and fibrinolytic and coagulation factors. Thus it raises blood pressure and increases the likelihood of migraine and the risk of thromboembolic disease in some women. Gall bladder disease is also more common because of the increased turnover of cholesterol by the liver, which raises the concentration of cholesterol in bile, making stones more likely.

A new class of drug for the treatment of menopause is currently being developed: selective oestrogen receptor modulators (SERMs). These drugs act on oestrogen receptors differently in different parts of the body. In bone and cardiovascular tissue they switch on receptors, thus preventing osteoporosis and cardiac disease. They switch off receptors in breast and uterine tissue and thus do not increase the risk of neoplasms. **Raloxifene hydrochloride**, a benzothiopine derivative originally developed to treat breast cancer 10 years ago, is undergoing trials for use in the treatment of osteoporosis. It appears effective in preventing bone reabsorption (Nursing Standard, 1996).

For those women with an intact uterus, the endometrial function is best preserved to reduce the risk of neoplasm. Endometrial tissue will hypertrophy if not sloughed off monthly. Progesterone is the treatment of choice but this hormone can cause breast tenderness, pelvic irritability and adverse blood lipid and carbohydrate levels. The effects of combination therapy will be reduced if it is taken orally in conjunction with phenytoin, carbamazepine, phenobarbitone, primidone, rifampicin or ampicillin, because these drugs interrupt the enterohepatic circulation of oral sex steroids. Hormone replacement therapy can also be administered in the form of skin gel, an implant, vaginal cream (for local effect) or a vaginal ring, or intra-nasally or sublingually.

16.1

The reproductive function of the female finishes naturally at menopause, approximately 50 years of age. Around this time the increasing pituitary stimulus of FSH and LH on the ovary devoid of ova can cause vasomotor effects, e.g. flushing and sweating. The long-term effects of reduced female hormones are many and varied; however, all females will eventually notice cessation of menses and changes in skin, hair and body shape. Internally, changes of the skeleton and cardiovascular system also occur. Elderly women may suffer atrophy of the vaginal mucosa and grow hair on their faces: distressing signs that can be alleviated with oestrogen therapy.

ENDOMETRIOSIS

In endometriosis ectopic deposits of endometrium appear in the fibres of the uterine muscle layer, but most commonly they are scattered throughout the peritoneal cavity. It is painful premenstrually and during menstruation; complications arise when endometrial deposits bleed in the pelvis cavity or in other organs, forming endometrial blood-filled cysts. Of women investigated for infertility, 30–70% have been found to have this condition.

Pathophysiology

Endometriosis has an unknown aetiology but three suggestions have been offered: first, that it is a reduced immune response to reflux menstruation; second, that ectopic endometrial cells are carried via vascular or lymphatic embolism to distant sites in the body; third, that endometrial cells are misplaced during embryological development and are activated by hormonal stimulation later in life (Biley, 1995).

Pharmacological management

The aim of treatment is to give pain relief, to resolve the ectopic deposits and to restore fertility if required. **Danazol** inhibits the output of gonadotrophins, which particularly affects the midcycle surge, and steroid synthesis in the ovary. It has adverse virilising and gastrointestinal tract effects, inducing weight gain and muscle cramps.

Gestrinone is a derivative of 19-nortestosterone. It interacts with the pituitary steroid receptors to decrease gonadotrophic secretion, which results in diminished follicular growth and anovulation. **Gonadotrophic releasing hormone analogues** desensitise the pituitary receptors for GnRH and are administered by injection or nasal spray. These drugs may cause pseudomenopausal effects of hot flushes, atrophy of the reproductive organs and bone loss. Laser treatments locally can result in a rise in conception rates.

INFERTILITY

Infertility is defined as 1 year of unprotected coitus without conception. Together with the medications, the couple are given counselling in relation to following correct protocols; the multifactorial nature of infertility requires that an holistic view of their lives be taken.

Pathophysiology

Of all infertile women, 30–50% have some anatomical abnormality as the root cause. Another 30–40% do not ovulate or ovulate inconsistently. There is no obvious cause in 20–30% and 10% have a cervical barrier to fertility (Herfindal and Gourlay, 1996).

Pharmacological management

Drugs used in the treatment of infertility are **clomiphene** and **danazol**. Clomiphene increases ovary function. Danazol, an androgen, inhibits gonadotrophins and has anti-oestrogenic and anti-progestogenic activity; 400 mg can be given daily in divided doses. It has no effect on blood coagulation. Its action is to decrease FSH and LH, but care should be given to its virilisation effect.

INFLAMMATORY DISORDERS

VULVAL INFLAMMATION

This is often caused by infection in the vagina, and physical and anatomical conditions in the area, for example being overweight, incontinence and proximity to the anus. Itching may be the result of more serious disease such as diabetes and jaundice, or an infestation such as scabies.

Vulval pruritus (acute contact dermatitis) may be caused by deodorants and washing powders. These irritants produce an unwanted immune response, termed allergic or hypersensitivity.

Pathophysiology

Type 1 hypersensitivity occurs when an antigenic material such as perfume evokes the production of antibodies of the IgE type, which fix to mast cells. Subsequent contact with the antigen causes the release of histamine, platelet-activating factor, eosinophil chemotactic factor and neutrophil chemotactic factor from mast cells, resulting in the inflammatory response.

Pharmacological management

The anti-inflammatory effect of **glucocorticoids** is to block the action of the intracellular enzymes that trigger the manufacture of the chemicals of inflammatory response in the mucous membrane. The effect of the **NSAIDs** is to block the action on mucous membrane cells of these same chemicals once they have been manufactured in the mast cells.

LICHEN PLANUS

This is a benign inflammatory disorder of unknown origin

Pathophysiology

Lichen planus results in the ulcerating form of dermatitis in the vulvovaginal area. The lesions are self-limiting and are present for 12–18 months; unfortunately, they often recur.

PERSON CENTRED STUDY 2

Marion tells you that she has an 'itch down there'. She says that she is very embarrassed because she feels that she smells and the deodorants she has been spraying on do not seem to help. What would you advise her?

Pharmacological management

Itching may be controlled with antihistamines, **terfenadine** and **cetirizine**. These are selective antagonists for H_1 receptors and thus reduce the increased vascular permeability caused by histamine.

BACTERIAL VAGINOSIS

This is a chronic inflammation of the vagina and is common in women who have had several sexual partners.

Pathophysiology

A pH of more than 4.5, foul-smelling milky or grey discharge and vaginal cells showing no lactobacilli and no inflammation is diagnostic.

Pharmacological management

Bacterial vaginosis is treated effectively with **metronidazole**, 400 mg twice daily orally for 7 days. However, a new treatment with **clindamycin** vaginal cream, 2% for 7 days, is proving useful. Clindamycin is an antibacterial agent that is active against Gram-positive cocci and many anaerobic bacteria and inhibits bacterial protein synthesis. However, reports say that careful microbiological examination reveals one constant feature: the tiny Gram-negative coccus bacillus, a facultative anaerobe *Gardnerella vaginalis*, which causes the stippling effect on the 'clue cell' of the vaginal squamae (Govan *et al.*, 1993). This thus explains the effectiveness of the antimicrobial chemotherapy.

INFECTIOUS DISORDERS

Sexually transmitted diseases (STDs) have been known since biblical times and their treatments, historically, have been bizarre and dangerous. Leeches in the scrotum and mercury orally have been documented (Cooper, 1991; Evans, 1994). Today there are more than 50 diseases and syndromes listed. In the twentieth century there has been an increase in adolescent sexual activity, which has led to younger patients suffering STDs; because of the immature anatomy of the cervix adolescents predispose themselves to cervical pathologies (Woolley, 1992). Sex education is now recommended in schools to change sexual behaviour. Practitioners would be well advised to recognise the various appearances of vaginal discharge to aid diagnosis.

In 1990, 578 000 new cases of STD were reported from genitourinary clinics in England. Sexually transmitted disease causes psychological and physical morbidity, infertility and neoplasms. Ulcerative states may facilitate the spreading of HIV and the development of AIDS. Some common conditions and their appropriate treatments are described.

GONORRHOEA

This is an increasingly common infection of the reproductive system in young people. It is symptomatic in 90% of men and asymptomatic in 80% of women.

Pathophysiology

Gonococcal infection is caused by *Neisseria gonorrhoeae*, which produces oropharynx, urethral, rectal and cervical inflammatory symptoms and tissue fibrosis.

Pharmacological management

Gonorrhoea is successfully treated using **penicillin with probenecid** in most cases, but because of the increasing prevalence of penicillinase-producing bacteria, 4-quinolone drugs such as **ciprofloxacin** are now first-line therapy. The adult dosage is 250 mg in a single dose and 500 mg in resistant cases (see Chapter 3 *Classes of drugs* for further information). The 4-quinolones act against bacterial DNA gyrase, inhibiting bacterial DNA supracoiling. They should not be used in pregnancy and they impair the metabolism of theophylline and warfarin. Gonococcal conjunctivitis is transmitted by direct inoculation during birth. The baby must be treated with systemic antibiotics. Ninety-five per cent of vulvovaginitis in prepubescent girls is now suspected to be caused by sexual abuse.

CHLAMYDIA TRACHOMATIS INFECTION

Chlamydia trachomatis infection is the commonest cause of nonspecific urethritis in women (Nelson and Daniels, 1993) and the commonest cause of pelvic inflammatory disease in the West (Bower, 1993). It is the leading cause of neonatal blindness and pneumonia in the developing world (Howe, 1996).

Pathophysiology

Chlamydia, a Gram-negative bacterium, has the properties of a bacterium but, like a virus, has to live within cells to survive (Priestley and Hicks, 1994a). It is an obligate intracellular parasite spread by sexual intercourse. It adheres to the columnar cells of the endocervix and facilitates endocytosis of the infectious but metabolically inert *Chlamydia* elementary body (EB) into the cytoplasm of the endocervical cells. The EB then changes into the larger vegetative reticulate body (RB), which multiplies by binary fission forming up to 10 000 RBs. These then condense to EBs and, with host cell lysis, the infective forms are released into the extracellular fluid to repeat the cycle. They spread upward through the tract causing acute endometriosis and acute salpingitis. Repeat infections cause scarring, because of a delayed hypersensitivity-type immune response in which pockets of chronic antigenic stimulation occurs. Secondary invasion occurs from endogenous flora from the lower genital tract and abscesses may occur. Tubal blockage occurs in 8% of patients after one episode, 19.5% after two and 45% after three. Ectopic pregnancy is six times more common. The chances of spontaneous abortion, intrauterine growth retardation, premature rupture of membranes, preterm birth, perinatal death and puerperal sepsis during pregnancy are increased. *Chlamydia* is a major cause of neonatal infection immediately after delivery. Chronic abdominal pain may be experienced with fever, purulent discharge, vaginal bleeding and a raised erythrocyte sedimentation rate above 30. Vulvovaginal infection with *Chlamydia* bacteria should raise the suspicion of sexual abuse if found in children under the age of 12 years (Priestley and Hicks, 1994a).

Pharmacological management

Treatment is with azithromycin 1 g for one dose, which shows better results than erythromycin (the formerly used macrolide antibiotic) and improved compliance (Nelson and Daniels, 1993; Bower, 1993; Howe, 1996). Macrolide antibiotics work by inhibition of protein synthesis within the cell, thus the bacterium dies. Other drugs are **oxytetracycline hydrochloride**, a bacteriostatic, 500 mg 12 hourly for 4 days, and **doxycycline**, 100 mg twice daily for 14 days; both are absorbed well from the gut and are completely excreted in the bile via the intestinal tract, unlike tetracycline, the older antibiotic of this group. **Cefuroxime**, a second-generation cephalosporin, interferes with bacterial cell wall synthesis. It is given with **probenecid**, which increases the plasma levels of the antibiotic. **Metronidazole** was introduced as an antiprotozoal agent, but is also active against anaerobic bacteria. It is given with the antibiotic for 14 days (Bevan and Ridgway, 1996).

HERPES SIMPLEX VIRUS TYPE 2

This viral disease appears to be increasing in the United Kingdom; figures for 1979–1985 show a substantial rise in the number of sufferers. It has been indicated in the aetiology of cervical carcinoma in women who have themselves had multiple sexual partners or whose partners have been promiscuous.

Pathophysiology

Viruses are intracellular parasites that use the DNA from the cells of their host to facilitate replication of their progeny. Herpes virus stimulates epidermal cells to produce an inflammatory response and the formation of vesicles. These vesicles dry, forming a crust; this exfoliates and spontaneously heals in 10 days if it is not secondarily infected with bacteria. As with many inflammatory responses, local lymphadenopathy is present. Because the mechanism of replication is by manipulation of genetic material, a trigger to malignant and premalignant states appears to exist. Herpes simplex virus type 2 (below the waist) causes multiple shallow painful ulcers of the genital skin and flu-like symptoms. Recurrences are usually less severe (Nelson and Daniels, 1993) and do not appear in 50% of those suffering an attack (Bower, 1993). A primary maternal infection poses a greater risk of complications: the fetus may be infected via the cervix and lack total protection from the maternal antibodies that may be low in the mother's first infection. Those patients who are immunosuppressed risk severe effects if they become infected.

Pharmacological management

Systemic analgesics and locally applied anaesthetic gels help with pain on urinating but the drug of choice is **acyclovir**, which inhibits viral synthesis; 400 mg can be given twice daily, and the dosage reduced appropriately after 3 months (Nelson and Daniels, 1993). Safety of this drug in pregnancy has not been established although no side effects have been reported (Dignan, 1996). Patients infected with HIV may be given the antiviral drug prophylactically.

HUMAN PAPILLOMA VIRUS

This causes the development of genital warts, the most common viral STD (Barton, 1994). It is also thought that human papilloma virus may contribute to the development of malignant and premalignant states in the cervix.

Pathophysiology

The pathophysiology is as for herpes, but instead of vesicles, the epidermal cells are manipulated to hypertrophy.

Pharmacological management

Topical cytotoxic therapy is the most commonly used treatment for human papilloma virus; **podophyllin** remains the drug of choice. The drug arrests cell division at metaphase, causing local necrosis of wart tissue and often accompanying ulceration of surrounding tissue. It is a non-homogenous, nonuniform mixture of chemically complex plant resins. The 20–25% solution may contain 2–10% podophyllotoxin, 0.5–2.5% other lignans and other harmful substances such as mutagen quercetin, which may become toxic if absorbed systemically in the treatment of large warts (Stevens and Lowe, 1995). Thus the maximum volume for treatment with podophyllin is 0.4–0.5 ml and it is contraindicated in pregnancy and breastfeeding; in these circumstances cryotherapy is the only feasible approach.

CANDIDA ALBICANS

Candida albicans, a yeast-like fungus, may exist as a normal commensal in the rectum and in small numbers in the acid environment of the vagina. It may produce symptoms of a curdy white discharge in pregnancy as the increased concentration of sex hormones in the blood maintains an increased glycogen formation in the vaginal epithelium and alters the local acidity. It also may occur in patients who are immunosuppressed, have glycosuria, are on antibiotic therapy or have chronic anaemia.

Pathophysiology

Candida is a commensal yeast-like fungus that lives in the mouth and vagina without doing any harm unless the individual's resistance is lowered by illness or stress. It is often kept in check by commensal bacteria living in the same place. Another reason the fungus may become

16.1 DEVELOPMENTAL REMINDERS

The reproductive structures in children are present but not functioning effectively until puberty. In girls body weight, chronological age and genetics appear to be important factors in the timing of menarche. Early sexual intercourse with multiple partners has been suggested as one cause of premalignant changes in the incomplete epithelialisation of the cervix in adolescent girls. A rise in androgen production at this time may be one reason for the increased libido and sexual experimentation in this age group.

active is because the bacteria have been killed by the use of antibiotics. Most fungi are saprophytes; they cause decay by secreting enzymes and digesting dead organic material. The fine thread-like hyphae secrete enzymes to digest the skin cells and it is these secretions that can cause an irritation and inflammatory response. The fungus produces reproductive bodies that are able to be transmitted from one person to the other by direct contact on clothing or towels.

Pharmacological management

Nystatin pessaries containing 100 000 i.u. of the antibiotic are inserted night and morning for 7 days followed by nightly for a further 2 weeks. Other topical medications used are **clotrimazole** and **miconazole**. Oral **fluconazole**, 150 mg as a single dose (Govan *et al.*, 1993), and **itraconazole**, 200 mg twice for 1 day, are more expensive but more acceptable to the patient.

TRICHOMONAS VAGINALIS

Trichomonas vaginalis is a protozoan that may be transmitted through intercourse or acquired from infected articles such as lavatory seats.

Pathophysiology

The organism attaches itself to the vaginal epithelium and takes glycogen from Döderlein's bacilli, which then disappear as the acidity rises to pH 5.5. There is a frothy yellow discharge, burning sensation, pruritus, dysuria and dyspareunia.

Pharmacological management

Treatment is always systemic with azoles that bind to DNA and prevent nucleic acid formation. **Metronidazole**, 200 mg, is given thrice daily for 1 week and **tinidazole**, 2 g, is given as a single dose with food (Bower, 1993).

NEOPLASTIC DISORDERS

OVARIAN TUMOURS

Most tumours arise from the ovarian stroma and germinal epithelium. Nearly 25% of ovarian neoplasms are malignant.

Pathophysiology

For a description of the pathophysiology of benign and malignant tumours, see Chapter 6 *Drugs and neoplastic disorders*.

Pharmacological management

Treatment is usually surgery, chemotherapy and radiotherapy. In the United Kingdom 5000 women develop ovarian tumours every year and 4400 die (Stevens and Lowe, 1995). **Paclitaxel** and **cisplatin** are the first-line chemotherapy drugs for these neoplasms. Paclitaxel binds to intracellular tubulin, enhancing its polymerisation into cytoskeletal microtubules and preventing microtubule disaggregation; this results in the arrest of mitosis after the synthesis phase and the death of sensitive cells. It is given intravenously over 3 hours with a premedication of corticosteroids plus H_1 and H_2 antihistamines. Every 3 weeks 175 mg/m^2 is given. It has a biphasic decline and half-life of 6.4–12.7 hours. To avoid a toxic reaction, it must be used with nonPVC equipment and there are severe side effects. **Hycamtin** is a new second-line chemotherapy treatment for patients who relapse. **Topotecan hydrochloride** kills cancer cells by inhibiting the enzyme topoisomerase 1, an enzyme essential in the replication of human DNA (Nursing Standard, 1997).

CONTRACEPTION, ABORTION AND LABOUR

CHEMICAL CONTRACEPTION

Hormonal contraception is the best method of fertility control, an effective oral contraceptive uses both an oestrogen and a progesterone, which stop ovulation by inhibiting synthesis of the hormones FSH and LH in the pituitary. The oestrogen content, ethinyloestradiol, ranges from 20 to 50 µg; the minimal dose that gives good cycle control and few side-effects should be prescribed. However, it is not suitable for breast-feeding women. Diarrhoea and vomiting will interfere with its absorption and drugs that interfere with hepatic enzyme activity, such as rifampicin, will reduce its effectiveness. **Oestrogen** inhibits FSH release, thus suppressing development of the ovarian follicle. The preparation commonly used is ethinyloestradiol or mestranol, synthetic agents, 30–35 µg daily. High doses are required for those patients also taking anti-epileptics or rifampicin as these increase liver metabolism of medications. **Progesterone** inhibits LH release and thus ovulation and cervical mucus change; the preparation of choice is levonorgestrel, norethisterone, ethynodiol, gestodene or desogestrel. The 'combined pill' action is to discourage implantation in the endometrium and interfere with the contractions of the reproductive organs that facilitate implantation. It is taken for 21 consecutive days followed by a 7-day break during which bleeding takes place as the progesterone effect is withdrawn. The progesterone-only pill, injection, pessary or implant is taken continuously and works as stated under *Sex steroids* above.

Patients should be seen regularly to monitor the oestrogen effect. Blood pressure and weight can rise. Cervical

16.1 DRUG MONITORING IN PREGNANCY

Heparin and curare do not cross the placenta, so the baby will not be affected by these agents if they are given to the mother. However, drug levels in the mother require careful monitoring, particularly in labour.

Anticonvulsants, lithium and ampicillin blood levels are reduced in pregnancy because fluid retention and decreased protein concentrations raise the blood volume thus lowering plasma concentration. Increased liver metabolism and renal blood flow also enhance excretion of medications. The mother taking any of these preparations needs careful monitoring.

Some drugs have teratogenic effects on fetal development: anticonvulsants, lithium, warfarin, retinoids, and diethylstilbestrol, which may lead to adenocarcinoma of the vagina in female infants.

16.2 DRUGS AND THEIR EFFECTS ON THE BREASTFED BABY

Laxatives: diarrhoea.
Amiodarone: affects neonatal thyroid.
Indomethacin: convulsions.
Barbiturates: drowsiness.
Benzodiazepines: associated with failure to thrive.
Lithium: hypotonia and cyanosis.
Carbimazole: reduced neonatal thyroid activity.
Alcohol: fetal alcohol syndrome (flat mid-face and nose, toxic action of metabolite acetaldehyde, vitamin B deficiency and protein malnutrition).
Smoking: intrauterine growth retardation because carbon monoxide reduces carriage of oxygen to cells.
Narcotic drugs: placental insufficiency and intrauterine growth retardation.

erosion and infection can occur as intercourse is unprotected by any barrier. Glucose tolerance is reduced because of the peripheral effect of lowered insulin action. Crohn's disease can be exacerbated as can gall bladder dysfunction. There may be changes in breast, liver, ovary and endometrial tissue. Because of the adverse oestrogen effect on the plasma lipoprotein profile, the contraceptive pill should be omitted 4 weeks before surgery and a barrier method used for that time. Smoking should be reduced as tobacco inhalation adds to the altered blood picture. Long-term contraception can be offered with the use of medroxyprogesterone acetate 150 mg/ml (one dose) given by deep intra-muscular injection in the first five days of the cycle. This gives protection for three months by inhibiting secretion of the pituitary gonadotrophins and thus ovulation. Implants are also available, for even longer-lasting protection, which can be placed subdermally. Six capsules, each containing 38 mg of levonorgestrel, will give protection for five years by inhibiting the secretion of pituitary gonadotrophin, thus preventing follicular maturation and ovulation. Unfortunately, irregular and prolonged bleeding are common side-effects.

Emergency contraception can also be given up to 72 hours after unprotected intercourse. Two tablets that contain 50 µg oestrogen and 250 µg levonorgestrel followed by 2 more tablets 12 hours later can inhibit implantation. Health care workers need to ensure a three-week follow-up check and ensure their client understands that a barrier method of contraception will be required until the next period which may be late or early.

Spermicides, **nonoxinols**, are surfactants that alter the permeability of the lipoprotein membrane of sperm. They can be used alone, introduced with an applicator, or with a barrier method such as a vaginal or cervical cap. They are available as pessaries, gels and foams.

New chemical contraceptives are being researched: vaccines to produce antibodies to sperm and an intranasal GnRH agonist, which would block pituitary FSH and LH release in both sexes.

MEDICAL INDUCTION OF ABORTION

Up to 12 weeks' gestation, suction termination is the method of choice.

Prostaglandin pessaries may be given a few hours before operation to soften the cervix. In the first 64 days of gestation 600 mg **mifepristone** (RU 486), an anti-progestogen, can be given orally with 1 mg **gemeprost** given by pessary 36 hours later. After this time abortion can be induced by a combination of prostaglandin E_2 applied to the cervix slowly at a rate of 2.5 ml/hour for 6–8 hours and **oxytocin** given intravenously at a dose of up to 150 µg/min (Govan *et al.*, 1993).

SOME MEDICATIONS USED IN LABOUR

Prostaglandins E_2 and $F_{2\alpha}$ stimulate myometrial activity and cause disaggregation of collagen fibres in the cervix:

they 'ripen' it. Dosage is decided locally but it is usually 1–2 mg depending on parity and stage of pregnancy. Given systemically these prostaglandins can cause hypothermia, gastrointestinal cramps, diarrhoea, nausea and vomiting.

Oxytocin is a peptide hormone of the posterior pituitary gland that stimulates rhythmic uterine activity after membranes have ruptured. It is used in the induction of labour; an intravenous infusion of 1–3 mU/min, increased every 10 minutes until contractions commence, is given. It is reflexively released from the pituitary in response to suckling and causes immediate contraction of the myoepithelium of the breast. Synthetic oxytocin (Syntocinon) is not contaminated with antidiuretic hormone (vasopressin), as the natural product is, so larger doses can be given. It is given in conjunction with **ergometrine maleate** to deliver the placenta and to control haemorrhage. Ergometrine, an α-adrenal receptor and dopamine receptor agonist, produces fast contractions superimposed on a tonic contraction. The dose is ergometrine 500 μU with 5 i.u. of oxytocin in 1 ml (Banister, 1997). The association with neonatal jaundice appears to be because the baby's increased erythrocyte fragility causes haemolysis. High doses lead to tachycardia and a lowered blood pressure.

Beta$_2$-adrenal receptor agonists suppress myometrial activity and are used in the treatment of preterm labour. **Ritodrine hydrochloride**, **salbutamol** and **terbutaline** raise the pulse and produce a peripheral vasodilatation and tremor. Serum glucose is raised but serum potassium is lowered. Ritodrine is given as an intravenous infusion of 50 μg/min and raised to 350 μg/min, and then given orally to maintain blood levels. It is necessary to monitor the maternal and fetal heart rate.

MALE DISORDERS

The male reproductive organs develop in the embryo and fetus stimulated by testosterone produced in response to the effect of the Y chromosome on developing tissues.

Young men experience ejaculation or 'wet dreams' at night as their reproductive system 'practices' its function. This is not to be confused with enuresis, a common developmental problem for boys until the age of 7 years, young children with infections of the urinary tract, or those with emotional lability. The developmental condition of the testes, cryptorchidism, is treated surgically to preserve spermatogenesis and prevent tumour development. Between the ages of 20 and 35 years germ cell tumours may also develop, perhaps caused by the surge in testosterone at this time in the male life cycle. It is interesting that these new growths secrete chorionic gonadotrophin and α fetal protein, thus the man would test positive for pregnancy (Nowak and Handford, 1994). Surgery, radiation and chemotherapy are the treatments of choice (see Chapter 6 *Drugs and neoplastic disorders*). In vigorous exercise the testes can twist on the spermatic cord; necrosis, haemorrhage and infarction ensue.

Infertility is a problem for 8% of men (Herfindal and Gourlay, 1996); 37% of these men have a varicocele or abnormality of the veins within the spermatic cord, which raises testes temperature and thus reduces sperm production. Spermatogenesis is low or absent in 9% of otherwise healthy men. Anatomical abnormalities account for a further 6% of infertility, semen abnormalities 10% and others are classified as unknown aetiology. The treatment depends on the individual cause. To enhance spermatogenesis (as in ovulation in the woman), stimulation of the hypothalamus and anterior pituitary is effective. The use of androgens is only useful if there is hypogonadism (**Fig. 16.4**).

In the elderly, all tissues begin to function less efficiently. In elderly men, as testosterone levels fall, physical features change; the male sex drive diminishes and erection becomes less frequent. Recent developments in medication to improve erectile function and libido are of considerable current public interest.

Recently, midlife crisis has been described in men; this may be caused by changes in hormone balance similar to those that occur in the female menopause. The psychological effects of this are acknowledged in behavioural treatment that are offered.

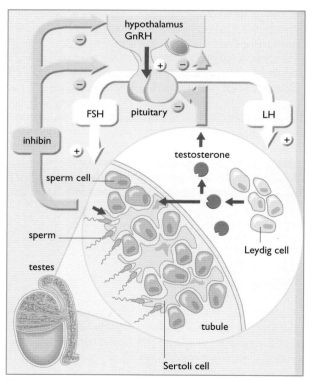

Fig 16.4 Hormonal control of Sertoli, Leydig and sperm cell function. FSH: follicle stimulating hormone; GnRH: gonadotrophin releasing hormone; LH: luteinising hormone. (From Page 1997, with permission.)

Sperm production continues until the eighth decade, thus octogenarians can become fathers.

BENIGN PROSTATIC HYPERTROPHY

Benign prostatic hypertrophy occurs in 90% of men over the age of 65 years. The prostate grows to 20 g by the age of 20 years, and this weight is maintained until the man reaches the age of about 45 years. Then a second period of slow growth commences, which ultimately results in some degree of obstruction of the urinary tract in most men over 50 years of age. This partial obstruction increases the incidence of infection and pyelonephritis as urine retention facilitates bacterial growth.

Pathophysiology

The term hypertrophy, the enlargement of existing cells, is in fact inaccurate. This condition is caused by hyperplasia: the production of new tissue. It is thought to be related to changing testosterone production associated with the ageing process.

Pharmacological management

The symptoms of urinary obstruction necessitate surgical removal, which has been the treatment of choice (Dickson, 1995). However, medical therapies are now available. Alpha-blockers such as **doxazosin** and **terazosin** work by relaxing smooth muscle in the prostate gland. Maximum effect is usual in about 2 weeks (Downey, 1997). An alternative treatment is 5α-reductase inhibitors such as **finasteride**, which is also used in prostatic tumour reduction. It improves symptoms in 6 months. Side effects include decreased libido, problems with ejaculation and impotence. Alpha-blockers have been shown to give significantly better results for men with moderately reduced peak urinary flow rates (Farmer and Noble, 1997).

TUMOURS OF THE PROSTATE

These are the second most common malignancy in men and may have both genetic and environmental aetiology.

Pathophysiology

Prostatic cancer growth is supported by testosterone (see Chapter 6 *Drugs and neoplastic disorders*).

Pharmacological management

Treatments for prostate cancer include alteration of the endocrine support. **Oestrogens** antagonise male hormone effect; GnRH analogues such as **buserelin** and **goserelin** and anti-androgens such as **finasteride** and **cyproterone acetate** are effective. Gonadotrophin releasing hormone in men is produced at a constant rate, rather than cyclically as in women, and in a pulsatile fashion. Its level in the bloodstream is normally controlled by negative feedback from the Leydig's cells in the testes, which produce testosterone. Giving buserelin, by subcutaneous injection 500 μg 8 hourly for 7 days, and then by nasal spray, 100 μg to each nostril 6 times per day, initially stimulates then progressively desensitises the pituitary and inhibits the release of FSH and LH and thus the stimulus to the testes to produce testosterone. **Goserelin**, 3.6 mg every 28 days by implant into the anterior abdominal wall, has the same effect. An unwanted rare effect is breast development. The disease flare at the start of treatment may result in ureteric obstruction, therefore an anti-androgen is often prescribed with this medication at the commencement of treatment (Joshua and King, 1996). Anti-androgens inhibit the enzymes that give rise to the active steroids or compete with the endogenous androgens for their receptors. **Finasteride**, 5 mg once a day, inhibits the enzyme 5α-reductase, which converts testosterone to dihydrotestosterone and has a great affinity for androgen receptors. Finasteride has a role in the treatment of benign prostatic hypertrophy as well as malignant prostate tumours. **Cyproterone**, 300 mg daily in a divided dose, is a derivative of progesterone and has weak progestational activity. It is a partial agonist at androgen receptors, competing with dihydrotestosterone for receptors in androgen-sensitive target tissue. In the hypothalamus, it depresses the synthesis of GnRH. It can cause liver changes and should not be taken with alcohol (**Fig. 16.5**).

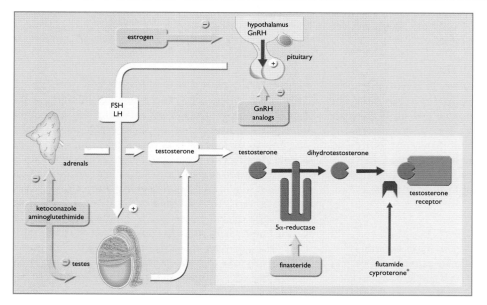

Fig 16.5 Prostate cancer can be controlled by reducing the action of testosterone on the prostate. FSH: follicle stimulating hormone; GnRH: gonadotrophin releasing hormone; LH: luteinising hormone. (From Page 1997, with permission.)

KEY POINTS

- Sex steroids regulate secretion of the hormones from the hypothalamus and pituitary that control gonad function.
- Puberty describes the phase during which the gonads mature.
- Many congenital and developmental abnormalities in both sexes can be treated in some way to address distressing symptoms.
- Dysfunction of menses may be caused by physical, psychological or social factors.
- Contraceptive medications interfere with the natural hormonal phases of the body.
- Failure of ovarian and testicular function may be caused by anatomical abnormality; if physiological, this imbalance can sometimes be redressed with medications.
- Premenstrual tension and menopause can be made more tolerable with a variety of nutritional, chemical and psychological treatments.
- Inflammatory conditions of the reproductive tracts in men and women respond to specific antibiotic therapy.
- Prostate hypertrophy can be treated conservatively but the medication does have side effects.

MULTIPLE CHOICE QUESTIONS

Choose all answers that apply.

1. Primary dysmenorrhoea may be treated with all of the following except
   a. ritodrine hydrochloride
   b. progestin
   c. anti-prostaglandin analgesia
   d. oestrogen
   e. salbutamol

2. Secondary amenorrhoea, which is the absence of menses for three cycles or 6 months in previously menstruating women may be caused by
   a. hyperprolactinaemia
   b. primary hypothyroidism
   c. Sheehan's syndrome
   d. follicular cystic disease
   e. severe diabetes mellitus

3. Infertility may be the result of
   a. elevated ovarian steroid hormones
   b. increased secretion of gonadotrophins
   c. Turner's syndrome
   d. Cushing's syndrome
   e. lowered ovarian steroid hormones

4. Side effects of chemical contraception include
   a. cervical mucus change
   b. gall bladder dysfunction
   c. inhibiting synthesis of hormones in the pituitary
   d. weight gain
   e. increased endometrial lining

5. Premenstrual tension is
   a. all in the head
   b. a survival mechanism
   c. caused by a vitamin deficiency
   d. related to antidepressive use
   e. caused by decreased levels of dopamine

6. Teratogenic effects on fetal development can be caused by
   a. diethylstilboestrol
   b. stanazolol
   c. heparin
   d. carbamazepine
   e. fluoxetine hydrochloride

7. Choose the true statements.
   a. anti-androgens such as finasteride and cyproterone acetate are effective against testicular tumours.
   b. benign prostatic hypertrophy occurs in 90% of men over the age of 65 years
   c. testosterone is only produced in the testes and adrenal glands
   d. synthetic androgens are more rapidly broken down than their natural counterparts
   e. anabolic steroids can cause coronary heart disease, testicular atrophy, sterility and gynaecomastia in men and hirsutism and acne in women

8. Gonadotrophin-releasing hormone (GnRH)
   a. is bound to plasma protein, the sex-steroid-binding globulin and inactivated in the liver
   b. is given in pulsatile fashion subcutaneously to induce ovulation
   c. can produce hypo-oestrogenism and hot flushes, decreased libido and osteoporosis in prolonged use
   d. can cause salt and water retention and lead to acne in children
   e. is used to treat Klinefelter syndrome

9. Women who take hormone replacement therapy at menopause must remember that certain other drugs will reduce its effect; these drugs include
   a. phenytoin
   b. insulin
   c. tetracycline
   d. ampicillin
   e. ACE inhibitors

10. *Chlamydia trachomatis* treatment is with
    a. antibiotics
    b. antiviral agents
    c. nystatin pessaries
    d. cisplatin
    e. yoghurt

REFERENCES

Banister C. *The midwife's pharmacopoeia*. Cheshire: BFM Press, 1997.

Barton S. New therapies for the treatment of genital warts. *Nurs Times* 1994; **90(20):**38-40.

Bevan C, Ridgway G. Pelvic inflammatory disease and *Chlamydia trachomatis*. *Maternal Child Health* 1996; **April:**91-5.

Biley A. Making sense of diagnosing and treating endometriosis. *Nurs Times* 1995; **91(9):**33-34.

Bonnar J, ed. *Recent advances in obstetrics and gynaecology*. Edinburgh: Churchill Livingstone, 1990.

Bower H. Be alert to STDs. *Practice Nurse* 1993; **June:**153-157.

Campbell S, Glasper EA, eds. *Whaley and Wong's children's nursing*. London: Mosby, 1995.

Chalmers C. Fertility and the menopause. *Br J Nurs* 1994; **3:**450-453.

Coleman J, Hendry L. *The nature of adolescence, 2nd ed*. London: Routledge, 1995.

Cooper V. Prevalence and prevention. *Practice Nurse* 1991; **June:**105-110.

Dickson C. Operative procedures for benign prostatic hypertrophy. *Nurs Times* 1995; **91(38):**34-35.

Dignan K. Genital herpes. *Prof Nurse* 1996; **11:**801-802.

Downey P. Benign prostatic hyperplasia. *Prof Nurse* 1997; **12:**501-506.

Evans G. A history of sexually transmitted disease. *Nurs Times* 1994; **90(18):**29- 31.

Farmer A, Noble J. Drug treatment for benign prostatic hyperplasia. *Br Med J* 1997; **314:**1215-1216.

Govan ADT, McKay Hart D, Callender R. *Gynaecology illustrated*. Edinburgh: Churchill Livingstone, 1993.

Herfindal ET, Gourlay DR. *Textbook of therapeutics: drug and disease management, 6th ed*. London: Williams and Wilkins, 1996.

Hewison A, van den Akker O. Dysmenorrhoea, menstrual attitude and GP consultation. *Br J Nurs* 1996; **5:**480-484.

Hinchliff S, Montague M. *Physiology for nursing practice*. London: Baillière Tindall, 1996.

Howe J. *Chlamydia trachomatis*: symptoms and consequences. *Nurs Stand* 1996; **11(10):**34-36.

Joshua A, King T. *Guy's Hospital nursing drug reference, 3rd ed*. London: Mosby, 1996.

Nelson M, Daniels D. New treatments for sexually transmitted diseases. *Maternal Child Health* 1993; **Aug:**229-233.

Nowak TJ, Handford AG. *Essentials of pathophysiology*. Oxford: WC Brown, 1994.

Nursing Standard. Innovations: a safer HRT alternative? *Nurs Stand* 1996; **10(47):**28.

Nursing Standard. Innovations. *Nurs Stand* 1997; **11(21):**28.

Page C. *Integrated Pharmacology*. London: Mosby, 1997.

Priestley C, Hicks D. *Chlamydia trachomatis* genital infection part 1. *Maternal Child Health* 1994a; **June:**188-192.

Priestley C, Hicks D. *Chlamydia trachomatis* infection in women and children part 2. *Maternal Child Health* 1994b; **July:**212-216.

Rang HP, Dale MM, Ritter JM. *Pharmacology, 3rd ed*. Edinburgh: Churchill Livingstone, 1995.

Rutishauser S. *Physiology and anatomy*. Edinburgh: Churchill Livingstone, 1994.

Stevens A, Lowe J. *Pathology*. London: Mosby, 1995.

Temple CA. Diagnosis and treatment of bacterial vaginosis. *Nurs Times* 1994; **90(37):**43-44.

Woolley P. Sexually transmitted diseases. *Practitioner* 1992; **236:**1156-1159.

World Health Organization. *Patterns and perceptions of menstruation*. New York: Croom Helm, 1983.

17 Sylvia Prosser & Pauline Runyard
DRUGS AND DERMATOLOGICAL DISORDERS

INTRODUCTION

The skin is a large and complex organ that forms the interface between the internal environment of the body and the external world. It is therefore not surprising that skin is subject to trauma, which results in wounds and infections. Excessive exposure to the sun causes sunburn. Insufficient exposure to ultraviolet rays means that the role of the skin in processing the precursor of vitamin D to its active form is lost and, as a consequence, the absorption of dietary calcium from the intestine is inhibited. The appearance of the skin may also alter as a result of changed internal health states, such as infection, or because of localised dysfunction (**Fig. 17.1**).

WOUND HEALING

Skin wounds require a specific environment in order to heal. With a simple cut, cleanliness and apposition of the wound edges will usually be sufficient for healing by first intention (uncomplicated bonding of cut edge of a clean wound) in a healthy person. For larger wounds and stasis ulcers, healing must take place by second intention and new granulation tissue must spread from the base of the wound. For this to occur, the tissue needs a moist environment that is not subjected to undue interference. In the past, nurses have unwittingly inhibited healing by 'cleaning' wounds that looked moist. In the process, the microenvironment for healing was damaged. The treatment of large wounds nowadays is by the use of occlusive dressings that are left undisturbed. Premature closure of deep cavitated wounds is prevented by the use of polyurethane foam plugs that conform to the shape of the cavity. Excessive slough is drawn away from the wound surface by osmotic agents such as hydrocolloid gels. Accurate assessment of wounds is important (Hampton, 1997; Tonge, 1997; Leaper, 1996) in order to select the optimum course of action to promote healing.

17.1 SKIN CHANGES

Changes in the skin with age largely involve the connective tissue and fat just below the epidermis. Collagen in the connective tissue becomes cross-linked, reducing the elasticity of the skin; fat deposits increase to a certain age then decrease. Sweat glands show diminished function and hair- and pigment-forming cells die (Brookbank, 1990). These changes may result from a reduction of the skin's protective function. The effect of medication may be altered by its changing structure and the physiological alterations that occur in any ageing individual. Many environmental effects, multiple systemic pathological conditions and/or their treatments and emotional stress leave their mark on 'our outside cover' (Baker, 1989). Thus the assessment of skin is an excellent guide to the history and health of older patients.

17.2 LEG ULCERS

An important problem for older people is the development of ulcerations on the legs. Skin needs a good blood supply to provide nourishment and oxygen (McCance and Huether, 1994). Multiple pathologies may inhibit this supply and the use of topical zinc may promote healing better than relying on that found in the diet. Zinc is important for deoxyribonucleic acid synthesis and protein synthesis and breakdown. It is also essential for tissue growth and repair. It activates several metalloenzymes and binds to the active site and takes part in the catalytic processes. A vehicle for zinc should hydrate, de-slough and lessen inflammation and the likelihood of infection so that granulation and epithelialisation can take place.

CHANGED INTERNAL HEALTH STATES

In addition to local alterations in function, the skin can be affected by systemic disorders. For example, childhood disorders such as chickenpox and measles produce a characteristic rash; malignant tumours may produce skin metastases, detectable as lumps in the skin; endocrine disorders that result in abnormal levels of adrenal androgens may cause an outbreak of acne among other problems. Hepatic obstruction or failure causes jaundice, in which the skin becomes coloured by deposited biliary pigments. People with long-standing lower limb oedema and poor circulation may develop dermatitis, with areas of pigmented skin that result from blood products exuding into the skin from the overloaded venous system. This tissue may become irritated and infected, and subsequently break down, forming an ulcer. Moistening creams are helpful to control the dryness and skin scaling, and hydrocortisone cream is helpful to control pruritus as long as the skin remains unbroken. Once an ulcer has developed, the main approach to treatment is to control the oedema and thus improve the oxygen supply to the cells. This is achieved by elevation of the limb, and by the use of compression stockings. It is inadvisable to apply hydrocortisone to ulcers, as this delays the healing process further.

Pharmacological preparations may therefore be prescribed for application to the skin for a variety of reasons. Skin is an absorptive tissue, so chemical agents will pass through the skin and may be taken into the capillary circulation of the dermis. Absorption rates vary according to the thickness of the stratum corneum at the area of application. Uptake from areas in which the stratum corneum is relatively thin, such as the face, scrotum or vulva is therefore more rapid than from areas such as the palms of the hands and soles of the feet. The stratum corneum may act, therefore, to regulate the speed of uptake and, additionally, serves as a slow release reservoir of pharmaceutical products applied topically. This principle is used for the administration of drugs such as glyceryl trinitrate to control angina pectoris, or for postmenopausal hormone replacement therapy via skin patches. In such cases, the preparation is applied through a rate-controlling membrane covered by an adhesive skin patch. Care should be exercised by users of such preparations to ensure that the patch does not become accidentally stuck to another person. If the skin is made moist, the absorption of topical drugs is enhanced. For this reason, waterproof dressings may be used to increase the rate of entry of a topical drug to the body, as the underlying skin sweats and the moisture is unable to evaporate.

DISORDERS OF THE SKIN

Although systemic disease can alter the appearance and function of the skin, these are dealt with in other more appropriate chapters; for example, skin metastases and malignant melanoma are more fully addressed in Chapter 6 *Drugs and neoplastic disorders*, in which the principles of cytotoxic chemotherapy are discussed. This chapter focuses on primary disorders of the skin. The appearance and texture of the skin is familiar, and so minor alterations

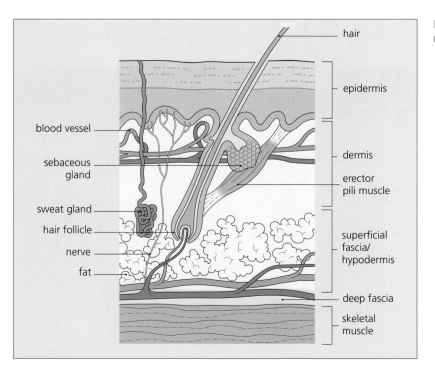

Fig 17.1 Cross section of the skin. (From Page 1997, with permission.)

hair

epidermis

blood vessel

dermis

sebaceous gland

erector pili muscle

sweat gland

hair follicle

superficial fascia/ hypodermis

nerve

fat

deep fascia

skeletal muscle

are quickly noticed. Although abnormal skin function may cause a variety of symptoms, these are generally perceived as not being life threatening. This may result in the individual resorting to home remedies, which may or may not have been scientifically tested, seeking over-the-counter remedies from a pharmacy or visiting their general practitioner.

COMMON MANIFESTATIONS OF SKIN DISORDER

The appearance of the skin may alter in numerous ways, and it is not always easy for insignificant lesions to be differentiated from more sinister manifestations of disease. Skin disorders may result in an outbreak of visible lesions, termed a rash, or symptoms, such as pruritus (itching), stinging sensations or pain. **Table 17.1** provides definitions of terms that are useful when discussing lesions of the skin.

DRUG REACTIONS AND THE SKIN

Skin reactions may occur as a result of medication. Drugs such as **penicillin**, **aspirin** and the radio-opaque substances used in radiological examinations may produce a hypersensitivity reaction caused by the activation of mast cells or of immunoglobulin E. The patient may complain of pruritus and skin wheals. There may be associated deep skin oedema (angioedema), and subsequent exposure to the agent may result in a potentially fatal anaphylactic reaction.

Light reactions

Some pharmacological preparations may cause the side effect of increased sensitivity to light, which may be the result of a toxic or a hypersensitivity effect. Phototoxicity may produce a reaction similar to that of sunburn on areas of skin exposed to light. Photoallergy appears to be a form of delayed hypersensitivity. Drugs that may provoke phototoxicity or photosensitivity reactions include:

- Chlorpromazine.
- Tetracycline.
- Non-steroidal anti-inflammatory drugs.

The symptoms subside when either the drug or exposure to ultraviolet irradiation is stopped, although it may take some time for the effects to disappear.

Altered pigmentation

Some drugs alter the skin's normal pigmentation, as shown by the following examples. Heavy metals that form components of some pharmacological compounds may be deposited in the skin, resulting in alteration of the skin colour. **Phenothiazines** may cause the skin to assume a grey colour; antimalarial preparations may cause the skin to become grey or yellow in colour. Some oral contraceptives and **adrenocorticotrophic hormone** may cause excessive melanisation of the skin. **Amiodarone** may cause

Terms commonly used to describe dermatological conditions	
Macule	A flat lesion, less than 2 cm in diameter, of a different colour from the surrounding skin. A good example of a macule is a freckle. Such a lesion, but more than 2 cm in diameter, is termed a **patch**.
Papule	A small raised solid lesion, such as occurs in the skin in a German measles infection.
Nodule	Similar to a papule but larger, between 1 and 5 cm in diameter.
Plaque	A flat-topped raised lesion of more than 1 cm in diameter. Plaques are seen in eczema and psoriasis, which will be described later.
Lichenification	Thickening or hardening of the skin.
Vesicle	A fluid-filled lesion, like a small blister, of less than 1 cm in diameter. An example is the lesion seen in the early stages of a cold sore.
Pustule	A vesicle filled with leucocytes. An example is a 'spot' that appears on the face.
Wheal	A raised papule or plaque, usually caused by localised increased blood flow and oedema to the area. An example of a wheal is the appearance of the skin after contact with stinging nettles, when white papules surrounded by a demarcated red area is evident.

Table 17.1 Terms commonly used to describe dermatological conditions

a violet pigmentation in skin exposed to the sun. Pituitary tumours may result in skin depigmentation because of the loss of the effect of melanocyte-stimulating hormone. This is particularly noticeable in people from black races.

SENSORY EFFECTS OF SKIN DISORDERS

If the sensory apparatus of the skin is affected by the lesion, symptoms are experienced consistent with the sensory nerves that are stimulated.

Remedies for such symptoms are commonly sought from within the home or from the local pharmacist. The sort of skin preparations that are routinely purchased over the counter may be classified into cosmetic preparations, in which a change in the skin's appearance is sought, and symptomatic preparations, in which an alteration to the sensory information coming from the nerves in the skin is required. Before discussing dermatological preparations further, it is helpful to consider the manner in which such preparations take their effect.

Transport through the skin

In order to be able to take effect internally, skin preparations need to be capable of being absorbed through the skin. The absorptive capacity of the skin depends upon whether it is intact or whether the surface is interrupted. In order to be absorbed through intact skin, substances must usually be soluble in water and fats, or they need to be able to combine with the fatty acids found in the skin. If a substance is not soluble in fat and water, it will be left on the skin surface. Skin that is diseased has a higher absorptive capacity, so toxic levels of the preparation may accumulate (Laurence and Bennett, 1992). Dermatological preparations are delivered to the skin in chemical 'vehicles'. Speed of delivery may be enhanced by the application of an occlusive covering to treated skin. The speed of delivery of the vehicle influences the effectiveness of the preparation. Once delivered into the skin, the active agent must leave the vehicle in order to influence the activity of the skin cells. The major modes of dermatological preparations are summarised in **Table 17.2**.

When it is intact, the keratin layer constitutes a barrier to substances diffusing across the epidermis. It also acts as a storage area, from which drugs gradually diffuse to the deeper layers of the skin. Active agents based in vehicles of

fat or oil may also pass into the deeper layers of the skin via the hair follicles and sebaceous glands. This is a point to consider when applying dermatological agents to different surfaces of the body; the rate of absorption of lipid-based agents is altered depending upon the varying distribution of hair follicles and sebaceous glands. Absorption via the palms of the hands and the soles of the feet is slower than via the scalp or axilla.

Protection against sunburn

The sun's rays are necessary for our health and wellbeing; for example, the skin uses ultraviolet irradiation to convert cholesterol molecules in the epidermal cells to vitamin D (Marieb, 1989). The shorter wavelengths of ultraviolet irradiation have a higher energy level than do the longer wavelengths, and are therefore potentially the more harmful. Normally, the structural proteins keratin and melanin protect the skin against ultraviolet irradiation. Most of us have probably in the past acquired varying degrees of sunburn. On exposure to UVB irradiation, vasoactive chemicals are released by the body cells, causing dermal vasodilatation and the other inflammatory changes associated with sunburn. Exposure to the sun's rays has now been implicated in premature ageing of the skin, premalignant actinic keratoses (dry scaly plaques of skin) and carcinoma of the skin. A case of sunburn sufficient to cause blistering has been associated with a doubled increase in the risk of development of malignant melanoma at the site of the burn (Bickers, 1991).

When the atmospheric ozone layer was more intact than it is now, wavelengths shorter than 320 nm, the potentially harmful frequencies, were absorbed by the ozone and therefore did not reach the skin of those exposed. Those who became sunburned resorted to cooling moisturising agents to relieve the burn symptoms, and looked forward to an enhanced suntan as the melanin layer increased as a protective response. The depletion of the ozone layer has increased the potential exposure to UVB short wavelength irradiation, and therefore the potential risk of solar skin damage is now greater. For these reasons, people who are likely to be exposed to the sun's rays without protection from sunscreens or clothing are now encouraged to purchase and use sun blockers. A new treatment being tried in response to the increasing incidence of sun-related malignancy of the skin is fluorouracil, which acts as a cytotoxic agent, reducing the rate of mitosis of skin cells.

Sun blockers

These preparations may be chemical or physical in their action and are graded according to their effectiveness in blocking the passage into the skin of the potentially harmful lower frequency UVB rays. Physical sunscreens consist of substances that are impermeable to light rays, such as **zinc oxide**, **titanium** compounds or **talc**. Their mode of

17.1 SKIN MEDICATION IN CHILDHOOD

Young children are cognitively immature; this affects their comprehension of and compliance with treatment. Medications applied to the skin may very well be eaten before they have had a chance to be effective.

action is to scatter light rays, rather than to allow them through into the skin.

Chemical sunscreens absorb UVB and, sometimes, UVA energy. This prevents the skin from absorbing photons from the sun. The Sun Protection Factor (SPF) signifies the ratio of the time taken to produce erythema (reddening of the skin) with and without the use of a sun-blocking agent. An SPF of more than 15 protects the skin against UVB irradiation and to a certain degree against UVA irradiation. Chemical sunscreens have as their active agents compounds such as para-aminobenzoic acid and salicylates. In addition to possessing light-blocking qualities, sunscreens need to have staying power, so that they remain on the skin for an acceptable length of time. They are commonly presented in some form of moisturising vehicle.

Those who have spent many years in the sun, with unprotected Caucasian fair complexions, will show in later life the itchy scaly lesions of solar keratosis, where there is loss of collagen and elastin, increasing the vulnerability of dermal venules to minor trauma because of the loss of their protective cover. Also **actinic lentigo** appear: large brown and white 'freckles' that arise from the irreversible damage to basal melanocytes. A controversial treatment option is to peel off this damaged skin with tretinoin to stimulate new collagen and elastin production, increase thickness of epidermal and granular layers, decrease melanin content and make the stratum corneum more compact (McHenry *et al.*, 1995). In the older person regeneration may not be as successful as with the young, although a pre-cancerous state may be postponed and a sense of wellbeing restored. Topical **glucocorticoids** in

Summary of the major modes of action of dermatological preparations	
ACTION	**EFFECT**
Alleviate symptoms	Soothe pruritus by cooling the skin and thus reducing the sensory information transmitted from the nerve receptors. Water-based preparations are useful for this purpose, because they cool the skin through the latent heat of evaporation. Constriction of skin capillaries through cooling may help to relieve pressure on skin receptors caused by hyperaemia or dermal oedema. Reduce pain by the use of similar measures to those described for the treatment of pruritus, or by introducing a local anaesthetic agent, as in the pain-relieving gels used in the treatment of mouth ulcers.
Protect	Reducing friction or by blocking entry of unwanted elements, such as some frequencies of ultraviolet light. Sunblocking agents. Dusting powders such as talc and zinc starch powder help to reduce friction between closely related skin surfaces. Lotions such as calamine lotion BP contain powder in a water-based vehicle, so a dual action, cooling plus reduction of friction, is achieved. Barrier creams are emulsions of oil and water particles, usually in conjunction with silicone, soaps or talc (Laurence and Bennett, 1992). They are used in nursing practice to protect the skin from secretions such as in cases of nappy rash, or for patients who are at risk of skin excoriation caused by the presence of fluids escaped from a stoma.
Improve appearance	Hiding blemishes – masking creams consist of an inactive opaque substance such as titanium oxide, with a suitable tinted colouring agent. They are useful for concealing extensive skin naevi (birthmarks). Removal of unwanted hair – depilatories are used by some to remove hair before surgery. Chemical depilatories work by breaking the disulphide bonds in the molecules that form the hairs. Osmotic pressure alterations within the hair shaft causes the hair to swell and assume a gelatinous structure, in which state it can be wiped away, removing a similar proportion of the hair as occurs in shaving (Laurence and Bennett, 1992).
Alter existing levels of functioning	Correct excessive dryness or oiliness. Introduce a biologically active substance. Reduce numbers of bacterial colonies.

Table 17.2 Summary of the major modes of action of dermatological preparations

creams and ointments speed the degradation of dermal collagen proteins, causing the skin to become more fragile and thinner. The lack of connective tissue support will further expose the friable blood capillaries to easy bruising. Applied for long periods, topical cortisone produces an unsightly plethoric complexion (Burton, 1990).

Before being exposed to these more radical treatments, elderly people should be advised to use conservative measures first, for example topical antipruritic agents. Also, maintenance care should be considered using 'high factor' sun screens and regular application of simple emollients such as petroleum jelly that soften the scaly eruptions.

INFECTION AND INFECTIVE DISORDERS

The concern is with disorders that are treated by dermatological products, so these are highlighted and are discussed further in this chapter.

DRUGS FOR THE TREATMENT OF INFECTIVE CONDITIONS

The skin is usually protected against infections by the presence of skin commensals, sebum and the immune mechanisms in the skin surfaces. Infections and infestations of the skin require the administration of a biologically active agent to poison the invading organism, either killing it or reducing its reproductive capacity. For a discussion of the mode of action of antibiotics and antifungal and antiviral agents see Chapter 3 *Classes of drugs*. Skin infections may be **primary** infections, in which the dermis or epidermis are directly invaded by a pathogenic organism, or a **secondary infection** may complicate a pre-existing dermatological condition, such as when pruritus induces scratching, following which the excoriations are colonised by microorganisms. As is the case elsewhere in the body, infection may be caused by bacteria, viruses, yeasts or fungi or as a sequel to parasitic infestation.

Prophylaxis

A common topical antimicrobial agent used for the prevention of bacterial colonisation of burn wounds or other raw infected areas is silver sulphadiazine. The silver ion produces structural changes in bacteria cell members and also binds to bacterial DNA to kill bacteria or prevent replication. This drug can produce optic or nasal irritation and a rash or itching if it comes into contact with healthy skin (Hazinski, 1992).

IMPETIGO

An example of a bacterial infection of the superficial layers of the skin is **impetigo**, in which the skin is infected by *Staphylococcus aureus* or β-haemolytic *Streptococcus*. It is a contagious condition, and is particularly transmissible between young children. The sequence of events in impetigo are outlined in **Figure 17.2**.

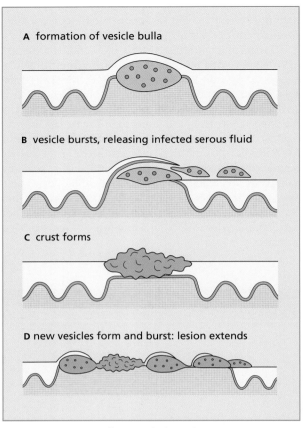

Fig 17.2 Sequence of events in impetigo.

Pathophysiology

The primary lesion of impetigo is a vesicle or bullae, which bursts, releasing yellow serous fluid that contains the microorganism. The exudate dries into a firmly fixed golden coloured crust and new vesicles rapidly develop, aided by skin excoriation subsequent to itching. The outbreaks are commonly located on the face (**Fig. 17.3**). If the infection is caused by β-haemolytic *Streptococcus*, the impetigo may precede glomerulonephritis (see Chapter 15 *Drugs and urological disorders*).

Impetigo now more commonly occurs as a result of *S. aureus* infection (Mattson Porth, 1994). In some cases of staphylococcal impetigo, there are large areas of skin excoriation, which provides its colloquial name of scalded skin syndrome. The condition is also known as Ritter's disease.

Pharmacological management

Treatment of impetigo is by removal of the crusts, plus the application of a biologically active agent, in this case a topical antibiotic, possibly in conjunction with systemic antibiotics.

FUNGAL INFECTIONS

In people with a normal immune response, fungal lesions involve only the superficial layers of the skin. The superficial

17.1 HEAD LICE

Pediculus capitus (head louse) could well be considered endemic in childhood; in some areas 10–20% of school children are affected. The female louse reproduces every 2 weeks and hundreds of 'nits' are laid attached to the hair shaft in warm parts of the scalp such as the nape of the neck and behind the ears. Lice secrete a toxic saliva while piercing the skin and sucking blood; together these actions produce a pruritic dermatitis, which can then become complicated by bacterial infection. Malathion and carbaryl lotions, rather than shampoos, ensure that the medication stays in contact with the hair and scalp for 12 hours. An aqueous base is preferable for children rather than alcohol, especially for those with asthma. After shampoo and combing out followed by a second application 7 days later, the treatment is considered complete.

Most health districts operate a rotating policy for head lice treatment to prevent the development of resistant strains (Spowart, 1995). However, recent studies in children in Ethiopia have shown absorption toxicity related to exposure to malathion and other organothiophosphate insecticides, repeated doses of which have resulted in respiratory and skin conditions (Yemaneberhan et al., 1997).

fungal organisms can only grow in the shell temperature, rather than in the warmer conditions of the body core. Skin fungi obtain their nutrition from the dead cells of the epidermis, and they secrete a digestive enzyme that enables them to break down keratin. As a result, the skin commonly appears scaly, and hair and nail structures may be damaged.

TINEA

A frequently occurring fungal infection of the skin is tinea, known more colloquially as ringworm. The fungus can affect the skin of the trunk, arms or legs (tinea corporis), scalp (tinea capitis) or feet (tinea pedis); the latter is known to the public as athlete's foot.

Pathophysiology

The tinea organism invades the stratum corneum; its initial appearance is as a red papule, which becomes larger and heals at its centre, producing a raised red annular (ring-shaped) lesion with distinct borders. The lesions may coalesce, and usually pruritus, burning and erythema is present. The condition is diagnosed by microscopic examination of skin scrapings. The fungus has a tendency to fluoresce under ultraviolet light.

Pharmacological management

Tinea corporis is treated by the administration of **antifungal agents**, either topical fungistats, which prevent cell division, such as **undecenoic acid** 1% and **griseofulvin** in doses

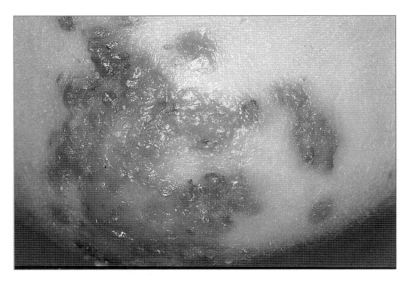

Fig 17.3 Impetigo. (From Stevens & Lowe 1995, with permission.)

of 10 mg/kg body weight for children and 500 mg for adults daily, or fungicides such as the synthetic agents **icetoconazole** or **fluconazole**, which kill the organisms by inhibiting fungal enzymes. The adult dose is 50 mg daily; its safety for children under 16 years is still to be established. A cheaper method of treating the infection is to bathe the feet in salt water as the organism does not tolerate hyperosmolar solutions.

Tinea infections of the scalp and feet are treated with similar preparations to those used for tinea corporis. The lesions of tinea capitis (ringworm of the scalp) may be characterised by balding or hairless regions caused by destruction of individual hairs. It is thought that the condition affects children more than adults because of the lack of the protective effect of the increased fatty acid content of sebum, which occurs subsequent to puberty. In the past, it was not uncommon to use harsh chemicals and to shave the heads of those affected, but these drastic remedies have ceased to be necessary since the development of antifungal agents in a fatty acid base that treat the infection and provide a substitute for the protection offered by adult sebum (Mattson Porth, 1994). Antibiotics are used if secondary bacterial infections occur as a result of scratching. In addition to antifungal agents, tinea pedis responds to the feet being kept clean and dry. Tinea of the nails is usually caused by tinea pedis. The fungus digests the keratin, producing opacity and yellow discoloration of the nails, which thicken and crack. The nail becomes distorted as it separates from the nail bed. Toenails are particularly resistant to pharmacological treatment: the sufferer may need to take oral **griseofulvin** for between 6 months and 1 year.

CANDIDIASIS

Changes in the internal environment of the skin may occur, predisposing the patient to infection of the skin by the yeast *Candida albicans*. Yeasts release toxins that irritate the skin. Those susceptible to yeast infection include those receiving long-term antibiotics, which alter the natural commensal colonies, those taking oral contraceptives, diabetics, pregnant women and malnourished or immunosuppressed individuals.

Pathophysiology

Candidiasis results in a red rash that commonly appears in moist areas such as in skin folds. The epidermis becomes eroded and scaly, vesicles and pustules may be present and the sufferer complains of pruritus and burning sensations of the skin and/or mucous membranes.

Pharmacological management

Candidiasis is commonly treated with **nystatin**, which, although ineffective against bacteria, is a useful antifungal agent because it binds to a molecule found specifically within the cytoplasm of fungi. Nystatin is available in the form of tablets containing 500 000 i.u., as oral suspension and powder, usually presented to constitute into a suspension of 100 000 i.u./ml, and as pessaries and cream. It is poorly absorbed from the alimentary tract, which makes it useful in the treatment of intestinal colonisation by fungi. Interestingly, for those with gynaecological candidiasis, nystatin gynaecological cream should not be used with latex diaphragms or condoms because the cream may damage the rubber, and reduce the effectiveness of the contraceptive (Walker, 1995).

SCABIES

Scabies is an infection of the skin by a burrowing mite, which is passed from host to host as a result of close body contact or exchange of infected clothing. The infection may affect those of any socioeconomic group, but it is particularly prevalent in the poorer social groups, and occurs most commonly in young people under 15 years old.

Pathophysiology

The female *Sarcoptes scabiei* mite is a four-legged turtle-shaped creature that burrows into the superficial layers of the epidermis where two to three eggs are laid daily until the mite dies 1–2 months later. The larvae hatch, mature on the skin surface and then reproduce in the epidermis. The mite is able to live independently of the host for

---

PERSON CENTRED STUDY 1

Giles has been backpacking around the world in his 'gap year' before going to university. On his return to the family home, he goes to see the local practice nurse complaining of an itchy rash between his fingers, on his wrists and in his axillae. He thoroughly enjoyed his travels, although he admits to having stayed in some 'pretty shaky' places. The practice nurse notes thread-like marks in the webs of the fingers, on the wrists and in the axillae. In places, the skin is broken and slightly infected. She suspects that Giles has an infection with *Sarcoptes scabiei*. This is confirmed by the family doctor. Giles asks if he needs to tell his mother as she will 'go up the wall' as Giles' young brothers and sisters are all just getting over measles.

1. Does Giles need to tell his mother about the outbreak?
2. Does the family need treatment, and are any special precautions necessary?
3. Giles asks whether he has to burn his sleeping bag, which he considers as an 'old friend' after all the miles it has travelled with him.

2–3 days, which is important to remember when handling the clothing of people infested with *S. scabiei*.

The burrows of the females appear as dark wavy lines of around 2 mm in length, with a vesicle at the end of the burrow indicating the position of the egg-laying female. They may appear on the flexor surfaces of the wrists, elbows or in the axilla, the webs of the fingers or in skin creases at the waist or around the gluteal muscle. Pruritus is caused by hypersensitivity to the presence of the mite, its larvae or their faeces, and scratching may cause bacterial infection. The presence of the mite or its excreta is confirmed by skin scrapings.

Pharmacological management

In addition to good personal hygiene and laundering of infested clothing and bedding, specific scabicides are ordered. These may include γ-**benzene hexachloride** cream or lotion, **benzyl benzoate**, **sulphur** ointment, **crotamiton** 10% cream or **permethrin** 5% cream. The use of γ-benzene hexachloride in babies, young children and pregnant women is contraindicated as there is a risk of toxicity. Gamma-benzene hydrochloride disables the creature, usually by poisoning its nervous system. For this reason, health professionals who regularly apply such preparations are advised to use gloves to prevent their own skin from absorbing the product, and to ensure that the product is not used for vulnerable groups (Plorde, 1991).

WARTS

There are more then 60 types of papillomavirus that result in an exaggeration of the normal structure, either of the skin or of the mucous membrane. One form of human papilloma virus is thought to be implicated in the development of carcinoma of the cervix (see Chapter 6 *Drugs and neoplastic disorders*). The organism responsible for the formation of skin warts is usually transmitted as a result of skin contact. The warts disappear when the body is able to mount an immune defence against the virus. However, this process may take up to 5 years, which helps to explain the persistence of warts and then their sudden disappearance even when no treatment is given.

Pathophysiology

Warts tend to produce thickening of the malpighian layer of the skin, irregular shaping of the epidermis, thickening of the horny layer and abnormalities of the nuclei in the epidermal cells. Seventy per cent of lesions are common warts (verruca vulgaris), which produce firm, rough structures, often on the backs of the hands or fingers, or on knees. Usually, they produce no symptoms (**Fig. 17.4**).

Pharmacological management

Warts used to be treated by excision. Now the overgrowths of keratin are removed by chemical means, by the use of caustic or keratolytic agents such as **liquid nitrogen** therapy or by the use of **silver nitrate** sticks or 2% **salicylic acid** paint, all of which break down the accumulated keratin layers. Care must be taken to direct the agent only to the area of hyperkeratinisation, otherwise damage to normal skin cells will occur.

HERPES INFECTIONS

There are two main forms of herpes virus: type 1 and type 2. Type 1 occurs above the waist and produces a herpes simplex infection. The type 2 virus more commonly causes genital herpes, although this is not invariably the case.

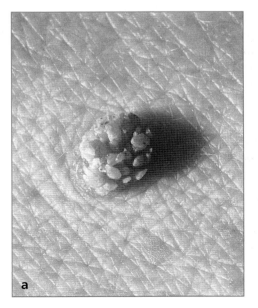

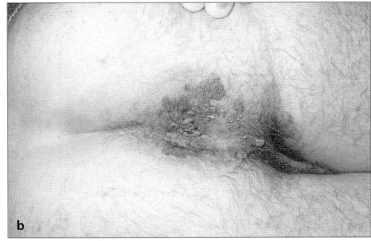

Fig 17.4 Skin warts. (From Stevens & Lowe 1995, with permission.)

Pathophysiology

The skin manifestations of the herpes viral infection include the presence of sensations of burning and tingling and the appearance of skin vesicles and erythema. The vesicles turn into pustules and small ulcers, and then develop crusts before healing. Outbreaks on the face, lips and mouth are particularly painful, and may take between 10 and 14 days to heal. Herpes infections tend to take a course that suggests the development of cell-mediated immunity; the effects at the time of first infection are marked, but those associated with any subsequent episode are considerably less severe, because of the rapid production of specific antibodies. Herpes simplex infections seem to recur more frequently in stressful circumstances, during menstruation and, for some reason, in conjunction with exposure to sunlight.

Pharmacological management

Mechanisms that reduce the pain associated with herpes viral infections are useful. These include applications of cold packs, the application of local anaesthesia such as oral gel containing **choline salicylate** 8.7% w/v and **cetalkonium chloride** 0.01% w/v for mouth ulcers and systemic analgesics such as **salicylic acid** are useful. In severe cases, topical applications of preparations such as **acyclovir** 5% in an aqueous cream base and **idoxuridine** 5% creams are used to inhibit viral reproductive cycles and thus limit the infective process.

HERPES ZOSTER

This painful condition, known colloquially as shingles, occurs when the herpes zoster virus is reactivated after a dormant period in a sensory dorsal nerve ganglion. The infection may be the sequel to an earlier infection of a sensory nerve by the chicken pox virus, varicella zoster. When the virus is reactivated, it travels to the area of skin served by the sensory nerve it formerly colonised, and a rash erupts along the tract of this tissue. The effects are more severe in immunosuppressed people.

Pathophysiology

A herpes zoster infection is characterised by skin lesions similar to but deeper than those of varicella zoster. Vesicles develop and form crusts; they dry and separate within 2–3 weeks, often leaving scars. A particularly unpleasant type of herpes zoster infection involves the trigeminal nerve, when the lesions follow a tract that may include the eye and cause ophthalmic involvement.

Pharmacological management

Herpes zoster infection produces severe pain. The effects are worse in older people, possibly because, as a result of the wear and tear of time, original large nerve tracts have become dysfunctional and have been supplemented by additional smaller nerve fibres, thus increasing the potential for the perception of pain. The skin symptoms of herpes zoster infections are treated with **acyclovir**, administered early so as to reduce the extent of the infection, with narcotic analgesics for the pain and with topical cooling applications such as **calamine lotion** to reduce the perception of pain from dermal pain fibres.

ACNE

This group of conditions provides an example in which, in severe forms, pharmacological treatment consists of measures to alter the activity of certain cells within the skin; to adjust the proportion of epidermal to dermal cells and to alter the nature of the bacterial colonies inhabiting the skin. Most of us may have experienced some degree of acne during our adolescent years. For the fortunate majority, this state of affairs resolves itself with the onset of adulthood. For some sufferers, acne may become a chronic problem, and some forms develop in later life. The discussion here is limited to acne vulgaris, the condition that commonly afflicts younger people, and extends to a discussion of persistent inflammatory acne, in which more than over-the-counter measures become necessary. For a more comprehensive examination of this topic, the reader is referred to specialist dermatological texts.

Acne is primarily a disorder of the sebaceous glands, which are found on all parts of the body with the exception of the palms of the hands and the soles of the feet. Sebaceous glands are found most commonly on the face, scalp, chest and back, which explains the characteristic distribution of acne when it is present. The events leading to the production and distribution of sebum are shown in **Figure 17.5**.

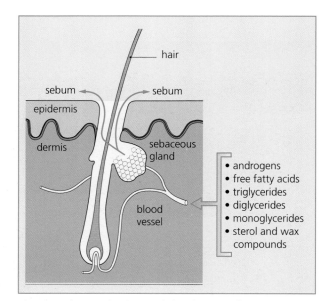

Fig 17.5 The production and distribution of sebum. (From Steven & Lowe 1995, with permission.)

Pathophysiology

The sebaceous cells break down and empty their contents into the hair follicle. The rate of sebum production depends upon the size of the sebaceous gland and the rate of sebaceous cell proliferation. This production is governed by the secretion of androgens from:

• The testes in the male.
• The ovaries and adrenal glands in the female.

Non-inflammatory acne is characterised by the presence of whiteheads (pale, slightly raised papules) and blackheads,

17.3 DERMATOLOGICAL CHANGES WITH ADOLESCENCE

All children will mature and experience adolescence; the pubescent growth 'spurt' results from the effect of changing hormone levels. Androgens, hormones that are highly specialised lipids derived from cholesterol, are constantly secreted from the adrenal cortex at this time in increased amounts. At the skin, this increased secretion is directly related to excess sebum production. Acne begins with accumulation that obstructs the pilosebaceous unit and allows proliferation of the bacterium *Propionibacterium acnes* (Yemaneberhan et al, 1997). Any treatments should take into consideration the adolescence self-image, which may be very fragile at this stage of development. A deformed face may lead to personality disturbance, physical self-harm or social distancing.

which are plugs of sebaceous material that have blocked the sebaceous glands. The pigmentation of blackheads is composed of melanin that has been released into the sebaceous glands. The lesions, which are collectively termed comedones, are distributed in the same manner as the sebaceous glands. Because of the influence of androgens, acne is more persistent in boys and men (**Fig. 17.6**).

With inflammatory acne it is thought that sebum migrates from the sebaceous glands into the dermis, where the component fatty acids cause inflammation in the tissues. Inflammatory acne is characterised by the presence of papules, pustules and sometimes cysts. The situation is exacerbated by the presence of *Propionibacterium acnes*, which secretes lipase. Free fatty acids are degraded and released, contributing to the inflammation.

Pharmacological management

The treatment of acne is directed towards the correction of the unbalanced skin physiology. Skin hygiene is important with water- rather than oil-based make-up or skin preparations – used to minimise the accumulation of lipids. Exposure to sunlight lessens symptoms, probably because of the drying effect of the sun, as does a balanced diet and avoidance of stress or fatigue.

Pharmacological treatment is directed towards:
• Drying and reducing the depth of the keratin layer by the use of keratolytic agents such as **resorcinol**, **salicylic acid** and **sulphur** compounds.
• Removing comedones.

Topical **Retin A**, a vitamin A derivative, is used to increase the rate of mitosis in the follicles. The increased rate of turnover has the effect of pushing the comedones out of the follicles, reducing the colonies of *P. acnes*. Low doses of

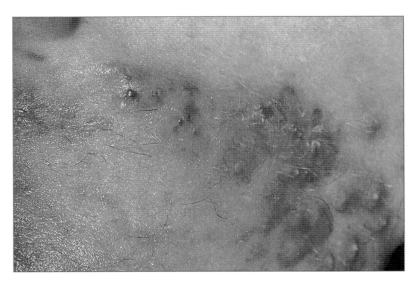

Fig 17.6 Acne vulgaris. (From Stevens & Lowe 1995, with permission.)

oral **tetracycline** reduce the levels of free fatty acids. Antibiotics **erythromycin** or **clindamycin** have been found to be useful, as has the antimicrobial agent **dapsin**. The oral synthetic acid form of **vitamin A** has the hormonal effects of reducing the activity of the sebaceous glands, decreasing inflammation and reducing the colonies of *P. acnes*. This latter preparation can, however, raise lipid levels in the liver and serum, and it is teratogenic so must not be given to pregnant women (Lawley and Yancey, 1991).

KERATINISATION

Keratinisation of the skin is caused by factors that trigger the increased rate of epidermal proliferation. Mild itching of the affected areas caused by the dry scales is common.

PSORIASIS

Psoriasis affects approximately 2% of the population, men and women equally. It can occur at any age but there is an increased incidence during the teens and 20s and again around the ages of 50–60 years. There is known to be a genetic tendency as 35% of sufferers have a family history of the condition. The basic defect of psoriasis is unknown but lymphocytic infiltration is often seen on histology, which suggests that immunological factors may play a part. Keratinisation of the skin is seen to occur and the skin is characterised by the formation of plaques of thickened scaly epidermis. Mild itching of affected areas, caused by the dry scales, is common in psoriasis. Leucotrienes (inflammatory agents and stimulators of keratinocyte proliferation) and chalones (inhibitors of mitosis) have been implicated in their role as cell division modulators. Other factors that trigger the increased rate of epidermal proliferation are prostaglandins and epidermal growth factor. Emotional stress is another factor that tends to exacerbate this inflammatory skin disease.

Pathophysiology

The pathological skin changes of psoriasis are the development of abnormal skin patches, caused by the proliferation of epidermal undifferentiated cells (Laurence and Bennett, 1992) and the whole process of skin formation occurring in 4 days because of a 30-fold increase in new epidermal cells (**Fig. 17.7**). This results in a much thicker epidermis as more cells are produced; these are less mature therefore they are not fully keratinized (this causes the scales). The scales heap up and dry; the keratin becomes hard, brittle, less pliable and can crack, causing painful fissures. There is capillary dilatation in the dermis and lymphocytic infiltration to the area, leading to the appearance of inflammation and redness of the skin (**Fig. 17.8**) (Venables, 1994).

Pharmacological management

The treatment for psoriasis is by topical application as this gives obvious intimate contact between the drug and the tissues that are targeted. The drug prescribed depends on

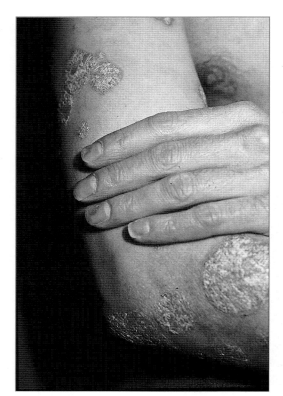

Fig 17.7 Psoriasis. (From Stevens & Lowe 1995, with permission.)

the patient's age, lifestyle (social activities, holidays and employment), the severity of the disease and the previous effects and responses to treatment (Richards, 1995). With mild psoriasis the outcome desired from the treatment is to ease itching, soreness and fissures by 'soothing, smoothing and hydrating' the affected skin (Marrs, 1991).

Skin rehydration

Rehydration of the skin is achieved by the use of emollients, which should be used daily or more frequently and come in the form of soap substitutes, bath additives and moisturisers. General moisturisers such as aqueous cream also reduce scaling and lichenification; they are best applied after a *warm* bath and left to soak into the skin for 45 minutes before application of treatment (Venables, 1994).

Removal of scales

The removal of scales is achieved by the use of keratolytic preparations (e.g. **coal tar 10% with or without salicylic acid**). This precipitates epidermal proliferation during the first 2 weeks of application, which is then followed by a prolonged reduction in skin thickness as a result of its antimitotic action. In addition, tar has been found to have antipruritic properties; it is also a photosensitising agent that is used to advantage in Ingram's method, in which a coal tar bath is given to descale and photosensitise the skin, followed by ultraviolet light exposure (UVB) and the application of **dithranol** 0.4%.

Descaling agents

To normalise the appearance of skin and allow access for further treatment to plaque, **coal tar cream** or **lotion** is used: 2% sulphur, 2% salicylic acid, 4% prepared coal tar, 25% emulsifying wax and liquid paraffin to 100% (for scalp).

Side effects can include acne-type eruptions and folliculitis, caused by a build-up of application of coal tar cream and infection of the hair follicle. It should also be noted that some preparations stain clothing and bedding.

Dithranol is another keratolytic preparation, which has tended to supersede the coal tar products and is a more potent antimitotic – achieving more lasting results upon the disease process itself – and often produces a true remission. Its action is to clear chronic plaque psoriasis in an average of 3 weeks; it is applied daily and left for 12–24 hours.

Dithrocream, a more concentrated preparation, is presented in a yellow soft paraffin vehicle. It is applied daily from 5 to a total of 30 minutes, according to strength (0.1–2.0%), and must then be washed off immediately after the time specified otherwise it damages the skin. The side effects are the same as those for dithranol. Special considerations are that gloves should be worn and surrounding skin protected with petroleum jelly when strong coal tar preparations, salicylic acid and dithranol are applied. These preparations must never be applied to red, raw or inflamed areas.

The aim of remission of pathology is to induce cell differentiation and inhibit proliferation of keratinocytes,

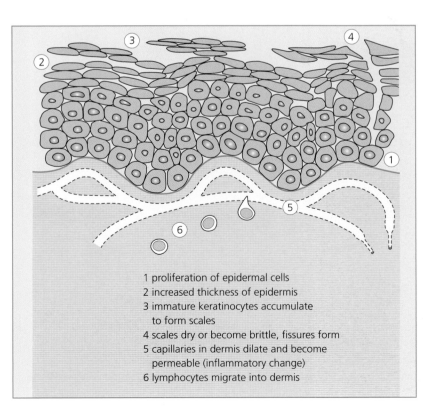

Fig 17.8 Pathological skin changes in psoriasis.

1 proliferation of epidermal cells
2 increased thickness of epidermis
3 immature keratinocytes accumulate
  to form scales
4 scales dry or become brittle, fissures form
5 capillaries in dermis dilate and become
  permeable (inflammatory change)
6 lymphocytes migrate into dermis

thereby normalising epidermal cell behaviour and reducing the psoriatic plaques (Richards, 1995). These effects occur with the use of **calcipotriol**, which is a vitamin D_3 analogue and comes as an ointment or cream containing 50 µg active agent per gram of vehicle. Calcipotriol reduces plaques but may not produce a remission of the psoriasis. The outcome is for plaques to be less red, smaller and lead to normal skin. The side effects are few but it may cause some skin irritation.

Reduction of epidermal cell division

A treatment that has been found to be beneficial for some severe psoriasis sufferers is PUVA (ultraviolet light therapy). The treatment is a combination of tablets (psoralens) and long-wave ultraviolet light therapy (UVA). In the presence of UVA the psoralens interact with DNA and RNA in the cell nucleus and inhibit DNA synthesis. Psoralens (obtained from citrus and other plants) induces photochemical reactions in the skin and is taken 2 hours before UVA exposure in a UVA cabinet.

The side effects are prickling and burning of the skin, nausea and malaise. Kidney, liver, and cardiac function may be affected. There is an increased risk of skin cancer, accelerated skin ageing and cataracts. Goggles are worn during treatment and protective spectacles should be worn for 12 hours afterwards, as the increased sensitivity to ultraviolet light causes cataracts.

Suppression of the immune response

Glucocorticoids control and improve some forms of psoriasis by their anti-inflammatory and immunosuppressant actions. However, not all the physiological and pharmacological properties of glucocorticoids are understood. When applied topically they are rapidly absorbed, and the more water soluble they are the more rapid their penetration is to below the level of the dermis. It is in the epidermis that keratinocytes and fibroblasts are to be found and, via cytoplasmic receptors in these cells, the glucocorticoids are transferred to the nuclei of the cells (Bowman, 1994). Here they inhibit the rate of DNA synthesis and epidermal cell mitosis (Richards, 1995), which occurs at a rapid rate in psoriasis. Suppression of the inflammatory action is thought to be brought about by inhibition of antigen-processing by

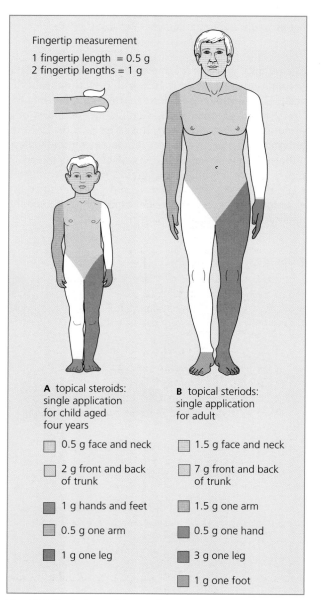

Fingertip measurement

1 fingertip length = 0.5 g
2 fingertip lengths = 1 g

A topical steroids: single application for child aged four years

- 0.5 g face and neck
- 2 g front and back of trunk
- 1 g hands and feet
- 0.5 g one arm
- 1 g one leg

B topical steriods: single application for adult

- 1.5 g face and neck
- 7 g front and back of trunk
- 1.5 g one arm
- 0.5 g one hand
- 3 g one leg
- 1 g one foot

Fig 17.9 Topical steroids: application recommendations for adults and children.

Treatment for severe psoriasis and eczema or dermatitis	
Generic name	**Comments**
Betamethasone dipropionate and betamethasone valerate	These products are fluorinated, need to be used sparingly and applied to affected areas only.
Triamcinolone acetonide	May be used with occlusive dressings.
Betamethasone 0.1% (as dipropionate) salicylic acid 3% is also obtainable as a lotion for use on the scalp.	Use 2–4 times per day for adults.
Special considerations: Fluorinated products should not be used on the face, as they may cause thinning and leave scars.	

Table 17.3 Treatment for severe psoriasis and eczema/dermatitis

A patient, John Green, is re-admitted with an exacerbation of psoriasis. While you are assessing him, he shows you his hands, pointing out reddened areas of skin. You note that it is the anterior surface of the finger tips that are sore and erythematous, particularly the first and second finger of the right hand. The boundary of the reddened areas is not well defined and seems irregular, merging unobtrusively with the surrounding, apparently healthy, skin.

On further examination, you find that there are multiple scaly psoriatic lesions on the torso, the scalp and on the extensor surfaces of his legs and left arm.

The current treatment regime includes 1% dithranol cream. John volunteers that he has had a bad sore throat recently, and has been taking penicillin tablets prescribed by his GP. He wonders whether the antibiotic might have something to do with the appearance of the hand lesions.

John has worked at the check-out of a supermarket for the past 5 years, and, as part of his job, he handles a variety of food stuffs. His hands are constantly on display to customers who have bought the food he then handles as he checks the food items through the till. John is worried that the psoriasis is spreading to affect his hands. If it is, he fears that customers may complain about his unsightly lesions and he may lose his job.

1. Do you think that John's contact with foodstuffs in the supermarket has any bearing upon his condition?
2. Do you think that the antibiotics John has been taking have any relation to the present state of his hands?
3. Is the state of his hands part of his psoriasis and therefore likely to be consistently visible to the customers in the store?
4. What advice might you give John to help minimise his current symptoms?

preparation that extends from the adult's fingertip to first joint (Bowman, 1994). This will give a weight of approximately 0.5 g, which is equal to 1 unit. The topical steroids (glucocorticoids) used are potent to very potent for severe manifestations of psoriasis and contain **betamethasone** or **triamcinolone**, to which is added valerate, diprorionate or acetonide to give increased penetration of the skin, thereby increasing potency.

Grease-based steroid ointments are more useful as a means of delivery, and are more potent than creams. Because of their emollient properties they also enhance absorption, thereby reducing the length of time of direct contact with the skin. Areas of action of topical skin preparations and steroids can be seen in **Figure 17.9** and **Table 17.3**.

Side effects of topical steroids can include skin atrophy, vascular effects, perioral dermatitis, the rebound phenomenon and systemic absorption.

Skin atrophy of the epidermal layer or dermis may produce thinning and affect collagen synthesis in the dermis. This may result in striae of skin flexures, thighs, breasts and abdomen; women are particularly prone to suffer this complication.

Vascular effects may involve fixed vasodilatation, which shows as reddening of the skin (plethoric complexion), and telangiectasia. This particularly affects the body image when it occurs on the face.

Perioral dermatitis Papules around the mouth and skin may occur when more potent steroids are used.

Purpura These reddened or purple eruptions may be seen particularly on the arms when skin already thinned is exposed to sunlight.

The **rebound phenomenon** occurs as a consequence of inappropriate use of topical steroids, leading to overdilatation of small blood vessels which then allows oedema and enhanced inflammation of the psoriasis.

Topical steroids are not normally used as first-line management because of the effect caused by the withdrawal or reduction in their potencies.

Systemic absorption – betamethasone used for prolonged periods could cause:
- Glucocorticoid-induced osteoporosis in children and post-menopausal women.
- Impairment of the growth rate in children through inhibition of the biological effects of insulin-like growth factor-1 (formerly somatomedin C).
- Adrenal insufficiency on withdrawal of the steroid preparation.

INFLAMMATION AND INFLAMMATORY DISORDERS

Inflammatory skin disorders tend to possess a complex aetiology. There may be genetic, psychological, dietary or environmental triggers. For this reason, an holistic

the macrophages and mediators of the inflammatory response (interleukins, cytokines and prostaglandins) within the dermis (Margionis, 1994).

To aid the application of topical steroid preparations the finger tip unit (FTU) was devised and is the amount of

approach may constitute the most appropriate method of management, although the use of pharmacological products is at present the most common form of treatment. Skin treatments that moisten, cool and soothe, oral sedatives, modifications to diet and complementary treatments such as acupuncture have been found useful by some. Inflammatory skin conditions tend to follow a fluctuating course, remitting and exacerbating with the changing effects of ageing and stress, and environmental alterations.

Inflammation of the skin can be described using the four cardinal signs of redness, swelling, heat and pain, which lead to loss of function. For example, the loss of protection against invasion by microorganisms produces increased susceptibility to infection. Systemic and topical medication is used to address these symptoms. In this inflammatory response, blood is diverted from the 'core' to the peripheral skin, so causing redness and heat. Wet wraps and cool baths (at around 37°C) with simple emollient preparations such as arachis (peanut) oil compound, liquid paraffin or lanolin are useful to counteract dry skin. Mast cells in skin produce histamine that dilates and makes more permeable superficial blood capillaries. Consequently, fluid escapes and swelling, 'weeping' and pain result. Topical steroids constrict these vessels and, in conjunction with antibiotics and/or pastes, prevent secondary infections. Long-term damage may result in acanthosis nigricans (patches of velvety hyperpigmentation) and lichenification, which can be controlled by using topical tar preparations or creams and ointments containing icthammol. Such preparations act as mild antiseptics and antipruritics and reduce areas of skin thickening. Damage to the horny layer of the skin allows antigens to pass through and may cause intense itching. The use of small doses of systemic antihistamines such as promethazine or trimeprazine help to provide sufficient sedation to allow the sufferer to obtain sleep. Complementary therapies, such as some types of herbal teas, are currently receiving attention as possible adjuncts to treatment.

DERMATITIS OR ECZEMA

The terms 'eczema', 'dermatitis' and 'eczematous dermatitis' are regarded as synonymous (Baker, 1989). Eczema from the Greek word *ekzein* means boiling out and dermatitis refers to inflammation of the skin (Donald, 1995). Both these terms require further explanation to make the diagnosis more exact. In practice, however, people often call an eczema 'dermatitis' when they think they know the cause, as in allergic contact dermatitis to metals such as nickel, and 'eczema' when they do not, as in atopic eczema. The incidence of eczema is high: 12% of children and 10% of the population as a whole suffer from it. The inflammatory skin response of eczema is caused by endogenous and exogenous agents. Endogenous eczemas include **atopic dermatitis**, in which there is a family history of asthma, allergic rhinitis and is the more common cause of eczema in children, and seborrhoeic dermatitis, which occurs at any age. Exogenous eczemas include **irritant dermatitis** caused by chemical irritants such as soaps and detergents and **allergic contact dermatitis**, which is a cell-mediated delayed hypersensitivity in response to allergens. Examples include nickel and chromate found in wet cement and plaster; medications such as antihistamines and anaesthetics if applied topically; lanolin; preservatives in creams and ointments; chemicals in rubber gloves; dyes and plants such as poison ivy and primula (**Fig. 17.10**).

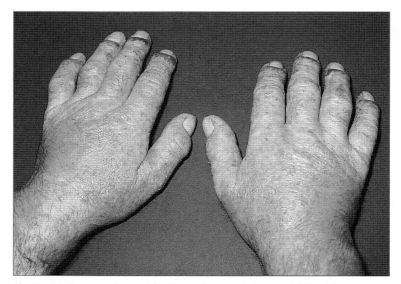

Fig 17.10 Contact dermatitis. (From Stevens & Lowe 1995, with permission.)

17.4 CHILDHOOD ECZEMA

The new baby has little fat beneath the epidermis, which is uncornified and thus poorly protected from drying out and invasion from microorganisms. In children with eczema the use of wet wraps is very effective in rehydrating the skin and allowing increased absorption of emollients and topical steroids (Margionis et al., 1994). Children also have an immature immune system and are prone to repeated skin infections if they suffer from atopic eczema. The use of unrestricted antibiotics can lead to allergic response and resistant organisms.

Pathophysiology

Atopic dermatitis is an activation of mast cells, T lymphocytes, monocytes and other inflammatory cells that release histamine, lymphokines and other inflammatory mediators as a result of an interaction of the allergen, for example common food, and events in the immune system, leading to chronic inflammation (Yemaneberhan et al., 1997). The inflammatory lesions often start as vesicles, which can result in exudation of serum and crusting of excoriated areas. Pruritus is often present. Dry skin (xeroderma) results in scratching, which leads to fissures developing, thickening of the skin (lichenification) and pinpoint bleeding of the skin (purpura) (**Fig. 17.11**).

Systemic drug therapy

H_1-antihistamines – of which there are two main types – may be administered. The first types inhibit the action of histamine and causes drowsiness, therefore they are recommended to be prescribed for the night. Examples of type

1 preparations are **promethazine hydrochloride 10–20 mg** 2–3 times daily or **in the adult dosage** 25 mg at night. For children, an elixir containing 1 mg/ml of promethazine is available. The second type dissociates very slowly from the receptor and exhibit insurmountable antagonism to the action of histamine. Because of their action they can be taken during the day. Examples of type 2 are **terfenadine**, which does not cross the blood–brain barrier, **120 mg daily (adult dosage)**, **15–30 mg twice daily (child dosage)** and **astemizole** 10 mg for adults with a maximum dose of 5 mg for children under 12 years. Because of their mode of action neither cause drowsiness.

Antibiotics are necessary when excoriation becomes infected; usually broad-spectrum antibiotics are used and may be given topically. Short courses are given to prevent resistant strains of staphylococci from developing.

Analgesia is taken when needed to relieve heat, tenderness and localised pain.

Topical therapy

Emollients are used to moisturise dry and scaly skin, improve skin tone and reduce pruritus. They also create a barrier for inflamed skin, thus preventing further fluid and heat loss. They should be used frequently and liberally, but intolerance is common. The section on psoriasis discusses the products that are available Other treatment is shown in **Table 17.4**.

Treatment for irritation and inflammation

Medicated bandages are applied overnight and provide a cooling effect and relieve irritation. The moist environment created aids absorption of emollients and steroid applications. They are particularly helpful in forming a mechanical barrier that prevents damage occurring from scratching at night by infants during sleep.

Mild topical steroids may be used such as hydrocortisone base or acetate 0.5–2% products. The preferred

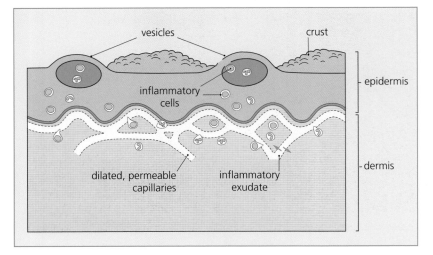

Fig 17.11 Pathophysiolgogy of atopic dermatitis.

Treatment for dermatitis	
Acute weeping stage	
Lotions – aluminium acetate, calamine	Cooling effect.
Soaks – potassium permanganate (1:8000)	Soothing lotion. Prevents secondary infection and tends to reduce weeping.
Caution: can cause dryness and cracking of skin if continued for too long.	

Table 17.4 Treatment for dermatitis

preparation is as ointment, except for babies. High-potency steroids are needed to control intolerable exacerbations. These are reduced when control is established (see *Pharmacological management* in *Psoriasis* section).

Rarely, in very severe atopic dermatitis, alternate-day oral prednisolone therapy is justifiable and has been found to be very effective (**Fig. 17.12**). It is usually used after growth has ceased (see Chapter 5 *Drugs and immune disorders* for the effects of oral steroids).

Severe atopic eczema that has not responded to emollients and mild topical steroids may be helped by essential fatty acids, which are cell wall precursors that assist immunity and anti-inflammatory prostaglandins. Essential fatty acids are to be found in fish oils or evening primrose oils and are administered orally (Laurence and Bennett, 1992; Burton, 1990).

ALLERGIC CONTACT DERMATITIS

Contact dermatitis is a commonly experienced condition. An area of skin that has been in contact with a substance capable of producing delayed hypersensitivity becomes red and itches and may become scaly and weep. Common sites include the area of the wrist in contact with the back of a wristwatch and, in women, areas on the back and thorax which have been in contact with the metallic parts of a brassiere. Soaps and detergents may provoke irritant contact dermatitis in susceptible people.

Pathophysiology

Contact dermatitis occurs when an allergen comes into contact with skin and becomes bound to a carrier protein, forming a sensitising antigen. The Langerhans cells, which migrate to the dermis from the bone marrow, initiate an immune response by processing the antigen and carrying it to the T lymphocytes, which become sensitised to the antigen (McCance, 1994). On re-exposure to the allergen the T cells then differentiate and secrete lymphokines that attract macrophages and initiate coagulation, and the inflammatory response results: erythema, swelling, vesicles, scaling, exudation of serum leading to the formation of crusts and pruritus. The pattern of distribution provides a clue to the source of the antigen. At this stage it is important to identify and remove the causative factor.

Pharmacological management

The first line of treatment for dry and scaly skin is to use an **emollient** to improve skin tone and reduce pruritus. This can be followed after 20 minutes with the application of a mild topical steroid of 1% hydrocortisone cream. Directions for use should be strictly adhered to, and consist of applying the cream to a small area sparingly twice a day for 7 days (see **Table 17.4**).

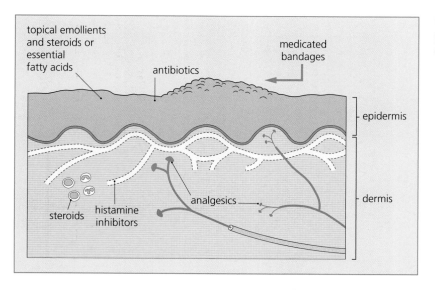

Fig 17.12 Summary of the pharmacological treatment of dermatitis or eczema.

🔑 KEY POINTS

- Skin disorders may cause a rash and symptoms such as pruritus, pain and stinging sensations.
- The skin can be affected by systemic disorders such as endocrine conditions, measles and hepatic failure.
- Drug therapy may cause hypersensitivity reactions, an increased sensitivity of the skin to light or an alteration to normal pigmentation.
- Skin preparations must be soluble in water and fats to be absorbed through the skin; the deeper layers of the skin are reached via the hair follicles or sebaceous glands.
- Dermatological agents may be used on the skin to alleviate symptoms, for protection, to improve appearance or to alter existing levels of functioning.

- The use of sun blockers is very important in the protection against UVB short wavelength irradiation.
- Skin infection may be primary or secondary and may be caused by bacteria, viruses, yeasts or fungi.
- Non-inflammatory acne is characterised by whiteheads and blackheads, whereas inflammatory acne is characterised by the presence of papules, pustules and cysts.
- Psoriatic lesions are red, inflamed and scaly and are caused by excessive proliferation of undifferentiated epidermal cells.
- Atopic dermatitis is a form of endogenous eczema that produces an inflammatory skin response.

MULTIPLE CHOICE QUESTIONS

Choose all those that apply.

1. Drugs that can alter the pigmentation of the skin include
   a. heavy metal compounds
   b. phenothiazines
   c. non-steroidal anti-inflammatory drugs
   d. antimalarial preparations
   e. diphenhydramine hydrochloride

2. The skin is protected from harmful UVB rays by the use of
   a. a sun protection factor (SPF) of 15
   b. zinc oxide, titanium compounds or talc
   c. para-aminobenzoic acid and salicylates
   d. petroleum jelly or baby oil
   e. coal tar cream or lotion

3. The skin can become thin from
   a. the use of betamethasone or triamcinolone
   b. the ageing process
   c. eczema
   d. psoriasis
   e. all of the above

4. The difference between whiteheads and blackheads is
   a. the amount of fatty acids in the sebum
   b. melanin in the sebum of blackheads
   c. an increase or decrease of vitamin D being formed in the skin
   d. whether you are tanned
   e. the presence of bacteria

5. A fluid-filled lesion is referred to as a
   a. wheal
   b. nodule
   c. vesicle
   d. pustule
   e. macule

6. Psoriasis is characterised by
   a. lymphocytic infiltration of the dermis
   b. undifferentiated cell proliferation
   c. swelling and exudate
   d. scaly, itching plaques
   e. inflammation and redness of the epidermis

7. The aim of treatment of psoriasis is to
   a. rehydrate the epidermis
   b. remove scale
   c. induce cell differentiation
   d. inhibit the rate of DNA synthesis
   e. inhibit inflammatory mediators

8. Scabies is treated by
   a. decontamination of all clothing and bedding for the whole family
   b. use of a topical antibiotic ointment
   c. cream, lotion or shampoos of lindane or malathion
   d. emollient or emulsifying creams to soften scales
   e. local anaesthetics to reduce pain

9. Topical preparations that are most penetrating to the skin
   a. are water soluble
   b. are soluble in fatty acids
   c. contain glucocorticoids
   d. contain dipropionate
   e. contain steroids

10. Cold compresses applied to itching skin work by
    a. reducing heat by evaporation
    b. increasing the sensory information from nerve receptors
    c. constricting skin capillaries to reduce hyperaemia
    d. reducing oedema and pressure on skin receptors
    e. all of the above

REFERENCES

Baker H. *Clinical dermatology*. London: Baillière Tindall, 1989.

Bickers DR. Photosensitivity and other reactions to light. In: Wilson JD, Braunwald E, Isselbacher KJ, Petersdorf RG, Martin JB, Fauci AS, Root RK. *Harrison's principles of internal medicine, 12th ed.* New York: McGraw Hill, 1991.

Bowman J. More than skin deep. *Nursing*

Brookbank J. *The biology of ageing.* New York: Harper and Row, 1990.

Burton J. *Essentials of dermatology.* Edinburgh: Churchill Livingstone, 1990.

Hampton S. Wound assessment. *Prof Nurs* 1997; **12(Suppl):**S5-S17.

Hazinski M. *Nursing care of the critically ill child, 2nd ed.* London: Mosby, 1992.

Laurence DR, Bennett PN. *Clinical pharmacology, 7th ed.* Edinburgh: Churchill Livingstone, 1992.

Lawley TJ, Yancey KB. Alterations in the skin. In: Wilson JD, Braunwald E, Isselbacher KJ, Petersdorf RG, Martin JB, Fauci AS, Root RK *Harrison's principles of internal medicine, 12th ed.* New York: McGraw Hill, 1991.

Leaper D. Antiseptics in wound healing. *Nursing Times* 1996 **92(39):** 63-64; 66-68.

Margionis A, Gravanis A, Chrousos G. Glucocorticoids and mineralocorticoids. In: Brody TM, Larner J, Minneman KP, Neu HC, eds. *Human pharmacology: molecular to clinical.* St Louis: Mosby, 1994: 473-481.

Marieb EN. *Human anatomy and physiology.* Redwood City, CA: Benjamin Cummings, 1989.

Marrs R. Motivation the key to control: nurses' role in treatment of psoriasis. *Prof Nurs* 1991; **7:**103-108.

Mattson Porth C. *Pathophysiology: concepts of altered health states.* Philadelphia: JB Lippincott, 1994.

McCance K, Huether S. *Pathophysiology, 2nd ed.* London: Mosby, 1994.

McHenry PM, *et al.* Management of atopic eczema. *Br Med J* 1995; **310:**843-847.

Page C. *Integrated Pharmacology.* London: Mosby, 1997.

Plorde JJ. Scabies, chiggers and other ectoparasites. In Wilson JD, Braunwald E, Isselbacher KJ, Petersdorf RG, Martin JB, Fauci AS, Root RK *Harrison's principles of internal medicine, 12th ed.* New York: McGraw Hill, 1991.

Richards C. The effects of psoriasis and its treatment: part 1. *Nurs Times* 1995; **91/21:**38-39.

Spowart K. Childhood skin disorders. *Paediatr Nurs* 1995; **7:**29-37.

Tonge H. Special focus: tissue viability, the management of infected wounds. *Nurs Stand* 1997; **12(12):**49-53.

Venables J. Knowledge needed to educate patients about psoriasis. *Nurs Times* 1994; 90(23) 33-35

Walker G. *ABPI data sheet compendium.* London: Datapharm Publications, 1995.

Yemaneberhan H, Bekele Z, Venn A, Lewis S, Parry E, Britton J. Prevalence of wheeze and asthma and relation to atopy in urban and rural Ethiopia. *Lancet* 1997; **350:**85-90.

18 Kate Dewar
PHARMACOLOGICAL MANAGEMENT OF PAIN

INTRODUCTION

Pain is useful as a signal that something is 'wrong', and is a common experience in illness. Its management depends on an understanding of the particular mix of psychological, sociological and physical features that influence an individual's experience of pain. In this chapter these features are described and based on this understanding, the use of pharmacological agents is explained.

DEFINITION OF PAIN

There are many definitions of pain, and the one offered here is chosen for its focus on the individual experience, as this forms a basis for any treatment plan. Pain is 'an unpleasant sensory or emotional experience associated with actual or potential tissue damage, or described in terms of such damage' (International Association for the Study of Pain, 1986).

TYPES OF PAIN

Classification of pain is a useful first step in assessment of pain before an appropriate management programme is planned and implemented. It can be classified in many ways but two commonly used categorisations are described: pain as acute or chronic, and pain as nociceptive or neurogenic.

Acute Pain

This is generally part of the body's normal 'fight or flight' defence mechanisms. By its presence it allows the individual to recognise danger. Acute pain may be mild or severe and usually runs a short course, lasting less than 3 months. It generally has a predictable intensity pattern, with the initial pain sensation diminishing during the course of the pain experience. This can be explained by the cause of the pain, which is usually the result of sudden trauma, whereas the diminution in pain intensity that follows is associated with healing.

Superficial acute pain results from sensation felt on the surface of the body. It lasts seconds or minutes rather than weeks. It may be mild or more severe and is often described as sharp or prickling in nature. The site of the pain is identified easily by sufferers.

Deep acute pain arises from sensations in deep layers of the skin or from other internal tissues such as joints, tendons, muscles and membranes. It is often described as a burning or aching pain. The site of the pain is often difficult for the sufferer to identify precisely and registers as a more diffuse location than the origin of superficial acute pain.

A single pathology may include both superficial acute and deep acute pain. For example after a burn, the initial pain can be precisely located and is a relatively short-lived sharp pain. It is followed by a more diffuse aching pain that persists for longer (Thomas, 1997).

Chronic pain

This type of pain lasts longer than 3 months; it persists after healing is complete and is unlikely to resolve spontaneously. It generally has no useful function and may actually have destructive sequelae as it can adversely effect the social, psychological and physical functioning of the individual. Chronic pain is dull, aching and/or burning in nature and is poorly localised, particularly when it arises from the viscera (McCaffery and Beebe, 1994).

Recurrent acute pain is a type of chronic pain that may recur repeatedly over months or years in episodes each with a predictable end, for example the pain of migraine or period pain.

Chronic malignant pain is long lasting and caused by a clearly defined pathology such as a cancer or degenerative joint disease.

Chronic non-malignant pain, or chronic benign pain, is a type of pain that may be the most disabling feature of the disease process. It can persist for the individual's lifetime and usually occurs every day. The cause is not life-threatening and the pain often responds poorly to ordinary pain control measures. Examples include low back pain and peripheral neuropathy.

An acute pain may progress to chronic pain because of a persistent underlying disease or because of changes within the nervous system. The pain event can 'imprint' itself on the neurons and synapses originally involved in the pain sensation. Consequently, the pain sensation is persistent, continuing after the original cause, and is often unpredictable in its intensity or duration. In addition to progression from one pain type to another, different types of pain can coexist in an individual and this is particularly common in the elderly (Thomas, 1997).

Neurogenic (or neuropathic) pain

This is a term used to describe pain resulting directly from damage to a nerve. As a consequence, abnormal spontaneous pain impulses are generated or are produced inappropriately in response to a minor stimulus. The individual perceives the pain to be on or near the surface of the body, whereas its real origin is the nervous system. Examples include the pain of cancer invading a nerve plexus and phantom limb pain. This type of pain is difficult to manage as it is generally highly resistant to common therapeutic

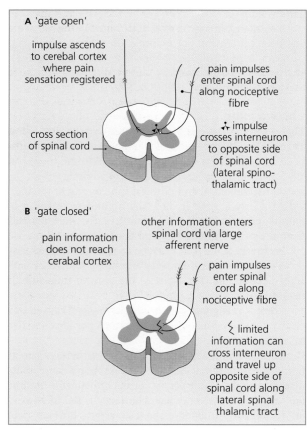

Fig 18.1 The 'gate theory' of pain transmission.

regimes. It often requires considerable resources, including the use of unconventional therapies, to bring this type of pain under control (McCaffery and Beebe, 1994).

Nociceptive pain

This category of pain is the result of damage to any tissue other than nervous tissue and it is transmitted via normal nerve pathways. Visceral pain is one type of nociceptive pain and arises from internal organs; examples include dysmenorrhoea and gastritis. This type of pain is not well understood and its management is therefore sometimes difficult. Somatic nociceptive pain arises from other internal tissues and examples include the pain of musculo-skeletal sports injuries and skeletal metastases. This type of pain is well understood and management can be precisely targeted to control it.

THEORY OF PAIN

Historically, ideas of pain were simplistic and failed to explain its complexity. It is only since Melzack and Wall (1965) developed their theory of pain that its complexity began to be revealed, although as yet our understanding remains incomplete. Identification of the different types of pain is the basis for an understanding of the different neurophysiological pathways involved in each (O'Hara, 1996).

THE GATE CONTROL THEORY

The gate control theory was developed by Melzack and Wall in 1965. It offers an explanation of the psycho-physiological components of pain. A central feature of this theory is the concept of a 'gate' in the central nervous system that can be opened or closed (**Fig. 18.1**). When open, pain messages are transmitted and can be perceived, when the gate is closed pain messages are blocked. The gate is operated by sensory nerve impulses originating from viscera and the periphery.

Pain impulses originate from nerve endings sensitive to pain stimuli called nociceptors. Mechanonociceptors are sensitive to heavy pressure sensations such as damage from sharp objects, whereas polymodal nociceptors react to a variety of other stimuli such as noxious chemicals, a change in pH and extremes of temperature. Chemicals released from damaged cells, such as bradykinin and prostaglandins, sensitise these nociceptors, triggering action potentials and the transmission of impulses along neurons. The pain intensity depends upon the number of nociceptors recruited and the severity of the initial stimulus.

Transmission of pain impulses depends on a variety of neurons. A-beta neurons have myelinated axons of large diameter and transmit impulses quickly. They are activated by vibration and light touch such as rubbing. A-delta neurons have slightly smaller, myelinated axons capable of fairly fast impulse relay, and transmit in response to sharp and heavy pressure stimuli. C neurons have small unmyelinated axons and so transmit electrical change from stimulation of polymodal nociceptors more slowly. C neurons have many neural connections so the pain messages transmitted are diffuse (dull, throbbing pain) and their site of origin is difficult to identify precisely.

The gate mechanism lies in the dorsal horn of the spinal cord and receives information from A-beta, A-delta and C neurons. Here there are neurons, which, when stimulated, block the passage of pain impulses. Similarly there are cells that, when stimulated, cause onward transmission of pain impulses.

A-beta neurons generally inhibit the transmission cells, thus preventing passage of pain information. C neurons and A-delta neurons carry impulses that bring about the transmission of pain messages.

Neurons descending from the brain also influence the activity of inhibitory and transmission cells. If the individual is relaxed, for example, neuronal impulses inhibit transmission of pain messages. On the other hand, in the individual who is distressed or tense, neurons from the brain stimulate transmission of pain messages at the gate.

There are also neurons that influence the ascending neurons carrying pain messages from the spinal cord to the brain. Neurons in the reticular formation of the brainstem can be stimulated by inputs from other sensory modalities such as the eyes and ears. They then inhibit or potentiate further transmission of the pain messages.

Cortical neurons influence perception of pain in several ways. For example, neurons from the limbic pathways affect the gate mechanism, causing transmission of pain messages, and can also enhance the individual's perception of pain. Frontal cortex and temporal lobe neurons allow individuals to define the pain experience in relation to past experiences. They, along with thalamic neurons, also enable it to be described in terms of time and place, that is, where the pain stimulus is and how long it lasts. Similarly, neurons involved in 'thinking' or cognitive activity can inhibit pain transmission, acting both within the brain and at the gate mechanism.

Melzack and Wall (1965) suggested that there are central coordinating mechanisms whereby all potential psychological influences on pain perception are activated and processed. Such influences include feelings of helplessness, control and excitement, the degree of attention, anxiety and arousal, and the learned effects of a particular culture as well as learned individual behavioural responses that have in the past minimised similar pain. Pain management therefore includes assessment of the particular influences operating on the individual (O'Hara, 1996).

On the basis of this theory, stimulation of, for example, A-beta neurons should minimise pain transmission, and this offers some explanation for the beneficial effects of acupuncture, massage and transcutaneous electrical nerve

18.1 USE OF TOPICAL AGENTS IN 'NEEDLEPHOBIA'

Most children and at least 10% of adults fear injections.

By application of eutectic mixture of local anaesthetics (EMLA) cream to intact skin under an occlusive dressing, anaesthesia of the surface tissues is achieved after 90 minutes.

Amethocaine gel may also be used and may have a quicker onset of action. Currently, it is not advised for use in children aged 3 months or younger as it is absorbed too readily into the circulation.

Use of these agents has prevented an enormous amount of pain and distress in children, and may also prevent these children becoming adult needlephobics. It is expected that in future such formulations will be used more frequently in the relief of injection pain and phobic responses in adults.

Transdermal agents that are suitable for neonates should also become available in the near future.

stimulation (TENS). Similarly, cognitive therapies that relax the individual, alter perception of the pain and give the sufferer some control over their pain may be useful.

Referred Pain

The phenomenon of referred pain occurs when pain from one site is experienced at another. It can be explained in terms of embryology and impulse transmission. The two 'sites' of pain may have been neighbours in the embryo or, alternatively, the two sites may share the same ascending pathways in the spinal cord. As a result the actual origin of the pain impulses arriving at the brain is perceived wrongly (McCaffery and Beebe, 1994).

NEUROTRANSMITTERS AND PAIN

Various chemicals are released from nerve endings and pass across the synaptic gap to lock into receptors on the post-synaptic neuron or effector cell. These neurotransmitters have an excitatory or an inhibitory effect. An excitatory neurotransmitter provokes an action potential, which enables the electrical charge to be transmitted along the post-synaptic neuron or through the effector cell. An inhibitory neurotransmitter prevents the generation of electrical charge, so that the impulse is not transmitted further. Each neuron synapses with many others, of which some may be sending inhibitory and others excitatory messages. If more excitatory than inhibitory neurotransmitter molecules are received, then the message will be relayed further; if more inhibitory signals are received the message will be blocked (see Chapter 7 *Drugs and psychological disorders* and Chapter 8 *Drugs and neurological disorders*).

Knowledge about the nature and effects of neurotransmitters involved in the transmission or inhibition of pain impulses is incomplete, but those known to be involved are substance P, somatostatin, serotonin (5-HT), noradrenaline and the endorphins (including encephalins and dynorphins), which are endogenous opioid peptides. Endorphins have been the subject of much research and are known to have an inhibitory effect on pain transmission; they are released on perception of pain and also in response to other stimuli such as major trauma, exercise, acupuncture and sexual activity. They have their effects at nerve endings in the cerebral cortex, the hypothalamus and thalamus, brainstem and spinal cord, where they bind to specific receptors, inhibiting the action of excitatory neurotransmitters such as substance P. Various types of opioid receptors, including mu (μ), kappa (κ) and sigma (σ), have been identified so far in these areas of the central nervous system. They are important in pain management as exogenous opioid drugs have effects similar to those of endorphins at these receptors (Brody *et al.*, 1994).

AGE AND PAIN MANAGEMENT

Health professionals tend to have mistaken beliefs about pain in the younger and older age groups (Horn and Munafo, 1997). As a result, pain management may be inadequate and unnecessary suffering may be caused.

Assessment of pain in individuals of any age using behavioural and physiological changes alone without an

18.1 PAIN MANAGEMENT AND THE YOUNG

Although young children cannot verbalise their painful experiences in the same way as adults they do feel pain.

Procedures that would produce a pain response in adults will also do so in children.

In addition, some treatments that are not painful to adults may be so to children.

Neonates and other children too young to talk should be carefully assessed for pain by observation of their facial and body movements, vocalisations and changes to physiological data such as heart rate.

Young children with some language skills are unable to describe the nature and site of their pain as adults would. Jerrett and Evans (1986) have identified a variety of words used by children to describe their pain, e.g. 'dizzy', 'snow' and 'sausage'.

Alternatively, sometimes children deny they have pain, or say that their pain is milder than it really is.

Health professionals caring for children must therefore maintain their research-based knowledge in order to become more expert in the way children view the world so that management of children's problems (including pain management) can become more effective. This is particularly important as there is considerable evidence suggesting that pain control is often inadequate (Lloyd, 1994: Davis, 1988).

18.1 PAIN MANAGEMENT AND THE OLDER PERSON

Health professionals may falsely believe that pain is an expected component of normal old age, and as a result pain may be undertreated in their elderly patients.

Similarly, nurses may believe that pain perception and sensitivity decreases with old age, and this can result in unnecessary suffering.

Also, although elderly people may be more sensitive to opioids, this is not a reason for withholding this type of analgesic or for underdosing. It is a safe therapy providing nurses monitor their patients' responses as thoroughly as they would if their patients were younger.

Older patients, particularly those who have suffered pain for some time, may have learnt to minimise behavioural expression of pain, believing that these are not appreciated by their friends and carers and they may therefore actually appear cheerful and comfortable.

understanding of the different characteristics of pain and influences upon it can result in inadequate treatment (Fordham and Dunn, 1994). For example, pain eventually leads to exhaustion and the patient will sleep as a result. Health professionals may mistakenly 'read' the sleep response as evidence that pain has diminished and treatments have been effective when in reality the patient's pain is unrelieved.

The most important source of information for assessment of pain in children and adults who can verbalise their feelings is the patient's self-report. Nurses should believe their patients and it is their self-report that should form the basis of a management programme (Thorn, 1997). Pain assessment protocols should be produced and used locally to act as an evidence-based tool for the delivery of consistent high-quality care.

However, there is much work yet to be done to improve pain relief services and before health professionals can deny the reality of Liebeskind and Melzack's assertion that '...pain is most poorly managed in those who are most defenceless against it – the young and the elderly...' (Liebeskind and Melzack, 1987).

CATEGORIES OF DRUGS USED IN THE MANAGEMENT OF PAIN

A variety of drugs may be useful in the relief of pain. They can be categorised as opioid (narcotic) analgesics, non-opioid analgesics and adjuvant drugs (**Table 18.1**). Each has different sites of action, side effects and degrees of effectiveness. Nurses' main responsibilities are to determine the appropriate drug or drugs, to evaluate their effects and advise doctors, patients and carers on modifications necessary to control the pain, and to recognise side effects and take appropriate action. Treatment of overdosage is discussed in Chapter 19 *Pharmacological management of medical emergencies*.

NON-OPIOID ANALGESICS

Some of these are available without prescription as over-the-counter drugs (**aspirin**, **paracetamol** and **ibuprofen**). Individuals often self-diagnose and prescribe these drugs for themselves, for relief of pain that the sufferer considers will be relatively benign and short lived (Seal, 1997).

Paracetamol

This is the most commonly used non-opioid analgesic and can be taken as tablet, capsule, liquid or as a rectal suppository. It acts centrally in the brain, reducing the individual's perception of pain; it also has an antipyretic action and some inhibitory effect on prostaglandin production. Paracetamol is useful for the control of mild pain and as an adjuvant drug in more severe pain, but it has a relatively minor anti-inflammatory effect (Seal, 1997). The adult dose is 1 g, and the maximum daily dose is 4 g. Its effects last for up to 4 hours only, so it is not useful as the sole treatment for continuous pain lasting longer than 16 hours. Side effects associated with paracetamol overdosage include liver and kidney failure, nausea and vomiting and skin rash. A dose of 12 g may be sufficient to cause liver cell necrosis.

Aspirin

Aspirin or acetylsalicylic acid is an equally important analgesic for mild pain and also acts as an anti-inflammatory, anti-platelet and antipyretic agent (see Chapter 12 *Drugs and cardiovascular disorders* for further information on its anti-platelet function). It is taken as a tablet, an enteric-coated tablet, a soluble tablet or as a rectal suppository. It shares many of the features of the non-steroidal anti-inflammatory drugs (NSAIDs), and is sometimes classified as such. Aspirin acts by blocking prostaglandin synthesis at the site of the pain stimulus. As a result, nociceptors are less responsive to stimuli so that a greater stimulus is required to generate an action potential. Analgesic effects last for a maximum of 6 hours and the adult dose is 300–900 mg 3–6 hourly up to 8 g/day for acute conditions or up to 4 g/day in chronic disease.

Main categories of drugs used in management of pain	
Drug category types	Causes of pain
Analgesics non-opioid Paracetamol Non-steroidal anti-inflammatory drugs (NSAIDs) Aspirin	Mild nociceptor pain. Inflammatory conditions. Bony metastases, musculoskeletal disease, postoperative.
Weak opioid Codeine Dextropopoxyphene Dihydrocodeine	As above As above As above
Strong opioid Morphine Diamorphine Pethidine Dextromoramide Oxycodone	Cancer pain Severe forms of nociceptive pain As above Short-term pain 'Background' pain relief in terminal care
Muscle relaxants Baclofen Orphenadrine	Muscle spasm pain
Corticosteroids Hydrocortisone Prednisone Dexamethasone	Cancer pain, compression of spinal cord, musculoskeletal disease
Psychotrophics	
Antidepressants Amitriptyline Doxepin	Depression associated with pain Neurogenic pain, sleep disturbance caused by pain
Anxiolytics Diazepam Chlordiazepoxide	Anxiety associated with pain
Anticonvulsants Phenytoin Carbamazepine	Neurogenic pain
Local anaesthetics Lignocaine Amethocaine	Chronic severe pain Injection pain

Table 18.1 Main categories of drugs used in management of pain

Side effects include bleeding as a result of its anti-prostaglandin action in the gastrointestinal tract, and tablets should therefore be taken with food. Rarely its anti-platelet action may cause a bleeding disorder (see Chapter 12 *Drugs and cardiovascular disorders*). Rash, tinnitus and bronchospasm are other rare side effects. Enteric-coated preparations should not be taken with antacids or milk as these may prematurely dissolve the coating. It should not be used for children under the age of 12 years, as it is known to cause Reye's syndrome, which is associated with a mortality of 54% (Seal, 1997).

Non-steroidal anti-inflammatory drugs

There are several categories of NSAIDs and all are useful in the treatment of mild to moderate pain. They act peripherally, inhibiting the production of the enzyme cyclo-oxygenase, necessary for the synthesis of prostaglandins, in a way similar to that of aspirin and as a result they have an anti-inflammatory effect. They also seem to have a separate analgesic property and an antipyretic action. Major uses are in musculoskeletal conditions such as osteoarthritis, rheumatoid arthritis, gout and ankylosing spondylitis along with migraine and dysmenorrhoea. More recently they have been used in postoperative pain control with effect, as operative trauma produces an inflammatory response (Day, 1997). They can be used as analgesic adjuncts to opioid drugs without increasing the risk of opioid side effects.

Side effects include gastrointestinal bleeding so tablets should be taken with food. More rarely, other systems may be affected on prolonged use, causing dizziness, insomnia, pruritus and rash, bleeding disorders, tinnitus and blurred vision, fluid retention and bronchospasm. They should not be taken in the third trimester of pregnancy or by those with hypersensitivity to other NSAIDs and aspirin, as cross hypersensitivity reactions can occur. As they can precipitate renal failure in patients with a compromised renal blood flow, they should be avoided in hypotensive patients or those with known renal disease. They may also slow new bone formation and should be used with caution after skeletal surgery (Thomas, 1997). Non-steroidal anti-inflammatory drugs may potentiate the effects of other NSAIDs, and of anticoagulant and anti-diabetic therapy; they may also inhibit diuretic action and the action of antihypertensive agents. There are several categories of NSAID: proprionic acid derivatives, oxicams, non-acetylated salicylates and indole acid derivatives.

Proprionic acid derivatives include **ibuprofen**, which is the only NSAID that can be taken without prescription as an over-the-counter drug. Adult dose by capsule or tablet is 200–400 mg up to a normal maximum of 1.2 g/day (2.4 g maximum for initial treatment of acute moderate pain). Modified release spansules are available that can be taken in one daily dose and there is also a topical formulation. Ibuprofen is the safest of this category of drugs and can be used as an analgesic and antipyretic for children (in divided doses up to 20 mg/kg daily). **Naproxen sodium** is available on prescription only in tablet and liquid formulation and adult dosage is 0.5–1 g/day in divided doses every 6–8 hours. Like ibuprofen, naproxen sodium has a quick onset of analgesic effect but the latter is generally better tolerated than other proprionic acid derivatives (McCaffery and Beebe, 1994).

Oxicams include **diclofenac sodium** and **piroxicam**. Diclofenac is available as a tablet, a sustained-release form, a suppository, a topical preparation and an intramuscular injection. Adult oral dose is 25–50 mg every 6–12 hours, with a maximum of 150 mg/day. In children, 1–3 mg/kg is given daily in divided doses. The intramuscular dose is 75 mg up to twice daily for a maximum of 2 days. It is used as the drug of choice in renal colic (rather than pethidine), given by deep intramuscular (intragluteal) injection (Thomas, 1997). Piroxicam is available in tablet, capsule and suppository formulations. The normal adult dosage is to a maximum of 30 mg/day in one or more doses, although 40 mg may be given for initial short-term treatment of acute pain. It may be given orally to children over the age of 6 years, in doses ranging from 5 to 20 mg daily, determined by body weight. Because of its long half-life, toxicity can develop, particularly in those with kidney or liver disease. It is generally better tolerated than aspirin, but its maximal anti-inflammatory effect is reached only after 2 weeks of treatment (McCaffery and Beebe, 1994).

Non-acetylated salicylates include **diflunisal**. In tablet form, adult dosage is up to 1.5 g/day in divided doses. It is better tolerated than aspirin and does not have the antipyretic or anti-platelet effects of aspirin. It is not recommended for use in children.

Indole acetic acid derivatives include **indomethacin**, available as tablet, suspension, modified-release capsule and suppository. Dosage is 8–12 hourly to a maximum of 200 mg/day. It is not recommended for use in children. Side effects are likely, particularly with use exceeding 4 weeks but therapeutic effects increase over time and may not reach maximum within 4 weeks. Indomethacin is likely to increase blood levels of lithium and may interact with concurrent steroid therapy. For unknown reasons it seems to be better tolerated if given by the rectal route and at night, so a nightly dose might be combined with a different type of analgesic during the day to avoid the high risk of side effects. Patients should be informed that urine and faeces may become green (McCaffery and Beebe, 1994).

OPIOID ANALGESICS

All opiates and opiate-like drugs are derived from opium and they are used in the relief of moderate to severe pain. They act in a similar way to endogenous opioids at one or more of the endogenous opioid receptors in the central nervous system, so inhibiting ascending pain impulses. Some are completely agonistic in effect whereas others act as agonist at one receptor and antagonist at others, or as partial agonists. These differences may help to explain the variations in analgesic and side effects associated with different types of opioids (Brody *et al.*, 1994).

Side effects

Endogenous opioid peptides regulate respiration, which offers an explanation for the respiratory depression associated with opioid drug therapy. Some opioid receptors are present in tissues outside the central nervous system, such as the bowel and bladder walls, and this accounts for the commonly occurring side effects of constipation and urinary retention with opioid administration. A summary of the main side effects of opioid therapy is given in **Table 18.2**. Reversal of unwanted dangerous respiratory effects can be achieved by administration of the opioid receptor antagonist, **naloxone**; an intravenous infusion of 2 mg in 500 ml achieves the desired effect. Naxolone occupies opioid receptor sites thus making them unavailable to the opioid. Because of the risk of nausea and vomiting, antiemetic therapy is often given as a prophylactic (see Chapter 14 *Drugs and gastrointestinal disorders*).

Because of the central nervous system action of these drugs, administration can cause side effects through interaction with other central nervous system agents. For example, the effects of alcohol, barbiturates and anxiolytics are potentiated and may result in severe respiratory depression. Concomitant monoamine oxidase inhibitor therapy may also produce respiratory depression and profound hypotension (see Chapter 7 *Drugs and psychological disorders*).

After regular opioid use for 2 weeks or more, physical dependence occurs as the body adapts to the pharmaco-dynamic effects of the drug. Tolerance then develops and the individual requires a larger dose to achieve the same analgesic effect. Nurses should be aware of this normal physiological response and ensure that doses are increased as required to adjust to the changed requirements. Physical dependence can elicit unpleasant effects when opioid therapy is suddenly stopped. The patient shows 'withdrawal' symptoms such as diaphoresis, rhinorrhoea, anxiety, nausea and vomiting, joint pain and painful cramps, irritability and extreme mood swings. Health professionals should therefore ensure that patients do not suffer from withdrawal, by slowly decreasing opioid doses after long-term therapy (Field and Parry, 1994).

Physical dependence is a normal physiological effect and is distinct from addiction (psychological dependence). Addiction arises in individuals with a psychological need to experience the euphoriant, 'wellbeing' side effects of these drugs, not the pain-relieving effects (see Chapter 7 *Drugs and psychological disorders*). Patients with long-lasting severe pain have rarely been known to become addicted. Health professionals tend to worry unduly about the risk of addiction and other side effects of opioids and as a result may fail to give adequate pain treatment (Liebeskind and Melzack, 1987). Nurses should also be aware that the addiction which occurs in patients taking opioids as palliative treatment for terminal disease is not a reason for modifying an effective pain relief regime.

WEAK OPIOID ANALGESICS

These agents can be used alone or in a combined formulation with a non-opioid. They are given for moderate pain and can also act as a 'step up' in analgesia when increasing pain is no longer controlled effectively by non-opioid therapy, or as a 'step down' from strong opioids when pain is diminishing (National Medical Advisory Committee, 1994). Combined formulations, such as **paracetamol 325 mg with dextropropoxyphene** 32.5 mg (**co-proxamol**), or **paracetamol 500 mg with dihydrocodeine 30 mg**, have the advantage of containing a reduced opioid dose so they are less likely to produce the side effects of opioids. However, nurses should check that patients are not allergic to the non-opioid content of the combined formulation before administration.

Codeine phosphate

Codeine is derived from opium and, although similar to morphine in its pharmacodynamic characteristics, has less analgesic effect. The adult dose is 30–60 mg 4 hourly to a maximum of 240 mg/day, given orally in tablet or syrup, or intramuscularly. Children aged 1–12 years are given 3 mg/kg daily in divided doses, orally. Codeine has a cough depressant effect and is therefore also used in cough linctus. Aside from its action in the central nervous system, codeine binds to opioid receptors in the bowel wall, and is more likely than morphine to produce nausea, vomiting and constipation as a consequence (McCaffery and Beebe, 1994).

Main adverse effects of opioid therapy	
System affected	**Adverse effect**
Integumentary (skin)	Rash, pruritus.
Gastrointestinal	Nausea, vomiting, constipation, spasm of bile ducts.
Urinary	Urinary retention.
Respiratory	Respiratory depression, bronchospasm.
Cardiovascular	Palpitations, hypotension.
Nervous	Sedation, euphoria, hallucinations, disorientation, tremors, lower threshold to convulsions.

Table 18.2 Main adverse effects of opioid therapy

Dextropropoxyphene

This is rarely prescribed alone because it has only a mild analgesic effect, but is commonly given orally in small doses (32.5 mg) in a combined formulation with paracetamol (co-proxamol).Through this combination, an additive analgesia is produced by central and peripheral action. However, there is little evidence of increased benefits from this type of combination and the mixture of side effects produced may make their recognition and treatment difficult (Joint Formulary Committee, 1997).

Dihydrocodeine

Its degree of analgesic effect is similar to that of codeine. Dihydrocodeine can be used for patients with head injury or after intracranial surgery as it has little respiratory or sedative effect (Field and Parry, 1994). Dosage is 30–60 mg 4 hourly in tablet, syrup or injection (intramuscular or intravenous), but a slow-release formulation is also available. In injection form it is a controlled drug (see Chapter 4 *Legal aspects of drug administration*). Analgesia is improved if the dose interval is reduced rather than if the dose is increased, for example 30 mg 2 hourly rather than 60 mg 4 hourly.

STRONG OPIOID ANALGESICS

These are given to treat severe acute and chronic pain arising from a variety of conditions (see **Table 18.1**). A common use of drugs such as pethidine and papaveretum used to be as preoperative medication. Their relatively long-lasting effects provided perioperative and intraoperative analgesia. Anaesthetists now more commonly use a short-acting opioid for intraoperative analgesia such as intravenous **fentanyl** 50–200 µg at induction of anaesthesia followed as required by maintenance doses of 50 µg (in children dosage is 3–5 µg/kg followed by 1 µg/kg as required) (Joint Formulary Committee, 1997).

Morphine

Formulations of morphine include tablet, modified-release tablet, suppository, injection and preservative-free solution for spinal or epidural injection. The oral dose is 30–60 mg given 4 hourly and is 3–6 times the intramuscular dose. Sustained-release preparations are available; these can be given once or twice daily. Effects are on receptors at brain and spinal cord levels. It is the most popular opioid analgesic and the analgesic effects of others are judged in comparison with morphine. Although nausea and vomiting are common side effects, they have not affected its popularity. In palliative terminal care, oral morphine is the analgesic of choice for severe pain and up to 500 mg or more may be required daily. If pain occurs before the next dose is due, an interim additional dose should be given and the next dose increased (Field and Parry, 1994).

Diamorphine

This is more soluble than morphine so it can be given in a smaller volume of fluid intramuscularly; this causes less injection discomfort, which is a particularly important consideration in the emaciated patient. Oral adult dose is 5–10 mg, depending on the size of the patient, 4 hourly if required, and intramuscular dosage is approximately one-half the oral one, with effects lasting for up to 4 hours. Continuous subcutaneous injection via syringe pump or driver can be used and it can also be given by slow intravenous injection (1 mg/min up to 5 mg). It generally causes less nausea and vomiting than morphine (McCaffery and Beebe, 1994). In concomitant therapy with cimetidine, domperidone or metoclopramide, they may have a reduced effect.

Pethidine

Pethidine is shorter acting than morphine; its analgesic effect is noticeable after 15 minutes and peaks 1 hour after oral administration. The adult oral dose is up to 150 mg 4 hourly and is four times the intramuscular dose. In children the dose is 0.5–2 mg/kg every 4 hours. Pethidine seems to have some muscle relaxant effect as well as an analgesic one and it is useful in labour and as operative premedication. An active metabolite, norpethidine, has a half-life of approximately 15 hours; accumulative toxicity can therefore occur and it causes hyperactivity that affects the nervous system. Naloxone increases rather than minimises the toxic effects of norpethidine (Thomas, 1997).

Dextromoramide

Dextromoramide is available in tablet, sublingual preparation or suppository form, and the adult oral dose is 5 mg, rising to a maximum of 20 mg if required. Profound analgesia is achieved, and the effect begins 20–30 minutes after sublingual administration but only lasts for a maximum of 3 hours. It is therefore not an appropriate choice when long-term analgesia is required, but dextromoramide is useful for the treatment of breakthrough pain or to give analgesic cover for painful procedures (McCaffery and Beebe, 1994).

Oxycodone

This is an example of a drug that can be prescribed under special order for patients requiring palliative care. It is given by rectal suppository, is longer acting than morphine and can be given once or twice daily (Joint Formulary Committee, 1997). Oxycodone is particularly useful as 'background' analgesia, for example during the night, to which short-acting analgesics can be added as required to individualise and maximise pain control.

Other strong opioid analgesics

There are many drugs in this category and if the examples given above produce unwanted effects in patients, other drugs may be used with more success as there is variation in the way individuals respond to different drugs. Some potent analgesics are not generally used in pain relief for various reasons, for example they have an unacceptably high level of side effects; **methadone** is one such drug. Although a potent opioid analgesic that is longer acting than morphine, methadone suffers from potential accumulation toxic effects so is not used in pain relief. It is most commonly used in the support of addicts withdrawing from opiate use (see Chapter 7 *Drugs and psychological disorders*).

ADJUVANT ANALGESIC DRUGS

The nature of the pain experience determines whether adjuvant therapy with non-analgesic drugs is appropriate. When given in appropriate conditions, in conjunction with analgesics, they potentiate the analgesic effect. **Table 18.1** contains some examples of conditions in which muscle relaxants, corticosteroids, psychotrophics, anxiolytics and anticonvulsants may be used as adjuvant- or co-analgesics (see relevant chapters for information about dosage and effects).

Examples of local anaesthetics are also included in **Table 18.1** and they can be used as co-analgesics in various ways (see Chapter 3 *Classes of drugs*). Drugs such as **lignocaine** or **bupivacaine** can be used, for example, by anaesthetists or specialists at pain control clinics for administration through the epidural route (National Medical Advisory Committee, 1994). Analgesia as part of anaesthesia is achieved over the area below the site of insertion, proving a useful tool for example in labour and in postoperative pain relief.

Lignocaine and bupivacaine can also be injected into or near spinal and autonomic nerves to achieve nerve block. Onset of effect relies on diffusion into the surrounding nerves and may take 20 minutes. Blockage of nerve transmission is an 'all or nothing' phenomenon. This is an important pain management consideration for nurses as, when this type of analgesia is withdrawn, the patient may suddenly become aware of unrelieved pain. Nurses should ensure therefore that adequate alternate pain relief is operating before nerve block is withdrawn.

Local anaesthetics can also be applied to the skin for analgesic purposes (see Chapter 2 *Introduction to pharmacology*).

Other adjuvant drugs

Currently, **cannabis** (Indian hemp) products such as marijuana can be prescribed only under special licence in the United Kingdom. As a mild hallucinogen with relatively little withdrawal or tolerance problems, it may be licensed in future for use in a variety of conditions, though as yet there is little evidence that its therapeutic advantage outweighs concern about its illegal use (Joint Formulary Committee, 1997).

Alcohol in amounts that do not produce inebriation has been found to offer effective co-analgesic effects. Researchers in one study discovered that 2 units of alcohol provide approximately the same analgesic effect as 10 mg morphine (Woodrow and Eltherington, 1988). Taken in moderate amounts alcohol does not produce respiratory depression so can be used as an adjunct in opioid and non-opioid regimes. Nurses should, however, ensure that patients are aware of the increased sedation produced by alcohol taken in combination with opioid therapy. Similarly patients should be informed of the potential for gastro-intestinal inflammation.

Caffeine may be safely combined with aspirin or paracetamol in chronic pain relief regimes. It has been found to reduce the analgesic dose required by up to 40% and may minimise the risk of aspirin or paracetamol toxicity that might result from using larger doses of analgesic without caffeine. Alternatively, in the shorter term, patients may be advised to take caffeine in the form of coffee or tea. An effective caffeine dose is 100–200 mg; a large cup of filter coffee contains approximately 125 mg, instant coffee contains 75 mg and strong tea 80 mg per cup (McCaffery and Beebe, 1994).

METHODS OF DELIVERY OF ANALGESICS

Analgesic agents can be delivered peripherally using common routes: via the mouth, or injection into subcutaneous tissue, muscle or directly into a vein. However, special routes may be used in the treatment of pain at specific loci. For example, an epidural technique can be used for acute pain relief in labour, and baclofen can be given intrathecally to relieve chronic pain associated with muscle spasm.

Transdermal patches are used for delivery of an increasing variety of drugs, anti-anginal drugs, for example (see Chapter 12 *Drugs and cardiovascular disorders*), and may become a common route of analgesic delivery in future (Thomas, 1997).

PATIENT-CONTROLLED ANALGESIA

It is increasingly recognised that most patients should be in control of their own pain relief. Health professionals' fears that patients would over-medicate themselves have proved groundless. Evidence suggests rather that patients who are in control of their own pain relief require less analgesics than patients who have analgesics administered by nurses. Explanations for this may lie in the nature of nurses' and doctors' work, the patient's role and in pain theory (Latham, 1994). Patients may be unwilling to ask for analgesia when pain is mild and would rather wait until pain is causing them great discomfort. Nurses in acute care settings may find it difficult to respond immediately to a patient's request for analgesia, as often there are many competing calls on their attention at one time. When pain relief is inadequate and requires a changed prescription, the doctor may be unable to carry this out immediately because of his other commitments. Patients' anxiety, as a result of these poor pain control experiences, may become a major influence in increasing their perception of pain, so setting up a spiral of more pain/less relief. Use of patient-controlled analgesia has resulted in increased patient satisfaction and quicker recovery (Thomas, 1997).

There are various systems that enable patients to self-administer bolus doses intravenously or via the epidural route. The equipment allows health professionals to pre-programme the amount of bolus and a minimal interval between bolus doses thus preventing overdose. It is a doubly safe method as patients, becoming drowsy with potent analgesia, cannot operate the machine to self-medicate in their sedated state.

There are similar efforts to allow patients control over delivery of all their drug therapy. Providing patients with bedside locked cabinets to store their own drugs has proved beneficial. As use of this process spreads it can be expected that oral pain relief will become more effective. If this system is to be used safely, assessment and selection of patients who can reliably self-medicate is obviously an important function of nurses and doctors (McCaffery and Beebe, 1994).

GOOD PAIN RELIEF PRACTICE

It may seem strange that despite the range of analgesic agents and alternative pain relief measures available to us, unrelieved pain remains a common and destructive experience for our patients (Working Party of the Commission on the Provision of Surgical Services, 1990). The explanation is likely to be multifaceted. For example, health professionals may have inappropriate goals; they may believe that pain prevention is not an appropriate goal and seek only to reduce pain thus providing, at best, ineffective therapy. False beliefs may also influence their choice of pain management strategies.

EQUIVALENT ANALGESIC EFFECTS
- As with all drugs, the effects of opioids are dose dependent.
- Health professionals may incorrectly assume that an opioid delivers 'better' pain relief than a non-opioid drug.
- Illustrated here is the equivalent analgesic response of various drugs:

Analgesic	Oral dose (mg)
Paracetamol	1000
Aspirin	600
Codeine	32
Pethidine	50

- So, for example, two aspirin tablets provide as much pain relief as 50 mg pethidine taken orally.
- Health professionals may tend to overestimate the analgesic effect of opioids in low doses and underestimate the effect of non-opioids.
- It is therefore important to ensure not only the type of analgesic chosen but also the dose given is appropriate to an individual's pain relief needs (McCaffery and Beebe, 1994).

Pain and analgesic therapy is complex, and nurses and other health professionals often lack up-to-date and detailed knowledge on which to base their judgements, particularly as use of valid pain assessment tools and protocols is not currently widespread. As a result, old myths and ineffective practices may be perpetuated.

An important duty of the nurse is to relieve suffering (International Council of Nurses, 1973). It is to be hoped that, with continuing education programmes in pain management for all nurses and an increased availability of pain specialists of all disciplines, standards of pain management will rise (Welsh Health Planning Forum, 1992). As a result nurses will be able to carry out their duty of care, and patients will receive pain control based on effective strategies that are oriented towards the prevention of pain.

PERSON CENTRED STUDY 1

Mr Alfred Storey aged 76 years developed a strangulated hernia, which was treated by an intestinal resection. He made a slow postoperative recovery and was discharged home 3 weeks later. A month later he suffered a myocardial infarction, from which he made a good recovery without complications. Unfortunately he has recently had increasing abdominal pain associated with nausea and vomiting. On admission 2 days ago, abdominal adhesions causing intestinal obstruction were diagnosed. A further intestinal resection was carried out with end-to-end anastomosis. He was returned to the ward from the High Dependency Unit earlier today. He has persistent paralytic ileus and his nasogastric tube is draining small amounts of bile-stained fluid. As a result he remains 'nil by mouth', with an intravenous clear fluid regime maintaining his fluid intake requirements.

1. What factors would you consider when assessing Mr Storey's pain?
2. Which analgesics are likely to prove most effective?
3. What dose and method of delivery would you judge appropriate?

KEY POINTS

- A given condition may be associated with a range of different types of pain. This may complicate a nursing assessment.
- The choice of analgesia will be influenced by the origin of the pain and the type of nociceptive pathway affected.
- The rate of transmission of pain sensation is influenced by how relaxed or anxious the patient is.
- Children are able to experience pain, although pain assessment poses a challenge as their descriptions of their pain may be difficult to understand.

- Old age and pain are not synonymous.
- Simple analgesics that may be bought over the counter may be life threatening if taken in overdose.
- Patients receiving opioid analgesia are likely to need the dose adjusted upwards as tolerance develops. This does not mean that they are addicted.
- Addiction to analgesia is rarely a problem in patients suffering severe persistent pain.

Any or none of the answer options provided may apply.

1. Pain is
a. usually perceived more clearly by health professionals rather than by the individual with pain
b. sometimes misjudged by health professionals
c. a personal experience
d. always the result of some degree of tissue damage
e. proportional to the degree of physical trauma that causes it

2. Aspects of pain are influenced by the sufferer's age in the following ways:
a. neonates are able to feel pain and show signs of distress as a consequence
b. children do not feel as much pain as adults
c. pain perception is decreased in the elderly
d. pain is a natural occurrence in old age
e. pain cannot be assessed in infants

3. Chronic pain
a. may be diffuse
b. identifies those patients who have psychiatric disease
c. involves stimulation of polymodal nerve endings
d. impulses are transmitted generally via C neurons
e. lasts less than 4 weeks

4. Opioid analgesics usually
a. are available on prescription only
b. produce tolerance on prolonged use
c. cause addiction after long-term therapy
d. are given in high intramuscular dose and lower dose by mouth
e. are prescribed for patients with severe pain

5. A patient's perception of pain depends on his or her
a. level of consciousness
b. past experiences of pain
c. beliefs about culturally acceptable behavioural responses
d. state of relaxation or anxiety
e. age

6. According to the gate control theory of pain
a. A-beta and C nerve fibres are involved in pain transmission
b. the gate is situated in the dorsal horn area of the spinal cord
c. activation of transmission may stimulate further transmission of pain impulses
d. inhibition of transmission may prevent further transmission of pain impulses
e. the gate can be 'opened' or 'closed' by descending nerve impulses from the brain

7. Some non-opioid analgesics may be used
a. as the primary treatment option for severe pain
b. as adjuvants to opioids for treatment of moderate to severe pain
c. more effectively if combined with alcohol
d. rarely as they are relatively ineffective analgesics
e. despite the almost certain risk of life-threatening toxic effects

8. Patient-controlled analgesia
a. has dangerous consequences for patients
b. increases patients' satisfaction with treatment
c. is an effective pain relief technique
d. uses a pre-programmed apparatus for delivery of epidural and intravenous analgesia
e. generally results in patients needing less analgesic than when its administered by nurses

9. On the first day after major surgery, pain is likely to be controlled by
a. an opioid treatment regime
b. a non-steroidal anti-inflammatory drug in conjunction with paracetamol
c. non-pharmacological therapies e.g. massage
d. use of a non-opioid analgesic alone
e. analgesia given orally rather than by intramuscular or intravenous injection

10. Adjuvant drugs useful in pain relief
a. have their effect at central opioid receptors
b. operate by inhibiting the action of opioids
c. may potentiate the action of other analgesic agents
d. include anxiolytics and antidepressants
e. are usually blocked by alcohol and caffeine

REFERENCES

Brody T, Larner J, Minneman K, Neu H. *Human pharmacology – molecular to clinical*. St. Louis: Mosby, 1994.

Davis P. Changing nurse practice for more effective control of post operative pain through a staff-initiated educational programme. *Nurse Educ Today* 1988; **8:**325-331.

Day R. A Pharmacological approach to acute pain. *Prof Nurse* 1997; **13(suppl):**9-12.

Field G, Parry J. Pain control: some aspects of day-to-day management. *Eur J Cancer Care* 1994; **3:**79-86.

Fordham M, Dunn V. *Alongside the patient in pain*. London: Baillière Tindall, 1994.

Horn S, Munafo M. *Pain – theory research and intervention*. Buckingham: Open University, 1997.

International Association for the Study of Pain, Subcommittee on Taxonomy. Classification of chronic pain. *Pain* 1986; **(suppl 3)**

International Council of Nurses. *Code for nurses: ethical concepts applied to nursing*. Geneva: International Council of Nurses, 1973.

Jerrett M, Evans K. Children's pain vocabulary. *J Adv Nurs* 1986; **11:**403-408.

Joint Formulary Committee. *British National Formulary, no 33*. London: British Medical Association and Royal Pharmaceutical Society of Great Britain, 1997.

Latham J. Assessment and measurement of pain. *Eur J Cancer Care* 1994; **3:**75-78.

Liebeskind J, Melzack R. The International Pain Foundation: meeting a need for education in pain management. *Pain* 1987; **30:**1-2.

Lloyd G. Nurses attitudes towards management of pain. *Nurs Times* 1994; **90(43):**40-43.

McCaffery M, Beebe A. (Ed. Latham, J) *Pain – clinical manual for nursing practice*. London: Mosby, 1994.

Melzack R, Wall PD. Pain mechanisms - a new theory. *Science* 1965; **150:** 971-978

National Medical Advisory Committee. *Working group report on the management of patients with chronic pain*. Scottish Home and Health Department: HMSO, 1994.

O'Hara P. *Pain management for health professionals*. London: Chapman and Hall, 1996.

Seal R. Choosing the right step on the analgesic ladder. Nurse Prescriber *Community Nurse* 1997; **3:**58-59.

Thomas VN. *Pain: its nature and management*. London: Baillière Tindall, 1997.

Thorn M. A survey of nurses' attitudes towards the assessment and control of post operative pain. *J Orthop Nurs* 1997; **1:**30-38.

Welsh Health Planning Forum. Protocol for investment in health gain: pain, discomfort and palliative care. Welsh Office: NHS Directorate, 1992.

Working Party of the Commission on the Provision of Surgical Services. *Report on pain after surgery*. London: Royal College of Surgeons of England and the College of Anaesthetists, 1990.

Woodrow KM, Eltherington LG. Feeling no pain, alcohol as an analgesic. *Pain* 1988; **32:**159-163.

19 Sylvia Prosser
PHARMACOLOGICAL MANAGEMENT OF MEDICAL EMERGENCIES

INTRODUCTION

In the context of this chapter, a clinical emergency is one in which homeostasis is so disrupted that, without rapid intervention, life is not sustainable. The drugs that are commonly used in prevention and treatment of cardiorespiratory arrest are considered here only in the context of their effect in emergency treatment, although some have many other uses, which are discussed in other chapters in this book. This chapter is arranged in sections; the first outlines drugs that are kept on resuscitation trolleys and commonly used as part of the cardiac arrest protocol. In this section, each drug is summarised before a more detailed description is given. It is important to remember that the conditions for which emergency drugs are used are highly complex, and in some cases, the treatment is contentious. The second section provides an overview of drugs that may also be used in a medical emergency. The aim of this chapter is to provide a simple rapid aide memoire, and the reader is encouraged to refer to dedicated texts such as Colquhoun *et al.* (1995) for more comprehensive information.

CARDIORESPIRATORY ARREST

Serious disruption of cardiovascular function results in the failure of oxygen delivery to the cells and the failure of carbon dioxide, electrolyte and metabolic acid removal from the extracellular fluid. Untreated respiratory arrest produces similar results. Whichever system fails first, if normal function is not resumed speedily, a full scale cardiorespiratory arrest will ensue, followed by death if the situation is not rescued. The aims of cardiopulmonary resuscitation are to support circulatory and respiratory function by mechanical and pharmacological means until recovery occurs or death is considered inevitable. For a full consideration of management of basic and advanced life support, the reader is referred to the manuals of the Resuscitation Council (Handley and Swain, 1996).

The use of pharmacological products within advanced life support is based upon the need to resume and support cardiac function so as to restore the circulation to the cells. This chapter considers some of the preparations regularly used to help this process.

Cardiac arrest may occur as a result of ventricular fibrillation, low output tachycardias or asystole. In ventricular fibrillation, the synchrony of myocardial contraction is lost, resulting in the heart losing its effectiveness as a pump. Fast tachycardias produce no effective cardiac output because there is insufficient myocardial contractility and inadequate cardiac filling. The result of asystole is that there is no myocardial electrical activity to produce muscular contraction and thus no cardiac output. The major drugs used in collapse and cardiac arrest are outlined below.

MAJOR DRUGS USED FOR RESUSCITATION

Adrenaline

- **Use:** administered to increase cardiac output. Increases cardiac rate, force and responsivity to nerve stimuli. Adrenaline is usually the first drug used in cardiac arrest protocols (Handley and Swain, 1996).
- **Side effect:** may cause tachyarrhythmias.
- **Dosage:** 1 mg intravenously in cardiac arrest; 2 mg by the same route may be given subsequently, or 5 mg via an endotracheal tube.

Adrenaline (named epinephrine in the USA) is a widely acting sympathomimetic drug. It activates all of the known adrenergic receptors (Moore, 1994), and so produces a wide range of effects upon physiological functioning.

The effect of adrenaline upon cardiac function is to activate β_1-adrenergic receptors and increase the rate and force of myocardial contraction. The heart rate is influenced by activation of the β_1 receptors on the pacemaker cells of the sinoatrial node. The increased contractility is achieved by activation of β_1 receptors on the myocardial cells. Adrenaline also causes the myocardial cells to relax more rapidly, which shortens the duration of the cardiac cycle and alters the proportion of duration of the systolic to the diastolic phase; the length of the diastolic phase is increased compared with systole. The result is that cardiac function is improved because of the increased filling time for the coronary arteries and the ventricles. Although the heart is driven to work harder, it is also enabled to function more effectively and to meet its increased metabolic demands by better perfusion of the myocardium. Adrenaline also increases the activation of the conduction pathways within the heart, so the response to nerve impulses is more rapid and the refractory time is less. Side effects of the increased sensitivity to nerve impulses are tachycardia, premature ventricular contractions and increasing the risk of provoking ventricular fibrillation.

Atropine

- **Use:** to treat asystole and bradycardias, which produce hypotension. Usually the second drug cited in cardiac arrest protocols.
- **Side effects:** nil relevant to the emergency situation, although atropine causes dilatation of the pupils, which should be remembered when assessing recovery from cardiac arrest.
- **Dosage:** 3 mg intravenously in cardiac arrest; 0.5–1 mg intravenously for bradycardia. May be given via an endotracheal tube when no vascular access is available.

Atropine inhibits the effect of the parasympathetic transmitter acetylcholine at muscarinic receptors (see Chapter 7 for an explanation of these). Atropine therefore blocks the effects of parasympathetic stimulation upon cardiac muscle. It also decreases secretion from the salivary glands and respiratory tract, so reduces the volume of secretions in the airways. The major parasympathetic nerve is the vagus nerve, which, when stimulated, slows the firing of the sinoatrial node. Use of atropine to inhibit this effect therefore increases the heart rate. Additionally, conductivity at the atrioventricular node is increased when the bradycardia results from excessive vagal stimulation. Use of atropine intravenously may cause acute confusional states. This should be remembered when assessing a patient's recovery from an episode involving emergency treatment with this drug.

Bretylium

- **Use:** as an antiarrhythmic agent for resistant ventricular tachycardia and as a chemical defibrillator in cardiac arrest caused by ventricular fibrillation.
- **Side effects:** transient stimulation then blockage of the adrenergic receptor system, causing brief hypertension then hypotension. Cardiac arrhythmia and angina may also occur.
- **Dosage:** 5 mg/kg body weight given intravenously.

Bretylium influences the release of catecholamines at adrenergic nerve terminals. It is absorbed by the chemical pump in the adrenergic neurons, displaces noradrenaline and then blocks further sympathetic activity in the neuron. At first catecholamine release is stimulated, then it is blocked, so the use of bretylium produces a transient sympathomimetic effect, followed by a sympathetic blockade. The duration of action potentials is increased and the length of the refractory period in the atria, ventricles and bundle of His and Purkinje fibres is prolonged (Hume, 1994). The antiarrhythmic effect takes approximately 20 minutes to become established.

Calcium

- **Use:** to treat electromechanical dissociation resulting from hyperkalaemia, hypocalcaemia or overdose of calcium-channel blockers.
- **Side effects:** progression of myocardial ischaemia, impaired central nervous system recovery after cardiac arrest. Interaction between calcium chloride and sodium bicarbonate results in precipitation if both substances are given in close succession into the same intravenous line without prior flushing.
- **Dosage:** 10 ml calcium chloride, 10%, intravenously.

Calcium is needed to enable neuromuscular transmission and muscle contraction to take place. When the serum calcium is low, or when the secretion of calcium ions is reduced by calcium-channel blockers, the myocardial contractility may be seriously impaired. This will result in circulatory collapse. Similarly, when hyperkalaemia of more than 6 mmol/l is present, the usual polarity of the neuromuscular membrane is disorganised and life-threatening cardiac arrhythmias may occur. Intravenous infusion of calcium chloride or calcium gluconate are used as a short-term measure to restore the membrane potential to a more stable state. Calcium promotes the entry of potassium ions into the cells. In hyperkalaemia, this is useful to reduce the serum potassium to safer levels. Insulin and glucose intravenously may also be used to promote a shift of potassium into the cells, thus reducing the dangerously high serum level.

Lignocaine

- **Use:** for the treatment of ventricular fibrillation and ventricular tachycardia with cardiac output, particularly after myocardial infarction.
- **Side effects:** may cause myocardial depression, drowsiness, confusion, convulsion and coma.
- **Dosage:** treatment for ventricular fibrillation is 100 mg by rapid intravenous infusion. For ventricular tachycardia, 1 mg/kg body weight is given, followed by an infusion of 2–4 mg/min if needed.

Lignocaine blocks the entry of sodium ions through the voltage-sensitive channels into the myocardial cell membrane. This reduces the generation and transmission of action potentials. Lignocaine slows depolarisation of myocardial cells and reduces the ability of the ventricular myocardium to respond to abnormal pacemakers. The ventricular myocardium is also made more resistant to fibrillation.

Sodium bicarbonate

- **Use:** to buffer the metabolic acidosis that accompanies circulatory or respiratory arrest. Sodium bicarbonate may also be used to reduce pre-existing hyperkalaemia by promoting the entry of potassium ions into the cells.
- **Side effects:** intracellular acidosis. Damage to previously ischaemic cells. Intracerebral vasoconstriction; cerebral oedema. Cellular hypoxia.
- **Dosage:** the amount given depends upon the patient's blood gases; 8.4% sodium bicarbonate is infused intravenously in small quantities and repeated as needed.

Sodium bicarbonate is used to buffer the metabolic acids that have accumulated as a result of anaerobic cellular metabolism in response to cardiorespiratory arrest. Sodium bicarbonate combines with the metabolic acids to form a weaker acid, which is eventually excreted via the lungs in the form of carbon dioxide. When sodium bicarbonate is given to a collapsed patient, it is important that ventilation – whether mechanical or via bag and mask – is adequate to enable excretion of the additional carbon dioxide.

The use of sodium bicarbonate is contentious as it can exacerbate cellular acidosis; the combination of the base and the metabolic acids causes the formation of weaker acids, which enter the cells. This further reduces the intracellular pH. Excessive infusion of sodium bicarbonate may contribute to cerebral oedema. Correction of intracerebral acidity may provoke vasoconstriction, which can compromise cerebral recovery from a hypoxic episode.

Rapid correction of metabolic acidosis may result in an inappropriate elevation of the arterial pH (metabolic alkalosis). The consequence of this is that the affinity of haemoglobin for oxygen is increased and unloading of oxygen molecules to the already hypoxic cells occurs less readily.

DRUGS USED TO STABILIZE THE HAEMODYNAMIC STATE OF THE PATIENT

Adenosine

- **Use:** diagnosis and treatment of paroxysmal tachycardias.
- **Side effects:** headache, dyspnoea, chest pain. Bronchospasm in asthmatics.
- **Dosage:** 3 mg by rapid intravenous injection.

Adenosine must be given by rapid injection as it is inactivated by the circulating enzyme adenosine deaminase. Adenosine slows conduction across the atrioventricular node. This is helpful in aiding diagnosis of tachyarrhythmias as it enables P waves to be visualised on the electrocardiogram. The agent is also useful for short-term eradication of paroxysmal supraventricular tachycardia. As adenosine is most commonly used to assist diagnosis, and the patient may be conscious having suffered myocardial infarction, it is important to note that the side effects of the drug can be confused with the symptoms of further myocardial infarction. The patient requires reassurance that these effects are short-term and drug-related, and not an indication that his or her condition is deteriorating.

Amiodarone

- **Use:** control of chronic ventricular and supraventricular dysrhythmias.
- **Side effects:** bradycardia, heart block, ventricular dysrhythmias. Potentiates the activity of warfarin and digoxin.
- **Dosage:** initially, 5 mg/kg diluted in 100 ml, 5% dextrose, given over 1–4 hours. May subsequently be given orally for 5–10 days in doses of around 200 mg daily.

Amiodarone lengthens the duration of action potentials and the refractory period in cardiac muscle. It reduces the influence of the sinoatrial node and ectopic pacemakers, and thus helps to re-establish sinus rhythm.

Beta-blockers

- **Use:** control of supraventricular tachycardias. Suppression of ventricular extrasystoles.
- **Side effects:** loss of sympathetic compensatory mechanisms, heart block, cardiac failure. Bronchospasm in known asthmatics.
- **Dosage:** depends upon the product used. Propranolol is given for the emergency treatment of cardiac arrhythmias in a dose of 1 mg, injected intravenously over 1 minute. The dose may be repeated at 2 minute intervals to a maximum of 10 mg if the patient is conscious.

The β-adrenergic blockers oppose the catecholamine response to stimulation of the sympathetic nervous system. For this reason, they constitute a useful treatment of unstable angina and supraventricular tachycardias. The agents used have varying degrees of selective action upon the heart.

Digoxin

- **Use:** control of atrial fibrillation; ventricular failure.
- **Side effects:** ventricular extrasystoles, heart block, paroxysmal supraventricular tachycardia.
- **Dosage:** 500 µg in 50 ml, 5% dextrose given over 1 hour, then oral digoxin to a maximum of 1 mg in 24 hours.

Digoxin influences the ATP-dependent sodium–potassium pumps in the myocardial cell membranes. As a result, intracellular sodium and calcium levels rise and intracellular potassium levels fall. Digoxin also enhances vagal stimulation and has some direct action on the atrioventricular node (Laurence and Bennett, 1992). The resulting effect is increased responsivity and contractility in the myocardial cells and decreased production and slower transmission of impulses within the sinoatrial node, atrioventricular node and the conducting fibres. Thus the cardiac rate is slowed, and the myocardial force is increased. The toxicity of digoxin is increased in the presence of hypokalaemia.

Isoprenaline
- **Use:** bradycardia that does not respond to atropine.
- **Side effects:** extension of existing myocardial infarctions; tachyarrhythmias.
- **Dosage:** 2 mg diluted in 500 ml, 5% dextrose given intravenously at a rate of 0.5–2.5 ml/min.

Isoprenaline (known in the USA as isoproterenol) is a general β-adrenoceptor agonist that is a potent cardiac stimulant. It increases both cardiac rate and force and also acts as a vasodilator, thus increasing the coronary artery blood flow and reducing peripheral resistance. The main use of isoprenaline is in the emergency treatment of complete heart block. Although isoprenaline increases coronary perfusion, it also increases the metabolic demands of the myocardium, which produces a risk of infarction in previously ischaemic muscle. Its general sympathomimetic effect may produce feelings of anxiety in conscious patients.

Verapamil
- **Use:** treatment of angina and supraventricular tachycardia.
- **Side effects:** hypotension; headaches.
- **Dosage:** 5–10 mg given intravenously over 2 minutes.

The action of verapamil is to block the entry of calcium ions into the cells. Verapamil works predominantly on the cells of the sinoatrial and atrioventricular nodes and the smooth muscle of the blood vessels of the peripheral and coronary arteries. The muscle cells in the blood vessel walls relax, and the stimulus from the sinoatrial and atrioventricular nodes is reduced. The major outcomes of treatment with verapamil are that the blood supply to the myocardium is increased and the myocardial metabolic needs are decreased, because of the slowing of the heart rate and the reduced force of the myocardial contraction. Thus, myocardial ischaemia and angina pectoris are reduced and supraventricular tachycardias slowed.

Dopamine
- **Use:** to correct hypotension when there is no deficit in blood volume.

- **Side effects:** cardiac arrhythmias; exacerbation of ischaemic heart disease.
- **Dosage:** is adjusted according to blood pressure. The dose on commencement of treatment is 2–5 μg/kg body weight per minute.

Dopamine enhances activation of natural dopamine receptors, producing a generalised sympathomimetic effect. The effect produced is dependent on the rate of intravenous administration. At an infusion rate of 2–5 μg/kg body weight per minute, the renal blood flow is increased, which should increase urinary output if oliguria is present. Further increase in the rate of administration produces an increase in the cardiac rate and force (Laurence and Bennett, 1992). The drug is useful to protect renal function during recovery after cardiovascular collapse. The rate of administration needs careful control to avoid cardiac failure as the peripheral resistance rises.

Dobutamine
- **Use:** treatment of hypotension when the intravascular volume is not depleted.
- **Side effects:** arrhythmias; ventricular extrasystoles, exacerbation of pre-existing ischaemic heart disease.
- **Dosage:** as small a dose as possible within a range of 2.5–20 μg/kg body weight per minute.

The effect of dobutamine is to increase myocardial contractility without producing an undue rise in the cardiac rate or alteration of the peripheral resistance (Moore, 1994). It is used in intensive care units to stabilise patients who have poor cardiac output and inadequate tissue perfusion.

Nitrates
- **Use:** to relieve angina pectoris; increase myocardial perfusion; improve cardiac output. Used in patients with established ischaemic heart disease to control angina pectoris.
- **Side effects:** palpitations, dizziness, hypotension, headache.
- **Dosage:** intravenously: 2–12 mg/hour as isosorbide mononitrate or dinitrate; sublingually 300–600 μg in tablet form or 400 μg via aerosol spray; between 1 and 5 mg via buccal mucosa.

Nitrates are altered in smooth muscle cells to release nitric oxide. Via a complex chemical chain reaction, nitric oxide alters the movement of calcium ions in smooth muscle cells, producing dilatation of venules and arterioles. The main coronary arteries dilate, peripheral resistance decreases and the cardiac preload diminishes.

Opioids
- **Use:** analgesia. Also to reduce preload in left ventricular failure.

- **Side effects:** hypotension; respiratory depression; nausea.
- **Dosage:** depends upon age and size of the patient and the agent selected. As examples, 2.5–10 mg diamorphine, or 5–20 mg morphine may be given. In the emergency context, they may be given by slow intravenous injection or intramuscular injection.

In emergency management, opioids may be used to relieve the pain of trauma or acute myocardial infarction. Additionally, by producing dilatation of venules and arterioles, opioids are helpful in reducing left ventricular workload when cardiac failure is present. Care must be taken to avoid shock because of hypotension and respiratory failure caused by inappropriate suppression of the respiratory centre. For a detailed discussion of opioids, see Chapter 18.

Naloxone
- **Use:** to counter respiratory depression that results from opioid analgesia.
- **Side effects:** increased perception of pain.
- **Dosage:** adults 0.8–2 mg intravenously; 2 mg may be diluted in 500 ml sodium chloride, 0.9%, or 5% dextrose or dextrose saline. This produces a concentration of 4 µg/ml. Children may be given 10 µg/kg body weight, intravenously (Walker, 1997).

Naloxone binds to opioid receptors, opposing the effect of opioid analgesia. Its effect is short acting, so the dose may need to be repeated. Acute withdrawal effects can be provoked if naloxone is given to people who are opioid dependent or who have taken large quantities of the opioid.

Thrombolytic agents
- **Use:** to reduce thrombus formation and minimise extent of infarction.
- **Side effects:** bleeding; hypersensitivity reactions; reperfusion syndrome.
- **Dosage:** see below.

Aspirin
This is used in low doses (75 mg enteric-coated tablets) as a prophylaxis in those at risk of thrombotic episodes.

Streptokinase
The dose for streptokinase is 1 500 000 i.u. given intravenously in 0.9% sodium chloride over 60 minutes (Handley and Swain, 1996). It is used to contain thrombus formation immediately after myocardial infarction. Ideally, streptokinase should be given within 1 hour of infarction occurring in order to salvage myocardial tissue (see Chapter 12 *Drugs and cardiovascular disorders* for a fuller discussion).

Tissue plasminogen activator
The dose for tissue plasminogen activator is 10 mg given intravenously over 1–2 minutes, 50 mg in 50 ml water for injection over 1 hour; or 40 mg in 40 ml water for injection over 2 hours. This is used as an alternative approach to thrombolytic therapy in those eligible for thrombolytic

---

PERSON CENTRED STUDY 1

Mr Tariq Haq was brought into hospital as an emergency after his GP diagnosed an acute myocardial infarction. His GP gave him intravenous cyclomorph, 10 mg at home, plus 150 mg aspirin. The paramedical technician noted a sinus tachycardia with occasional ventricular extrasystoles on the cardiac monitor during the ambulance journey to hospital. Some cyanosis of the nail beds was present. His blood pressure was 115/80 mmHg. Mr Haq was given oxygen in the ambulance and the paramedic established intravenous access via a peripheral cannula. During the journey, Mr Haq became dyspnoeic and anxious. The paramedic noted short bursts of ventricular tachycardia that reverted spontaneously. On arrival at the hospital, Mr Haq was admitted directly to the Coronary Care Unit where streptokinase therapy was commenced. Three hours after admission, Mr Haq suddenly became unconscious and pulseless. The cardiac monitor showed ventricular fibrillation. A 'precordial thump' was given, he was ventilated by the use of a bag valve mask device and defibrillation was attempted by giving Mr Haq a sequence of direct current shocks. These being unsuccessful, cardiopulmonary resuscitation was commenced, he was intubated and intravenous adrenaline given. During the next sequence of defibrillating shocks, Mr Haq responded and his cardiac monitor indicated a sinus rhythm.

By the time his wife, a psychiatrist who had been at a conference in another city, reached his bedside, he was breathing spontaneously, extubated but drowsy, and had a blood pressure of 100/75 mmHg.

1. Dr Haq asks whether the adrenaline her husband has received will increase the risk of his myocardial infarction extending?
2. How did the initial actions of the GP and the paramedic and the staff of the Coronary Care Unit give Mr Haq the best chance of recovering from this incident?

therapy for whom treatment with streptokinase is inadvisable (see Chapter 12 *Drugs and cardiovascular disorders* for a fuller discussion).

Plasma volume expanders

These are used to restore blood volume in shock caused by fluid loss from the intravascular compartment. Choice of replacement fluid depends upon the nature of the fluid lost: blood to replace lost blood, plasma to treat burns and electrolyte solutions for losses from the gastrointestinal tract (Laurence and Bennett, 1992).

The molecular size of the intravenous replacement fluid determines the extent to which it is likely to remain within the intravascular compartment. Solutions of small molecular weight such as electrolyte solutions (crystalloids) are inexpensive and readily available, but rapidly leave the circulatory system. Solutions with comparatively large molecules (colloids) are retained in the blood vessels for longer and therefore are a more effective treatment than crystalloids. Colloid solutions may consist of large molecules of glucose (dextran), gelatine or complex starch, in combination with electrolytes.

Side effects include hypersensitivity reactions. Glucose colloids may alter blood clotting mechanisms and impede the cross-matching of blood (Laurence and Bennett, 1992).

TREATMENT OF ANAPHYLACTIC SHOCK

In this condition, an extreme inflammatory reaction occurs, resulting in widespread vasodilatation, increased capillary permeability and bronchoconstriction. As a result, fluid from the circulatory system is lost into the extracellular compartment and the circulatory system becomes haemodynamically unstable. If anaphylactic shock is untreated, cardiovascular collapse is likely to result. An explanation of the pathophysiology of anaphylaxis is presented in Chapter 5.

Anaphylactic shock constitutes a medical emergency. The main principles of treatment are to give adrenaline, plasma volume expanders and steroids and antihistamines. Adrenaline is given intravenously over 2–3 minutes. The dose is repeated, if needed, up to three times every 15–20 minutes (Haak *et al.*, 1994). The aim of this treatment is to reverse the vasodilatation and bronchoconstriction. Plasma volume expanders are given to restore the blood pressure; steroids and antihistamines are given to halt the inflammatory reaction.

PHARMACOLOGICAL TREATMENT OF POISONING

When poisoning occurs, the main aims of treatment are to support vital functions until the poison can be excreted naturally from the body or, in specific cases, to accelerate removal of the poison from the body by chemical or other means.

CHELATING AGENTS

Poisoning with heavy metals such as arsenic, lead, mercury, copper or iron is treated by using the chemical that acts as a chelating agent for the substance taken. Chelating agents bind the toxic metal into their own molecular structure, forming a relatively harmless compound that can then be excreted using normal physiological processes.

PERSON CENTRED STUDY 2

Brian Clarke, a 38-year-old prison officer, was riding his motorbike home one evening when he was in collision with a car. The attending ambulance personnel found him to be alert and orientated and indicating considerable pain from his right thigh and his pelvic area. On examination, Brian was found to have a closed fracture of his right femur and his pelvis was found to be unstable, with bruising and abrasions. Brian's blood pressure was 110/60 mmHg, and his pulse 140 bpm; he was pale, diaphoretic (sweating) and his capillary fill was delayed. Oxygen therapy was commenced, the fractured femur was stabilised with the assistance of entonox administration and he was loaded into the ambulance. Once inside and en route to hospital, the paramedic inserted two wide-bore cannulae into Brian's arms and commenced an infusion of Hartmann's solution into each, titrating the flow rate against blood pressure readings.

Ten minutes into the journey it was found that Brian's blood pressure had fallen to below 90 mmHg and the paramedic increased the infusion rate to compensate for this. On arrival at the Accident and Emergency Department, Brian's blood pressure, despite the rapid infusion of intravenous fluids, had continued to fall to 80/60 mmHg, with a pulse rate of 160 bpm. As whole blood was not available, gelofusine infusions were set up as the Hartmann's infusions were completed and after rapid assessment of his condition and injuries by the trauma team he was taken to the operating theatre in an attempt to control the bleeding from his fractured pelvis and to stabilise his fractured femur.

1. Why were intravenous fluids given in the pre-hospital care and why were both crystalloid and colloid infusions used?
2. How did the actions of the paramedics and the trauma team ensure that the casualty had the best chance of surviving his traumatic injuries ?

Examples of chelating agents include dimercaprol (arsenic), sodium calcium edetate [calcium EDTA] (lead), penicillamine (lead, copper) and desferrioxamine (iron).

FORCED ALKALINE DIURESIS

Alteration of the normal pH of urine can in some cases aid excretion of a toxic chemical by causing it to ionise. This causes chemicals that are difficult to excrete because they are lipid soluble in their de-ionised state to remain in the tubular filtrate and to be excreted in the urine.

Examples of substances removed by making the urinary pH alkaline include salicylates and phenobarbitone.

Alkalinisation of the urine is achieved by the administration of sodium bicarbonate by intravenous infusion.

Examples of substances that could be removed by making the urinary pH more acidic include amphetamine and quinine.

USE OF ADSORBANTS

Poisoning with phenobarbitone or carbemazepine may be treated with activated charcoal. This binds any drug that remains in the gastrointestinal tract, and removes any of the substance that has already been absorbed and is in the intestinal blood vessels or has entered the bile by diffusion from the bloodstream.

Poisons may also be removed by haemoperfusion or haemodialysis.

KEY POINTS

- Cardiac arrest may occur as a result of ventricular fibrillation, low output tachycardias or asystole.
- The first drug used in a cardiac arrest is usually adrenaline, which increases the rate and force of myocardial contraction.
- Atropine is used to treat asystole and profound bradycardias.
- Bretylium may cause the patient to experience the symptoms of angina.
- Calcium is necessary for normal neuromuscular transmission and myocardial contractility. It can also be used to control hyperkalaemia.
- Side effects of intravenous lignocaine are myocardial depression, drowsiness, convulsion, confusion and coma.

- Ill advised use of intravenous sodium bicarbonate can extend damage to hypoxic cells.
- If an alkalotic state is produced during resuscitation, the affinity of haemoglobin for oxygen is increased and oxygen is unloaded less readily to cells that are already ischaemic.
- Use of β-adrenergic blockers results in a loss of the sympathetic compensatory mechanisms, which protect against the effects of shock.
- Anaphylactic shock constitutes a medical emergency. Treatment is with adrenaline, plasma volume expanders and steroids and antihistamines.
- The removal of poison from the body may be accelerated by chelating agents, for heavy metals, and forced alkaline diuresis.

MULTIPLE CHOICE QUESTIONS

1. When a patient has a cardiorespiratory arrest, the MOST IMPORTANT aim of resuscitation is to
a. give drugs to restore the heart to sinus rhythm
b. raise the blood pressure
c. ensure adequate renal perfusion
d. restore intracellular homeostasis
e. remove carbon dioxide from the bloodstream

2. Cardiac arrest may occur as a result of
a. ventricular tachycardia
b. respiratory arrest
c. hyperkalaemia
d. anaphylaxis
e. all of the above

3. In a cardiac arrest, adrenaline is used to
a. increase myocardial responsivity
b. produce vasoconstriction
c. slow and strengthen the heart rate
d. reduce myocardial irritability
e. prevent ventricular extrasystoles

4. When given intravenously, adrenaline has the effect of
a. decreasing filling time in the coronary arteries
b. increasing cardiac filling time
c. decreasing myocardial energy requirements
d. decreasing the activation of the conduction pathways
e. increasing the activation of the conduction pathways

5. In a cardiac emergency, atropine is given to
a. stimulate the vagus nerve
b. reduce the firing rate of the sinoatrial node
c. decrease vagal tone
d. increase conductivity at the atrioventricular node
e. stimulate the sympathetic receptors

6. Intravenous calcium is used during cardiac arrest to
a. protect against myocardial ischaemia
b. reduce hyperkalaemia
c. prevent ventricular fibrillation
d. reverse heart block
e. restore myocardial contractility

7. During a cardiac arrest, intravenous lignocaine would be given in order to
a. treat profound bradycardia
b. increase myocardial responsiveness
c. suppress response to ventricular pacemakers
d. increase transmission in the Purkinje fibres
e. stimulate the sinoatrial node

8. Adenosine must be given with care in a cardiac emergency because it may produce
a. severe angina
b. supraventricular tachycardia
c. ventricular tachycardia
d. bronchospasm
e. hypertension

9. Diamorphine may be given to patients in acute left ventricular failure because it
a. reduces anxiety
b. is a potent analgesic
c. reduces the cardiac work
d. prevents shock
e. stimulates respiration

10. A patient with anaphylactic shock is likely to require which of the following treatments?
a. intravenous steroids
b. adrenaline
c. antibiotics
d. plasma volume expanders
e. diuretics

REFERENCES

Colquhoun M, Handley AJ, Evans TR. *ABC of resuscitation*. London, BMJ Publishing Group, 1995.

Haak SW, Richardson SJ, Davey SS, Parker-Cohen PD. Alterations of cardiovascular functions. In: McCance KL, Huether SE, eds. *Pathophysiology: the biologic base for disease in adults and children*. St Louis: Mosby, 1994. 1000-1084

Handley AJ, Swain A, eds. *Advanced life support manual, 2nd ed*. London: Resuscitation Council, 1996.

Hume JR. Cardiac electrophysiology and antiarrhythmic drugs. In: Brody TM, Larner J, Minneman KP, Neu HC, eds. *Human pharmacology; molecular to clinical*. St Louis: Mosby, 1994. 173-187

Laurence DR, Bennett PN. *Clinical pharmacology*. Edinburgh: Churchill Livingstone, 1992.

Moore KE. Drugs affecting the sympathetic nervous system. In: Brody TM, Larner J, Minneman KP, Neu HC, eds. *Human pharmacology; molecular to clinical*. St Louis: Mosby, 1994. 113-137

Walker G. *ABPI Compendium of Data Sheets*. London: Datapharm Publications, 1997.

Appendix I

STANDARDS FOR THE ADMINISTRATION OF MEDICINES

United Kingdom Central Council for Nursing, Midwifery and Health Visiting

October 1992 (Reprinted with permission of the UKCC)

List of Contents

Introduction

1 This standards paper replaces the Council's advisory paper 'Administration of Medicines' (issued in 1986) (1) and the supplementary circular 'The Administration of Medicines' (PC 88/05) (2). The Council has prepared this paper to assist practitioners to fulfil the expectations which it has of them, to serve more effectively the interests of patients and clients and to maintain and enhance standards of practice.

2 The administration of medicines is an important aspect of the professional practice of persons whose names are on the Council's register. It is not solely a mechanistic task to be performed in strict compliance with the written prescription of a medical practitioner. It requires thought and the exercise of professional judgement which is directed to:

2.1 confirming the correctness of the prescription;

2.2 judging the suitability of administration at the scheduled time of administration;

2.3 reinforcing the positive effect of the treatment;

2.4 enhancing the understanding of patients in respect of their prescribed medication and the avoidance of misuse of these and other medicines and

2.5 assisting in assessing the efficacy of medicines and the identification of side effects and interactions.

3 To meet the standards set out in this paper to honour, in this aspect of practice, the Council's expectation (set out in the Council's 'Code of Professional Conduct') (3) that:
"As a registered nurse, midwife or health visitor you are personally accountable for your practice and, in the exercise of your professional accountability, must:

3.1 act always in such a manner as to promote and safeguard the interests and well-being of patients and clients;

3.2 ensure that no action or omission on your part, or within your sphere of responsibility, is detrimental to the interests, condition or safety of patients and clients;

3.3 maintain and improve your professional knowledge and competence;

3.4 acknowledge any limitations in your knowledge and competence and decline any duties or responsibilities unless able to perform them in a safe and skilled manner;"

4 This extract from the 'Code of Professional Conduct' applies to all persons on the Council's register irrespective of the part of the register on which their name appears. Although the content of pre-registration education programmes varies, dependent on the part and level of the register involved, the Council expects that, in this area of practice as in all others, all practitioners will have taken steps to develop their knowledge and competence and will have been assisted to this end. The word 'practitioner' is, therefore, used in the remainder of this paper to refer to all registered nurses, midwives and health visitors, each of whom must recognise the personal professional accountability which they bear for their actions. The Council therefore imposes no arbitrary boundaries between the role of the first level and second level registered practitioner in this respect.

Treatment with medicines

5 The treatment of a patient with medicines for therapeutic, diagnostic or preventative purposes is a process which involves prescribing, dispensing, administering, receiving and recording. The word 'patient' is used for convenience, but implies not only a patient in a hospital or nursing home, but also a resident of a residential home, a client in her or his own home or in a community home, a person attending a clinic or a general practitioner's surgery and an employee attending a workplace occupational health department. 'Patient' refers to the person receiving a prescribed medicine. Each medicine has a product licence, which means that authority has been given to a manufacturer to market a particular product for administration in a particular dosage range and by specified routes.

Prescription

6 The practitioner administering a medicine against a prescription written by a registered medical practitioner, like the pharmacist responsible for dispensing it, can reasonably expect that the prescription satisfies the following criteria:

6.1 that it is based, whenever possible, on the patient's awareness of the purpose of the treatment and consent (commonly implicit);

6.2 that the prescription is either clearly written, typed or computer-generated, and that the entry is indelible and dated;

6.3 that, where the new prescription replaces an earlier prescription, the latter has been cancelled clearly and the cancellation signed and dated by an authorised registered medical practitioner;

6.4 that, where a prescribed substance (which replaces an earlier prescription) has been provided for a person residing at home or in a residential care home and who is dependent on others to assist with the administration,

information about the change has been properly communicated;

6.5 that the prescription provides clear and unequivocal identification of the patient for whom the medicine is intended;

6.6 that the substance to be administered is clearly specified and, where appropriate, its form (for example tablet, capsule, suppository) stated, together with the strength, dosage, timing and frequency of administration and route of administration;

6.7 that, where the prescription is provided in an out-patients or community setting, it states the duration of the course before the review;

6.8 that, in the case of controlled drugs, the dosage is written, together with the number of dosage units or total course if in an out-patient or community setting, the whole being in the prescriber's own handwriting;

6.9 that all other prescriptions will, as a minimum, have been signed by the prescribing doctor and dated;

6.10 that the registered medical practitioner understands that the administration of medicines on verbal instructions, whether she or he is present or absent, other than in exceptional circumstances, is not acceptable unless covered by the protocol method referred to in paragraph 6.11;

6.11 that it is understood that, unless provided for in a specific protocol, instruction by telephone to a practitioner to administer a previously unprescribed substance is not acceptable, the use of fascimile transmission (fax) being the preferred method in exceptional circumstances or isolated locations and

6.12 that, where it is the wish of the professional staff concerned that practitioners in a particular setting be authorised to administer, on their own authority, certain medicines, a local protocol has been agreed between medical practitioners, nurses and midwives and the pharmacist.

Dispensing

7 The practitioner administering a medicine dispensed by a pharmacist in response to a medical prescription can reasonably expect that:

7.1 the pharmacist has checked that the prescription is written correctly so as to avoid misunderstanding or error and is signed by an authorised prescriber;

7.2 the pharmacist is satisfied that any newly-prescribed medicines will not dangerously interact with or nullify each other;

7.3 the pharmacist has provided the medicine in a form relevant for administration to the particular patient, provided it in an appropriate container giving the relevant information and advised appropriately on storage and security conditions;

7.4 where the substance is prescribed in a dose or to be administered by a route which falls outside its product licence, unless to be administered from a stock supply, the pharmacist will have taken steps to ensure that the prescriber is aware and has chosen to exceed that licence;

7.5 where the prescription for a specific item falls outside the terms of the product licence, whether as to its route of administration, the dosage or some other key factor, the pharmacist will have ensured that the prescriber is aware of this fact and, mindful of her or his accountability in the matter, has made a record on the prescription to this effect and has agreed to dispense the medicine ordered;

7.6 if the prescription bears any written amendments made and signed by the pharmacist, the prescriber has been consulted and advised and the amendments have been accepted and

7.7 the pharmacist, in pursuit of her or his role in monitoring the adverse side-effects of medicines, wishes to be sent any information that the administering practitioner deems relevant.

Standards for the administration of medicines

8 Notwithstanding the expected adherence by registered medical practitioners and pharmacists to the criteria set out in paragraphs 6 and 7 of this paper, the nurse, midwife or health visitor must, in administering any medicines, in assisting with administration or overseeing any self-administration of medicines, exercise professional judgement and apply knowledge and skill to the situation that pertains at the time.

9 This means that, as a matter of basic principle, whether administering a medicine, assisting in its administration or overseeing self-administration, the practitioner will be satisfied that she or he:

9.1 has an understanding of substances used for therapeutic purposes;

9.2 is able to justify any actions taken and

9.3 is prepared to be accountable for the action taken.

10 Against this background, the practitioner, acting in the interests of the patients, will:

10.1 be certain of the identity of the patient to whom the medicine is to be administered;

10.2 ensure that she or he is aware of the patient's current assessment and planned programme of care;

10.3 pay due regard to the environment in which that care is being given;

10.4 scrutinise carefully, in the interests of safety, the prescription, where available, and the information provided on the relevant containers;

10.5 question the medical practitioner or pharmacist, as appropriate, if the prescription or container information is illegible, unclear, ambiguous or incomplete or where it is believed that the dosage or route of administration falls outside the product licence for the particular substance and, where believed necessary, refuse to administer the prescribed substance;

10.6 refuse to prepare substances for injection in advance of their immediate use and refuse to administer a medicine not placed in a container or drawn into a syringe by her or him, in her or his presence, or prepared by a pharmacist, except in the specific circumstances described in paragraph 40 of this paper and others where similar issues arise and

10.7 draw the attention of patients, as appropriate, to patient information leaflets concerning their prescribed medicines.

11 In addition, acting in the interests of the patient, the practitioner will:

11.1 check the expiry date of any medicine, if on the container;

11.2 carefully consider the dosage, method of administration, route and timing of administration in the context of the condition of the specific patient at the operative time;

11.3 carefully consider whether any of the prescribed medicines will or may dangerously interact with each other;

11.4 determine whether it is necessary or advisable to withhold the medicine pending consultation with the prescribing medical practitioner, the pharmacist or a fellow professional colleague;

11.5 contact the prescriber without delay where contra-indications to the administration of any prescribed medicine are observed, first taking the advice of the pharmacist where considered appropriate;

11.6 make clear, accurate and contemporaneous record of the administration of all medicines administered or deliberately withheld, ensuring that any written entries and the signature are clear and legible;

11.7 where a medicine is refused by the patient, or the parent refuses to administer or allow administration of that medicine, make a clear and accurate record of the fact without delay, consider whether the refusal of that medicine compromises the patient's condition or the effect of other medicines, assess the situation and contact the prescriber;

11.8 use the opportunity which administration of a medicine provides for emphasising, to patients and their carers, the importance and implications of the prescribed treatment and for enhancing their understanding of its effects and side-effects;

11.9 record the positive and negative effects of the medicine and make them known to the prescribing medical practitioner and the pharmacist and

11.10 take all possible steps to ensure that the replaced prescription entries are correctly deleted to avoid duplication of medicines.

Applying the standards in a range of settings

Who can administer medicines?

12 There is a wide spectrum of situations in which medicines are administered ranging, at one extreme, from the patient in an intensive therapy unit who is totally dependent on registered professional staff for her or his care to, at the other extreme, the person in her or his own home administering her or his own medicines or being assisted in this respect by a relative or another person. The answer to the question of who can administer a medicine must largely depend on where within that spectrum the recipient of the medicines lies.

Administration in the hospital setting

13 It is the Council's position that, at or near the first stated end of that spectrum, assessment of response to treatment and speedy recognition of contra-indications and side-effects are of great importance. Therefore prescribed medicines should only be administered by registered practitioners who are competent for the purpose and aware of their personal accountability.

14 In this context it is the Council's position that, in the majority of circumstances, a first level registered nurse, a midwife, or a second level nurse, each of whom has demonstrated the necessary knowledge

and competence, should be able to administer medicines without involving a second person. Exceptions to this might be:

14.1 where the practioner is instructing a student;

14.2 where the patient's condition makes it necessary and

14.3 where local circumstances make the involvement of two persons desirable in the interests of the patient (for example, in areas of specialist care, such as paediatric unit without sufficient specialist paediatric nurses or in other acute units dependent on temporary agency or other locum staff).

15 In respect of the administration of intravenous drugs by practitioners, it is the Council's position that this is acceptable, provided that, as in all other aspects of practice, the practitioner is satisfied with her or his competence and mindful of her or his personal accountability.

16 The Council is opposed to the involvement of persons who are not registered practitioners in the administration of medicines in acute care settings and with ill or dependent patients, since the requirements of paragraphs 8 to 11 inclusive of this paper cannot then be satisfied. It accepts, however, that the professional judgement of an individual practitioner should be used to identify those situations in which informal carers might be instructed and prepared to accept a delegated responsibility in this respect.

Administration in the domestic or quasi-domestic setting

17 It is evident that in this setting, on the majority of occasions, there is no involvement of registered practitioners. Where a practitioner engaged in community practice does become involved in assisting with or overseeing administration, then she or he must observe paragraphs 8 to 11 of this paper and apply them to the required degree. She or he must also recognise that, even if not employed in posts requiring registration with the Council, she or he remains accountable to the Council.

18 The same principles apply where prescribed medicines are being administered to residents in small community homes or in residential care homes. To the maximum degree possible, though related to their ability to manage the care and administration of their prescribed medicines and comprehend their significance, the residents should be regarded as if in their own home. Where assistance is required, the person providing it fills the role of an informal carer, family member or friend. However, as with the situation described in

paragraph 17, where a professional practitioner is involved, a personal accountability is borne. The advice of a community pharmacist should be sought when necessary.

Self-administration of medicines in hospitals or registered nursing homes

19 The Council welcomes and supports the development of self-administration of medicines and administration by parents to children wherever it is appropriate and the necessary security and storage arrangements are available.

20 For the hospital patient approaching discharge, but who will continue on a prescribed medicines regime following the return home, there are obvious benefits in adjusting to the responsibility of self-administration while still having access to professional support. It is accepted that, to facilitate this transition, practitioners may assist patients to administer their medicines safely by preparing a form of medication care containing information transcribed from other sources.

21 For the long stay patient, whether in hospital or a nursing home, self-administration can help foster a feeling of independence and control in one aspect of life.

22 It is essential, however, that where self-administration is introduced for all or some patients, arrangements must be in place for the appropriate, safe and secure storage of the medicines, access to which is limited to the specific patient.

The use of monitored dosage systems

23 Monitored dosage systems, for the purpose of this paper, are systems which involve a community pharmacist, in response to the full prescription of medicines for a specific person, dispensing those medicines into a special container with sections for days of the week and times within those days and delivering the container, or supplying the medicines in a special container of blister packs, with appropriate additional information, to the nursing home, residential care home or domestic residence. The Council is aware of the development of such monitored dosage systems and accepts that, provided they are able to satisfy strict criteria established by the Royal Pharmaceutical Society of Great Britain and other official pharmaceutical organisations, that substances which react to each other are not supplied in this way and that they are suitable for the intended purpose as judged by the nursing profession, they have a valuable place in the administration of medicines.

24 While, to the present, their use has been primarily in registered nursing homes and some community or residential care homes, there seems no reason why, provided the systems can satisfy the standards referred to in paragraph 25, their use should not be extended.

25 In order to be acceptable for use in hospitals or registered nursing homes, the containers for the medicines must:

25.1 satisfy the requirements of the Royal Pharmaceutical Society of Great Britain for an original container;

25.2 be filled by a pharmacist and sealed by her or him or under her or his control and delivered complete to the user;

25.3 be accompanied by clear and comprehensive documentation which forms the medical practitioner's prescription;

25.4 bear the means of identifying tablets of similar appearance so that, should it be necessary to withhold one tablet (for example digoxin), it can be identified from those in the container space for the particular time and day;

25.5 be able to be stored in a secure place and

25.6 make it apparent if the containers (be they blister packs or spaces within a container) have been tampered with between the closure and sealing by the pharmacist and the time of administration.

26 While the introduction of a monitored dosage system transfers to the pharmacist the responsibility for being satisfied that the container is filled and sealed correctly so as to comply with the prescription, it does not alter the fact that the practitioner administering the medicines must still consider the appropriateness of each medicine at the time administration falls due. It is not the case, therefore, that the use of a monitored dosage system allows the administration of medicines to be undertaken by unqualified personnel.

27 It is not acceptable, in lieu of a pharmacist-filled monitored dosage system container, for a practitioner to transfer medicines from their original containers into an unsealed container for administration at a later stage by another person, whether or not that person is a registered practitioner. This is an unsafe practice which carries risks for both practitioner and patient. Similarly it is not acceptable to interfere with a sealed section at any time between its closure by the pharmacist and the scheduled time of administration.

The role of nurses, midwives and health visitors in community practice in the administration of medicines

28 Any practitioner who, whether as a planned intervention or incidentally, becomes involved in administering a medicine, or assisting with or overseeing such administration, must apply paragraphs 8 to 11 of this paper to the degree to which they are relevant.

29 Where a practitioner working in the community becomes involved in obtaining prescribed medicines for patients, she or he must recognise her or his responsibility for safe transit and correct delivery.

30 Community psychiatric nurses whose practice involves them in providing assistance to patients to reduce and eliminate their dependence on addictive drugs should ensure that they are aware of the potential value of short term prescriptions and encourage their use where appropriate in the long term interests of their clients. They must not resort to holding or carrying prescribed controlled drugs to avoid their misuse by those clients.

31 Special arrangements and certain exemptions apply to occupational health nurses. These are described in Information Document 11 and the Appendices of 'A Guide to an Occupational Health Nursing Service; A Handbook for Employers and Nurses'; published by the Royal College of Nursing (4).

32 Some practitioners employed in the community, including in particular community nurses, practice nurses and health visitors, in order to enhance disease prevention, will receive requests to participate in vaccination and immunisation programmes. Normally these requests will be accompanied by specific named prescriptions or be covered by a protocol setting out the arrangements within which substances can be administered to certain categories of persons who meet the stated criteria. The facility provided by the 'Medicines Act 1968' (5) for substances to be administered to a number of people in response to an advance 'direction' is valuable in this respect. Where it has not been possible to anticipate the possible need for preventive treatment and there is no relevant protocol or advance direction, particularly in respect of patients about to travel abroad and requiring preventive treatment, a telephone conversation with a registered medical practitioner will suffice as authorisation for a single administration. It is not, however, sufficient as a basis for supplying a quantity of medicines.

Midwives and midwifery practice

33 Midwives should refer to the current editions of both the Council's 'Midwives Rules' (6) and 'A Midwife's Code of Practice' (7), and specifically to the sections concerning administration of medicines. At the time of publication of this paper, 'Midwives Rules' sets out the practising midwife's responsibility in respect of the administration of medicines and other forms of pain relief. 'A Midwife's Code of Practice' refers to the authority provided by the 'Medicines Act 1968' and the 'Misuse of Drugs Act 1971' (8), and regulations made as a result, for midwives to obtain and administer certain substances.

What if the Council's standards in paragraphs 8 to 11 cannot be applied?

34 There are certain situations in which practitioners are involved in the administration of medicines where some of criteria stated above either cannot be applied or, if applied, would introduce dangerous delay with consequent risk to patients. These will include occupational health settings in some industries, small hospitals with no resident medical staff and possibly some specialist units within larger hospitals and some community settings.

35 With the exception of the administration of substances for the purpose of vaccination or immunisation described in paragraph 32 above, in any situation in which a practitioner may be expected or required to administer 'prescription-only medicines' which have not been directly prescribed for a named patient by a registered medical practitioner who has examined the patient and made a diagnosis, it is essential that a clear local policy be determined and made known to all practitioners involved with prescribing and administration. This will make it possible for action to be taken in patients' interests while protecting practitioners from the risk of complaint which might otherwise jeopardise their position.

36 Therefore, where such a situation will, or may apply, a local policy should be agreed and documented which:

36.1 states the circumstances in which particular 'prescription-only medicines' may be administered in advance of examination by a doctor;

36.2 ensures the relevant knowledge and skill of those to be involved in administration;

36.3 describes the form, route and dosage range of the medicines so authorised and

36.4 wherever possible, satisfies the requirements of Section 58 of the 'Medicines Act 1968' as a 'direction'.

Substances for topical application

37 The standards set out in this paper apply, to the degree to which they are relevant, to substances used for wound dressing and other topical applications. Where a practitioner uses a substance or product which has not been prescribed, she or he must have considered the matter sufficiently to be able to justify its use in the particular circumstances.

The administration of homoeopathic or herbal substances

38 Homoeopathic and herbal medicines are subject to the licensing provisions of the 'Medicines Act 1968', although those on the market when that Act became operative (which means most of those now available) received product licenses without any evaluation of their efficacy, safety or quality. Practitioners should, therefore, make themselves generally aware of common substances used in their particular area of practice. It is necessary to respect the right of individuals to administer to themselves, or to request a practitioner to assist in the administration of substances in these categories. If, when faced with a patient or client whose desire to receive medicines of this kind appears to create potential difficulties, or if it is felt that the substances might either be an inappropriate response to the presenting symptoms or likely to negate or enhance the effect of prescribed medicines, the practitioner, acting in the interests of the patient or client, should consider contacting the relevant registered medical practitioner, but must also be mindful of the need not to override the patient's rights.

Complementary and alternative therapies

39 Some registered nurses, midwives and health visitors, having first undertaken successfully a training in complementary or alternative therapy which involves the use of substances such as essential oils, apply their specialist knowledge and skill in their practice. It is essential that practice in these respects, as in all others, is based upon sound principles, available knowledge and skill. The importance of consent to the use of such treatment must be recognised. So, too, must the practitioner's personal accountability for her or his professional practice.

Practitioners assuming responsibility for care which includes medicines being administered which were previously checked by other practitioners

40 Paragraph 10.6 of this paper referred to the unacceptability of a practitioner administering a substance drawn into a syringe or container by another practitioner when the practitioner taking over responsibility for the patient was not present.

An exception to this is an already established intravenous infusion, the use of a syringe pump or some other kind of continuous or intermittent infusion or injection apparatus, where a valid prescription exists, a responsible practitioner has signed for the container of fluid and any additives being administered and the container is clearly and indelibly labelled. The label must clearly show the contents and be signed and dated. The same measures must apply equally to other means of administration of such substances through, for example, central venous, arterial or epidural lines. Strict discipline must be applied to the recording of any substances being administered by any of the methods referred to in this paragraph and to reporting procedures between staff as they change and transfer responsibility for care.

Management of errors or incidents in the administration of medicines

41 In a number of its Annual Reports, the Council has recorded its concern that practitioners who have made mistakes under pressure of work, and have been honest and open about those mistakes to their senior staff, appear often to have been made the subject of disciplinary action in a way which seems likely to discourage the reporting of incidents and therefore be to the potential detriment of patients and of standards.

42 When considering allegations of misconduct arising out of errors in the administration of medicines, the Council's Professional Conduct Committee takes great care to distinguish between those cases where the error was the result of reckless practice and was concealed and those which resulted from serious pressure of work and where there was immediate, honest disclosure in the patient's interest. The Council recognises the prerogative of managers to take local disciplinary action where it is considered to be appropriate but urges that they also consider each incident in its particular context and similarly discriminate between the two categories described.

43 The Council's position is that all errors and incidents require a thorough and careful investigation which takes full account of the circumstances and context of the event and the position of the practitioner involved. Events of this kind call equally for sensitive management and a comprehensive assessment of all of the circumstances before a professional and managerial decision is reached on the appropriate way to proceed.

Future arrangements for prescribing by nurses

44 In March 1992 the Act of Parliament entitled the 'Medicinal Products: Prescription by Nurses etc Act 1992' (9) became law. This legislation is to come into operation in October 1993. The legislation will permit nurses with a district nursing or health visiting qualification to prescribe certain products from a Nurse Prescribers' Formulary. The statutory rules, yet to be completed, will specify the categories of nurses who can prescribe under this limited legislation. The Council will issue further information concerning this important new legislation prior to it becoming operative.

45 Enquiries in respect of this Council paper should be directed to the:

Registrar and Chief Executive
United Kingdom Central Council for Nursing, Midwifery and Health Visiting
23 Portland Place
London W1N 3AF

References

1 United Kingdom Central Council for Nursing, Midwifery and Health Visiting, 'Administration of Medicines; A UKCC Advisory Paper; A framework to assist individual professional judgement and the development of local policies and guidelines', April 1986.

2 United Kingdom Central Council for Nursing, Midwifery and Health Visiting, 'The Administration of Medicines', PC 88/05, September 1988.

3 United Kingdom Central Council for Nursing, Midwifery and Health Visiting, 'Code of Professional Conduct for the Nurse, Midwife and Health Visitor', Third Edition, June 1992.

4 Royal College of Nursing, 'A Guide to an Occupational Health Nursing Service; A Handbook for Employers and Nurses', Second Edition 1991.

5 'Medicines Act 1968', Her Majesty's Stationery Office, London, Reprinted 1986.

6 United Kingdom Central Council for Nursing, Midwifery and Health Visiting, 'Midwives Rules', March 1991.

7 United Kingdom Central Council for Nursing, Midwifery and Health Visiting, 'A Midwife's Code of Practice', March 1991.

8 'Misuse of Drugs Act 1971', Her Majesty's Stationery Office, London, Reprinted 1985.

9 'Medicinal Products: Prescription by Nurses etc Act 1992', Her Majesty's Stationery Office, London, 1992.

Appendix 2

EXCERPT FROM MIDWIVES' RULES AND CODE OF PRACTICE (UKCC, 1998)

Administration of medicines and other forms of pain relief

1 A practising midwife shall only administer those medicines, including analgesics, in which she has been trained as to use, dosage and administration.

2 A practising midwife shall only administer medicines including inhalational analgesics by mean of apparatus if she is satisfied that the apparatus has been properly maintained and:
   a. it has a CE marking or, if it does not have such a marking,
   b. it is of a type for the time being approved by the UKCC as suitable for use by a midwife and in this paragraph, CE marking has the meaning assigned to it in the *Medical Devices Regulations 1994 No 3017.*

3 In a situation in which clinical trials involving new medicines including inhalation analgesics, or new apparatus are taking place, a practising midwife may only participate under the direction of a registered medical practitioner.

Reproduced with the permission of the United Kingdom Central Council for Nursing, Midwifery & Health Visiting

Source: United Kingdom Central Council for Nursing, Midwifery and Health Visiting. *Midwives' Rules and Code of Practice.* London: UKCC, 1998

Appendix 3

PROPRIETARY AND GENERIC NAMES OF DRUGS

Proprietary	Generic	Group/Indication
Abelcet	amphotericin B	antifungal
Accupro	quinapril	ACE inhibitor
Accuretic	quinapril	ACE inhibitor
Achromycin	tetracycline	antibacterial
Acnisal	salicylic acid	acne topical preparation
Actilyse	alteplase	fibrinolytic drugs
Actrapid	insulin	diabetes
Adalat	nifedipine	calcium channel blocker
Adenocor	adenosine	arrhythmias
Adipine	nifedipine	calcium channel blocker
adrenaline	adrenaline	cardiopulmonary resuscitation/anaphylaxis
AeroBec	beclomethasone	corticosteroid
Aerolin Autohaler	salbutamol	asthma
Afrazine	oxymetazoline	decongestant
Aldactone	spironolactone	diuretic
Aldomet	methyldopa	hypertension
AlfaD	alfacalcidol	vitamin D supplement
Alkeran	melphalan	alkylating drug
Alomide	lodoxamide	anti-inflammatory
Alu-Cap	aluminium hydroxide	antacid
aluminium acetate	aluminium acetate	otitis externa
AmBisome	amphotericin B	antifungal
Ametop	amethocaine	local anaesthetic
Amikin	amikacin	antibacterial
amiloride	amiloride	diuretic
Amoxil	amoxycillin	antibacterial
Amphocil	amphotericin B	antifungal
Anafranil	clomipramine	depression
Ancotil	flucytosine	antifungal
Androcur	cyproterone	anti-androgen
Angiopine	nifedipine	calcium channel blocker
Angitak	isosorbide dinitrate	angina
Antepsin	sucralfate	ulcers
Anturan	sulphinpyrazone	gout
Apresoline	hydralazine	hypertension
Aredia	disodium pamidronate	osteoporosis

Proprietary	Generic	Group/Indication
Arimidex	anastrozole	hormone antagonist
Arpicolin	procyclidine	antimuscarinic; parkinsonism
Arthrotec	diclofenac	non-steroidal anti-inflammatory (NSAID) drug
Asmasal Clickhaler	salbutamol	asthma
Atromid-S	clofibrate	lipid regulation
Augmentin	clavulanic acid	antibacterial
Aureomycin	chlortetracycline	antibacterial
Avloclor	chloroquine	malaria; disease modifying anti-rheumatic drugs (DMARDs)
Avoca	silver nitrate	warts
Axid	nizatidine	H2 receptor antagonists
Axsain	capsaicin	rheumatic disease
Baxan	cefadroxil	antibacterial
Becotide	beclomethasone	corticosteroid
bendrofluazide	bendrofluazide	diuretic
Benemid	probenecid	gout
Benoral	benorylate	non-steroidal anti-inflammatory (NSAID) drug
Benoxinate	oxybuprocaine	local anaesthetic
benserazide	benserazide	dopamine receptor stimulant; parkinsonism
benzyl benzoate	benzyl benzoate	antiparasitic
Beta-Adalat	atenolol	beta-blocker
Betagen	levobunolol	beta-blocker (glaucoma)
Betaloc	metoprolol	beta-blocker
Betim	timolol	beta-blocker (glaucoma)
Betnelan	betamethasone	glucorticoid
Betnesol	betamethasone	glucorticoid
Betoptic	betaxolol	beta-blocker (glaucoma)
BCNU	carmustine	alkylating drug
Biocadren	timolol	beta-blocker (glaucoma)
Biorphen	orphenadrine	muscle relaxant; antimuscarinic used in parkinsonism
bisacodyl	bisacodyl	laxative
bleomycin	bleomycin	cytotoxic antibiotic
Bretylate	bretylium	arrhythmias
Brevinor	ethinyloestradiol	combination contraceptives
Brexidol	piroxicam	non-steroidal anti-inflammatory (NSAID) drug
Bricanyl	terbutaline	asthma
Britaject	apomorphine	dopamine receptor stimulant; parkinsonism
Broflex	benzhexol	antimuscarinic; parkinsonism
Brufen	ibuprofen	non-steroidal anti-inflammatory (NSAID) drug
Burinex	bumetanide	diuretic
Buscopan	hyoscine butyl bromide	antispasmodic
Butacote	phenylbutazone	non-steroidal anti-inflammatory (NSAID) drug
Cabaser	cabergoline	dopamine receptor stimulant; parkinsonism
Cacit	ergocalciferol	vitamin D supplement
Caelyx	doxorubicin	cytotoxic drug
Cafergot	ergotamine	migraine
caffeine	caffeine	CNS stimulant
calamine	calamine	pruritus
Calceos	ergocalciferol	vitamin D supplement
Calcichew	ergocalciferol	vitamin D supplement
Calcijex	calcitriol	vitamin D supplement
Calciparine	heparin	anticoagulants
calcium carbonate	calcium carbonate/acetate	anatacid
Calcort	deflazacort	glucocorticoid therapy
Calsynar	salcatonin (calcitonin)	bone metabolism
Camcolit	lithium	mania
Capoten	captopril	ACE inhibitor
Caprin	aspirin (acetyl salicylic acid)	analgesic
Carace	lisinopril	ACE inhibitor
carbidopa	carbidopa	dopamine receptor stimulant; parkinsonism
carbocisteine	carbocysteine	mucolytic

Proprietary	Generic	Group/Indication
Cardene	nicardipine	calcium channel blocker
Cardilate	nifedipine	calcium channel blocker
Cardura	doxazosin	alpha-adrenoreceptor blocker
Carobel	carob	vomiting
Carylderm	carbaryl	antiparasitic
Catapres	clonidine	migraine
Cedocard	isosorbide dinitrate	angina
Celance	pergolide	dopamine receptor stimulant; parkinsonism
CellCept	mycophenolate	immunosuppressants
Ceporex	cephalexin	antibacterial
chlordiazepoxide	chlordiazepoxide	anxiolytic
Chlorohex	chlorhexidine	antibacterial
chlorpropamide	chlorpropamide	diabetes
Cidomycin	gentamicin	antibacterial
Cinobac	cinoxacin	antibacterial
Ciproxin	ciprofloxacin	antibacterial
cisplatin	cisplatin	antineoplastic drug
Claforan	cefotaxime	antibacterial
Clarityn	loratadine	antihistamine
Clinoril	sulindac	non-steroidal anti-inflammatory (NSAID) drug
clioquinol	clioquinol	otitis externa
Clomid	clomiphene citrate	antioestrogen
Clotam	tolfenamic acid	non-steroidal anti-inflammatory (NSAID) drug
clotrimazole	clotrimazole	antifungal
Clozaril	clozapine	antipsychotic
Co-codamol	paracetamol	analgesic
Co-danthramer	danthron	faecal softeners
codeine	codeine	analgesic; anti diarrhoea
Cogentin	benztropine	antimuscarinic; parkinsonism
colchicine	colchicine	gout
colecalciferol	cholecalciferol	vitamin D supplement
Colestid	colestipol	lipid regulation
Colomycin	colistin	antibacterial
Comegen Lyovac	dactinomycin (actinomycin D)	cytotoxic antibiotic
Condyline	podophyllin	warts
Convulex	sodium valproate	convulsions
Coracten	nifedipine	calcium channel blocker
Cordarone X	amiodarone	arrhythmias
Cordilox	verapamil	calcium channel blocker
Corgard	nadolol	beta-blocker
Corsodyl	chlorhexidine	antibacterial
Cortisyl	cortisone	glucocorticoid therapy
Coversyl	perindopril	ACE inhibitor
Cozaar	losartan	angiotensin II receptor antagonists
Creon	pancreatin	cystic fibrosis
Crixivan	indinavir	antiviral drug
Crystapen	benzylpenicillin	antibacterial
Crystapen	penicillin	antibacterial
Cyklokapron	tranexamic acid	antifibrinolytic agent
Cymevene	ganciclovir	antiviral drug
Cystrin	oxybutinin	urinary incontinence
Cytostar	cytarabarine	antimetabolite
Cytotec	misoprostol	prostaglandin analogue
Daktarin	miconazole	antifungal
Dalacin	clindamycin	antibacterial
Danol	danazol	gonadotrophin inhibition
Dantrium	dantrolene sodium	muscle relaxant
Daonil	glibenclamide	diabetes
Daraprim	pyrimethamine	malaria
DaunoXome	daunorubicin	cytotoxic antibiotic
DDAVP	desmopressin	posterior pituitary antagonists
debrisoquine	debrisoquine	adrenergic neurone blockers

Proprietary	Generic	Group/Indication
Decadron	dexamethasone	glucocorticoid therapy
Deca-Durabolin	nandrolone	anabolic steroid
Delfen	nonoxinols	spermicide
De-Noltab	bismuth chelate	ulcers
Deponit	glyceryl trinitrate	angina
Depo-Provera	progesterone	contraceptive
Derbac	malathion	parasiticidal preparations
Desferal	desferrioxamine	poisoning treatment
Desmospray	desmopressin	posterior pituitary antagonists
Desmotabs	desmopressin	posterior pituitary antagonists
Destolit	ursodeoxycholic acid	gallstone dissolution
Deteclo	tetracycline	antibacterial
Dexedrine	dexamphetamine sulphate	CNS stimulant
dextropropoxyphene	dextropropoxyphene	analgesic
DF 118 Forte	dihydrocodeine	analgesic
DHC Continus	dihydrocodeine	analgesic
Diamicron	gliclazide	diabetes
diamorphine	diamorphine	analgesic
Diamox	acetazolamide	epilepsy/glaucoma/diuretic
diazepam	diazepam	anxiolytic; muscle relaxant
Diclomax	diclofenac	non-steroidal anti-inflammatory (NSAID) drug
Didronel	disodium etidronate	osteoporosis
Diflucan	fluconazole	antifungal
Dimetriose	gestrinone	gonadotrophin inhibition
Dioctyl	docusate sodium	faecal softeners
Diovan	valsartan	angiotensin II receptor antagonists
Dirythmin	disopyramide	arrhythmias
Disipal	orphenadrine	muscle relaxant; antimuscarinic used in parkinsonism
Disprin	aspirin (acetyl salicylic acid)	analgesic
Distamine	penicillamine	disease modifying anti-rheumatic drugs (DMARDs)
Ditropan	oxybutinin	urinary incontinence
Dixarit	clonidine	migraine
Dobutrex	dobutamine	cardiac stimulants
Docusol	docusate sodium	faecal softeners
Dolobid	diflunisal	non-steroidal anti-inflammatory (NSAID) drug
dopamine	dopamine	cardiac stimulants
Double Check	nonoxinols	spermicide
Dovonex	calcipotriol	psoriasis
Dozic	haloperidol	antipsychotic
Dramamine	dimenhydramine	antihistamine
Drogenil	flutamide	hormone antagonist
Droleptan	droperidol	antipsychotic
DTIC-Dome	dacarbazine	antineoplastic drug
Duragel	nonoxinols	spermicide
Durogesic	fentanyl	analgesic
Dyspamet	cimetidine	H2 receptor antagonists
Dytac	triamterene	diuretic
Edicrin	ethacrynic acid	diuretic
edrophonium	edrophonium	skeletal muscle relaxants
Efcortesol	hydrocortisone	glucocorticoid therapy
Efudix	fluorouracil	antimetabolite
Eldepryl	selegiline	dopamine receptor stimulant; parkinsonism
Emcor	bisoprolol	beta-blocker
Eminase	anistreplase	fibrinolytic drugs
Emla	lignocaine	local anaesthetic
Endoxana	cyclophosphamide	cytotoxic drug
Epanutin	phenytoin	convulsions
ephedrine	ephedrine hydrochloride	nasal decongestant
Epilim	sodium valproate	convulsions
Epivir	lamivudine	antiviral drug
Eprex	epoetin-beta	erythropoetin

Proprietary	Generic	Group/Indication
Erymax	erythromycin	antibacterial
Erythrocin	erythromycin	antibacterial
Erythroped	erythromycin	antibacterial
Eskamel	resorcinol	acne
Estring	dienoestrol	topical oestrogens
ethambutol	ethambutol	tuberculosis
Etopophos	etoposide	antineoplastic drug
Eudemine	diazoxide	diabetes
Euglucon	glibenclamide	diabetes
Eurax	crotamiton	pruritus
Evista	raloxifene	osteoporosis
Famvir	famciclovir	antiviral drug
Fasigyn	tinidazole	antifungal
Feldine	piroxicam	non-steroidal anti-inflammatory (NSAID) drug
Femulen	ethynodiol	contraceptive
Fenbid	ibuprofen	non-steroidal anti-inflammatory (NSAID) drug
Fenopron	fenoprofen	non-steroidal anti-inflammatory (NSAID) drug
Feospan	ferrous sulphate	anaemia
Ferrogard	ferrous sulphate	anaemia
Fibro-Vein	sodium tetradecyl sulphate	sclerotherapy of varicose veins
Flagyll	metronidazole	amoebicides
Flamazine	silver sulphadiazine	antibacterial
Flixotide	fluticasone	corticosteroid
Florinef	fludrocortisone	corticosteroid
Floxapen	flucloxacillin	antibacterial
Fluanxol	flupenthixol	depression
folic acid	folic acid	megaloblastic anaemia
Fortipine	nifedipine	calcium channel blocker
Fortovase	saquinavir	antiviral drug
Fosamax	alendronic acid	osteoporosis
Foscavir	foscarnet	antiviral drug
Froben	flurbiprofen	non-steroidal anti-inflammatory (NSAID) drug
Fucidin	fusidic acid	antibacterial
Fulcin	griseofulvin	antifungal
Fungilin	amphotericin B	antifungal
Fungizone	amphotericin B	antifungal
Furadantin	nitrofurantoin	urinary tract infections
Galpseud	pseudoephedrine	decongestant
Gammaglobulin	human normal immunoglobin (HNIG)	immunoglobulins
Ganda	guanethidine	sympathomimetic
gemeprost	gemeprost	prostaglandin
Genotropin	somatotrophin	human growth hormone
genticin	gentamicin	antibacterial
Glibenese	glipizide	diabetes
Glucobay	acarbose	diabetes
Glucophage	metformin	diabetes
glycerol	glycerine	laxative
Glypressin	terlipressin	posterior pituitary anatagonists
Gopten	trandolapril	ACE inhibitor
Grisovin	griseofulvin	antifungal
Gynol II	nonoxinols	spermicide
Haldol	haloperidol	antipsychotic
Halfan	halofantrine	malaria
Heminevrin	clomethiazole	hypnotic
Herpid	idoxuridine	antiviral drug
Hismanal	astemizole	antihistamine
Hivid	zalcitabine	antiviral drug
HRF	gonadorelin	gonadotrophin-releasing hormone
Humalin	insulin	diabetes
Humalog	insulin lispro	diabetes
Humatrope	somatotrophin	human growth hormone

Proprietary	Generic	Group/Indication
Humilin I	isophane insulin	diabetes
Hyalase	hyaluronidase	enzyme
Hycamtin	topotecan	antineoplastic drug
Hydrocortone	hydrocortisone	glucocorticoid therapy
HydroSaluric	hydrochlorothiazide	diuretic
Hypovase	prazosin	alpha-adrenoreceptor blocker
Hypurin	insulin	diabetes
Hypurin Bovine Isophane	isophane insulin	diabetes
Hytrin	terazosin	alpha-adrenoreceptor blocker
Ikorel	nicorandil	potassium channel activator
Ilosone	erythromycin	antibacterial
Imigran	sumatriptin	migraine
Imodium	loperamide	antimotility
Imunovir	inosine pranobex	antiviral drug
Imuran	azathioprine	cytotoxic immunosuppressant
Inderal	propranolol	beta-blocker
indometacin	indomethacin	non-steroidal anti-inflammatory (NSAID) drug
Innovace	enalapril	ACE inhibitor
Instillagel	lignocaine	local anaesthetic
Insulatard	isophane insulin	diabetes
Intron A	interferon alpha	antiviral drug
Invirase	saquinavir	antiviral drug
iodine	iodine	hyperthyroidism
Isocard	isosorbide dinitrate	angina
Isoket	isosorbide dinitrate	angina
isoniazid	isoniazid	tuberculosis
Isordil	isosorbide dinitrate	angina
Isotopo Atropine	atropine	antimuscarinic
Isotrexin	isotretinoin	acne
Kabiglobulin	human normal immunoglobin (HNIG)	immunoglobulins
Kabikinase	streptokinase	thrombolytic agents
Kalten	atenolol	beta-blocker
Kannasyn	kanamycin	antibacterial
kaolin	kaolin	absorbents; antimotility
Kapake	paracetamol	analgesic
Keflex	cephalexin	antibacterial
Kemadrin	procyclidine	antimuscarinic; parkinsonism
Kemicetine	chloramphenicol	antibacterial
Kenalog	triamcinolone	glucocorticoid therapy
Klaricid	clarithromycin	antibacterial
Kytril	granisertron	nausea; vomiting
lactulose	lactulose	faecal softeners
Lamictal	lamotrigine	convulsions
Lanoxin	digoxin	heart failure
Lanvis	thioguanine	antimetabolite
Largactil	chlorpromazine	antiemetic
Lariam	mefloquine	malaria
Laryng-O-jet	lignocaine	local anaesthetic
Lasix	frusemide	diuretic
Lasma	theophylline	bronchodilator
Lederfen	fenbufen	non-steroidal anti-inflammatory (NSAID) drug
Lentaron	formestan	hormone antagonist
Lentizol	amitriptyline	depression
Leukeran	chlorambucil	alkylating drug
levodopa	levodopa	dopamine receptor stimulant; parkinsonism
Lingraine	ergotamine	migraine
Lioresal	baclofen	muscle relaxant
Lipostat	pravastain	lipid regulation
liquid paraffin	liquid paraffin	faecal softeners
Liskonium	lithium	mania
Litarex	lithium	mania

Proprietary	Generic	Group/Indication
Livial	tibolone	osteoporosis
Livostin	levocabastine	anti-inflammatory
Locorten-Viaform	flumetasone	otitis externa
Lodine SR	etodolac	non-steroidal anti-inflammatory (NSAID) drug
Loestrin	ethinyloestradiol	combination contraceptives
Logynon	ethinyloestradiol	combination contraceptives
Loniten	minoxidil	hypertension
Lopid	gemfibrozil	lipid regulation
loprazolam	loprazolam	hypnotic
Lopresor	metoprolol	beta-blocker
lorazepam	lorazepam	antiemetic; anxiolytic
lormetazepam	lormetazepam	hypnotic
Losec	omeprazole	proton pump inhibitors
Lyclear	permethrin	parasiticidal preparations
Maalox	aluminium hydroxide	antacid
Macrobid	nitrofurantoin	urinary tract infections
Macrodantin	nitrofurantoin	urinary tract infections
magnesium sulphate	magnesium sulphate	constipation
magnesiun trisilicate	magnesium trisilicate	anatacid
Manevac	senna	laxative
mannitol	mannitol	diuretic
Marcain	bupivacaine	local anaesthetic
Maxolon	metoclopramide	antiemetic
meclozine	meclozine	antihistamine
Medrone	methylprednisolone	glucocorticoid therapy
mefenamic acid	mefenamic acid	non-steroidal anti-inflammatory (NSAID) drug
Megace	megestrol acetate	progestogens
Melleril	thioridazine	antipsychotic
Mercilon	ethinyloestradiol	combination contraceptives
Metenix 5	metolazone	diuretic
Methadose	methadone	opioid dependence treatment
methtrexate	methotrexate	antimetabolite
Metipranolol	metipranolol	beta-blocker (glaucoma)
Metopirone	metyrapone	Cushings syndrome
Metrodin	urofollitropin	gonadotrophin inhibition
Metrolyl	metronidazole	amoebicides
Miacalcic	salcatonin (calcitonin)	bone metabolism
Micanol	dithranol	psoriasis
Microgynon	ethinyloestradiol	combination contraceptives
Micronor	ethynodiol	contraceptive
Micronor	norethisterone	contraceptive
Microval	ethynodiol	contraceptive
Mictral	nalidixic acid	urinary tract infections
Mifegyne	mifepristone	pregnancy termination
Migril	ergotamine	migraine
Minihep	heparin	anticoagulants
Minims	phenylephrine	sympathomimetic
Minocin	minocycline	antibacterial
Minodiab	glipizide	diabetes
Mintezol	thiabendazole	strongyloidiasis
Mirena	levonorgestrel	contraceptive
Mitomycin C	mitomycin	cytotoxic antibiotic
Mitoxana	ifosfamide	alkylating drug
Mobic	meloxicam	non-steroidal anti-inflammatory (NSAID) drug
Mobiflex	tenoxicam	non-steroidal anti-inflammatory (NSAID) drug
Modecate	fluphenazine	antipsychotic
Moditen	fluphenazine	antipsychotic
Moducren	timolol	beta-blocker (glaucoma)
Monocor	bisoprolol	beta-blocker
Monoparin	heparin	anticoagulants
Monotrim	trimethoprim	antibacterial

Proprietary	Generic	Group/Indication
Monovent	terbutaline	asthma
Monphytol	undecenoates	antiviral drug
Morcap	morphine	analgesic
Motifene	diclofenac	non-steroidal anti-inflammatory (NSAID) drug
Motilium	domperidone	antiemetic
Motipress	nortryptyline	depression
Motval	nortryptyline	depression
MST Continus	morphine	analgesic
Mucogel	aluminium hydroxide	antacid
Multiparin	heparin	anticoagulants
MXL	morphine	analgesic
Mycifradin	neomycin	antibacterial
Mycota	undecenoates	antiviral drug
Myleran	busulphan	alkylating drug
Myocrisin	sodium aurothiomalate	rheumatic disease
Mysoline	primidone	epilepsy
nabilone	nabilone	antiemetic
Naprosyn	naproxen	non-steroidal anti-inflammatory (NSAID) drug
Narcan	naloxone	anatagonist for central and respiratory depression
Nardil	phenelzine	monamine-oxidase inhibitor
Nasonex	mometasone	allergic rhinitis
Nebcin	tobramycin	antibacterial
Negram	nalidixic acid	urinary tract infections
Neogest	ethynodiol	contraceptive
Neo-mercazole	carbimazole	hyperthyroidism
Neoral	cyclosporin	immunosuppressants
NeoRecormon	epoetin-beta	erythropoetin
nicotinic acid	nicotinic acid	lipid regulation
nitrazepam	nitrazepam	hypnotic
Nitromin	glyceryl trinitrate	angina
Nitronal	glyceryl trinitrate	angina
Nivaquine	chloroquine	malaria; disease modifying anti-rheumatic drugs (DMARDs)
Nivaten	nifedipine	calcium channel blocker
Nivemycin	neomycin	antibacterial
Nizoral	ketoconazole	antifungal
Nolvadex	tamoxifen	hormone antagonist
Norditropin	somatotrophin	human growth hormone
Norgeston	ethynodiol	contraceptive
Noriday	ethynodiol	contraceptive
Noristerat	progesterone	contraceptive
Norvir	ritonavir	antiviral drug
Nuelin	theophylline	bronchodilator
Nurofen	ibuprofen	non-steroidal anti-inflammatory (NSAID) drug
Nutrizyme	pancreatin	cystic fibrosis
Nycipren	naproxen	non-steroidal anti-inflammatory (NSAID) drug
Nystan	nystatin	antifungal
Ocusert	pilocarpine nitrate/hydrochloride	miotic
Odrik	trandolapril	ACE inhibitor
oestrogen	oestrogen	hormone replacement therapy (HRT)
Oncovin	vincristine	antineoplastic drug
One Alpha	alfacalcidol	vitamin D supplement
Optilast	azelastine	anti-inflammatory
Oramorph	morphine	analgesic
Orimeten	aminoglutethemide	hormone antagonist
Orovite	pyridoxine	vitamin B6
Ortho Gynest	dienoestrol	topical oestrogens
OrthoCreme	nonoxinols	spermicide
Orudis	ketoprofen	non-steroidal anti-inflammatory (NSAID) drug
Oruvail	ketoprofen	non-steroidal anti-inflammatory (NSAID) drug
Otrivine-Antistin	antazoline	anti-inflammatory
Ovestin	dienoestrol	topical oestrogens

Proprietary	Generic	Group/Indication
Ovranette	ethinyloestradiol	combination contraceptives
oxycodone	oxycodone	analgesic
Palfium	dextromoramide	analgesic
Paludrine	proguanil	malaria
Pamergan	pethidine	analgesic
Pancrease	pancreatin	cystic fibrosis
Pancrex	pancreatin	cystic fibrosis
Paraplatin	carboplatin	antineoplastic drug
Parlodel	bromocriptine mesylate	dopamine receptor stimulant; parkinsonism
Parnate	tranylcypromine	monamine-oxidase inhibitor
Pendramine	penicillamine	disease modifying anti-rheumatic drugs (DMARDs)
pentazocaine	pentazocine	analgesic
Pepcid	famotidine	H2 receptor antagonists
Perdix	moexipril	ACE inhibitor
Periactin	cyproheptadine	antihistamine
Permitabs	potassium permanganate	astringent, oxidiser
Persantin	dipyridamole	antiplatelet
Phenergan	promethazine	antihistamine/antiemetic
phenoxymethylpenicillin	phenoxymethylpenicillin	antibacterial
phosphate	phosphate	supplement
Pilogel	pilocarpine nitrate/hydrochloride	miotic
Pipril	piperacillin	antibacterial
Piriton	chlorpheniramine	antihistamine
Pitressin	vasopressin	posterior pituitary anatagonists
Posiject.	dobutamine	cardiac stimulants
Precortisyl	prednisolone	corticosteroid
Prednesol	prednisolone	corticosteroid
Premarin	dienoestrol	topical oestrogens
Prepulsid	cisapride	antispasmodic
Preservex	aceclofenac	non-steroidal anti-inflammatory (NSAID) drug
Prestim (Timoptol)	timolol	beta-blocker (glaucoma)
Priadel	lithium	mania
Primolut N	norethisterone	contraceptive
Prioderm	malathion	parasiticidal preparations
Pripsen	piperazine	anthelmintics
Pro-Banthine	propantheline	antispasmodic
Prograf	tacrolimus	immunosuppressants
promazine	promazine	antipsychotic/antiemetic
Pronestyl	procainamide	arrhythmias
Propine	dipivefrine	sympathomimetic
propylthiouracil	propylthiouracil	hyperthyroidism
Proscar	finasteride	anti-androgen
Prostap	leuprorelin	hormone antagonist
Prothiaden	dothiepin	depression
Protium	pantoprazole	proton pump inhibitors
Provera	medroxyprogesterone	menstrual problems
Pro-Viron	mesterolone	male sex hormones
proxymetacaine	proxymetacaine	local anaesthetic
Prozac	fluoxetine	selective serotonin re-uptake inhibitor (SSRI)
Psorin	dithranol	psoriasis
Pulmicort	budesonide	corticosteroid
Pyralvex	choline salicylate	local anaesthetic
Pyrogastrone	carbenoxolone	ulcers
Quellada	malathion	parasiticidal preparations
Questran	colestyramine	lipid regulation
quinine	quinine	malaria
Qvar		
Rapitil	nedocromil sodium	anti-inflammatory
Relifex	nabumetone	non-steroidal anti-inflammatory (NSAID) drug
Resonium A	calcium resonium	potassium removal
Retrovir	zidovudine	antiviral drug
Rheumox	azapropazone	non-steroidal anti-inflammatory (NSAID) drug

Proprietary	Generic	Group/Indication
Ridaura	gold (sodium aurothiomalate)	disease modifying anti-rheumatic drugs (DMARDs)
Rifadin	rifampicin	antibacterial
Rifater	rifampicin	antibacterial
Rifinah	rifampicin	antibacterial
Rimactane	rifampicin	antibacterial
Rimactazid	rifampicin	antibacterial
Rinatec	ipratropium	antimuscarinic
Risperdal	risperidone	antipsychotic
Ritalin	methylphenidate	CNS stimulant
Rocaltrol	calcitriol	vitamin D supplement
Rocephin	ceftriaxone	antibacterial
Roferon A	interferon alpha	antiviral drug
Rynacrom	sodium cromoglycate	allergic rhinitis
Rythmodan	disopyramide	arrhythmias
Sabril	vigabatrin	convulsions
Saizen	somatotrophin	human growth hormone
Salazopyrin	sulphasalazine	colitis; Crohn's disease
Sandimmum	cyclosporin	immunosuppressants
Sandostatin	octreotide	somatostatin
SangCya	cyclosporin	immunosuppressants
Sanomigran	pizotifen	migraine
Saventrine	isoprenaline	cardiac stimulants
Scopoderm	hyoscine	antiemetic
Securon	verapamil	calcium channel blocker
Semprex	acrivastine	antihistamine
Senokot	senna	laxative
Septrin	cotrimoxazole	antibacterial
Serc	betahistine	Ménière's disease
Serenace	haloperidol	antipsychotic
Seretide	fluticasone	corticosteroid
Serophene	clomiphene citrate	antioestrogen
Sevredol	morphine	analgesic
Sinequan	doxepin	depression
Slow-Fe	ferrous sulphate	anaemia
sodium bicarbonate	sodium bicarbonate	anatacid
Soframycin	framycetin	antibacterial
Solpadol	paracetamol	analgesic
Solu-Cortel	hydrocortisone	glucocorticoid therapy
Sorbichew	isosorbide dinitrate	angina
Sporanox	itraconazole	antifungal
Stemitel	prochlorperazine	antipsychotic/antiemetic
Stilnoct	zolpidem	hypnotic
streptomycin	streptomycin	antibacterial
Stretase	streptokinase	thrombolytic agents
Stromba	stanozolol	anabolic steroid
Stugeron	cinnarizine	antihistamine
Sudafed	pseudoephedrine	decongestant
Suleo	malathion	parasiticidal preparations
sulphadiazine	sulphadiazine	antibacterial
Suprefact	buserelin	hormone antagonist
Surgam	tiaprofenic acid	non-steroidal anti-inflammatory (NSAID) drug
Survanta	beractant	pulmonary surfactant
Suscard	glyceryl trinitrate	angina
Sustanon	testosterone enanthate/propionate	male sex hormones
Symmetrel	amantadine	antiviral drug; dopaminergic drug used in parkinsonism
Synarel	nafarelin	gonadorelin analogues
Synflex	naproxen	non-steroidal anti-inflammatory (NSAID) drug
Syntaris	flunisolide	allergy
Syntocinon	oxytocin	labour induction
Tagamet	cimetidine	H2 receptor antagonists
Tambocor	flecainide	arrhythmias

Proprietary	Generic	Group/Indication
Tampovagen	dienoestrol	topical oestrogens
Targocid	teicoplanin	antibacterial
Tarivid	ofloxacin	antibacterial
Taxol	paclitaxel	cytotoxic drug
Taxotere	docetaxel	cytotoxic drug
Tazocin	piperacillin	antibacterial
Tegretol	carbamazepine	convulsions
Telfast	fexofenadine	antihistamine
Temazepam	temazepam	hypnotic
Tenben	atenolol	beta-blocker
Tenif	atenolol	beta-blocker
Tenoret	atenolol	beta-blocker
Tenormin	atenolol	beta-blocker
Teoptic	carteolol	beta-blocker (glaucoma)
Teril	carbamazepine	convulsions
Terramycin	oxytetracycline	antibacterial
Theo-Dur	theophylline	bronchodilator
thymol	thymol glycerine	mouthwash
thyroxine	thyroxin	thyroid disease
Tiloryth	erythromycin	antibacterial
Timonil	carbamazepine	convulsions
Tofranil	imipramine	depression
Tolanase	tolbutamide	diabetes
Tomudex	raltitrexed	antimetabolite
Toradol	ketorolac	analgesic
Triapin	ramipril	ACE inhibitor
triclofos	triclofos	hypnotic
tri-iodothyronine	liothyronine sodium	thyroid disease
Triludan	terfenadine	antihistamine
Trimopan	trimethoprim	antibacterial
Tritace	ramipril	ACE inhibitor
Trobicin	spectinomycin	antibacterial
troglitazone	troglitazone	diabetes
Tylex,	paracetamol	analgesic
Ubretid	distigmine bromide	myasthenia gravis
Uirben	nalidixic acid	urinary tract infections
Uniparin	heparin	anticoagulants
Univer	verapamil	calcium channel blocker
Urdox	ursodeoxycholic acid	gallstone dissolution
Ursofalk	ursodeoxycholic acid	gallstone dissolution
Ursogal	ursodeoxycholic acid	gallstone dissolution
Utinor	norfloxacin	antibacterial
Utovlan	norethisterone	contraceptive
Vagifem	dienoestrol	topical oestrogens
Valoid	cyclizine	antiemetic
Valtrex	valaciclovir	antiviral drug
Vancocin	vancomycin	antibacterial
Vascace	cilazapril	ACE inhibitor
Velbe	vinblastine	antineoplastic drug
Ventide	beclomethasone	corticosteroid
Ventolin	salbutamol	asthma
Vepesid	etoposide	antineoplastic drug
Verapress	verapamil	calcium channel blocker
Vertab	verapamil	calcium channel blocker
Vibramycin	doxycycline	antibacterial
Videx	didanosine	antiviral drug
Viraferon	interferon alpha	antiviral drug
Virormone	testosterone enanthate/propionate	male sex hormones
Visclair	mecysteine	mucolytic
Vivalan	viloxazine	depression
Volmax	salbutamol	asthma
Voltarol	diclofenac	non-steroidal anti-inflammatory (NSAID) drug

Proprietary	Generic	Group/Indication
warfarin	warfarin	antiplatelet
Welldorm	chloral hydrate	hypnotic
Wellferon	interferon alpha	antiviral drug
Xylocaine	lignocaine	local anaesthetic
xylometazoline	xylometazoline	nasal decongestant
Yutopar	ritodrine hydrochloride	myometrial relaxant
Zacin	capsaicin	rheumatic disease
Zantac	ranitidine	H2 receptor antagonists
Zelapar	selegiline	dopamine receptor stimulant; parkinsonism
Zerit	stavudine	antiviral drug
Zestril	lisinopril	ACE inhibitor
Zinamide	pyrazinamide	tuberculosis
Zirtek	cetirizine	antihistamine
Zithromax	azithromycin	antibacterial
Zocor	simvastatin	lipid regulation
Zofran	ondansetron	antiemetic
Zoladex	goserelin	hormone antagonist
Zomacton	somatotrophin	human growth hormone
Zomorph	morphine	analgesic
Zoton	lansoprazole	proton pump inhibitors
Zovirax	aciclovir	antiviral drug
Zyloric	allopurinol	gout
Zymovane	zopiclone	hypnotic

Generic	Proprietary	Group/Indication
acarbose	Glucobay	diabetes
aceclofenac	Preservex	non-steroidal anti-inflammatory (NSAID) drug
acetazolamide	Diamox	epilepsy/glaucoma/diuretic
aciclovir	Zovirax	antiviral drug
acrivastine	Semprex	antihistamine
adenosine	Adenocor	arrhythmias
adrenaline	adrenaline	cardiopulmonary resuscitation/anaphylaxis
alendronic acid	Fosamax	osteoporosis
alfacalcidol	AlfaD/One Alpha	vitamin D supplement
allopurinol	Zyloric	gout
alteplase	Actilyse	fibrinolytic drugs
aluminium acetate	aluminium acetate	otitis externa
aluminium hydroxide	Alu-Cap/Maalox/Mucogel	antacid
amantadine	amantadine; Symmetrel	antiviral drug; dopaminergic drug used in parkinsonism
amethocaine	Ametop	local anaesthetic
amikacin	Amikin	antibacterial
amiloride	amiloride	diuretic
aminoglutethemide	Orimeten	hormone antagonist
amiodarone	Cordarone X	arrhythmias
amitriptyline	Lentizol	depression
amlodipine	Cordarone X	arrhythmias
amoxycillin	Amoxil	antibacterial
amphotericin B	Fungilin, Fungizone, Abelcet, AmBisome, Amphocil	antifungal
anastrozole	Arimidex	hormone antagonist
anistreplase	Eminase	fibrinolytic drugs
antazoline	Otrivine-Antistin	anti-inflammatory
apomorphine	Britaject	dopamine receptor stimulant; parkinsonism
aspirin (acetyl salicylic acid)	Caprin; Disprin	analgesic
astemizole	Hismanal	antihistamine
atenolol	Tenormin; Kalten; Tenben; Tenoret; Beta-Adalat; Tenif	beta-blocker
atropine	Isotopo Atropine	antimuscarinic

Generic	Proprietary	Group/Indication
auranofin	Ridaura	rheumatic disease
azapropazone	Rheumox	non-steroidal anti-inflammatory (NSAID) drug
azathioprine	Imuran	cytotoxic immunosuppressant
azelastine	Optilast	anti-inflammatory
azithromycin	Zithromax	antibacterial
baclofen	Lioresal	muscle relaxant
beclomethasone	AeroBec; Becotide; Qvar; Ventide	corticosteroid
bendrofluazide	bendrofluazide	diuretic
benorylate	Benoral	non-steroidal anti-inflammatory (NSAID) drug
benserazide	benserazide	dopamine receptor stimulant; parkinsonism
benzhexol	Broflex	antimuscarinic; parkinsonism
benztropine	Cogentin	antimuscarinic; parkinsonism
benzyl benzoate	benzyl benzoate	antiparasitic
benzylpenicillin	Crystapen	antibacterial
beractant	Survanta	pulmonary surfactant
betahistine	Serc	Ménière's disease
betamethasone	Betnelan; Betnesol	glucocorticoid
betaxolol	Betoptic	beta-blocker (glaucoma)
bisacodyl	bisacodyl	laxative
bismuth chelate	De-Noltab	ulcers
bisoprolol	Emcor; Monocor	beta-blocker
bleomycin	bleomycin	cytotoxic antibiotic
bretylium	Bretylate	arrhythmias
bromocryptine mesylate	Parlodel	dopamine receptor stimulant; parkinsonism
budesonide	Pulmicort	corticosteroid
bumetanide	Burinex	diuretic
bupivacaine	Marcain	local anaesthetic
buserelin	Suprefact	hormone antagonist
busulphan	Myleran	alkylating drug
cabergoline	Cabaser	dopamine receptor stimulant; parkinsonism
caffeine	caffeine	CNS stimulant
calamine	calamine	pruritus
calciferol (see ergocalciferol)		
calcipotriol	Dovonex	psoriasis
calcitonin (see salcalcitonin)		
calcitriol	Calcijex/Rocaltrol	vitamin D supplement
calcium carbonate/acetate	calcium carbonate	anatacid
calcium resonium	Resonium A	potassium removal
capsaicin	Axsain; Zacin	rheumatic disease
captopril	Capoten	ACE inhibitor
carbamazepine	Tegretol; Teril; Timonil	convulsions
carbaryl	Carylderm	antiparasitic
carbenoxolone	Pyrogastrone	ulcers
carbidopa	carbidopa	dopamine receptor stimulant; parkinsonism
carbimazole	Neo-mercazole	hyperthyroidism
carbocysteine	carbocisteine	mucolytic
carboplatin	Paraplatin	antineoplastic drug
carmustine	BCNU	alkylating drug
carob	Carobel	vomiting
carteolol	Teoptic	beta-blocker (glaucoma)
cefadroxil	Baxan	antibacterial
cefotaxime	Claforan	antibacterial
ceftriaxone	Rocephin	antibacterial
cefuroxime	Zinacef/Zinnat	antibacterial
cephalexin	Ceporex/Keflex	antibacterial
cetirizine	Zirtek	antihistamine
chloral hydrate	Welldorm	hypnotic
chlorambucil	Leukeran	alkylating drug
chloramphenicol	Kemicetine	antibacterial
chlordiazepoxide	chlordiazepoxide	anxiolytic
chlorhexidine	Chlorohex; Corsodyl	antibacterial

Generic	Proprietary	Group/Indication
chloroquine	Avloclor; Nivaquine	malaria; disease modifying anti-rheumatic drugs (DMARDs)
chlorpheniramine	Piriton	antihistamine
chlorpromazine	Largactil	antiemetic
chlorpropamide	chlorpropamide	diabetes
chlortetracycline	Aureomycin	antibacterial
cholecalciferol	colecalciferol	vitamin D supplement
choline salicylate	Pyralvex	local anaesthetic
cilazapril	Vascace	ACE inhibitor
cimetidine	Dyspamet; Tagamet	H2 receptor antagonists
cinnarizine	Stugeron	antihistamine
cinoxacin	Cinobac	antibacterial
ciprofloxacin	Ciproxin	antibacterial
cisapride	Prepulsid	antispasmodic
cisplastin	cisplatin	antineoplastic drug
clarithromycin	Klaricid	antibacterial
clavulanic acid	Augmentin	antibacterial
clindamycin	Dalacin	antibacterial
clioquinol	clioquinol	otitis externa
clofibrate	Atromid-S	lipid regulation
clomethiazole	Heminevrin	hypnotic
clomiphene citrate	Clomid; Serophene	antioestrogen
clomipramine	Anafranil	depression
clonidine	Dixarit; catapres	migraine
clotrimazole	clotrimazole	antifungal
clozapine	Clozaril	antipsychotic
codeine	codeine	analgesic; anti diarrhoea
colchicine	colchicine	gout
colestipol	Colestid	lipid regulation
colestyramine	Questran	lipid regulation
colistin	Colomycin	antibacterial
cortisone	Cortisyl	glucocorticoid therapy
cotrimoxazole	Septrin	antibacterial
crotamiton	Eurax	pruritus
cyclizine	Valoid	antiemetic
cyclophosphamide	Endoxana	cytotoxic drug
cyclosporin	Neoral; Sandimmum; SangCya	immunosuppressants
cyproheptadine	Periactin	antihistamine
cyproterone	Androcur	anti-androgen
cytarabarine	Cytostar	antimetabolite
dacarbazine	DTIC-Dome	antineoplastic drug
dactinomycin (actinomycin D)	Comegen Lyovac	cytotoxic antibiotic
danazol	Danol	gonadotrophin inhibition
danthron	Co-danthramer	faecal softeners
dantrolene sodium	Dantrium	muscle relaxant
dapsin		
daunorubicin	DaunoXome	cytotoxic antibiotic
debrisoquine	debrisoquine	adrenergic neurone blockers
deflazacort	Calcort	glucocorticoid therapy
desferrioxamine	Desferal	poisoning treatment
desmopressin	DDAVP; Desmotabs; Desmospray	posterior pituitary antagonists
dexamethasone	Decadron	glucocorticoid therapy
dexamphetamine sulphate	Dexedrine	CNS stimulant
dexfenfluramine	withdrawn	
dextromoramide	Palfium	analgesic
dextropropoxyphene	dextropropoxyphene	analgesic
diamorphine	diamorphine	analgesic
diazepam	diazepam	anxiolytic; muscle relaxant
diazoxide	Eudemine	diabetes
dichlorphenamide		
diclofenac	Voltarol/Diclomax/Motifene/Arthrotec	non-steroidal anti-inflammatory (NSAID) drug

Generic	Proprietary	Group/Indication
didanosine	Videx	antiviral drug
dienoestrol	Ortho Gynest; Ovestin; Premarin; Tampovagen; Vagifem; Estring	topical oestrogens
diflunisal	Dolobid	non-steroidal anti-inflammatory (NSAID) drug
digoxin	Lanoxin	heart failure
dihydrocodeine	DF 118 Forte, DHC Continus	analgesic
dimenhydramine	Dramamine	antihistamine
dipivefrine	Propine	sympathomimetic
dipyridamole	Persantin	antiplatelet
disodium etidronate	Didronel	osteoporosis
disodium pamidronate	Aredia	osteoporosis
disopyramide	Rythmodan/Dirythmin	arrhythmias
distigmine bromide	Ubretid	myasthenia gravis
dithranol	Micanol; Psorin	psoriasis
dobutamine	Dobutrex; Posiject.	cardiac stimulants
docetaxel	Taxotere	cytotoxic drug
docusate sodium	Dioctyl; Docusol	faecal softeners
domperidone	Motilium	antiemetic
dopamine	dopamine	cardiac stimulants
dothiepin	Prothiaden	depression
doxazosin	Cardura	alpha-adrenoreceptor blocker
doxepin	Sinequan	depression
doxorubicin	Caelyx	cytotoxic drug
doxycycline	Vibramycin	antibacterial
droperidol	Droleptan	antipsychotic
edrophonium	edrophonium	skeletal muscle relaxants
enalapril	Innovace	ACE inhibitor
ephedrine hydrochloride	ephedrine	nasal decongestant
epoetin-beta	Eprex; NeoRecormon	erythropoetin
ergocalciferol	Cacit/Calceos/Calchichew	vitamin D supplement
ergotamine	Cafergot; Lingraine; Migril	migraine
erythromycin	Erymax/Erythrocin/Erythroped/ Ilosone/Tiloryth	antibacterial
ethacrynic acid	Edicrin	diuretic
ethambutol	ethambutol	tuberculosis
ethinyloestradiol	Loestrin; Mercilon; Logynon; Microgynon;Brevinor;Ovranette	combination contraceptives
ethynodiol	Femulen; Micronor; Microval; Neogest; Norgeston; Noriday	contraceptive
etodolac	Lodine SR	non-steroidal anti-inflammatory (NSAID) drug
etoposide	Etopophos; Vepesid	antineoplastic drug
famciclovir	Famvir	antiviral drug
famotidine	Pepcid	H2 receptor antagonists
fenbufen	Lederfen	non-steroidal anti-inflammatory (NSAID) drug
fenfluramine	withdrawn	
fenoprofen	Fenopron	non-steroidal anti-inflammatory (NSAID) drug
fentanyl	Durogesic	analgesic
ferrous sulphate	Feospan; Ferrogard; Slow-Fe	anaemia
fexofenadine	Telfast	antihistamine
finasteride	Proscar	anti-androgen
flecainide	Tambocor	arrhythmias
flucloxacillin	Floxapen	antibacterial
fluconazole	Diflucan	antifungal
flucytosine	Ancotil	antifungal
fludrocortisone	Florinef	corticosteroid
flumetasone	Locorten-Viaform	otitis externa
flunisolide	Syntaris	allergy
fluorouracil	Efudix	antimetabolite
fluoxetine	Prozac	selective serotonin re-uptake inhibitor (SSRI)
flupenthixol	Fluanxol	depression
fluphenazine	Moditen; Modecate	antipsychotic
flurbiprofen	Froben	non-steroidal anti-inflammatory (NSAID) drug

Generic	Proprietary	Group/Indication
flutamide	Drogenil	hormone antagonist
fluticasone	Flixotide; Seretide	corticosteroid
folic acid	folic acid	megaloblastic anaemia
formestan	Lentaron	hormone antagonist
foscarnet	Foscavir	antiviral drug
framycetin	Soframycin	antibacterial
frusemide	Lasix	diuretic
fusidic acid	Fucidin	antibacterial
ganciclovir	Cymevene	antiviral drug
gemeprost	gemeprost	prostaglandin
gemfibrozil	Lopid	lipid regulation
gentamicin	Cidomycin/genticin	antibacterial
gestrinone	Dimetriose	gonadotrophin inhibition
glibenclamide	Daonil; Euglucon	diabetes
gliclazide	Diamicron	diabetes
glipizide	Glibenese; Minodiab	diabetes
glycerine	glycerol	laxative
glyceryl trinitrate	Nitromin; Suscard; Nitronal; Deponit	angina
gold (sodium aurothiomalate)	Myocrisin; Ridaura	disease modifying anti-rheumatic drugs (DMARDs)
gonadorelin	HRF	gonadotrophin-releasing hormone
goserelin	Zoladex	hormone antagonist
granisertron	Kytril	nausea; vomiting
griseofulvin	Fulcin, Grisovin	antifungal
guanethidine	Ganda	sympathomimetic
halofantrine	Halfan	malaria
haloperidol	Dozic; Haldol; Serenace	antipsychotic
heparin	Calciparine; Minihep; Monoparin; Multiparin; Uniparin	anticoagulants
human normal immunoglobin (HNIG)	Gammaglobulin; Kabiglobulin	immunoglobulins
hyaluronidase	Hyalase	enzyme
hydralazine	Apresoline	hypertension
hydrochlorothiazide	HydroSaluric	diuretic
hydrocortisone	Efcortesol; Hydrocortone; Solu-Cortel	glucocorticoid therapy
hyoscine	Scopoderm	antiemetic
hyoscine butyl bromide	Buscopan	antispasmodic
ibuprofen	Brufen/Nurofen/Fenbid	non-steroidal anti-inflammatory (NSAID) drug
idoxuridine	Herpid	antiviral drug
ifosfamide	Mitoxana	alkylating drug
imipramine	Tofranil	depression
indinavir	Crixivan	antiviral drug
indomethacin	indometacin	non-steroidal anti-inflammatory (NSAID) drug
inosine pranobex	Imunovir	antiviral drug
insulin	Hypurin; Actrapid; Humalin	diabetes
insulin lispro	Humalog	diabetes
interferon alpha	Roferon A; Intron A; Viraferon; Wellferon	antiviral drug
iodine	iodine	hyperthyroidism
ipratropium	Rinatec	antimuscarinic
isoniazid	isoniazid	tuberculosis
isophane insulin	Insulatard; Humilin I; Hypurin Bovine Isophane	diabetes
isoprenaline	Saventrine	cardiac stimulants
isosorbide dinitrate	Angitak; Isordil; Sorbichew; Isoket; Isocard; Cedocard	angina
isotretinoin	Isotrexin	acne
itraconazole	Sporanox	antifungal
kanamycin	Kannasyn	antibacterial
kaolin	kaolin	absorbents; antimotility
ketoconazole	Nizoral	antifungal
ketoprofen	Orudis/Oruvail	non-steroidal anti-inflammatory (NSAID) drug

Generic	Proprietary	Group/Indication
ketorolac	Toradol	analgesic
lactulose	lactulose	faecal softeners
lamivudine	Epivir	antiviral drug
lamotrigine	Lamictal	convulsions
lansoprazole	Zoton	proton pump inhibitors
leuprorelin	Prostap	hormone antagonist
levobunolol	Betagen	beta-blocker (glaucoma)
levocabastine	Livostin	anti-inflammatory
levodopa	levodopa	dopamine receptor stimulant; parkinsonism
levonorgestrel	Mirena	contraceptive
lignocaine	Xylocaine/Emla/Instillagel/ Laryng-O-jet	local anaesthetic
liothyronine sodium	tri-iodothyronine	thyroid disease
liquid paraffin	liquid paraffin	faecal softeners
lisinopril	Carace; Zestril	ACE inhibitor
lithium	Camcolit; Liskonium; Priadel; Litarex	mania
lodoxamide	Alomide	anti-inflammatory
loperamide	Imodium	antimotility
loprazolam	loprazolam	hypnotic
loratadine	Clarityn	antihistamine
lorazepam	lorazepam	antiemetic; anxiolytic
lormetazepam	lormetazepam	hypnotic
losartan	Cozaar	angiotensin II receptor antagonists
magnesium sulphate	magnesium sulphate	constipation
magnesium trisilicate	magnesiun trisilicate	anatacid
malathion	Derbac; Prioderm; Quellada; Suleo	parasiticidal preparations
mannitol	mannitol	diuretic
meclozine	meclozine	antihistamine
mecysteine	Visclair	mucolytic
medroxyprogesterone	Provera	menstrual problems
mefenamic acid	mefenamic acid	non-steroidal anti-inflammatory (NSAID) drug
mefloquine	Lariam	malaria
megestrol acetate	Megace	progestogens
meloxicam	Mobic	non-steroidal anti-inflammatory (NSAID) drug
melphalan	Alkeran	alkylating drug
mesterolone	Pro-Viron	male sex hormones
metergoline		
metformin	Glucophage	diabetes
methadone	Methadose	opioid dependence treatment
methotrexate	methtrexate	antimetabolite
methyldopa	Aldomet	hypertension
methylphenidate	Ritalin	CNS stimulant
methylprednisolone	Medrone	glucocorticoid therapy
metipranolol	Metipranolol	beta-blocker (glaucoma)
metoclopramide	Maxolon	antiemetic
metolazone	Metenix 5	diuretic
metoprolol	Betaloc; Lopresor	beta-blocker
metronidazole	Flagyl; Metrolyl	amoebicides
metyrapone	Metopirone	Cushings syndrome
miconazole	Daktarin	antifungal
mifepristone	Mifegyne	pregnancy termination
minocycline	Minocin	antibacterial
minoxidil	Loniten	hypertension
misoprostol	Cytotec	prostaglandin analogue
mitomycin	Mitomycin C	cytotoxic antibiotic
moexipril	Perdix	ACE inhibitor
mometasone	Nasonex	allergic rhinitis
morphine	Oramorph, Sevredol, Morcap, MST Continus, MXL, Zomorph	analgesic
mycophenolate	CellCept	immunosuppressants
nabilone	nabilone	antiemetic

Generic	Proprietary	Group/Indication
nabumetone	Relifex	non-steroidal anti-inflammatory (NSAID) drug
nadolol	Corgard	beta-blocker
nafarelin	Synarel	gonadorelin analogues
nalidixic acid	Mictral; Negram; Uirben	urinary tract infections
naloxone	Narcan	anatagonist for central and respiratory depression
nandrolone	Deca-Durabolin	anabolic steroid
naproxen	Naprosyn/Nycipren/Synflex	non-steroidal anti-inflammatory (NSAID) drug
nedocromil sodium	Rapitil	anti-inflammatory
neomycin	Mycifradin/Nivemycin	antibacterial
nicardipine	Cardene	calcium channel blocker
nicorandil	Ikorel	potassium channel activator
nicotinic acid	nicotinic acid	lipid regulation
nifedipine	Adalat; Adipine; Angiopine; Cardilate; Coracten; Fortipine; Nivaten	calcium channel blocker
nitrazepam	nitrazepam	hypnotic
nitrofurantoin	Furadantin; Macrobid; Macrodantin	urinary tract infections
nizatidine	Axid	H2 receptor antagonists
nonoxinols	Delfen; Double Check; Duragel; Gynol II; OrthoCreme	spermicide
norethisterone	Primolut N; Utovlan; Micronor	contraceptive
norfloxacin	Utinor	antibacterial
nortryptyline	Motipress, Motval	depression
nystatin	Nystan	antifungal
octreotide	Sandostatin	somatostatin
oestrogen	oestrogen	hormone replacement therapy (HRT)
ofloxacin	Tarivid	antibacterial
omeprazole	Losec	proton pump inhibitors
ondansetron	Zofran	antiemetic
orphenadrine	Biorphen; Disipal	muscle relaxant; antimuscarinic used in parkinsonism
oxybuprocaine	Benoxinate	local anaesthetic
oxybutinin	Cystrin; Ditropan	urinary incontinence
oxycodone	oxycodone	analgesic
oxymetazoline	Afrazine	decongestant
oxymetholone		
oxytetracycline	Terramycin	antibacterial
oxytocin	Syntocinon	labour induction
paclitaxel	Taxol	cytotoxic drug
pancreatin	Creon; Nutrizyme; Pancrease; Pancrex	cystic fibrosis
pantoprazole	Protium	proton pump inhibitors
paracetamol	Co-codamol, Kapake, Solpadol, Tylex,	analgesic
paradichlorparabenzene		
pemoline		
penicillamine (DMARDs)	Distamine; Pendramine	disease modifying anti-rheumatic drugs
penicillin	Crystapen	antibacterial
pentazocine	pentazocaine	analgesic
pergolide	Celance	dopamine receptor stimulant; parkinsonism
perindopril	Coversyl	ACE inhibitor
permethrin	Lyclear	parasiticidal preparations
pethidine	Pamergan	analgesic
phenelzine	Nardil	monamine-oxidase inhibitor
phenoxymethylpenicillin	phenoxymethylpenicillin	antibacterial
phenylbutazone	Butacote	non-steroidal anti-inflammatory (NSAID) drug
phenylephrine	Minims	sympathomimetic
phenytoin	Epanutin	convulsions
phosphate	phosphate	supplement
physostigmine		
pilocarpine nitrate/hydrochloride	Ocusert, Pilogel	miotic
piperacillin	Pipril/Tazocin	antibacterial

Generic	Proprietary	Group/Indication
piperazine	Pripsen	anthelmintics
piroxicam	Feldine/Brexidol	non-steroidal anti-inflammatory (NSAID) drug
pizotifen	Sanomigran	migraine
podophyllin	Condyline	warts
potassium permanganate	Permitabs	astringent, oxidiser
pravastatin	Lipostat	lipid regulation
prazosin	Hypovase	alpha-adrenoreceptor blocker
prednisolone	Precortisyl; Prednesol	corticosteroid
primidone	Mysoline	epilepsy
probenecid	Benemid	gout
probucol		
procainamide	Pronestyl	arrhythmias
prochlorperazine	Stemitel	antipsychotic/antiemetic
procyclidine	Arpicolin, Kemadrin	antimuscarinic; parkinsonism
progesterone	Depo-Provera; Noristerat	contraceptive
progestin		
proguanil	Paludrine	malaria
promazine	promazine	antipsychotic/antiemetic
promethazine	Phenergan	antihistamine/antiemetic
propantheline	Pro-Banthine	antispasmodic
propranolol	Inderal	beta-blocker
propylthiouracil	propylthiouracil	hyperthyroidism
proxymetacaine	proxymetacaine	local anaesthetic
pseudoephedrine	Galpseud; Sudafed	decongestant
pyrazinamide	Zinamide	tuberculosis
pyridoxine	Orovite	vitamin B6
pyrimethamine	Daraprim	malaria
quinapril	Accupro; Accuretic	ACE inhibitor
quinine	quinine	malaria
raloxifene	Evista	osteoporosis
raltitrexed	Tomudex	antimetabolite
ramipril	Tritace; Triapin	ACE inhibitor
ranitidine	Zantac	H2 receptor antagonists
reserpine	withdrawn	
resorcinol	Eskamel	acne
rifampicin	Rifadin; Rimactane; Rifater; Rifinah; Rimactazid	antibacterial
risperidone	Risperdal	antipsychotic
ritodrine hydrochloride	Yutopar	myometrial relaxant
ritonavir	Norvir	antiviral drug
salbutamol	Ventolin; Volmax; Aerolin Autohaler; Asmasal Clickhaler	asthma
salcatonin (calcitonin)	Calsynar; Miacalcic	bone metabolism
salicylic acid	Acnisal	acne topical preparation
saquinavir	Fortovase/Invirase	antiviral drug
selegiline	Eldepryl; Zelapar	dopamine receptor stimulant; parkinsonism
senna	Manevac; Senokot	laxative
silver nitrate	Avoca	warts
silver sulphadiazine	Flamazine	antibacterial
simvastatin	Zocor	lipid regulation
sodium aurothiomalate	Myocrisin	rheumatic disease
sodium bicarbonate	sodium bicarbonate	anatacid
sodium cromoglycate	Rynacrom	allergic rhinitis
sodium tetradecyl sulphate	Fibro-Vein	sclerotherapy of varicose veins
sodium valproate	Epilim; Convulex	convulsions
somatotrophin	Genotropin; Humatrope; Norditropin; Saizen; Zomacton	human growth hormone
spectinomycin	Trobicin	antibacterial
spironolactone	Aldactone	diuretic
stanozolol	Stromba	anabolic steroid
stavudine	Zerit	antiviral drug
streptokinase	Kabikinase/Stretase	thrombolytic agents

Generic	Proprietary	Group/Indication
streptomycin	streptomycin	antibacterial
sucralfate	Antepsin	ulcers
sulindac	Clinoril	non-steroidal anti-inflammatory (NSAID) drug
sulphadiazine	sulphadiazine	antibacterial
sulphasalazine	Salazopyrin	colitis; Crohn's disease
sulphinpyrazone	Anturan	gout
sumatriptin	Imigran	migraine
tacrolimus	Prograf	immunosuppressants
tamoxifen	Nolvadex	hormone antagonist
teicoplanin	Targocid	antibacterial
temazepam	Temazepam	hypnotic
tenoxicam	Mobiflex	non-steroidal anti-inflammatory (NSAID) drug
terazosin	Hytrin	alpha-adrenoreceptor blocker
terbutaline	Bricanyl; Monovent;	asthma
terfenadine	Triludan	antihistamine
terlipressin	Glypressin	posterior pituitary anatagonists
testosterone enanthate/propionate	Sustanon, Virormone	male sex hormones
tetracycline	Achromycin/Decteclo	antibacterial
theophylline	Nuelin; Lasma; Theo-Dur	bronchodilator
thiabendazole	Mintezol	strongyloidiasis
thioguanine	Lanvis	antimetabolite
thioridazine	Melleril	antipsychotic
thymol glycerine	thymol	mouthwash
thyroxin	thyroxine	thyroid disease
tiaprofenic acid	Surgam	non-steroidal anti-inflammatory (NSAID) drug
tibolone	Livial	osteoporosis
timolol	Betim; Biocadren; Moducren; Prestim (Timoptol)	beta-blocker (glaucoma)
tinidazole	Fasigyn	antifungal
tobramycin	Nebcin	antibacterial
tolbutamide	Tolanase	diabetes
tolcapone	withdrawn	
tolfenamic acid	Clotam	non-steroidal anti-inflammatory (NSAID) drug
topotecan	Hycamtin	antineoplastic drug
trandolapril	Gopten; Odrik	ACE inhibitor
tranexamic acid	Cyklokapron	antifibrinolytic agent
tranylcypromine	Parnate	monamine-oxidase inhibitor
triamcinolone	Kenalog	glucocorticoid therapy
triamterene	Dytac	diuretic
triclofos	triclofos	hypnotic
trimethoprim	Monotrim/Trimopan	antibacterial
troglitazone	troglitazone	diabetes
undecenoates	Monphytol; Mycota	antiviral drug
urofollitropin	Metrodin	gonadotrophin inhibition
ursodeoxycholic acid	Destolit; Urdox; Ursofalk; Ursogal	gallstone dissolution
valaciclovir	Valtrex	antiviral drug
valsartan	Diovan	angiotensin II receptor antagonists
vancomycin	Vancocin	antibacterial
vasopressin	Pitressin	posterior pituitary anatagonists
verapamil	Cordilox; Securon; Univer; Verapress;Vertab	calcium channel blocker
vigabatrin	Sabril	convulsions
viloxazine	Vivalan	depression
vinblastine	Velbe	antineoplastic drug
vincristine	Oncovin	antineoplastic drug
warfarin	warfarin	antiplatelet
xylometazoline	xylometazoline	nasal decongestant
zalcitabine	Hivid	antiviral drug
zidovudine	Retrovir	antiviral drug
zolpidem	Stilnoct	hypnotic
zopiclone	Zymovane	hypnotic

Answers: person centred studies and multiple choice questions

CHAPTER FIVE

Person Centred Study 1

1. The health visitor will need to explain how passive and active immunity is formed in a very simple but clear way, for example that prenatal maternal antibodies and those provided by breastfeeding can help while the baby is small but will disappear and the baby must begin to provide her own active immunity through vaccination.

2. The health visitor needs to explain the protocols about vaccination and how babies who should not be vaccinated for any reason are screened out of the programme. Without alarming Mrs Bailey, the health visitor needs to make it clear to her that many diseases are on the increase and antibiotic resistance is increasing, which makes treating many infections secondary to a viral infection more difficult. In addition, foreign travel has meant that diseases that were rare in the United Kingdom are now becoming more prevalent. General global warming has also meant warmer winters recently and an upsurge in children's viral infections, particularly because a scare campaign by a local paper has frightened many mothers away from immunisation clinics.

3. Mr and Mrs Bailey could be told about EMLA cream for Mr Bailey. This is a local anaesthetic, which unfortunately cannot be used for infants under 1 year of age but could enable Mr Bailey to have vaccinations to prevent his bringing home anything 'nasty' from abroad to his family. It is important to emphasise to both parents that if they remain calm and reassuring, their little girl is unlikely to remember the temporary pain of the injection and should not develop the fear of needles that Mr Bailey has.

Person Centred Study 2

1. The nurse's task is to explain to George the need for protease inhibitors, their mode of action, and, specifically, the importance of keeping to the regime. Protease inhibitors in combination with nucleoside analogues offer hope in progressive or advanced HIV infection. As George has had so many problems with changes of treatment, it will take a very positive view on the part of the nurse to help him to accept the difficulties of protease inhibitors, such as nausea, as necessary to his future wellbeing. Regular check-ups may help George to discuss any side effects that may occur and to monitor his progress.

2. George also needs preparation for the nausea that is likely to accompany protease inhibitors as there is treatment that may help. Protease inhibitors can be started at low doses, taking 3 months to reach the treatment dose to try and avoid the sickness. Access to complementary therapies is available for many patients, which may also help with the nausea. Metoclopramide then ondansetron can be prescribed and he will need to be on a maintenance dose of ondansetron during the treatment.

3. George needs a more realistic idea of the severity of his prognosis without treatment, without threatening his coping mechanism. The nurse must explore George's feelings about the disease to discover how realistic and aware he is. New treatments, especially the latest combination of drugs, appear to be able to reduce the virus so that, because the viral load is literally so small as to be uncountable, it may, for practical purposes, be seen by some as a cure. However, treatment and follow-up will be necessary for the rest of his life. Therefore, compliance and a hopeful attitude will improve his long-term chance of survival as research moves on. New treatments to boost the immune system are evolving and there is much hope if George can be helped to take a positive, realistic and proactive role in his treatment.

1. b, c, e
2. a, c
3. b, d, e
4. a, c, d
5. b
6. e
7. b, c, d
8. a
9. a, e
10. c, d, e

CHAPTER SIX

Person Centred Study 1

1. You might first think of damage to the epithelium lining the upper part of the digestive tract caused by the combined cytotoxic action of the chemotherapeutic regime as a cause of Jean's sore mouth and throat. Because these agents are not cell cycle specific, they can damage 'normal' epithelial cells: the fast-replicating cells in the basal layers of gastrointestinal tract epithelium as well as the more superficial ones in G0. The result may be an inflammatory reaction and may lead to ulceration, which is very painful. Once ulceration has occurred, superimposed infection is more likely.

   A further cause might be bone marrow suppression. Each of these drugs is associated with a moderate risk of bone marrow suppression, particularly granulocyte production inhibition, but together they have synergistic toxic effects. As a result of the reduction in white blood cell production, Jean is more likely to succumb to infection. The mouth is a particularly vulnerable site as it has a large population of transient microorganisms. Viral, bacterial or fungal infection is possible.

   Another cause might be anaemia resulting from suppression of erythropoiesis in the bone marrow. Because of the long life of red blood cells (120 days), the effects of the first course of chemotherapy on erythropoiesis may now be causing symptoms.

   An indirect contributory cause may be the tiredness often associated with chemotherapy (and with anaemia), although Jean has not complained of this. Tiredness may lead to a less meticulous oral hygiene routine than normal, which in turn predisposes to infection in the area. Nausea, an adverse effect of this regime, may have prevented Jean from drinking enough to maintain hydration and this would dry the mouth, contributing to the likelihood of superimposed infection.

2. You could check the nature of the cause(s) by first carefully inspecting Jean's mouth, with the aid of a torch, to identify areas of redness that would indicate inflammation or obvious ulceration. This examination may also identify overgrowth of microorganisms as small patches or a 'coating' on the tongue or palate and/or oropharynx. Associated with this, Jean's breath may smell. Nasal and throat swabs sent to the laboratory for culture and sensitivity tests may give you evidence of the infective agent(s).

   On examination of her skin and nail beds you may find that Jean appears abnormally pale or has a cyanotic tinge to the periphery, suggesting she may be anaemic; on questioning, Jean may admit to feeling increasingly tired over the past few days. By checking the latest full blood count result and comparing it with previous ones, you might identify a pattern of decreasing white and/or red blood cell counts, suggesting that bone marrow suppression is having an effect. A further full blood count would aid the diagnosis.

   On assessment of her body temperature you may find it is raised, suggesting an infection. However, pyrexia may not be present, as localised infection may not yet have produced systemic symptoms; alternatively, it may be because some microorganisms do not necessarily cause a pyrexial response. If Jean is apyrexial but has a raised pulse, this may suggest, among other causes, incipient systemic response to infection or a degree of anaemia sufficient to cause an adaptive cardiovascular response (see Chapter 1 *Introduction to the nature and causation of disease* and Chapter 5 *Drugs and immunological disorders*).

3. Other adverse effects associated with cisplatin, apart from the nausea mentioned above, include kidney, ear and peripheral nerve damage, leading to water and electrolyte imbalance, partial deafness and tingling or reduced sensation in the hands and feet. Similarly, liver and cardiovascular damage may be present, associated with doxorubicin. If Jean has a tachycardia, its cause may lie here rather than relate to an infection or anaemia.

   If the infusing solution should extravasate, you will find evidence of local erythema and swelling caused by cisplatin and blistering caused by doxorubicin. On questioning, or, more likely, spontaneously, Jean would tell you that the area around the cannula is very painful.

   As Jean is only 42 years old, she was probably premenopausal at the time of her operation. She may now be suffering from the symptoms associated with menopause such as hot flushes and sweats. Infection may mistakenly be assumed as the cause of these.

MCQs

1. all
2. a, b, d
3. a, b, e
4. a, c, d
5. b, d
6. a, d, e
7. a, c, e

8. a, b, c, e
9. a, b, d
10. a, c, d, e

CHAPTER SEVEN

Person Centred Study 1

1. Marjorie's abdominal symptoms may be the result of the 'fright or flight' mechanism associated with heightened sympathetic arousal. In order to ready the body to face or remove itself from danger, blood is diverted from the gut to the musculoskeletal system and to provide a greater flow to the brain, lungs and heart. The result is a sense of nausea and abdominal discomfort.

2. Marjorie's family doctor prescribed dothiepin rather than fluoxetine probably because her symptoms included anxiety and she needed the anxiolytic effect of dothiepin, which is not a feature of fluoxetine.

3. Marjorie would have been advised that dothiepin takes around 10 days to build up to therapeutic levels in the central nervous system and therefore it will take time before she feels the benefit of medication. Additionally, dothiepin produces antimuscarinic side effects, which may cause blurring of vision, dry mouth and hesitancy in initiating micturition. She may feel drowsy, and if this is so, she should not drive a car.

Person Centred Study 2

1. Edward's early symptoms of absent mindedness may have been influenced at this point by the acetylcholine depletion at the central nervous system synapses. His worsening symptoms would have developed as the structural changes surrounding the neurons developed; neurofibrillary tangles, tau protein and plaque deposition would impede nerve impulse transmission in the central nervous system.

2. Edward may have been prescribed tacrine in an attempt to augment the acetylcholine levels in the synapses and to halt the progress of the disease.

3. Edward's wife is likely to have been told that effective cure or containment of Alzheimer's disease has not yet been achieved. Symptomatic relief may be obtained from the use neuroleptics, antidepressants and anxiolytics, but improvements are likely to be of a temporary nature. The disease follows a degenerative pathway over a period of years, but although at present the prognosis is poor, knowledge about the pathology of this disease is increasing and new products may become available to help patients such as Edward. She will at some appropriate stage need to be made aware of respite help that is available for her and Edward.

MCQs

1. d
2. c
3. e
4. a
5. b
6. c, e
7. e
8. c, d
9. c, e
10. a

CHAPTER EIGHT

Person Centred Study 1

1. The inflammatory response causes vascular oedema, and increased permeability of the vessel walls. Purulent exudate then forms, which leads to increased pressure within the brain, causing compression of the meninges that surround all parts of the brain and spinal cord. The outcome of this is compression of the optic nerve, which results in photophobia, and general compression of the neural tissue; this increases the pressure in the cerebral spinal fluid, which thus irritates and compresses the meninges surrounding all parts of the brain and spinal cord. The consequent irritation of the nerve endings in the meninges caused Lana to experience the headache and for her normal behaviour to alter as a result of feeling ill.

2. The toxins from the multiplying bacteria cause inflammation of the walls of the capillaries and blood leaks into the intercellular spaces.

3. Antibiotics will be given intravenously to counteract the bacteria multiplying and dexamethasone will be administered to reduce the inflammation in the skull and reduce the pressure there so that tissue does not get damaged. These drugs are given intravenously so that therapeutic blood levels may be reached quickly.

Person Centred Study 2

1. These symptoms are classic of an overdose of levodopa and carbidopa. There is an increase in the level of levodopa that results in increased deposition in the peripheral tissues and gut. This leads to the side effects of nausea, vomiting and postural hypotension. The hypotension is brought about by the collection of dopamine in the noradrenaline nerve terminal where it acts as a false transmitter, leading to vasodilatation. The effects of extra dopamine within the body results in the development of temporary psychosis.

2. Later, when questioned, Mr Simons reveals that he was not sure that he had taken his morning dose and took

another. It is important to advise Mr Simons that if in future he is not sure whether he has taken his medication he should miss that dose in order to avoid the side effects he had experienced.

MCQs

1. b, c, e
2. a, c
3. a, c, e
4. b, e
5. b, e
6. c, d, e
7. a, d
8. a
9. a, c
10. a, d, e

CHAPTER NINE

Person Centred Study 1

1. As Leslie's optician discovered the beginnings of glaucoma, it is important to explain that initially glaucoma is asymptomatic but if left untreated can cause progressive loss of peripheral vision as the light sensitive cells of the retina are damaged by the back pressure from the aqueous humour on the lens and backwards onto the vitreous humour and thus the retina. Treatment is necessary to ensure that he continues to have minimal problems with his eyes.

2. It has long been recognised that glaucoma tends to 'run in families'. Because of this, eye tests are free to those with family members with the condition. Leslie will not have to pay for any more eye tests.

3. The doctor has ordered timolol, which is a beta-blocker. This can enter the systemic circulation as well as the eye and can make the symptoms of bronchial asthma worse by inducing bronchospasm, so it is important first to check the patient's medical history.

4. Although the eyes have natural immunoglobulins to help protect them against infections in the environment, contamination of his drops with bacteria could cause a serious eye infection. Microorganisms can proliferate at room temperature and over time the drops can deteriorate, which is why they must be refrigerated and disposed of by the date on the label. Leslie could administer an infection along with the acetazolamide drops and cause a serious intraocular infection, which, apart from causing intense pain, could put his eyesight at further risk.

MCQs

1. c
2. c, d

3. d
4. d
5. all
6. all
7. all
8. all
9. e
10. c

Person Centred Study 2

1. You could explain to Danielle that the reason for the recurrent earache is the anatomy of a small child's ear, which predisposes to infection ascending from upper respiratory tract infections. He probably gets these from the coughs and colds the other members of the family bring home from school and work. The middle ear directly communicates with the nose by the Eustachian tube to the pharynx, the throat, and is very small in a young child. Pressure differences between the external and middle ear are equalised through this passage. Inflammation, whether caused by infection or allergy, can swell the membranes, blocking the tube and causing earache, which is called otitis media, that is, inflammation of the middle ear.

2. Insertion of grommets is not recommended in the case of occasional otitis media. The middle ear can, with repeated and chronic infection, become filled with fluid as a result of the inflammatory exudate. This exudate eventually becomes thickened and the condition is termed glue ear. The thickened exudate that remains in the middle ear from persistent infection prevents the little bones of the middle ear from moving and causes loss of hearing as sound cannot get from the ear drum to the inner ear. After repeated audiometry, if the hearing loss is considered severe enough, then the decision to put grommets in is made. The 'glue' is sucked out under anaesthetic and grommets are inserted to act as a drain and 'air' the ear.

3. Although it is now debatable whether antibiotics are given for red ear or earache, this doctor may have prescribed a broad-spectrum antibiotic because of the fever, indicating a systemic viral or bacterial infection. He may also have been able to see a red ear drum, indicating that enough inflammation is present to make it likely that a secondary infection will develop. Because of this, even if it is a viral infection and is not amenable to antibiotics, a broad-spectrum antibiotic is necessary to prevent a secondary infection with a bacterium or to treat a bacterial infection if present. Other doctors, of course, might treat Dean differently.

4. Dean's grandmother is right in that children tend to 'outgrow' earache and ear infections because the middle

ear structures, as well as all of the anatomy of the head and neck, increase in size, therefore making it less likely for infections to travel upwards. His immune system will also have matured and developed immunity to many of the germs he is contacting now and will be able to deal with viruses and bacteria in a more efficient manner.

CHAPTER TEN

Person Centred Study 1

1. It would be important to know whether Mary is receiving steroids for medication, as the symptoms are classic of Cushing's syndrome with an iatrogenic cause.

2. Ask her whether she has noticed thinning of her legs (due to muscle loss), and whether she finds it difficult to stand from the sitting position. Look at her face to see if there is rounding of the cheeks (moon face) and plethora visible. Another question you could ask is whether she has any problems with sleep. Iatrogenic Cushing's syndrome is the type most commonly seen in clinical practice and nurses need to be aware of the problems it can give rise to.

Person Centred Study 2

1. Because Eileen is using human insulin, injecting into the same spot repeatedly can lead to hypertrophy of the subcutaneous layer of fat. This then slows the absorption of the injected insulin. Unfortunately, a hypertrophied site is painless, which encourages further usage. Animal insulin leads to atrophy of the subcutaneous fat, which produces the same effect on the rate of insulin absorption.

2. It matters whether insulin is injected intramuscularly or subcutaneously. This is because the insulin is absorbed more quickly by active muscles. Eileen is a slim lady and therefore does not have much subcutaneous tissue, so when she first gave her injection into her arm, the insulin entered the muscle, rather than the subcutaneous layers. If consumption of food were to be delayed, the insulin would lower the blood glucose levels too rapidly, which would result in hypoglycaemic symptoms of the type that Eileen experienced.

3. It is important to explain to Eileen that when she rotates a site, this does not only mean moving to thigh or abdomen; she also needs to find a new location within that anatomical site. It is also important to inform her that the abdomen absorbs insulin at a faster rate than the thighs and to ensure that blood glucose levels are maintained, it is best for her to use the abdominal site before eating the main meal of the day. Eileen needs

also to be given the reassurance that, if the lumpiness does not gradually disappear then it is possible to remove it surgically.

MCQs

1. a, b, c, d, e
2. c, d, e
3. a, c, d
4. d
5. b, d
6. c
7. a
8. c, e
9. c, d
10. b

CHAPTER ELEVEN

Person Centred Study 1

1. Mr Thresher has irritated his lungs for many years so now the mucus-secreting glands are hypertrophied in their effort to protect the bronchial passages. This over secretion leads to plugging of the smaller bronchioles that lead to the alveoli and this results in chronic infection. As the alveoli are damaged and their septa are broken down, elastic recoil is lost and Mr Thresher cannot cough out the infected debris that lies over the gas exchange membrane. Carbon dioxide is retained as it cannot diffuse out of the blood and oxygen cannot reach these end passages for exchange, so chronic hypoxia is inevitable. The infected residue in the lower lung lobes moves up towards the pharynx when Mr Thresher lies horizontal in bed; he is experiencing postural drainage. Gravity pulls the thick fluid from the alveoli sacs. When he sits up in the morning the movement of fluid in his respiratory airways stimulates his cough reflex and he is able to expel the sputum.

2. Ipratropium bromide antagonises acetylcholine at receptor sites on the bronchial smooth muscle, resulting in bronchodilatation. It is a preventative treatment rather than for control of bronchospasm. Mr Thresher would have to understand that it could make him dry mouthed but the constant use would keep his airways dilated so that he could experience better gas exchange all the time and perhaps reduce the periods of breathlessness.

Person Centred Study 2

1. Salbutamol works on the β receptors in the respiratory smooth muscle to reduce spasm. It is usually used to dilate the bronchioles when expiratory wheeze is evident. It produces tachycardia, shakiness, vasodilatation and headache if used frequently as it has sympathetic nerve stimulation properties. In children, hyperactivity may be apparent and this may be the effect on Jamie. By

understanding these frightening effects the nurse will be more able to prepare mother and child to give the medication and to understand Jamie's reactions.

2. In an asthma attack, the smooth muscle of the bronchioles goes into spasm in response to some irritant stimulus, for example particles from Jamie's father's mink pelts. The lumen of the bronchioles then closes and mucus production increases to protect the passage lining. This mucus is sticky and plugs the small airways as it drops down towards the alveoli. Expiration of carbon dioxide is inhibited so the alveoli expand and become over inflated so that elastic recoil is lost to push air out of the lungs. Jamie will keep taking lots of small breaths in and will need to be encouraged to breathe out; it is a frightening feeling and it increases panic as the sympathetic nervous system is stimulated. As the airway lining becomes more irritated it swells. The small capillaries in the mucosa leak fluid under the effect of histamine, which is released when tissue cells are damaged. Jamie's chest will feel very tight and he may feel sick and dry mouthed.

MCQs

1. a, b, c, d, e
2. b, c
3. b, d, e
4. c, d, e
5. b
6. a, b, c
7. a, d
8. a
9. b, c, d
10. c, d

CHAPTER TWELVE

Person Centred Study 1

1. One of the contraindications to administering a fibrinolytic agent such as streptokinase is active peptic ulceration. A frequent and undesirable effect of thrombolytic therapy is internal and superficial bleeding. Therefore after the administration of streptokinase Mr Thomas will be at great risk of bleeding from the site of ulceration.

2. The nurse's priority is to monitor Mr Thomas for possible systemic reactions during therapy and for 24 hours after therapy; these reactions include the major complications of thrombolysis such as anaphylaxis, haemorrhage, acute hypotension, cardiac arrhythmias and coronary artery occlusion. Baseline observation and continuous cardiac monitoring provide objective knowledge from which to determine a change in Mr Thomas' condition. Drugs for managing anaphylaxis, sudden bleeding or cardiac arrythmias must be readily accessible.

Mr Thomas's pulse and blood pressure should be recorded every 15 minutes while the infusion is in progress. He will need to be observed carefully for signs of bleeding, more specifically haematemesis, given his history of peptic ulceration. The physician should be notified immediately if bleeding occurs or is suspected, and treatment discontinued. The less obvious indications of bleeding such as redness, bruising and haematoma must also be watched for and Mr Thomas' cannula must be inspected regularly as this is the most common bleeding point. Mr Thomas' urine should be tested for haematuria.

Mr Thomas' temperature should also be recorded every 15 minutes while the infusion is in progress. This is to enable the early detection of possible febrile reactions caused by an inflammatory response to the streptococcal bacteria from which streptokinase is derived. The nurse should also monitor Mr Thomas for signs of anaphylaxis such as skin rash, nausea, flushing, bronchospasm and hypotension. If anaphylaxis is suspected the infusion should be discontinued immediately.

Person Centred Study 2

1. Atenolol is a β-adrenoceptor blocking agent. Although beta-blockers are effective anti-hypertensive agents, their mode of action is not completely understood. Atenolol is a cardioselective beta-blocking drug, which means that it tends to block the β_1 cardiac sites rather than β_2 peripheral sites. The blocking of the β_1 adrenoceptors causes a decrease in heart rate and cardiac output, which in turn reduces the blood pressure.

blood pressure = cardiac output × peripheral resistance

Some beta-blockers depress the plasma renin level, which would lead to a decrease in peripheral resistance through vasodilatation and a decrease in blood volume.

Bendrofluazide is a thiazide diuretic and they are effective anti-hypertensive agents because they promote salt and water loss; this reduces blood volume and causes arteriolar dilatation. Both vasodilatation and a reduction in blood volume reduce the peripheral resistance and therefore the blood pressure.

2. Paul Sandford should be given the following information about taking his drugs:

- To take his medication as prescribed, no more and no less.
- Not to stop taking the medication abruptly; rebound hypertension or chest pain may occur if he suddenly stops taking the atenolol.
- To contact his doctor if he becomes ill and is unable to take the prescribed doses.
- He may notice a decrease in exercise tolerance and dizziness or fainting may occur with increased activity.

- Not to take any non-prescription medications without first checking with the doctor.
- Alcohol may enhance the hypotensive effect.

  The side effects that Mr Sandford may experience as a result of taking atenolol are

- Cold extremities.
- Muscle fatigue.
- Gastrointestinal disturbances, which may be reduced if the drug is taken just before meals.
- A skin rash.
- Dry, burning eyes.

  Paul has been prescribed a low dose of bendroflu-azide, which should minimise the incidence of adverse side effects. However, he should be encouraged to include potassium-rich foods in his diet such as bananas, oranges, dates, raisins, fresh vegetables, pota-toes (especially the skins), meat and fish to prevent the development of hypokalaemia. He should be made aware of the early signs of hypokalaemia, which are apathy, muscle weakness, abdominal distension and an overall feeling of lethargy.

3. Paul Sandford could be given the following information about non-pharmacological measures he could adopt to help lower his blood pressure.

   - If he is overweight Paul should be encouraged to lose weight. He may need dietary advice as to an appropriate calorie intake for his weight and level of activity.
   - Paul should carefully assess his alcohol intake (a heavy alcohol consumption is associated with high blood pressure). If he normally drinks more than the recommended amount (21 units/week) he should be advised to reduce his alcohol intake.
   - There is overwhelming evidence that lowering salt intake lowers blood pressure. To reduce his salt intake Paul should not add salt to his food and not cook with salt. He should avoid very salty foods and processed food. He may also like to consider salt-free bread. If Mrs Sandford does most of the cooking she will need to be involved in the discussions related to diet.
   - There is evidence that an increase in potassium intake is associated with lower blood pressure. Mr Sandford could increase his level of potassium intake by increasing the amount of vegetables (i.e. greens, pota-toes), legumes (peas, lentils, beans) and fruit he eats.
   - Regular physical exercise helps in lowering the blood pressure. Paul should be encouraged to take up a form of aerobic exercise such as swimming, running, cycling or jogging. The amount of exercise should be approximately 20–30 minutes, three times per week, to maintain a level of fitness and to lower blood pressure.

4. Mr Sandford should be given the following information about captopril:

   - Not to discontinue the drug abruptly.
   - Not to use non-prescribed (cough, cold or allergy) products unless directed by a doctor.
   - To continue to take the prescribed dose even if he thinks that his blood pressure has returned to within normal limits and medication is no longer necessary.
   - To inform the doctor if mouth ulcers, sore throat, fever, palpitations, chest pain or ankle oedema occur.
   - He may experience dizziness or fainting during the first few days of therapy.
   - To rise from a sitting position slowly to reduce the effects of postural hypotension.

MCQs
1. c
2. c
3. a
4. e
5. b
6. c
7. d
8. c
9. e
10. a

CHAPTER THIRTEEN

Person Centred Study 1

1. An NSAID such as naproxen can be a very effective treatment for rheumatoid arthritis because in regular full dosage it has an analgesic and an anti-inflammatory effect.

2. Jane needed to continue taking the naproxen for 2–3 months after beginning the gold therapy because the auranofin has a slow action, only starting to work after 4–6 weeks and taking up to 6 months to produce the full effect. It is important that Jane realises that there may be a delay in order that good compliance is maintained during the early treatment period.

3. The most common side effect that Jane may experience is diarrhoea. This can be reduced by encouraging her to eat lots of bran to add bulk to the stools. Other common side effects are nausea and abdominal pain. Adverse effects that Jane should be informed to report to her doctor immediately include ulceration of the mouth (a possible sign of haematological toxicity), a metallic taste sensation, bleeding, skin reactions, peripheral neuritis, breathlessness, alopecia and jaundice.

4. Corticosteroids produce many side effects, especially if given in high doses or for prolonged periods. Two of the side effects associated with corticosteroid treatment that may particularly affect Jane are

- Altered glucose metabolism, with the possible precipitation of diabetes. If Jane were to take steroids they would reduce the hypoglycaemic effect of the insulin she is required to take and her blood sugar levels would rise, thus affecting her diabetic control.
- Altered calcium–phosphorus balance, producing osteoporosis and a tendency towards bone fracture. If Jane was prescribed steroids for her rheumatoid arthritis, it may be necessary, given her age, to monitor her bone mass, as she would be at increased risk of developing osteoporosis.

Person Centred Study 2

1. Mr Rudge should be reassured that the indomethacin will relieve his pain within 24–48 hours of starting to take the drug. It is unlikely that Mr Rudge will experience any serious side effects as he has only been prescribed a 4-day course. However, he should also be made aware of the possible side effects he may experience, which are headaches, dizziness, blurred vision and gastrointestinal disturbances. The gastrointestinal disturbances may include nausea, anorexia, vomiting, diarrhoea or constipation. Mr Rudge should be informed to report any of these effects to his GP who can then review the medication.

2. As Mr Rudge has only suffered one attack of gout he will not be prescribed any preventative treatment. He should, however, be encouraged to alter certain aspects of his lifestyle in an attempt to prevent further attacks. He should be encouraged to lose weight by altering his diet. He could be referred to a dietician who would be able to provide him with the appropriate advice and diet sheets. Mr Rudge should also be made aware of the foods containing high levels of purine such as offal, sardines, salmon, pulses, gravies and game, so that he can exclude them from his diet. Mr Rudge should be encouraged to reduce his alcohol intake as it increases uric acid levels. It will also help to reduce his weight. More specifically, lager has a high purine content and should be avoided. Mr Rudge should be encouraged to take more exercise. A sensible and appropriate regime could be discussed with his GP.

3. Mr Rudge has been taking bendrofluazide for his hypertension. This is a thiazide diuretic, which causes hyperuricaemia and may therefore have contributed to Mr Rudge's attack of gout. Hence the need to change his anti-hypertensive therapy to a different class of drug.

4. Mr Rudge is prescribed another dose of indomethacin because when treatment with allopurinol is commenced the blood urate level is likely to fall and this change in blood urate level may lead to an acute attack of gout. To prevent this from occurring, prophylactic indomethacin is prescribed concomitantly.

MCQs

1. d
2. c
3. b
4. e
5. d
6. a
7. b
8. c
9. e
10. c

CHAPTER FOURTEEN

Person Centred Study 1

1. Phosphate enemas increase water absorption in the colon by osmotic action. This increases the osmotic pressure within the colon after bacterial degradation and stimulates peristalsis. (A nurse should also address the fluid balance of their patient as the cause of the constipation.) It should be given at room temperature and gently so as not to shock or damage the elderly lady's colon mucosa. It can cause abdominal cramps and make the patient nauseous, so Mrs Davies should not be left alone until a result is evident. Glycerine suppositories also draw water into the colon, so there is a possibility that Mrs Davies may have expelled them too quickly, before they could have effect. They may have started the treatment and the phosphate enema, being a fluid rather than a solid entity, was able to build on drawing of water into the gut to increase the lumen pressure. Some persistent constipation may need regular enema use. This medication may need to continue after the problem has been addressed to rehabilitate the call to stool; however, the prolonged use of phosphate enemas may lead to the development of poor bowel tone and more resistant constipation, with irritation of the lower bowel mucosa.

2. Mrs Davies may also have been relieved to have been helped, so her sympathetic response to the gut muscles reduced, which allowed the faeces to move as parasympathetic nerve fibres increased activity. She may also have listened to the nurse and increased her fluid intake, and her activity round the flat. Thus, after 2 days she would have been less dehydrated and the use of her abdominal muscles would have had a massage action on the large intestine. As the body ages the muscles

become weaker, both skeletal and smooth, thus any function that relies on their strength is reduced. In the gastrointestinal tract, the ageing gut secretes less fluid to the lumen. Increase in dietary fibre and exercise may be of long-term benefit to many patients; improvement of inappropriate toilet facilities may be necessary for elderly people with poor mobility.

Person Centred Study 2

1. Hydrocortisone enemas daily would help decrease inflammation in the colon by suppressing migration of polymorphonuclear leucocytes and fibroblasts, and reverse the increased capillary permeability that is causing excess mucus production and bleeding. This would need to be done for a short duration only as this young lady may be anxious with her new situation rather than unsure of her treatment requirements.

2. The difference in the two conditions is the part of the gut that is affected. Crohn's disease results in inflammation throughout the gastrointestinal tract whereas ulcerative colitis is usually restricted to the sigmoid colon and the rectum. However, the distribution definition is disputed. Chronic ulceration is a feature of Crohn's disease that develops insidiously over time. There is granuloma formation and mucus surface erosion, which leads to bowel strictures and perforation. Malabsorption becomes evident in the sufferer but stools, although loose and foul smelling, do not show blood loss. More acute onset and superficial mucosa ulceration is seen in ulcerative colitis, the stools are thus watery and blood stained. Anaemia is common. Many sufferers control symptoms with diet and medication that calms the mucosa inflammation response. Abscess formation is a risk but sufferers often have long periods in remission.

MCQs

1. a, c
2. a, b
3. a, b, c, e
4. a, b, d
5. a, c, d
6. a, b, c, e
7. a, b, c, d, e
8. a, c, d, e
9. a, b, d
10. a, b, c, d

CHAPTER FIFTEEN

Person Centred Study 1

1. In acute tubular necrosis, there is a risk of potassium retention as a result of impaired renal excretion. Grapes and chocolate both have a high potassium content, and could contribute to hyperkalaemia and the risk of cardiac arrest.

2. Pratiba would receive 500 ml in addition to the volume of her previous day's urinary output. For this reason, it is important that her total urinary output is collected and measured. It will probably be collected continuously for biochemical analysis of creatinine clearance and urea and electrolyte excretion over 24 hours.

3. The main reason for the need to practise deep breathing and coughing is likely to be that, as a part of her renal failure, her acid–base balance has become disordered. The kidneys are part of the homeostatic mechanism for acid–base excretion. If her kidneys' ability to excrete hydrogen ions is decreased, she is at risk of becoming acidotic. Acid excretion also takes place as a result of exhaling carbon dioxide during breathing, so avoidance of pulmonary stasis and chest infection enables better pH control. In addition, she is likely to be inactive while she is ill, and therefore at risk of thromboemboli. Deep breathing exercises, in conjunction with leg exercises, reduce the risk of formation of deep vein thrombosis.

4. If Pratiba's renal dysfunction is fairly mild, she may not have had a urinary catheter inserted because of the risk of urinary tract infection. The apparent increase in her urinary output should be visible on her fluid balance chart, and her fluid intake should have automatically increased to correspond with the increased output. The increased urine output may mean that she has entered a 'convalescent' diuretic phase, in which the accumulated excess water load is excreted. However, during this phase of recovery, the distal tubule may not be fully responsive to the effect of antidiuretic hormone, so there is a risk that she will become dehydrated and it is most important that she keeps to the stated fluid intake; dehydration is likely to cause her renal failure to become worse. If Pratiba's urine output is satisfactory and her renal function is recovering, the medical team will probably consider tailing off the diuretic treatment.

Person Centred Study 2

1. The renal risk factors associated with John's condition include mild hypotension, which produces a risk of poor renal perfusion. Radio contrast medium can be nephrotoxic. There is a risk of obstructive uropathy if the ureteric obstruction is not relieved.

2. John needs to have venepuncture to obtain a specimen to estimate blood, urea and electrolytes, which is needed to establish a baseline of his renal function. Other blood chemical tests may help to establish the likely chemical composition of the calculus and the best mode of treatment for him.

3. John would be observed for pain to ensure adequate analgesia is given and to assess whether any alteration has occurred in the location of the calculus within the urinary tract. Blood pressure would be monitored to ensure that mild pain-related shock does not persist. Urinary output would be measured to assess whether particulate debris is being passed from the urinary tract, also to ensure that the lower urinary tract (urethra) does not become blocked by debris, resulting in urinary retention; urinalysis would be undertaken to test for blood (sign of damage to endothelium of urinary tract). Urine would be collected for biochemical analysis to detect the likely composition of calculus in order to assist possible selection of medication to prevent further occurrences.

4. The likelihood of further formation of calculi depends upon the cause. The risk of recurrence would be minimised by his avoiding becoming dehydrated, particularly in hot weather and when undertaking heavy work. Depending on the composition of the calculus, he might be advised to moderate his diet.

MCQs

1. e
2. a
3. a with Z; b with Y; c with Y; d with X; e with Z
4. c
5. a, b, d
6. d
7. d
8. b, d
9. d
10. The most suitable option is probably b

CHAPTER SIXTEEN

Person Centred Study 1

1. The pain is caused by physical changes such as abnormal contractibilty of the myometrium, age changes and cigarette smoking. These are mediated through the actions of prostaglandins E_2 and $F_{2\alpha}$, which are formed from the phospholipids of dead cell membranes in the menstruating uterus. Prostaglandin E_2 causes degregration of platelets and is a vasodilator, whereas prostaglandin $F_{2\alpha}$ mediates or potentiates pain sensations and stimulates smooth muscle contraction. Oestrogens can also stimulate synthesis and/or release of prostaglandin $F_{2\alpha}$ and antidiuretic hormone, which cause uterine hyperactivity, so Ms Jones will be taking a progesterone dominant oral contraceptive, which will reduce the amount of endometrium formed and consequently the amount of prostaglandins formed.

2. Mefenamic acid is an NSAID that inhibits prostaglandin synthesis by inhibiting an enzyme needed for biosynthesis. It possesses analgesic and anti-inflammatory properties. The dosage is 500 mg three times a day after food as it may have an irritant effect on the stomach lining. It has a half-life of 3 hours. By acting on the prostaglandins, this medication targets the cause of the problem rather than having other system side effects. Codeine phosphate acts on central nervous system opiate receptors and inhibits ascending pain pathways in the central nervous system. Unfortunately it also reduces gut motility. Ms Jones' abdominal comfort will not be enhanced by being chronically constipated as her diet and lifestyle will add to the symptoms produced with regular use of codeine.

Person Centred Study 2

1. There are many reasons for irritation, you should start with the simple ones. She may have been bathing in preparations to which she has become allergic. Some of the bath gels alter the skin pH and their perfume irritates the tender mucosa of the vaginal opening. Simple soothing creams may be beneficial (see Chapter 17 *Drugs and dermatological disorders*). Your advice here is for her to shower in plain water rather than soak in the bath – perhaps she bathes or swims very frequently and is drying out her skin too much. She may be wearing nylon underwear that retains perspiration, this will encourage growth of fungus and bacteria in the perineal area if she is also wearing nylon panty-hose. Perhaps she could purchase some cotton pants and wear suspenders and stockings. She may not have very good hygiene habits, on the other hand, and may need to be advised to wash between her legs and to wear clean pants daily. Spraying on deodorants does not remove the bacteria and fungus from the skin surface, it only seals them in. You would have to ask some careful questions about her diet, fluids and sexual habits. Lemon or cranberry juice and increase in fluid intake will change the pH of the urine and help to alter the environment that bacteria are growing in and the increase in fluid will keep the bladder flushed.

2. These symptoms may be caused by *Candida albicans*, a yeast that usually exists as a normal commensal in the rectum and in small numbers in the acid environment of the vagina. *Lactobacillus acidophilus* microbes are normally present in the stratified squamous epithelium of the vagina, where they secrete lactic acid to maintain the pH between 4.9 and 3.5. This acidity level inhibits the growth of most microbes that may enter the vagina from the perineum. The oestrogens present in some contraceptive medications change this flora of the vagina so the yeast *Candida albicans* is able to flourish in the less acid situation. Nystatin pessaries 100 000 units for 7 days or oral fluconazole 150 mg as a single dose may be required. Interestingly, live yoghurt application has been known to calm this irritation by altering

the pH of the mucosal surface; many women will self-medicate to avoid going to the doctor and having an examination before treatment is prescribed.

MCQs

1. d
2. all of them
3. all of them
4. b, d
5. b, e
6. a, b, d
7. a, b, e
8. b, c
9. a, d
10. a

CHAPTER SEVENTEEN

Person Centred Study 1

1. Giles does need to tell his mother about the outbreak because the family may have contracted the infection from contact with freshly infested clothing.

2. It would be safest for the whole family to be treated with a scabicide. Giles has young brothers and sisters, so the family doctor will probably avoid the use of γ-benzene hexachloride cream because of their susceptibility to toxic effects from this preparation.

3. Giles does not have to burn the sleeping bag, but he should not sleep in it until it has been washed! The scabies mite can only maintain an independent existence for a matter of days, so thorough laundering and airing should render it quite safe. If the sleeping bag has to be dry cleaned, it should be kept somewhere safe for sufficient time to lapse for the mites to have died, as the assistants in the dry cleaners will not appreciate an infection! It is important to stop the young members of the family from playing with it until it has been thoroughly washed.

Person Centred Study 2

1. It is possible that John has developed contact dermatitis from foods he has touched. However, this is an unlikely cause in this case, because John has been handling foodstuffs for 5 years so any abnormal response would probably have been obvious some time ago.

2. Some antibiotics photosensitise the skin but penicillin is not one of them, so would not provoke an erythematous response when the skin is exposed to sunlight. Even if penicillin had this potential, the site of the affected skin makes it highly unlikely that it could be the cause in this case. Skin surfaces most exposed to the sun are the extensor ones of the hands.

3. There are several types of psoriasis, classified according to the nature of individual lesions and their distribution. John's psoriasis is scaly and it is on the torso and extensor surfaces, rather than the flexor ones. New lesions can develop on other areas of the body, and hand and sole plaques are erythematous and without scales like John's. However, unlike John's they have well defined, obvious boundaries. It is unlikely, therefore, that his finger tip problem is caused by an extension of psoriasis.

4. To help you focus on the probable cause, you might decide to ask John whether he is left or right handed. Given that the majority of the population is right handed, he is also likely to be. You know that, as part of the treatment regime, he has been applying a potent dithranol cream to his lesions. You will remember that dithranol causes a painful irritation and redness if it is applied to 'normal' skin. It may be that John has not used a protective glove when applying the cream, and, as a result, he has developed this adverse reaction. You could check your findings by further questioning of John about his cream application technique.

MCQs

1. a, b, c
2. a, b, and c
3. a, b
4. b
5. c
6. all except c
7. all
8. a, c and, if bacterial infection is present, b
9. a, b, d
10. a, c, d

CHAPTER EIGHTEEN

Person Centred Study

1. It would be important to be aware of Mr Storey's history of pain and good or bad past experiences of pain relief measures. These will influence his pain perception and his expectations of pain management, including analgesia, and may ultimately affect dosage requirements. His own assessment of his pain (its nature, site, severity) should be monitored frequently and would act as the basis for your judgement about pain relief measures.

The results of physiological measurements and observations based on nursing charts and written reports should be checked. Of particular concern are his respiratory and cardiovascular functions and his state of mental alertness. It should be remembered that postoperative complications may develop as a result of the trauma of surgery such as internal bleeding, dehydration and electrolyte imbalance; these may destabilise cardiovascular, respiratory and central nervous system functions. Remember you may be tempted to overestimate the danger of these problems, so look for changes indicating a pattern or trend in physiological parameters rather than short-term 'blips'. In order to pick these up frequent monitoring and recording of such information is necessary. Mr Storey's height and weight data are also important considerations in determining dose and dosing intervals.

Although smaller dosage may be required because of his age this is not necessarily the case and underdosage must be avoided for Mr Storey has as much right to a pain-free postoperative recovery as a younger patient. Idiosyncratic responses to medication are more likely in the older patient so you should be alert to this possibility without allowing it to adversely influence Mr Storey's pain relief. His self-report and the reports of nurses in the High Dependency Unit will help you to decide whether his current analgesic schedule (analgesic agent, dose and dose intervals) is appropriate.

You should remember that your own attitudes and beliefs about pain and your own cultural expectations of 'normal' pain behaviour will influence your perception of Mr Storey's situation. Reflection on these beliefs will help minimise any adverse effect they might have on your professional ability to judge his pain relief needs.

Using all this data, you should attempt to unravel the cause(s) of destabilisation and recognise when the effects are attributable to unrelieved pain or to analgesic therapy rather than to other causes, so that you can take appropriate action.

2. At this early postoperative stage, opioid analgesics such as morphine are likely to provide the best pain relief. Pethidine may cause problems such as confusion or hallucinations, because of build-up of its long-lasting metabolite, and should be avoided.

Assertion of a 'correct' or 'appropriate' dosage is impossible, as it depends on your judgement of the relative importance of the factors identified above. However, Mr Storey's self-assessment and other nurses' reports (as above) would offer a sound basis on which to titrate the dose against the occurrence of pain (adjusting it up or down as required).

3. He is unable to absorb oral medication, but as he has an intravenous infusion *in situ*, analgesia may be infused or injected using this site. Alternatively, a separate intravenous cannula may be used and continuous relief afforded using a syringe driver. Intramuscular injections should probably be avoided as absorption may be delayed, resulting in unpredictable plasma levels, particularly if haemodynamic functions are not yet stabilised. The aim is to maintain pain relief by obtaining consistent plasma levels rather than peaks and troughs. If intermittent injections are given then it may be difficult to achieve this consistency, particularly if the analgesic dose is prescribed as 'prn'.

Patient-controlled analgesic methods may be appropriate, although this is unlikely as Mr Storey was originally admitted as an emergency in acute pain. As a result he is unlikely to have been able to understand preparatory, explanatory information about PCA, and patient understanding is particularly important for this type of delivery method.

MCQs

1. b, c
2. a
3. a, c, d
4. a, b, e
5. a, b, c, d
6. a, b, c, e
7. b, c
8. b, c, d, e
9. a
10. c, d

CHAPTER NINETEEN

Person Centred Study 1

1. Mr Haq is likely to be in an unstable condition for a while, but the action of adrenaline, although it 'drives' the heart and produces tachycardia, alters the length of time spent in the diastolic phase, so it is thought that there is enhanced coronary artery (and therefore myocardial) perfusion. Overall, therefore, the present thinking is that adrenaline is a helpful drug to have given in the circumstances.

2. The cyclomorph was beneficial as, by relieving the pain associated with the infarction, stress-related catecholamine release was reduced and the myocardial oxygen demands were less. This helps to prevent further infarction of ischaemic tissue. Aspirin reduces platelet activity and inhibits thrombus formation at the infarction site. Diamorphine is also used to reduce the cardiac preload, so is helpful in acute cardiac failure. The administration of oxygen ensures that satisfactory oxygen saturation of arterial blood occurs, which, again, helps to preserve viable myocardium. The paramedic established intravenous access early, before cardiovascular collapse made cannulation difficult, so there was a route for emergency intravenous medication. The staff of the coronary care unit commenced thrombolytic therapy rapidly, which, once again, helped to minimise the extent of the infarction. Most importantly, all parties diagnosed Mr Haq's changing condition rapidly and accurately, and instituted the appropriate actions.

Person Centred Study 2

1. Intravenous fluid infusion assists in the management of the trauma patient who is suffering from shock. It is a temporary measure to try and stabilise the cardiovascular system until the patient arrives in hospital when, for example, the bleeding present in hypovolaemic shock is controlled by surgery. The infusion rate is carefully controlled as rapid and large volume infusion can result in increased bleeding, and pre-hospital fluids cannot carry oxygen.

   Crystalloids and colloids are used when whole blood is not available and each has advantages and disadvantages. Crystalloid solutions are isotonic and remain isotonic, therefore they act as effective volume expanders for short periods. Filling the vascular space with such solutions improves preload and cardiac output, thus assisting with the control of the patient's shocked state. They are used in the pre-hospital setting as whole blood is not available and colloid infusions, although they achieve similar results, have their disadvantages, for example a shorter shelf life.

   Colloids provide a volume expansion for a longer period and unlike crystalloids (which require an infusion of three times the amount of blood lost to achieve fluid replacement), replace blood loss on an equal basis.

2. The ambulance personnel made effective assessment of his injuries, performing interventions while en route and making a rapid transfer to hospital, thus reducing pre-hospital time.

- Stabilising the femur and pelvis reduced pain and attempted to use pressure to reduce the bleeding at the fracture sites.
- The paramedic established intravenous access early before cardiovascular collapse made cannulation difficult or impossible to achieve. Intravenous access achieved a route for fluid infusion. The infusions attempted to stabilise the patient's shocked state and prevent even more rapid deterioration in his condition
- The administration of oxygen ensures that satisfactory oxygen saturation of arterial blood occurs, which helps to prevent tissue hypoxia.

By achieving a rapid assessment and rapid transfer to theatre, the trauma team facilitated surgical intervention before the patient's condition worsened to the point at which his chances of survival would have been significantly reduced.

MCQs

1. d
2. e
3. a
4. b, e
5. c, e
6. b, e
7. c
8. a, d
9. a, c
10. a, b, d

SUBJECT INDEX